The Internal Medicine Casebook

Real Patients, Real Answers

Second Edition

The Internal Medicine Casebook

Real Patients, Real Answers

Second Edition

Edited by

Robert W. Schrier, M.D.
Professor and Chairman of Medicine, University of
Colorado School of Medicine, Denver, Colorado

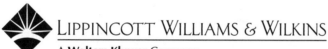

LIPPINCOTT WILLIAMS & WILKINS
A **Wolters Kluwer** Company
Philadelphia · Baltimore · New York · London
Buenos Aires · Hong Kong · Sydney · Tokyo

Acquisitions Editor: Richard Winters
Developmental Editor: Selina Bush
Production Editor: Aureliano Vázquez, Jr.
Manufacturing Manager: Kevin Watt
Cover Designer: Mark Lerner
Compositor: PRD Group
Printer: R. R. Donnelly, Crawfordsville

© **2000 by LIPPINCOTT WILLIAMS & WILKINS**
227 East Washington Square
Philadelphia, PA 19106-3780 USA
LWW.com

Printed in the USA

Library of Congress Cataloging-in-Publication Data

The internal medicine casebook : real patients, real answers / editor,
    Robert W. Schrier. — 2nd ed.
            p.   cm.
        Includes bibliographical references and index.
        ISBN 0-7817-2029-X
        1. Internal medicine Case studies.   I. Schrier, Robert W.
        [DNLM: 1. Internal Medicine Case Report.   2. Diagnostic Techniques
and Procedures Case Report.   WB 293 I61 1999]
RC66.I554   1999
616′.09—dc21
DNLM/DLC
for Library of Congress   99-31881
                                                                              CIP

10 9 8 7 6 5 4 3 2 1

Contents

Contributing Authors

Unless otherwise noted, all affiliations are with University of Colorado School of Medicine and University Hospital, Denver

Tomas Berl, M.D.
Professor of Medicine and Head
Division of Renal Diseases and
   Hypertension

Michael R. Bristow, M.D.
Professor of Medicine and Head
Division of Cardiology

William R. Brown, M.D.
Professor of Medicine
Division of Gastroenterology
Veterans Administration Medical Center
Denver, Colorado

Henry N. Claman, M.D.
Professor of Medicine
Division of Allergy and Clinical
   Immunology

Robert W. Janson, M.D.
Associate Professor of Medicine
Chief, Rheumatology Section
Veterans Administration Medical Center
Denver, Colorado

JoAnn Lindenfeld, M.D.
Professor of Medicine
Division of Cardiology

David E. Mann, M.D.
Professor of Medicine
Division of Cardiology

Jane E. Reusch, M.D.
Assistant Professor of Medicine
Division of Endocrinology
Veterans Administration Medical Center
Denver, Colorado

E. Chester Ridgway, M.D.
Professor of Medicine and Head
Division of Endocrinology

Laurence J. Robbins, M.D.
Associate Professor of Medicine
Associate Chief, Geriatrics Division
Veterans Administration Medical Center
Denver, Colorado

Robert T. Schooley, M.D.
Professor of Medicine and Head
Division of Infectious Diseases

Marvin I. Schwarz, M.D.
Professor of Medicine and Head
Division of Pulmonary Diseases and
   Intensive Care Medicine

Paul A. Seligman, M.D.
Professor of Medicine
Division of Hematology

Isaac Teitelbaum, M.D.
Associate Professor of Medicine
Division of Renal Diseases and
   Hypertension

Preface

The basis for an internal medicine casebook originated several years ago, born of my conviction that house staff and students are stimulated and motivated best when their learning is focused on real patients. Steps were taken, therefore, to augment the patient-oriented instruction of our house staff and students. This was accomplished in large part by our in-house publication of a large number of patient cases covering a variety of diseases that formed the curriculum for medical students and the house staff rotating on the medical wards and taking subspecialty electives. These studies became the basis for the first edition of *The Internal Medicine Casebook: Real Patients, Real Answers.* Since the first edition has been so well received, I am even more convinced of the need for such a patient-oriented educational tool.

In this second edition of the *Casebook,* we have revised and updated the patient-oriented cases, which cover approximately 90 areas of internal medicine. First, the pertinent aspects of the patient's history and physical exam are presented. Questions are then posed about the appropriate diagnostic work-up and treatment. This sets the stage for a Socratic approach to learning between the attending physician and the house officer or medical student. The format of the *Casebook* also lends itself to self-instruction with this question-and-answer approach.

The Internal Medicine Casebook: Real Patients, Real Answers should prove an invaluable learning tool to students and house officers, and also a teaching aid to anyone involved in the education of future physicians. I am grateful for the expertise and support of the authors, each of whom is an eminently qualified educator and highly regarded leader in his or her field. I also thank Shirley Artese for her editorial assistance.

R.W.S.

The Internal Medicine Casebook

Real Patients, Real Answers

Second Edition

1 Allergy and Clinical Immunology

Henry N. Claman

Anaphylaxis

1. What is the clinical presentation in a typical case of anaphylaxis?
2. What is the underlying pathophysiologic process?
3. What conditions should be considered in the differential diagnosis?

Discussion

1. *What is the clinical presentation in a typical case of anaphylaxis?*

In the most severe cases, the clinical presentation consists of sudden hypotension, with or without bronchospasm or laryngeal obstruction. This may occur within minutes after the injection of an antigen (e.g., an antibiotic) or an insect sting, and may be fatal. A less rapid onset can begin with shortness of breath, hoarseness, urticaria, and moderate hypotension. If the offending substance has been ingested, there can be abdominal cramps, vomiting, and diarrhea. There is no reason not to diagnose anaphylaxis if the symptoms described appear over the course of an hour. The blood pressure need not drop—that is, there can be anaphylaxis without shock.

2. *What is the underlying pathophysiologic process?*

Most of the signs and symptoms of anaphylaxis can be mimicked by intravenously (IV) administered histamine. Histamine (and other mediators) is released by the rapid and massive activation of tissue mast cells and blood basophils. If the mast cells are activated because an antigen (e.g., penicillin) has combined with antibodies to, for example, penicillin of the immunoglobulin E (IgE) isotype on the mast cell, this represents true immunologic anaphylaxis. If, however, the mast cell is activated by non-IgE mechanisms, such as may be triggered by radiocontrast dye injections, this is called an *anaphylactoid*

1

reaction, but the basic physiologic characteristics and treatment are the same as those of IgE-mediated anaphylaxis.

3. *What conditions should be considered in the differential diagnosis?*

The differential diagnosis list is not long. Collapse from a cardiac arrhythmia or asystole must be considered. The most common problem is vasovagal syncope. In this situation, the patient's pulse is slow and there is no urticaria, edema, or dyspnea. The pulse is always rapid in the setting of anaphylaxis unless the patient is taking a β-adrenergic blocker. Patients with hyperventilation do not wheeze or have hypotension or urticaria.

Case A 26-year-old white woman is seen in a local emergency room (ER) complaining of acute shortness of breath. Three hours before her symptoms began, she took 50 mg of indomethacin for the treatment of an acute migraine headache, as well as 20 mg of propranolol, which she takes daily for migraine prophylaxis. One hour before her arrival in the ER, she was attending a business meeting where lunch was served (consisting of salad, rice, and shrimp). After the meal, she began to deliver a speech, but soon started to feel flushed, itchy, and short of breath, and noted the sensation of an enlarging lump in her throat. In the ER, she reports that she has experienced similar symptoms (although much milder) on two prior occasions during episodes of emotional stress; she does not recall whether these episodes occurred after meals or the ingestion of particular medications. She appears anxious and diaphoretic; her vital signs are remarkable for a respiratory rate of 32 per minute and a pulse rate of 108 per minute. She is noted to be diffusely flushed, and careful examination of her skin reveals two small urticarial lesions on her trunk. Inspiratory stridor is noted over her throat and appears to radiate over both lung fields. The remainder of her examination findings are normal.

1. What might be the cause or causes of her reaction?
2. How should she be treated?
3. What follow-up should be recommended?

Case Discussion

1. *What might be the cause or causes of her reaction?*

There are a number of factors that might have triggered this reaction.

Aspirin and nonsteroidal antiinflammatory drugs (NSAIDs) such as indomethacin are potent inhibitors of the cyclooxygenase pathway of arachidonic acid metabolism, reportedly causing serious reactions in up to 10% of people with asthma and 1% of the general population. In asthmatic patients, the reaction consists of severe bronchospasm; people who do not have asthma may have urticaria, angioedema, and anaphylaxis. Reactions to these drugs are not mediated by IgE and the mechanism responsible for causing them is poorly understood, but is possibly related to the inhibition of cyclooxygenase and the shifting of arachidonate metabolism to the lipoxygenase pathway. There are no immunologic tests that can detect this sensitivity, and challenge tests, which require the use of strict precautions, remain the only reliable method to identify aspirin- and NSAID-sensitive patients.

Sodium and potassium **metabisulfite** are used as food fresheners and preservatives in dried fruits, wines, and some restaurant foods. Although the Food and Drug Administration has banned their use on fresh fruits and vegetables in restaurants, their use is still allowed for other foods; they are particularly commonly used on shellfish. Reactions to sulfites are often associated with positive reactions to sulfite skin tests, suggesting that the sensitivity may be IgE mediated. Although this additive can cause a variety of reactions, including anaphylaxis, it most commonly affects asthmatic patients, causing acute bronchospasm.

An **IgE-mediated allergy to foods** is a common cause of anaphylaxis in all age groups. The foods most commonly implicated include shellfish, legumes, nuts, milk, and eggs, but virtually any food is a potential cause in a sensitized person.

Finally, a few patients have **idiopathic anaphylaxis**, that is, they have one or more episodes of anaphylaxis that remain unexplained after a thorough evaluation. Severe, recurrent episodes respond well to long-term antihistamine and oral corticosteroid prophylaxis.

In this particular case, any of the diagnoses mentioned are possible explanations for the patient's recurrent episodes. However, either shrimp or sulfite sensitivity is especially likely because the shrimp (probably treated with sulfites) was ingested immediately before the anaphylactic episode. Because the indomethacin ingestion occurred a few hours before the symptoms began, it is a less likely cause. In the event that the results of all future diagnostic evaluations are negative, these recurrent events may indeed be idiopathic.

Although the list of potential causes of anaphylaxis is long and continues to expand, agents that deserve special mention include (by etiologic category) IgE-mediated reactions; antibiotics; injection of allergy extracts, latex, immunotherapy, chymopapain, and corticotropin (adrenocorticotropic hormone); immune complexes; blood products and IV immunoglobulin; mast cell degranulators; opiates and radiocontrast media; and physical allergy exercise-induced anaphylaxis and exercise-induced plus food-related anaphylaxis.

2. *How should she be treated?*

There is a generally accepted protocol for treating anaphylactic syndromes.

Epinephrine is the mainstay of treatment in anaphylaxis; it acts by inhibiting mediator release from mast cells and basophils, relaxing bronchial smooth muscle, and bolstering blood pressure. Often, all of the signs and symptoms of anaphylaxis resolve completely within minutes after a single injection of epinephrine. A starting dose of 0.3 mL of a 1:1,000 solution given subcutaneously is reasonable in an adult; however, asthmatic adults are often less sensitive to adrenergic stimuli and may therefore receive up to 0.5 mL per dose. If no untoward side effects occur, the patient may receive repeated doses every 10 minutes until the symptoms improve. IV bolus injections should be avoided because they may cause potentially fatal cardiac arrhythmias. In a patient whose primary site of involvement is the upper airway (such as the one described here), inhaled 2% racemic epinephrine is a valuable adjunct to parenteral therapy (at a dose of 0.5 mL). In addition, an **H₁ antagonist** (e.g., diphenhydramine, 50 mg) should be given slowly by the IV route. The use of **H₂ blockers**, such as cimetidine 300 mg by slow IV infusion, is controversial. It is used routinely in many emergency departments. The rationale is that there are **H₂** receptors on vascular smooth muscle that mediate vasodilation. A retrospective study indicated that the addition of cimetidine to a prednisone, diphenhydramine, and ephedrine regimen did not improve the prophylaxis of radiocontrast media reactions. If the patient has severe airway obstruction at presentation (cyanosis) or the obstruction worsens despite the prompt use of epinephrine, endotracheal intubation should be performed promptly using a small-bore tube (no. 4 or 5). If this is not possible because of the degree of edema, cricothyrotomy should be performed.

Anaphylaxis in patients who are taking β-adrenergic antagonists may be particularly difficult to treat. If wheezing does not respond to initial epinephrine or inhaled β-agonist therapy, IV aminophylline and inhaled atropine sulfate, along with IV antihistamines, should be administered. Patients with hypotension refractory to treatment with subcutaneous epinephrine, antihistamines, and parenteral fluids may require parenteral norepinephrine, isoproterenol, and occasionally glucagon therapy.

In patients who have significant symptoms affecting any target organ system, IV **corticosteroids** should be given immediately, followed by an oral dose 6 hours later. Patients who have a prolonged clinical course should continue to receive corticosteroids every 6 hours.

Initial therapy consisting of the interventions just described brings about complete and sustained relief of the signs and symptoms of anaphylaxis in 50% of patients. However, one fourth of the patients remain partially resistant to therapy for several hours and occasionally several days (protracted anaphylaxis). The remaining 25% of the patients respond to initial therapy, but after a variable interval (up to 8 hours) without signs or symptoms, they experience recurrence of life-threatening complications (biphasic anaphylaxis). There is no reliable way to predict which patients will have such a relapse. Therefore, all patients with significant anaphylaxis should be observed by medical personnel for at least 8 hours after the onset of the episode.

3. *What follow-up should be recommended?*

All patients with a previous history of anaphylactic reaction, no matter what the cause, should be given a kit containing epinephrine for self-administration (e.g., Anakit, Bayer Corp., Spokane, Washington; Epipen 0.3 mg Autoinjector, Dey Inc., Napa, California). Before they leave the ER, the patient and family members should be trained in how to administer it. Another important general measure to implement is the discontinuation of β-blocking drugs (unless the drug cannot be replaced by an alternative medication) in those people who are at possible risk for reexposure to the inciting agent.

After acute treatment of the anaphylactic episode, the most likely cause of the reaction should be determined so that recommendations on future avoidance can be made. In the patient described here, food skin tests to all of the ingredients in the meal preceding her reaction, particularly shellfish, should be performed by a physician with experience in allergic diseases. If the skin test results are positive to one or more foods, carefully monitored, graded, double-blinded, placebo-controlled (DBPC) food challenges should be performed to identify which food is the etiologic agent. In the event that the food challenge results are negative, it is not necessary for the patient to avoid shrimp or any of the other implicated foods. If a food allergy is excluded, skin testing followed by a graded, DBPC oral sulfite challenge should be carried out to determine whether metabisulfites are the offending agents.

Patients with recurrent episodes of idiopathic anaphylaxis have been shown to benefit from the daily administration of antihistamine and oral corticosteroid therapy. This type of therapy, however, is unwarranted in patients who have known avoidable causes of anaphylaxis.

Suggested Readings

Corren J, Schocket AL. Anaphylaxis: a preventable emergency. *Postgrad Med* 1990;87:167.

Greenberger PA, Patterson R, Tapio CM. Prophylaxis against repeated radiocontrast media reaction in 857 patients: adverse experience with cimetidine and safety of beta-adrenergic antagonists. *Arch Intern Med* 1985;145:2197.

Niklas, RA et al., eds. The diagnosis and management of anaphylaxis. *J Allergy Clin Immunol* 1998;101:S465.

Sullivan TJ. Systemic anaphylaxis. In Lichtenstein LM, Fauci AS, eds. *Current therapy in allergy and immunology.* St. Louis: Mosby-Year Book, 1988, p. 640.

Wiggins CA, Dykewicz MS, Patterson R. Idiopathic anaphylaxis: classification, evaluation, and treatment of 123 patients. *J Allergy Clin Immunol* 1988;82:849.

Angioedema

1. What are the clinical pictures associated with angioedema?
2. What pathophysiologic processes underlie angioedema?
3. How is hereditary angioedema (HAE) diagnosed?

Discussion

1. *What are the clinical pictures associated with angioedema?*

Angioedema can present with several different clinical pictures. It can include an exaggerated form of urticaria, with itching and swelling of soft tissues that can arise anywhere in the body and appear within a few minutes or over the course of hours. It may involve the bronchial mucosa or the vocal cords, leading to airway obstruction. Other forms of angioedema do not include itching or urticaria. They may be local or may result from trauma. In these cases, the swollen tissues may hurt, but do not itch.

2. *What pathophysiologic processes underlie angioedema?*

In angioedema that includes urticaria, the underlying mechanism is the same as that operating in anaphylaxis—the release of mast cell mediators such as histamine. In the setting of angioedema without urticaria, the mechanism responsible consists of the unbridled activation of the complement system due to lack of a major complement control protein, C1 inhibitor (**C1 INH**).

3. *How is HAE diagnosed?*

The clinical clue to HAE is a history of repeated bouts of angioedema arising anywhere in the body, such as the face, tongue, and extremities. The airway can be compromised. Some patients experience diffuse abdominal pain and may have had laparotomies at which only bowel edema is found. These lesions do not itch, and urticaria is not one of the symptoms of HAE. HAE is transmitted as an autosomal dominant trait. Nevertheless, the family history is negative in 50% of the patients. The laboratory clues point to the complement system, with a deficiency of complement control proteins at fault.

Case   A 25-year-old white woman presents to the ER with complaints of severe facial swelling resulting in difficulty swallowing arising on the day after she had undergone an endoscopic procedure. She noted mild facial swelling on awakening in the morning. Throughout the ensuing day, the swelling has worsened to involve her left cheek, upper and lower lips, and tongue. Approximately 6 hours before coming to the ER, she noted she was becoming hoarse. She had undergone the endoscopy as part of an evaluation for intermittent abdominal pain. Previous investigations include a barium swallow and enema, and the results of both were negative. Since the 19 years of age, she has had abdominal pain, which she describes as crampy and occasionally associated with nausea, vomiting, or diarrhea. These symptoms usually resolve within 3 to 4 days with no specific medical intervention and are not associated with her menstrual periods. The symptoms began when she started using birth control pills. She has had one other episode of facial swelling 3 years before, after a tooth extraction (although it was much less intense and not associated with difficulty swallowing). The swelling resolved spontaneously after approximately 3 days. There is no family history of similar syndromes.

1. What is the most likely diagnosis in this woman?
2. What laboratory tests for complement are useful in making a diagnosis of HAE?
3. How should an acute attack of HAE be treated?
4. What prophylactic measures are available for HAE?

Case Discussion

1. *What is the most likely diagnosis in this woman?*

The most likely diagnosis is HAE. Although local anesthetics can rarely cause an allergic reaction that includes angioedema, a diagnosis of HAE is much more consistent with this patient's case history. HAE characteristically presents as swelling of the submucosal and subcutaneous tissues. Although virtually any body part can be involved, usually the face and extremities are affected. Mucosal edema may occur. This can cause abdominal pain when the small bowel is affected, or a change in voice or even stridor when the larynx is affected. This patient had both of these symptoms. Urticaria is not a part of the HAE syndrome.

The angioedema associated with HAE frequently occurs after local trauma (including dental procedures and endoscopy), illness, or emotional stress, but can also arise in the absence of a specific trigger. HAE episodes usually begin during childhood, but the onset can occur at virtually any age. Attacks vary greatly in intensity and frequency. Most patients experience self-limited facial or extremity swelling, but others can have life-threatening laryngeal edema. Attacks usually last for 1 to 4 days. They may increase in the premenstrual or postpartum periods. This disease exhibits an autosomal dominant hereditary pattern, but the family history is negative in 50% of patients.

2. *What laboratory tests for complement are useful in making a diagnosis of HAE?*

A serum C4 level represents the *screen* for this disease because it is low during or between attacks.

Measurement of serum C1 esterase inhibitor is a laboratory test that can be performed to establish the diagnosis. HAE is caused by a decrease in the level of **C1 INH**, which is the inhibitor of the activated first component of complement (C1q or C1s). When the level of this inhibitor is low or absent, the early classic complement pathway is activated and various complement components are then used up faster than they can be synthesized. In 85% of patients, the level of the C1 INH protein is decreased, whereas in 15% of the patients the protein is dysfunctional. Thus, in a subgroup of these patients, the C1 INH *level* is normal and the nature of the disease cannot be detected unless the C1 INH *function* is assessed. The actual cause of the symptoms appears to be edema generated by the formation of kinin. Histamine release is not part of this condition.

3. *How should an acute attack of HAE be treated?*

Neither antihistamines nor corticosteroids have a role in the treatment of an acute attack of HAE, although they are effective in the treatment of allergic urticaria that includes angioedema. Because the medical treatment of HAE is not always effective, and if upper airway compromise is present or pending, a *stat* ear, nose, and throat consultation should be obtained because a tracheostomy may be required to prevent airway closure. The only alternative to tracheostomy is nasotracheal intubation, which should be performed only in an operating room with a surgeon present in the event an emergent tracheostomy is required. Treatment with fresh frozen plasma is somewhat controversial because this substance provides further proteins that, when activated secondary to a decrease in C1 INH, might worsen the angioedema. Nevertheless, many physicians routinely administer two units of fresh frozen plasma. Purified **C1 INH** is not yet generally available. As mentioned earlier, these diseases can present as crampy abdominal pain, sometimes misinterpreted as an acute abdominal condition, but this disease can be differentiated from an acute abdominal condition by the lack of abdominal rigidity, lack of fever, and absence of an elevated white blood cell count with a leftward shift. This abdominal pain can be relieved by narcotics such as meperidine. Some experienced physicians treat the abdominal or extremity pain associated with these angioedema attacks (which, in general, are self-limited) using meperidine. They reserve fresh frozen plasma (which supplies C1 1NH) and, of course, tracheostomy for threatened airway closure.

4. *What prophylactic measures are available for HAE?*

Chronic prophylaxis for this life-threatening disease is important. We use an attenuated androgen (such as stanozolol or danazol). These "impeded" androgenic steroids cause an increase in synthesis of C1 INH. High doses bring about correction of both the C1 INH as well as C4 levels. Unfortunately, unacceptable side effects may arise at these doses, including weight gain, headaches, muscle cramping, menometrorrhagia, androgenic effects, and mild increases in the serum aspartate and alanine aminotransferase levels. HAE can usually be controlled with lower doses of these androgens, which do not entirely correct these laboratory abnormalities, but produce fewer side effects. Thus, the androgen dose is adjusted to achieve symptomatic relief, not to correct the laboratory abnormalities. Androgens are not helpful in managing acute exacerbations of this disease, and neither corticosteroids nor antihistamines have a prophylactic effect.

Women with HAE frequently note a worsening of their disease when they start taking birth control pills. Possibly this is due to their antiandrogenic effect. Pregnant women with HAE, however, do well in late pregnancy and delivery.

Suggested Readings

Huran RF, Schneider LC, Sheffer AL. Allergic skin disorders and mastocytosis. *JAMA* 1992;268:2858.

Sheffer AL, Fearon DR, Austen KF. Hereditary angioedema: a decade of management with stanozolol. *J Allergy Clin Immunol* 1987;80:855.

Chronic Urticaria

1. What is the definition of chronic urticaria?
2. What is the pathogenesis of chronic urticaria?

Discussion

1. *What is the definition of chronic urticaria?*

Chronic urticaria is defined as urticaria that persists for 6 weeks or more.

2. *What is the pathogenesis of chronic urticaria?*

The pathogenesis of chronic urticaria includes a spectrum of events. Commonly, there is simple local edema and itching caused by the release of histamine from mast cells. Some other, more severe cases have an inflammatory component, such as vasculitis or perivasculitis, that is revealed by biopsy specimens. In these cases, the responsible mechanism may be either tumor necrosis factor-α, released from activated mast cells, or antigen–antibody complexes, which in turn activate complement and lead to the production of anaphylatoxins. These substances trigger local mast cell activation, with subsequent itching, erythema, and wheal formation.

Case   A 25-year-old woman is seen because of a pruritic rash characterized by multiple, circumscribed, raised areas of erythema varying in size from 2 mm to 3 cm and occurring over the skin. Each lesion lasts 1 or 2 days, but new ones arise as old ones fade. The rash has persisted for 9 weeks. She does not smoke or drink alcohol, nor has she taken any medications in the past 10 weeks, including antibiotics or aspirin, although she is sexually active and on birth control pills. She returned from trekking in Nepal 3 months ago, but has felt well since, except for the rash. Her family history is negative for atopic diseases such as allergic rhinitis, asthma, or eczema. Her physical examination findings are normal except for the presence of erythematous, papular wheals located over her trunk, back, and arms that blanch with pressure. The lesions are 5 to 25 mm in diameter and often overlap. She exhibits dermatographism. Her complete blood count (CBC) is normal and the erythrocyte sedimentation rate (ESR) is 11 mm per hour.

1. What causes of urticaria should be considered in this woman?
2. What diagnostic approach should be taken in this patient?
3. What therapeutic approach is desirable?
4. What is the prognosis in this patient if no specific allergen is identified?

Case Discussion

1. *What causes of urticaria should be considered in this woman?*

The most common cause of *acute* urticaria is an allergic reaction to a food or drug. By contrast, usually no cause is found in 80% to 90% of the patients with *chronic* urticaria. As a group, these patients are not atopic; that is, the prevalence of eczema, allergic rhinitis, or asthma is not increased. The presence of dermatographism indicates a general increase in the sensitivity of the mast cells and blood vessels in the skin, but the cause of dermatographism is unknown. Nevertheless, it is important to take a careful history to uncover any underlying cause, if present. Almost any medication can cause urticaria. Birth control pills as well as over-the-counter preparations such as aspirin, vitamins, and cold tablets should be considered as possible culprits.

Foods sometimes cause chronic urticaria and should be considered if indicated by the patient's history. Sensitivity to food dyes, natural salicylates, or benzoic acid derivatives is a rare cause of chronic urticaria, and diets specifically eliminating these materials may occasionally be helpful.

Urticaria can also be associated with underlying systemic illnesses such as systemic lupus erythematosus, Sjögren's syndrome, rheumatoid arthritis, and hyperthyroidism or hypothyroidism. However, these patients have elevated ESRs, and skin biopsy specimens reveal the presence of true vasculitis with polymorphonuclear infiltrates and the deposition of immunoglobulins and complement. Infections are also rare causes of urticaria, including viral infections, such as prodromal infectious hepatitis or infectious mononucleosis, as well as helminthic infections.

Certainly, any symptoms or signs of infection should be pursued and treated; however, it is not worthwhile to do a specific workup in pursuit of cryptic infections.

2. *What diagnostic approach should be taken in this patient?*

In diagnosing the cause of the urticaria in this patient, a good medical history and complete physical examination are important to exclude any underlying systemic disease. Some special tests may be done to investigate any clues revealed by the history. These might include food skin tests for a suspected food sensitivity or an "ice-cube test" of the skin if cold urticaria is suspected. If no cause is apparent, any underlying systemic disease can be ruled out by a CBC, urinalysis, ESR, blood chemistry profile, and chest radiographic study.

If the presence of an elevated ESR suggests the possibility of vasculitis, the following tests should be considered: CH_{50}, (total hemolytic complement), C_3 (third component of complement), C_4 (fourth component of complement), skin biopsy with immunofluorescent staining, hepatitis B surface antigen and antibody (HBsAg and HBsAb), cryoglobulins, anti-nuclear antibody, and circulating immune complexes.

In this patient, it is not unreasonable to obtain stool to test for ova and parasites because of her recent trip to Nepal.

If none of these approaches is successful in revealing a cause, have the patient stop taking birth control pills for a month and observe the urticaria, *untreated*. (Except for penicillin sensitivity, skin tests for drugs are usually unreliable.)

3. *What therapeutic approach is desirable?*

There is no known "cure" for urticaria unless the allergen is identified and eliminated. Otherwise, treatment is aimed at providing symptomatic relief. Antihistamines such as diphenhydramine [Benadryl (Parke-Davis, Morris Plains, NJ); 25 mg three times daily] or hydroxyzine [Atarax (Roerig, New York, NY); 10 to 25 mg two or three times daily] are commonly used first. For longer-term treatment, four nonsedating antihistamines are available: fexofenadine [Allegra (Hoechst Marion Roussel, Kansas City, MO); 60 mg twice daily], loratidine [Claritin (Schering-Plough, Madison, NJ); 10 mg once per day], cetirizine [Zyrtec (Pfizer, New York, NY); 10 mg once per day], and astemizole [Hismanal (Janssen Pharmaceutica, Titusville, NJ); 10 mg once per day]. This form of treatment is based on the concept that mast cells release histamine, and histamine is the primary offender in urticaria.

Combining H_1 and H_2 antihistamines has also been helpful in some patients. Short courses of corticosteroids may be used in severe, poorly controlled cases; however, the long-term use of steroids should be avoided if possible because of the severe side effects associated with these agents. Finally, some allergists may attempt an elimination diet or a fast in severely affected patients to rule out a food or preservative allergy, even when no specific agent is suspected.

4. *What is the prognosis in this patient if no specific allergen is identified?*

Assuming that no cause has been found, and there is no autoimmune disease present, the prognosis is quite good. The signs and symptoms almost always disappear within 2 years, but the reason for this is not known.

Suggested Readings

Champion RH. Urticaria: then and now. *Br J Dermatol* 1988;129:427.
Huran RF, Schneider LC, Sheffer AL. Allergic skin disorders and mastocytosis. *JAMA* 1992;268:2858.

Monoclonal Gammopathy

1. What is the definition of a monoclonal gammopathy?
2. What clinical pictures are seen in patients with monoclonal gammopathies?

Discussion

1. *What is the definition of a monoclonal gammopathy?*

A monoclonal gammopathy is defined as the overproduction of a particular immunoglobulin protein by a single clone of overactive or malignant B cells. This clone can produce a whole immunoglobulin, composed of both heavy and light chains, or it can produce just heavy chains, just light chains, or a combination of whole immunoglobulin plus excess light chains. The monoclonal light chains are called *Bence Jones protein*.

2. *What clinical pictures are seen in patients with monoclonal gammopathies?*

Some monoclonal serum immunoglobulins are discovered incidentally. These are usually small (<2 g/dL) and there are no associated signs, symptoms, or laboratory abnormalities. Patients with plasma cell (multiple) myeloma usually present with back pain (vertebral fracture or compression), anemia, and hypercalcemia, and often renal disease. The clinical picture of Waldenstrom's macroglobulinemia resembles that of a lymphoma, and consists of fever, lymphadenopathy, and sometimes hepatosplenomegaly. Hyperviscosity can be a component of this syndrome. Light chain disease can present as amyloidosis.

Case   A 62-year-old black man is seen in the ER because of right upper quadrant abdominal pain of 5 days' duration. The pain radiates around to his back and is worse with movement and coughing. He denies nausea, vomiting, or a change in his bowel habits but admits to having intermittent epigastric pain, frequent night sweats, a feeling of "weakness," general malaise, and a 15-pound (6.75-kg) weight loss over the past year. His past medical history is remarkable for a back injury incurred from a motor vehicle accident 10 years before and the presence of mild hypertension. His physical examination findings are unremarkable, except for the following. His blood pressure is 150/110 mm Hg. He has a grade I/VI systolic ejection murmur that can be heard along the left sternal border. Rectal examination reveals a 2+ prostate. His stool is heme negative. A slight kyphosis is noted and there is questionable decreased sensation to pinprick along the right lower rib cage (T-9 distribution). A chest radiographic study, CBC, and chemistry panel are performed. The chest radiograph shows no infiltrates, but a compression fracture of undetermined age is noted at T-9. His hemoglobin is 10 g/dL; hematocrit, 31%; and platelet count, 275,000. His chemistry panel shows creatinine, 2.2 mg/dL; blood urea nitrogen, 22 mg/dL; total protein, 10.2 mg/dL (normal, 6.8 to 8.4 mg/dL); albumin, 3.1 mg/dL (normal, 3.7 to 4.9 mg/dL); and calcium, 11.0 mg/dL (normal, 8.5 to 10.0 mg/dL). You conclude that his pain is most likely due to the T-9 compression fracture. Because of concern about his renal insufficiency, you avoid prescribing NSAIDs but instead prescribe acetaminophen with codeine. You order some additional laboratory studies on the extra tubes of blood before the patient is discharged.

1. If you were considering a diagnosis of a monoclonal gammopathy (which you should have), what screening test would you order?
2. What further immunologic tests should be ordered?
3. What further tests are important in this case?
4. What is the immunologic capability of this patient who has excess gamma globulin?
5. What is the current treatment for such a patient?
    While you are evaluating this patient, your colleague learns of your expertise in this field and asks you about a 61-year-old man with atopic dermatitis. A screening serum protein electrophoresis (SPEP) has shown a monoclonal band, which has been identified as immunoglobulin M (IgM) κ on immunofixation electrophoresis (IFE).
6. What course of action do you recommend in the 61-year-old patient?
7. What is the diagnosis in the patient described in question 6, and what is the prognosis?

Case Discussion

1. *If you were considering a diagnosis of a monoclonal gammopathy (which you should have), what screening test would you order?*
    The screening test that should be ordered in this patient is an SPEP, which shows a monoclonal spike in most cases. The clinical suspicion for myeloma should be high because he exhibits the classic triad of anemia, back pain, and renal insufficiency, which is associated with multiple myeloma. The most common presenting complaint is back pain. Multiple myeloma is the most common lymphoreticular neoplasm in nonwhite men and the third most common in whites. Its annual incidence is 3 in 100,000, and more than 90% of all affected patients are older than 40 years of age. Other factors in this case that implicate

multiple myeloma are the elevated total serum protein content and the relatively decreased albumin level. These suggest that there is an increase in the globulin fraction.

2. *What further immunologic tests should be ordered?*

   Further immunologic tests that should be done include an IFE, which can identify the heavy and light chains in the monoclonal protein. A urine electrophoresis can identify the spilling of light chains (Bence Jones protein) or, if the glomerulus is damaged, the presence of complete monoclonal protein.

3. *What further tests are important in this case?*

   A skeletal survey is an important additional test to document the extent of bone disease. It is better in this situation than a bone scan. The skeletal survey should include the skull, complete spine (both anteroposterior and lateral views), the pelvis, and the chest. A computed tomographic scan of the abdomen would be useful only if a solitary extramedullary plasmacytoma is suspected.

   A bone marrow aspiration is essential to clinch the diagnosis. In all but the rarest cases, clumps and sheets of plasma cells are seen.

   A serum calcium determination is needed because hypercalcemia can produce such symptoms as lethargy, nausea, and vomiting.

4. *What is the immunologic capability of this patient who has excess gamma globulin?*

   The immunologic capability in this patient is probably compromised, such that he is susceptible to high-grade bacterial pathogens. The excess immunoglobulin represented by the spike on SPEP is useless in fighting infection, and it is likely that he is severely depleted of normal polyclonal gamma globulins. In fact, these patients are functionally hypogammaglobulinemic. They are prone to infections with pyogenic organisms, and they do not make adequate antibodies after ordinary prophylactic immunizations. They should be carefully watched for early signs of infection. Some physicians have given monthly intravenous gamma globulin.

5. *What is the current treatment for such a patient?*

   Melphalan and prednisone constitute the chemotherapy most often used to treat myeloma. Bone marrow transplantation is being used more frequently.

6. *What course of action do you recommend in the 61-year-old patient?*

   You recommend that first lymphadenopathy, hepatosplenomegaly, anemia, hypercalcemia, holes in his bones, and Bence Jones protein be looked for. The monoclonal spike is IgM and is less than 2 g/dL. Because it is IgM, a protein that predisposes to hyperviscosity, you recommend that the serum viscosity be determined. This, too, proves to be normal.

7. *What is the diagnosis in the patient described in question 6, and what is the prognosis?*

   This is the clinical picture of monoclonal gammopathy of undetermined significance, which consists of a small monoclonal serum spike without other signs, symptoms, or laboratory indications of myeloma or macroglobulinemia. The prognosis in these patients is unclear. Some patients progress to frank disease; others do not. The best plan is to observe the patient by performing a physical examination and a screening SPEP every 6 to 12 months.

Suggested Readings

Barlogie B, Jaganath S, Tricot G, Desikan KR, Fassas A, Siegel D, et al. Advances in the treatment of multiple myeloma. *Adv Intern Med* 1998;43:279.

Gandera D, Mackenzie MR. Differential diagnosis of monoclonal gammopathies. *Med Clin North Am* 1988;72:5.

Penicillin Allergy

1. What are the clinical pictures that can result from an allergy to penicillin?
2. What are the immunologic mechanisms responsible for the clinical syndromes associated with penicillin allergy?

Discussion

1. *What are the clinical pictures that can result from an allergy to penicillin?*

   There are two categories of clinical pictures that can result from penicillin allergy: acute and subacute. Penicillin allergies can be mediated by IgE or immunoglobulin G (IgG) antibodies. The acute allergic reaction can arise immediately or rapidly, within a matter of minutes to an hour or two. It can include sudden anaphylaxis with hypotension, or asthma, rhinitis, and urticaria (see question 1 under the section on Anaphylaxis). Continued penicillin administration can cause continued symptoms. A less dramatic picture may occur 7 to 10 days after penicillin treatment starts, or after 1 to 2 days of repeat therapy. In this setting, the picture is subacute and can include urticaria, fever, and arthralgias or arthritis, and rarely nephritis or neuritis.

2. *What are the immunologic mechanisms responsible for the clinical syndromes associated with penicillin allergy?*

   Acute reactions result from penicillin reacting with preformed IgE to penicillin, left over from previous penicillin treatment that may have produced no visible allergic reaction itself. The IgE is present on mast cells and basophils. When the penicillin hapten binds to the IgE, the mast cells and basophils degranulate, releasing histamine and other mediators. These substances are responsible for producing the signs and symptoms. The subacute reaction is caused by preformed IgG to penicillin, also left over from previous penicillin treatment. IgG fixes complement. The combination of penicillin and the IgG antibody form an immune complex. When this is deposited in tissue, complement is activated and the complement breakdown products produce inflammation. The inflammation is responsible for the signs and symptoms in the organs where the immune complexes lodge, such as the skin, joints, and kidneys.

Case   A 26-year-old woman who has mitral stenosis requires extensive dental surgery. Penicillin prophylaxis against streptococci is indicated, but the patient is allergic to penicillin. She states that 15 years ago she had hives and wheezing 30 minutes after she had taken oral penicillin.

1. How would you determine whether the patient is likely to have an allergic reaction if she is treated with penicillin now?
2. What do you do if the skin test result to penicillin is positive?
3. What is the prevalence of allergic cross-sensitivity between penicillin and cephalosporins?
4. If the patient's skin test result to penicillin proves to be negative, how certain is it that she is *not* allergic?
5. If the skin test to penicillin is positive, could you avoid a reaction by giving penicillin orally instead of by injection?
6. If penicillin must be used because there is no acceptable alternative, can this patient be rapidly desensitized?

Case Discussion

1. *How would you determine whether the patient is likely to have an allergic reaction if she is treated with penicillin now?*

Skin testing for penicillin is an extremely useful procedure for determining whether a patient, who has a history of penicillin allergy and in whom an IgE-mediated immunologic mechanism is suspected, is likely to have an allergic reaction to a later exposure to penicillin. The reliability of these tests has been as high as 96% in studies of patients who had a history of allergy, whose skin test results were negative, and who were subsequently challenged with penicillin. The testing should be done by someone familiar with the procedure. The reagents used include histamine (the positive control), saline (the negative control), penicilloylpolylysine (Prepen, Kremers-Urban, Jacksonville, Florida), and penicillin G. For the test result to be positive, the patient must show a positive reaction to histamine, a negative reaction to saline, and a positive reaction to Prepen or penicillin G, or both. The positive reaction consists of a wheal and flare that appears in 15 minutes.

2. *What do you do if the skin test result to penicillin is positive?*

First, you *always* look for an effective nonpenicillin drug substitute and use it. If one is not found, you search for an effective penicillin relative (i.e., a second- or third-generation cephalosporin). If one still is not found, you consider desensitizing the patient to penicillin.

3. *What is the prevalence of allergic cross-sensitivity between penicillin and cephalosporins?*

The cephalosporins resemble the penicillins chemically, but the true prevalence of cross-reactivity between semisynthetic penicillins and cephalosporins is not known because investigators cite discordant results. A reasonable estimate is that 5% of penicillin-allergic patients are sensitive to third-generation cephalosporins.

4. *If the patient's skin test result to penicillin proves to be negative, how certain is it that she is not allergic?*

Assuming that the skin tests (including the controls) were properly done and the results properly interpreted, a negative skin test result is a reliable indicator that an acute IgE-mediated reaction will *not* occur. However, the skin test has no bearing on IgG-mediated reactions.

5. *If the skin test to penicillin is positive, could you avoid a reaction by giving penicillin orally instead of by injection?*

   No. Oral penicillin can also sensitize and elicit an acute reaction in already sensitized people.

6. *If penicillin must be used because there is no acceptable alternative, can this patient be rapidly desensitized?*

   Yes. However, this is a potentially dangerous and always time-consuming procedure. It should be done in the intensive care unit by an experienced allergist using published protocols.

Suggested Readings

deShazo RD, Kemp SF. Allergic reactions to drugs and biological reagents. *JAMA* 1997;278:1895.

Lin R. A perspective on penicillin allergy. *Arch Intern Med* 1992;152:930.

Sullivan TJ. Drug allergy. In Middleton E Jr, et al, eds. *Allergy: principles and practice*, 4th ed. St. Louis: Mosby-Year Book, 1993 p. 1726.

2 Cardiology

*JoAnn Lindenfeld, David E. Mann, and
Michael R. Bristow*

Acute Pericarditis and Cardiac Tamponade

1. What are the most common causes of acute pericarditis?
2. What is cardiac tamponade?
3. How is the echocardiogram helpful in the diagnosis of pericarditis or tamponade?
4. What is the treatment of cardiac tamponade?

Discussion

1. *What are the most common causes of acute pericarditis?*
   The most common causes of acute pericarditis are idiopathic, viral infection, uremia, and myocardial infarction (MI).
2. *What is cardiac tamponade?*
   Cardiac tamponade is the compression of the cardiac chambers by fluid accumulating in the pericardial space. This increased intrapericardial pressure limits filling of the heart, resulting in a reduced stroke volume.
3. *How is the echocardiogram helpful in the diagnosis of pericarditis or tamponade?*
   The echocardiogram is the most accurate and easily available tool to detect and quantify pericardial fluid. However, it often is not of diagnostic value in acute pericarditis because the absence of pericardial fluid does not exclude the diagnosis, especially in idiopathic or viral pericarditis. In patients with

pericarditis due to neoplasms, bacterial infections, trauma, or cardiac surgery, the echocardiogram may provide helpful information.

The echocardiogram is the most commonly used technique for the diagnosis of tamponade. Typical findings in addition to the presence of pericardial fluid include right atrial and right ventricular diastolic collapse, abnormal inspiratory increases in tricuspid valve flow or abnormal inspiratory decreases in mitral valve flow, and plethora of the inferior vena cava. Findings of tamponade may be detected by echocardiogram before the classically described clinical triad of hypotension, paradoxical pulse, and increased systemic venous pressure.

4. *What is the treatment for cardiac tamponade?*

The treatment for cardiac tamponade consists of withdrawal of fluid from the pericardial space, a procedure called *pericardiocentesis*. Pericardiocentesis may be performed using echocardiographic guidance or in the cardiac catheterization laboratory with fluoroscopic guidance.

Case   A 78-year-old man with a past history remarkable only for gout is seen because of the acute onset of chest pain. He describes a 4-day prodrome of rhinorrhea, nonproductive cough, myalgias, and anorexia. On the evening he is seen, he has experienced the gradual onset of sharp substernal chest pain, which is worse with inspiration, relieved by sitting up, and associated with diaphoresis but not dyspnea, and has lasted for 1 hour before his arrival in the emergency room (ER).

The pain is slightly worse with exertion but is not relieved by sublingual nitroglycerin (NTG) administered in the ER, although morphine sulfate and oxygen do seem to alleviate his discomfort. His temperature is 101°F (38.5°C), his heart rate is 105 beats per minute and regular, his respiratory rate is 17 per minute, and his blood pressure is 105/65 mm Hg. Physical examination findings are normal. The electrocardiogram (ECG) is interpreted by the ER staff to show "sinus tachycardia with ST segment elevations inferiorly and nonspecific ST and T-wave changes elsewhere." An arterial blood gas determination performed on room air shows normal arterial oxygenation with an alveolar-arterial oxygen gradient of 6. The chest radiographic study is normal.

The ER staff administers tissue plasminogen activator and then starts an intravenous (IV) heparin drip for the treatment of a presumed inferior MI. An IV NTG infusion and oxygen therapy are instituted but, despite these measures, the pain continues. Antacid therapy also does not relieve the pain. Only morphine sulfate seems to offer relief.

When the patient is transferred to the coronary care unit, the ECG shows continued "evolution" with ST segment elevations in leads I, II, III, aVL, aVF, and V_2 to V_6 that do not respond to IV NTG. The patient's chest pain persists. Blood tests reveal mildly elevated total creatine phosphokinase (CPK) levels (195 and 230 IU/L), but no increase in the CPK-MB isoenzyme level, normal electrolyte values, and normal renal function.

Further increments of NTG are given in an IV infusion and the patient's blood pressure begins to decrease. After 2 hours, the patient continues to writhe in pain, complains of feeling dizzy and having a severe headache, and vomits after the fifth dose of IV morphine sulfate. You are asked to see the patient and your examination reveals sinus tachycardia, a blood pressure of 92/50 mm Hg (no pulsus paradoxus), a respiratory rate of 16 per minute, a temperature of 101°F (38.5°C), fine rales at the lung bases, and no elevation in the jugular venous pressure, but a two-component pericardial friction rub is heard. The hemoglobin level is stable.

1. What is the most likely clinical diagnosis of this patient's chest pain?
2. Based on your clinical impression of this patient's presentation, what features would be expected on the ECG?
3. What is the most likely cause of the hypotension in this patient?

Case Discussion

1. *What is the most likely clinical diagnosis of this patient's chest pain?*

    The most likely clinical diagnosis of this patient's chest pain is acute idiopathic or viral pericarditis.

    The pertinent features of the history and physical examination that lead to this diagnosis are that the pain was preceded by a viral prodrome and was very clearly positional and pleuritic. Pericardial pain does not improve with NTG, but the lack of response to NTG does not exclude an acute MI. The patient's vital signs were stable except for a slight fever and tachycardia. The absence of tachypnea, together with the normal examination findings and a normal alveolar-arterial oxygen gradient, make acute pulmonary embolization unlikely. Acute costochondritis is often positional but associated with exquisite pain on palpation of the involved costochondral junction, and is not associated with ECG changes. If the examination and chest radiographic findings are normal and there is no past history of smoking or trauma, the likelihood of acute pneumothorax is low.

    The remaining two diagnoses, acute pericarditis versus MI, can still be differentiated on the basis of the history and physical examination findings. The sharp quality of the substernal chest pain, which is associated more with the recumbent position, deep breathing, and coughing, and which is relieved by sitting up, is atypical for MI but a classic symptom of pericarditis.

2. *Based on your clinical impression of this patient's presentation, what features would be expected on the ECG?*

    Sinus tachycardia and ST segment elevation are often the earliest findings, although the absence of ECG changes does not exclude the diagnosis of pericarditis. The typical changes of acute pericarditis often evolve over hours or days and are thought to be caused by a myocardial current of injury due to inflammation. There is early diffuse ST segment elevation. This differs from the ST segment elevation of acute MI, which usually is localized (anterior, inferior, or lateral), with the ST segments convex upward. In pericarditis, the ST segment elevation is concave upward and usually involves all the leads except aVR and V_1. PR segment depression is also common in the early phases of acute pericarditis. An important exception is in pericarditis after acute MI, in which typical ECG changes of pericarditis may not be present or may be atypical. The ECG changes of pericarditis evolve slowly over days, often with a phase of normalization of the ST segments followed by diffuse T-wave inversion.

3. *What is the most likely cause of the hypotension in this patient?*

The hypotension in this patient is most likely due to the cumulative effects of the medications he has been given (morphine and NTG). The accumulation and potentiation of medications, especially in the elderly, is a common clinical problem in the acute care setting. The combination of morphine and NTG in this patient induced sufficient vasodilation to cause hypotension.

Bleeding is also a possible cause of the hypotension. Thrombolytic agents would be contraindicated if the patient had a history of active peptic ulcer disease or a recent history of upper or lower gastrointestinal bleeding or melanotic stools. A more worrisome possibility is hemorrhagic pericarditis, especially because a new friction rub is heard. If the hypotension does not resolve quickly with discontinuation of NTG and morphine, an echocardiogram is indicated to exclude tamponade.

Suggested Readings

Levine MJ, Lorell BH, Diver DJ, Come PC. Implications of echocardiographically assisted diagnosis of pericardial tamponade in contemporary medical patients: detection prior to hemodynamic embarrassment. *J Am Coll Cardiol* 1991;17:59.

Lorell BH. Pericardial diseases. In: Branuwald E, ed. *Heart disease: a textbook of cardiovascular medicine.* Philadelphia: WB Saunders, 1997:1478.

Oliva PB, Hammill SC, Edwards WD. Electrocardiographic diagnosis of postinfarction regional pericarditis: ancillary observations regarding the effect of reperfusion on the rapidity and amplitude of T wave inversion after acute myocardial infarction. *Circulation* 1993;88:896.

Tsang TS, Freeman WK, Sinak LJ, et al. Echocardiographically guided pericardiocentesis: evolution and state-of-the-art technique. *Mayo Clin Proc* 1998;73:647.

Watkins MW. Physiologic role of the normal pericardium. *Annu Rev Med* 1993;44:171.

Acute Pulmonary Edema

1. What are the two most common underlying mechanisms of pulmonary edema?
2. What are the most common causes of acute cardiogenic pulmonary edema?
3. What is the immediate treatment for acute cardiogenic pulmonary edema?

Discussion

1. *What are the two most common underlying mechanisms of pulmonary edema?*

Pulmonary edema is usually caused by an imbalance of the Starling forces in the lung (cardiogenic pulmonary edema), by a disruption in the alveolar-capillary membrane (noncardiogenic pulmonary edema), or by a combination of these conditions.

With acute cardiogenic pulmonary edema, a sudden increase in pulmonary venous pressure results in increased pulmonary interstitial and alveolar fluid, and pulmonary lymphatic drainage cannot compensate acutely to remove the fluid. In noncardiogenic pulmonary edema, lymphatic drainage cannot compensate for the increased lung water caused by the disrupted alveolar-capillary membrane.

2. *What are the most common causes of acute cardiogenic pulmonary edema?*

A sudden increase in left ventricular end-diastolic pressure resulting from acute ischemia is the most common cause of acute cardiogenic pulmonary edema. The acute ischemia results in a stiff left ventricle and limited filling (diastolic dysfunction) and may also cause systolic dysfunction. The acute ischemia, if persistent, may result in an MI or may resolve without infarction (unstable angina). Other causes include malignant hypertension, new-onset atrial fibrillation (with loss of atrial contraction and a rapid ventricular response) or other arrhythmias, and acute mitral regurgitation such as might result from acute ischemia, endocarditis, or ruptured chordae tendineae.

3. *What is the immediate treatment for acute cardiogenic pulmonary edema?*

The immediate treatment for acute cardiogenic pulmonary edema should consist of oxygen therapy, IV diuresis with loop diuretics, and IV morphine. The patient should be sitting upright unless hypotension is present. If the patient has an acute MI or unstable angina, appropriate therapy should be instituted. Hypertension should be treated with IV nitroprusside or another acute agent such as labetalol.

Case   A 65-year-old man with a history of hypertension, diabetes mellitus, and exertional chest pressure is seen in the ER complaining of the sudden onset of chest pain and severe dyspnea at rest. He is currently taking enalapril (5 mg twice a day) to control his blood pressure. Physical examination reveals a pale white man in acute respiratory distress who is anxious and diaphoretic. His blood pressure is 180/100 mm Hg, his apical pulse is 170 beats per minute and irregularly irregular, and his respiratory rate is 40 per minute. Examination of the lungs reveals wet rales extending two thirds up from the basal lung fields bilaterally. Examination of the heart reveals a jugular venous pressure of 7 cm H_2O, a third sound (S_3) heard at the apex, and a grade II/VI holosystolic murmur heard at the apex. Arterial blood gas determinations performed on room air show a partial pressure of oxygen of 50 mm Hg, a partial pressure of carbon dioxide of 30 mm Hg, and a pH of 7.48. A chest radiograph shows an enlarged heart and pulmonary edema. The ECG reveals atrial fibrillation with a ventricular response of 170 beats per minute, a loss of R waves, and ST elevation anteriorly, findings that are consistent with an acute anterior MI. A diagnosis of acute anterior wall MI complicated by atrial fibrillation and pulmonary edema is made.

1. What is causing the pulmonary edema in this patient?
2. What medical therapy should be used to treat this patient acutely, and why?

Case Discussion

1. *What is causing the pulmonary edema in this patient?*

There are several causes of the pulmonary edema in this patient.

Myocardial infarction impairs both the systolic and diastolic function of the left ventricle. A loss of the contractile function of the large anterior wall of the left ventricle (systolic dysfunction) and acute stiffening of the damaged myocardium (diastolic dysfunction) lead to elevated filling pressures of the left ventricle and the left atrium. This causes the pulmonary venous and pulmonary capillary pressures to be elevated, producing an imbalance in the Starling forces and the transudation of fluid into the interstitium and then into the alveolar space.

Atrial fibrillation with a rapid ventricular response (170 beats per minute) is contributing to the left ventricular dysfunction because (a) a loss of atrial systolic contraction impairs left ventricular filling, which further elevates the left atrial pressure; (b) the rapid ventricular rate further impairs filling of the left ventricle; and (c) the rapid ventricular rate increases myocardial oxygen demands, which may increase ischemia, which in turn worsens the pulmonary edema.

Hypertension, especially when chronic and poorly controlled, produces a stiff, hypertrophied myocardium affected by elevated filling pressures. In a setting of MI, an acute increase in blood pressure caused by anxiety, pain, a catecholamine surge, and peripheral vasoconstriction augments the afterload against which the already compromised left ventricle has to work. This leads to a further elevation in the filling pressures, and worsens any mitral regurgitation already present.

Anxiety secondary to the pain and breathlessness is likely to increase the heart rate and blood pressure, thereby contributing to pulmonary edema by increasing the afterload.

A systolic murmur in this setting most likely represents mitral regurgitation secondary to ischemia or dysfunction or, less commonly, rupture of papillary muscle, a ventricular septal defect (VSD). These produce a systolic murmur, usually at the apex and radiating into the axilla in the presence of mitral regurgitation, and usually at the left lower sternal border in the presence of a VSD. When mitral regurgitation is acute and severe, the systolic murmur may be soft and may not be holosystolic because the left atrial pressure increases so rapidly in systole.

2. *What medical therapy should be used to treat this patient acutely, and why?*

There are several components to the acute treatment of this patient's pulmonary edema. The administration of **100% oxygen** is important because the alveolar edema interferes with adequate oxygen diffusion. **Morphine** (1-3 mg at a time in an IV push) diminishes anxiety and decreases central sympathetic outflow, thus reducing both venous and arterial vasoconstriction, resulting in decreases in ventricular preload and afterload, respectively. Morphine should not be given to patients with diminished sensorium or respiratory drive or hypercapnia because it may precipitate respiratory arrest. **Furosemide** (20 to 80 mg in a slow IV push) or other loop diuretics cause immediate venodilation, followed by diuresis within approximately 5 to 10 minutes. IV sodium nitroprusside may be used to reduce blood pressure if hypertension is present. **NTG**, administered in sublingual tablets or by IV drip, relieves the pulmonary edema by producing venodilation and treating acute ischemia, if hypotension is not present. **Digoxin** is not used to treat acute pulmonary edema except when atrial fibrillation with a rapid ventricular response is a contributing factor. (Digoxin slows the ventricular rate.) The total dose may approximate 1.0 to 1.5 mg IV in the first 24 hours, starting with 0.5 mg IV. IV diltiazem or a β blocker may be used to reduce the ventricular response if the patient can tolerate a negative inotropic agent.

Several new studies suggest that NTG, either intravenously or orally, may be superior to the standard treatment of morphine and furosemide in patients who are not hypotensive. Additional studies suggest that oral angiotensin-converting enzyme (ACE) inhibitors (in the absence of hypotension) may improve outcome when added to oxygen, morphine, and diuretics. Additional trials are needed before these recommendations can be made for routine care.

Suggested Readings

Beltrame JF, Zeitz CJ, Unger SA, et al. Nitrate therapy is an alternative to furosemide/morphine therapy in the management of acute cardiogenic pulmonary edema. *J Card Fail* 1998;4:271.

Bernard GR, Brigham KL. Pulmonary edema: pathophysiologic mechanisms and new approaches to therapy. *Chest* 1986;89:594.

Cotter G, Metzkor E, Kaluski E, et al. Randomised trial of high-dose isosorbide dinitrate plus low-dose furosemide versus high-dose furosemide plus low-dose isosorbide dinitrate in severe pulmonary oedema. *Lancet* 1998;351:389.

Gropper MA, Wiener-Kronish JP, Hashimoto S. Acute cardiogenic pulmonary edema. *Clin Chest Med* 1994;15:501.

Hamilton RJ, Carter WA, Gallagher EJ. Rapid improvement of acute pulmonary edema with sublingual captopril. *Acad Emerg Med* 1996;3:205.

Aortic Dissection

1. What is acute aortic dissection?
2. What is the most common cause of aortic dissection in the general population, in men younger than 40 years of age, and in women younger than 40 years of age?
3. What is the most sensitive initial diagnostic test for aortic dissection?
4. Where are the most common points of origin for aortic dissections?

Discussion

1. *What is acute aortic dissection?*

    Acute aortic dissection results from a tear in the aorta. Arterial blood driven by high pressure enters the diseased medial layer through the intimal tear and forms a plane in the media—"dissecting" the medial layer of the aortic wall. The area of dissection filled with blood is called the *false lumen*. Because of the shear forces of the dissecting blood, additional intimal tears may result. The false lumen may compress the true lumen or may cause the intimal flap to compress the true lumen, resulting in obstruction of major arteries.

2. *What is the most common cause of aortic dissection in the general population, in men younger than 40 years of age, and in women younger than 40 years of age?*

    The most common cause of aortic dissection in the general population is atherosclerosis associated with hypertension. The most common cause in men younger than 40 years of age is Marfan's syndrome; in women younger than 40 years of age, it is pregnancy. Fifty percent of all aortic dissections in women younger than 40 years of age occur in the third trimester of pregnancy. Women who have a dilated aortic root due to Marfan's syndrome are at particularly high risk for acute aortic dissection during pregnancy.

3. *What is the most sensitive initial diagnostic test for aortic dissection?*

    The preferred initial diagnostic test in most hospitals is transesophageal echocardiography (TEE). However, the best initial test may vary in different hospitals depending on the availability of and expertise with various diagnostic tests.

4. *Where are the most common points of origin for aortic dissections?*

    The most common point of origin for ascending aortic aneurysms is in the ascending aorta just above the aortic valve. The most common point of origin for descending aortic aneurysms is at the ligamentum arteriosum, which is just beyond the takeoff of the left subclavian artery.

Case   A 63-year-old man with a history of coronary artery disease and previous inferior MI has the following cardiac risk factors: 30 years of moderately controlled hypertension, 75 pack-years of tobacco use, type II non–insulin-dependent diabetes mellitus, and a family history of coronary artery disease. His cholesterol level 6 months before this admission was 260 mg/dL.

The patient has been experiencing his usual exertional angina, which is relieved with NTG and rest, without a change in pattern or character the month before presentation. At 11:00 a.m. on the day of admission, the patient was lifting a 50-pound bag of fertilizer when he acutely experienced a severe (10/10), tearing left precordial chest pain without radiation, but with diaphoresis, nausea, and lightheadedness. The pain was similar to his angina, but he obtained no relief with NTG (0.4 mg sublingually). He comes to the ER, where the physical examination reveals a right arm blood pressure of 80/40 mm Hg, a pulse rate of 110 per minute, and a respiratory rate of 24 per minute. He is a diaphoretic elderly man who is writhing in bed and complaining of left chest pain, which is now radiating to the throat and interscapular area. The cardiovascular examination reveals a tachycardia. The first (S_1) and second (S_2) sound are normal and a fourth sound (S_4) is present. There is a grade III/IV diastolic murmur consistent with aortic insufficiency heard at the left sternal border. Examination of the peripheral pulses reveals a diminished right radial pulse, a normal left radial pulse, and normal femoral pulses.

1. What tests would you do first to establish a working diagnosis?
2. How are aortic dissections classified, what are the causes, and what are the common signs and symptoms?
3. What initial therapy is indicated to stabilize this patient's condition?
4. Because aortic dissection is thought to be present, what imaging techniques should be done to confirm the diagnosis and assist in planning further therapy?
5. What definitive therapy should be instituted?
6. What long-term care is indicated for this patient?

Case Discussion

1. *What tests would you do first to establish a working diagnosis?*

   The first procedure to perform is a careful physical examination. Your examination in this patient confirms the ER findings, but the blood pressure in the left arm is 190/110 mm Hg, and the right arm blood pressure is still 80/40 mm Hg. The discrepancy in pulse and blood pressure between the right and left arms is strongly suggestive of aortic dissection involving the proximal aortic arch and ascending aorta. The finding of aortic insufficiency is consistent with involvement of the proximal ascending aorta. A chest radiograph should also be obtained, and in this patient it shows a widened mediastinum with aortic knob intimal calcium separated from the adventitial border by 1.2 cm. The calcium sign is defined as a separation that exceeds 1.0 cm, and it is pathognomonic for aortic dissection. An ECG should also be obtained to help determine whether there is evidence for an acute MI, which may result from occlusion of the coronary artery due to dissection. In this patient, there are diffuse, nonspecific ST segment and T-wave changes, but no acute ischemic ST segment changes. Based on the history and these findings, the likelihood of aortic dissection is deemed to be high in this patient.

2. *How are aortic dissections classified, what are the causes, and what are the common signs and symptoms?*

   Several classifications for aortic dissection have been proposed, but the most commonly used one is the DeBakey classification:

   Type I: Dissection originating in the ascending aorta, extending to or beyond the aortic arch
   Type II: Dissection limited to the ascending aorta

Type III: Dissection originating in the descending aorta and extending distally down the aorta or, rarely, extending retrograde into the aortic arch and ascending aorta

Another classification is the Daily or Stanford scheme, which is simpler:

Type A: All dissections involving the ascending aorta, whether the originating site is proximal or distal
Type B: All dissections not involving the ascending aorta

Thus, DeBakey types I and II and Stanford A both involve the ascending aorta and are termed *proximal dissections*, and DeBakey III and Stanford B involve the descending aorta and are termed *distal dissections*.

In reality, therapy is based on whether the dissection involves the ascending aorta or is distal to the ascending aorta. The clinical manifestations are determined by what arterial branches of the aorta are involved (the right brachiocephalic artery in this patient) and whether the aortic valve (aortic insufficiency in this patient) or coronary arteries, or both, are involved. Approximately two thirds of aortic dissections are proximal, whereas one third are distal.

The etiology of nontraumatic aortic dissection involves degeneration of the collagen and elastin fibers of the media of the aorta, which usually occurs in patients experiencing a chronic arterial stress, such as hypertension. A specific type of medial degeneration called cystic medial necrosis occurs in patients with Marfan's and Ehlers-Danlos syndromes.

Other predisposing factors for dissection include congenital coarctation of the aorta, bicuspid aortic valve, atherosclerosis, Noonan's and Turner's syndromes, and giant cell arteritis. Direct external trauma may lead to dissection and intravascular trauma from intraarterial catheterization and intraaortic balloon pumps; trauma during cardiac surgery may also result in dissection.

The incidence of aortic dissection peaks in the sixth and seventh decades, and it exhibits a male predominance, with a male-to-female ratio of 2:1; it can occur at any age, however. Most patients with aortic dissection between 40 and 70 years of age are hypertensive.

The predominant clinical manifestation of acute aortic dissection, seen in more than 90% of the patients, is a severe pain at onset. The pain is unbearable, and described as a tearing, ripping, or stabbing sensation. Unlike the pain of a MI, which is often crescendo in nature, the pain associated with aortic dissection is maximal at onset. In 70% of patients, the pain migrates, following the path of dissection. An anterior chest pain heralds a **proximal dissection**, whereas an interscapular pain indicates a **distal dissection** in over 90% of the patients with such dissections. The differential diagnosis of aortic dissection includes MI or ischemia, a thoracic nondissecting aneurysm, musculoskeletal pain, mediastinal tumors, and pericarditis.

Other signs and symptoms of acute aortic dissection depend on whether major arterial branches or the aortic valve, or both, are involved. Aortic insufficiency occurs in one half to two thirds of all cases of proximal dissections and is due to dilatation of the aortic root, hematoma interfering with leaflet coaptation, tearing of the annulus or leaflet, or a combination of these. Neurologic deficits, which are more common with proximal lesions, include stroke, ischemic peripheral neuropathy, or altered consciousness. Other complications include Horner's syndrome resulting from superior cervical ganglion compression, left recurrent laryngeal nerve paralysis causing hoarseness, and heart block (aortic annulus involvement). The involvement of major arterial branches can lead to myocardial, mesenteric, or renal infarctions.

Rupture of an aortic dissection is more common with the proximal type, and can cause acute pericardial effusion with cardiac tamponade or a left pleural effusion. Rupture into the airways or esophagus can result in hemoptysis or hematemesis.

3. *What initial therapy is indicated to stabilize this patient's condition?*

Medical therapy is indicated initially to stop the progression of the dissection. The patient should be admitted to an intensive care unit with hemodynamic monitoring. Medical therapy is aimed at reducing the mean arterial blood pressure and reducing the velocity of the left ventricular ejection (arterial dP/dt) to minimize arterial shear forces.

Sodium nitroprusside is a direct vasodilator and decreases arterial pressure in a dose-dependent manner. The aim is to reduce systolic arterial pressure to 100 to 120 mm Hg. However, dP/dt is increased as the result of a reflex tachycardia. dP/dt is best reduced by the administration of β-blocking agents. If there are no contraindications to β blockers, they should be given intravenously to reach a heart rate of 60 to 80 beats per minute. Esmolol, a short-acting IV β blocker, may be particularly useful because it can be titrated minute-to-minute to reduce heart rate. Labetalol is also a good choice for the treatment of acute aortic dissection because it is both an α- and β-blocking drug. In patients who have a contraindication to β blockers, calcium channel blockers such as verapamil or diltiazem delivered IV could be used to decrease heart rate and blood pressure.

4. *Because aortic dissection is thought to be present, what imaging techniques should be done to confirm the diagnosis and assist in planning further therapy?*

A **transthoracic echocardiogram** can be performed quickly and noninvasively to confirm aortic insufficiency, assess segmental left ventricular systolic function, and assess the proximal aortic root for the presence of dilatation. However it is poorly sensitive, especially for distal dissections. In general, TEE, computed tomography (CT), or magnetic resonance imaging (MRI) is indicated if dissection is suspected.

A more sensitive echocardiographic technique for the detection of thoracic and ascending aortic dissection is **TEE (transesophageal echocardiography)**. This technique can assess the ascending arch and proximal aorta. It is also capable of evaluating aortic insufficiency, left ventricular segmental wall function, and pericardial effusion, and often permits visualization of the proximal coronary arteries. Therefore, this technique achieves a more complete evaluation of the potential complications and can determine whether an aortic dissection is present. In hemodynamically stable patients, this test is as useful diagnostically as other imaging modalities when done by experienced TEE sonographers. Another benefit is that TEE can be carried out at the patient's bedside.

Magnetic resonance imaging is probably the most complete assessment tool for aortic dissection when spin-echo and ciné imaging protocols are used. The large field of view afforded by MRI can visualize the entire aorta from oblique angles, which is often necessary to assess the extent of dissection and the involvement of major branch vessels (i.e., the subclavian or carotid artery). Ciné MRI techniques provide noncontrast assessment of flowing blood to identify flow into a false lumen or an intimal flap, as well as significant aortic insufficiency (diastolic flow into the left ventricle with turbulence) and coronary artery flow. Often, proximal coronary artery involvement can be evaluated by both spin-echo images and ciné MRI flow within the arteries. Therefore, because of the large field of view it provides and because it is a less operator dependent imaging modality, MRI is the best imaging tool for the assessment of aortic dissection. The primary limitations are related to the emergent on-site availability of the modality and the hemodynamic stability of the patient, which needs to be sufficient to allow isolation and confinement for as long as 30 to 40 minutes.

A contrast CT scan is very good for defining the extent of an aortic dissection, that is, proximal versus distal. However, it does not define the site of the intimal tear or show whether the coronary arteries are involved.

The gold standard in the past for evaluating an acute aortic dissection has been angiography, including both coronary and aortic studies. Angiography may define the site of the intimal tear, the severity of aortic insufficiency, whether the coronary arteries are involved, and the extent of the dissection—proximal versus distal. However, comparisons of different imaging modalities have demonstrated that the sensitivity of angiography in the detection of aortic dissection is less than that of other modalities. Thus, the gold standard for the diagnosis of aortic dissection is probably changing to TEE in the acute and unstable patient and MRI in the chronic stable patient.

5. *What definitive therapy should be instituted?*

If left untreated, acute aortic dissection carries a 25% 24-hour mortality rate that progresses to 90% at 1 year. In general, surgical repair is better than medical therapy for the management of acute proximal dissections, and medical therapy (reducing the blood pressure and dP/dt) is better for uncomplicated acute distal dissections. Surgical repair is indicated in patients with acute distal dissections when there is vital organ compromise, rupture, expansion, saccular aneurysm formation, the presence of Marfan's syndrome, or continued pain. When dissection is chronic (present >2 weeks), medical therapy may be indicated in both proximal and distal dissections because the *highest* mortality risk is past.

6. *What long-term care is indicated for this patient?*

It is essential to control the patient's hypertension and decrease his dP/dt, preferably with β blockers. The long-term prognosis in survivors is good, with an actuarial survival rate only a little worse than that for age-matched control subjects. Once the patient is discharged, there is no difference in outcome between proximal and distal dissections, acute and chronic dissection, or medical and surgical therapy. Follow-up should include physical examination and chest radiographic studies. Other imaging modalities such as MRI, TEE, or CT scanning should be used for serial aortic imaging. However, studies evaluating their cost-effectiveness are not available.

Suggested Readings

Cigarroa JE, Isselbacher EM, De Sanctis RW, et al. Diagnostic imaging in the evaluation of suspected aortic dissection. *N Engl J Med* 1993;328:35.

Glower DD, Fann JI, Speier RH, et al. Comparison of medical and surgical therapy for uncomplicated descending aortic dissection. *Circulation* 1990;82[Suppl IV]:IV-39.

Kouchoukos NT, Dougenis D. Surgery of the thoracic aorta. *N Engl J Med* 1997;336:1876.

Pretre R, Von Segesser LK. Aortic dissection. *Lancet* 1997;349:1461.

Smith JA, Fann JI, Miller DC, et al. Surgical management of aortic dissection in patients with the Marfan syndrome. *Circulation* 1994;90[Suppl II]:II-235.

Congestive Heart Failure

1. What are the most common underlying diseases causing chronic congestive heart failure (CHF) in the U.S. population?

2. Can either systolic or diastolic dysfunction result in signs and symptoms of heart failure?

3. What is myocardial remodeling and what are its consequences?

4. Which drug classes have been shown to prolong life in patients with heart failure?

5. Which drug classes have been shown to lead to worsened survival in patients with heart failure?

Discussion

1. *What are the most common underlying diseases causing chronic congestive heart failure (CHF) in the U.S. population?*

In the United States and most developed countries, hypertension and ischemic heart disease are the most common underlying diseases in patients with heart failure. Valvular heart disease and cardiomyopathy are less common causes, but are still frequently encountered.

2. *Can either systolic or diastolic dysfunction result in signs and symptoms of heart failure?*

Systolic dysfunction is defined as a decrease in contractile function most commonly measured as a decrease in ejection fraction (EF). Diastolic dysfunction results when the heart is stiff and ventricular filling is impaired, resulting in increased end-diastolic pressures. Patients may have diastolic dysfunction with or without systolic dysfunction. Typical signs and symptoms of heart failure may result with either systolic or diastolic dysfunction. Typically, the prevalence of diastolic function as a cause of heart failure is increased in the elderly and in women.

3. *What is myocardial remodeling and what are its consequences?*

After myocardial injury with resulting systolic dysfunction, there is usually a progressive deterioration in the structure and function of the ventricular myocardium—a process termed *myocardial remodeling.* This progressive deterioration is partially responsible for the high mortality rates in patients with heart failure. Although the specific molecular and cellular events that lead to remodeling are not entirely understood, many factors that promote remodeling have been described. These mechanisms include increased wall stress and activation of the renin–angiotensin and β-adrenergic systems. Blockade of these mechanisms would be expected to slow or prevent myocardial remodeling and improve survival in patients with heart failure and systolic dysfunction.

4. *Which drug classes have been shown to prolong life in patients with heart failure?*

Those drug classes that have been found to prolong life in patients with heart failure are ACE inhibitors (CONSENSUS [Cooperative New Scandinavian Enupril Survival Trial], SOLVD [Studies of Left Ventricular Dysfunction], SAVE [Survival and Ventricular Enlargment], as well as other trials), hydralazine and isordil (VHeFT-1 [Vasodilator Heart Failure Trial] trial), and β blockers (Carvedilol trials, MERITHF [Metoprolol CR/XL Randomized Intervention Trial in Conjestive Heart Failure], CIBIS-II, BEST [Cardiac Insufficiency Bisoprolol Study] trials).

5. *Which drug classes have been shown to lead to worsened survival in patients with heart failure?*

Several drugs with positive inotropic action have resulted in an adverse effect on survival. These include several phosphodiesterase inhibitors (milrinone, vesnarinone, and possibly pimobendan and enoximone), xamoterol (a β-adrenergic receptor agonist), and ibopamine (a dopamine agonist). The exception is digoxin, which had a neutral effect on survival and a small beneficial effect on repeat hospitalizations in patients with heart failure. Surprisingly, two vasodilators (flosequinan and prostacyclin) have also increased the mortality rate in patients with systolic dysfunction and heart failure.

Case   A 42-year-old white man is seen in the ER with a chief complaint of shortness of breath that has lasted for 1 week. He reports having had a viral syndrome approximately 3 weeks before admission. Subsequently, he noted the development of lower extremity edema, a 15-pound (6.75-kg) weight gain, dyspnea on exertion, and orthopnea. Physical examination reveals his heart rate is 140 per minute and irregularly irregular, his blood pressure is 90/60 mm Hg, and his respiratory rate is 22 per minute. Examination of the jugular venous pressure demonstrates a mean pressure of 12 to 14 cm H_2O. Lung examination reveals bibasilar dullness with rales extending one fourth of the way up from the basal lung fields bilaterally. Cardiac examination findings are significant for a diffuse point of maximal impulse, which is displaced to the anterior axillary line. The S_1 and S_2 are of variable intensity, and a prominent S_3 gallop over the displaced cardiac apex is appreciated. There is a grade II/VI holosystolic murmur that is heard best at the cardiac apex, with prominent radiation to the axilla. On examination of the abdomen, an enlarged, tender liver is found. The extremities are cool and exhibit 2+ pitting edema. The ECG shows atrial fibrillation with nonspecific ST-T–wave changes and occasional ventricular premature beats. Arterial blood gas measurements performed with the patient on 4 L of oxygen per minute by nasal cannula reveal a pH of 7.46, a P_{O_2} of 52 mm Hg, a P_{CO_2} of 32 mm Hg, and a bicarbonate (HCO_3^-) concentration of 26 mmol/L.

1. Does this patient have left, right, or biventricular failure?
2. An S_3 is heard, but no S_4. Why?
3. What chest radiographic findings would you expect to see in this patient?
4. What neurohormonal mechanisms are activated in this patient?
5. What treatment options would likely be beneficial in this patient?
6. Which renal indices would be expected to be abnormal in this patient (before diuretic treatment)?

   After diuresis and stabilization on medical therapy, the patient continues to have dyspnea at rest, an S_3 gallop, and bibasilar rales.
7. In which New York Heart Association (NYHA) class would you categorize this patient's symptoms?
8. What is this patient's expected mortality rate in his current condition?

Case Discussion

1. *Does this patient have left, right, or biventricular failure?*

   This patient has findings indicating both right and left ventricular failure (biventricular failure). The cool extremities, tachycardia, and narrow pulse pressure suggest poor forward cardiac output and could reflect either right or left ventricular failure. A left ventricular S_3 gallop and pulmonary rales are signs of left ventricular failure. The bibasilar dullness suggests the presence of bilateral pleural effusions, which may be seen in the setting of either right or left ventricular dysfunction. The apical murmur most likely represents mitral regurgitation. We do not know from the history whether the patient had a preexisting valvular disorder. Secondary mitral or tricuspid regurgitation may occur due to distortion of the supporting structures of the atrioventricular valves, and occur commonly in the setting of left or right ventricular failure, respectively. Valvular regurgitation further decreases the effective forward cardiac output. Mitral regurgitation usually causes a large V wave in the left atrial or pulmonary capillary wedge pressure tracing, and tricuspid regurgitation causes a large V wave in the jugular venous pressure.

There are many signs of right ventricular failure in this patient. The cardinal finding of elevated central venous pressure is apparent from the patient's jugular venous distention. Kussmaul's sign is an absent fall in the jugular venous pressure with inspiration and is due to the right ventricle's inability to handle the augmented venous return. It may be encountered in patients with right ventricular failure or constrictive pericardial disease. The patient's enlarged liver is the result of hepatic congestion stemming from increased back pressure on the hepatic vein. The pitting edema in the lower extremities is caused by elevated hydrostatic pressure in the venous system, resulting in extravasation of fluid into the interstitial space of the ankles, where the forces of gravity are the greatest.

2. *An S_3 is heard, but no S_4. Why?*

An S_3 is a low-frequency sound heard 0.13 to 0.16 second after S_2. An S_3 occurs at the end of the rapid phase of ventricular filling and is most likely due to the vibration of the chordae tendineae or the left ventricular wall with rapid filling, and may arise from the right or left ventricle. A left ventricular S_3 is best heard with the bell of the stethoscope at the cardiac apex, at the end of inspiration. A right ventricular S_3 is also best heard with the bell, but is most audible at the lower left sternal border or over the epigastrium. An S_3 is a normal finding in children or young adults, but in middle-aged or older patients it is usually a sign of volume overload due to CHF or other problems.

An S_4 is a presystolic atrial sound (gallop) that is heard when the ventricle is poorly compliant. Given the patient's volume overload, it is likely that both ventricles are poorly compliant. However, the patient is in atrial fibrillation, and therefore there are no truly effective atrial systoles to give rise to an S_4 (rarely, an S_4 may be heard even in atrial fibrillation because of the high left atrial pressure and increased flow in late diastole).

3. *What chest radiographic findings would you expect to see in this patient?*

The likely findings on a chest radiography stem from the effects of volume overload and elevated pulmonary venous pressure. Cardiomegaly, which is defined as a cardiac-to-thoracic diameter ratio exceeding 0.5, is present in most cases in which there is depressed left ventricular systolic function. Cephalization of the pulmonary blood flow occurs and is evidenced by the enlarged pulmonary vessels in the superior portion of the pulmonary tree. The haziness of the central vasculature is a result of the increased hydrostatic pressure and subsequent transudation of fluid into the tissue surrounding the vessels. Kerley's B lines are horizontal, thin, sharp lines that extend inward from the periphery of the lungs. They represent edema formation within and hypertrophy of the interlobular septa. Pleural effusions may be found in the setting of right or left ventricular failure. When pulmonary congestion is severe and alveolar edema is present, a "butterfly" or "batwing" infiltrate may be seen centered over the main pulmonary artery.

4. *What neurohormonal mechanisms are likely to be activated in this patient?*

The two neurohormonal mechanisms most likely to be activated in this patient are the **renin–angiotensin–aldosterone axis** and the **adrenergic nervous system**. The serum norepinephrine level has been shown to correlate inversely with the EF and patient survival in patients with chronic CHF. Cardiac adrenergic activation occurs even earlier than systemic adrenergic activation. Other hormones that may be activated include vasopressin, endothelin, and cytokines such as tumor necrosis factor-α and interleukin-1.

5. *What treatment options would likely be beneficial in this patient?*

The general goals for the medical treatment of heart failure are:

(1). Identify and treat the underlying condition.

(2). Eliminate any precipitating factors.

(3). Treat the symptoms.

(4). Improve survival.

The first step is to identify the underlying cause of heart failure. This may be hypertension, coronary artery disease, cardiomyopathy, valvular heart disease, or many other causes. Examples of treatment include medical treatment for hypertension, coronary angiography and coronary angioplasty or coronary bypass surgery for coronary disease, and valve replacement or repair for valve disease.

In patients with chronic or acute heart failure, it is important to eliminate precipitating factors (e.g., dietary or medication noncompliance, arrhythmias, anemia). Excess alcohol use may cause a cardiomyopathy, but may also exacerbate heart failure of other causes.

Symptomatic improvement is usually achieved by relieving the excess salt and water retention with diuretics and by improving preload and afterload with vasodilators—particularly the ACE inhibitors. Diuretics help relieve the salt and water retention characteristic of CHF. Loop diuretics such as furosemide or bumetanide are most often used because they are more effective than thiazide diuretics when renal perfusion is decreased. Care must be taken to avoid overdiuresis and to replace potassium because hypokalemia may promote ventricular arrhythmias. Spironolactone, an aldosterone antagonist, has been reported to decrease the mortality rate in patients with heart failure due to systolic dysfunction. ACE inhibitors are the cornerstone of therapy for patients with systolic dysfunction. There are many ACE inhibitors now available (captopril, enalapril, lisinopril, quinapril, ramipril, benazepril, trandolapril, fosinopril, moexipril), and there does not appear to be a clear therapeutic advantage to the use of one over another. By decreasing the conversion of angiotensin I to angiotensin II, these drugs reduce preload and afterload, improve symptoms, and prolong survival in patients with systolic dysfunction. Cough is the most common side effect of ACE inhibitors, but cough is also a common symptom of heart failure. Care should be taken to exclude heart failure as a cause of the cough before these drugs are discontinued. Hypotension, renal insufficiency, and hyperkalemia are less frequent but serious side effects of the ACE inhibitors. In general, these occur in patients with severe heart failure or preexisting renal insufficiency. In patients with severe heart failure or intrinsic renal insufficiency, the ACE inhibitors must be started in very low doses, and the blood pressure and serum potassium and creatinine must be monitored carefully. Angiotensin II receptor blockers (ARBs) such as losartan, candesartan, irbesartan, and valsartan block the angiotensin II receptor directly. They appear to have beneficial effects in patients with heart failure, but it is not clear if the effects are equivalent to those of the ACE inhibitors. These drugs may be used in patients who cannot take ACE inhibitors because of cough or an allergy, but are as likely as the ACE inhibitors to cause hyperkalemia, hypotension, or renal insufficiency. Several clinical trials are evaluating the role of ARBs in patients with heart failure to determine if they should be used instead of, or in addition to, the ACE inhibitors. In patients who have severe symptoms despite therapy with ACE inhibitors or ARBs, the combination of hydralazine and isordil may be beneficial. Another option is the use of digoxin, which results in an improvement in symptoms and a reduction in hospital admissions.

The β-adrenergic blockers have also been shown to improve survival in patients with systolic dysfunction and heart failure. Although the benefit on symptoms is less clear than with ACE inhibitors, β blockers appear to produce a larger improvement in remodeling and EF. Because the β blockers reduce heart rate and initially decrease contractility, introduction of treatment or up-titration may result in worsening of symptoms. These drugs therefore must be started in low doses and up-titrated slowly, and patients must be monitored carefully. Patients with decompensated heart failure usually should not be given β blockers. Several β blockers (carvedilol, metoprolol, and bisoprolol) have been shown to reduce mortality in patients with heart failure. It is not yet clear if there are advantages of one over another. Implantable cardioverter-defibrillators improve survival in patients who have had a sustained episode of ventricular tachycardia or ventricular fibrillation. Studies are underway to define other subsets of patients for whom implantable cardioverter-defibrillators may improve survival.

Sodium restriction is an essential part of any program designed to treat patients in heart failure. Patients should avoid excess salt and water, weigh themselves daily, avoid nonsteroidal antiinflammatory drugs, and report any increase in symptoms or weight gain promptly to their physicians.

6. *Which renal indices would be expected to be abnormal in this patient (before diuretic treatment)?*

Several renal indices would be abnormal in this patient. Patients with CHF routinely exhibit a picture of decreased glomerular filtration, which leads to a prerenal state. Despite the increase in the total-body sodium and water content, the diminished effective forward cardiac output causes arterial underfilling. Compensatory mechanisms are then activated. The ultimate effect of these mechanisms is to conserve water and sodium through the operation of renal tubular mechanisms. This results in concentrated urine with an elevated urine osmolality, an elevated blood urea nitrogen/creatinine ratio, and low urine sodium concentration. The fractional excretion of sodium [defined as (urinary sodium/urinary creatinine×plasma creatinine/plasma sodium) × 100] usually is low, with values less than 1% common in the absence of diuretics. In general, the urine sediment is benign in nature. Hyaline and nonpigmented casts may be seen, but red blood cell casts are not seen in prerenal states due to CHF. If the renal perfusion is diminished to such a degree as to produce acute tubular necrosis, muddy brown granular casts and epithelial cells may be seen.

7. *In which NYHA class would you categorize this patient's symptoms?*

By definition, patients with symptoms (dyspnea) at rest are classified as NYHA class IV. The four categories that make up the NYHA classification, and their definitions, are

Class I: No symptoms with any level of exercise
Class II: Symptoms on more than ordinary activity
Class III: Symptoms on activities of daily living
Class IV: Symptoms at rest

8. *What is this patient's expected mortality rate in his current condition?*

An NYHA class IV designation in the general CHF population carries a 1-year mortality rate approaching 50% when management consists of medical therapy only. Cardiac transplantation has dramatically improved the 1-year survival rate to 80% to 90%. In general, life expectancy closely parallels the functional status. Therefore, as the functional status improves, so does longevity. In patients with NYHA class II to III heart disease who are treated medically, the 5-year mortality rate is 50%.

The predominant causes of death in these patients are progressive left ventricular dysfunction and dysrhythmias. The combination of ventricular tachycardia and fibrillation has been accepted as the predominant dysrhythmic cause of sudden death in these patients, but there is some evidence that bradycardic arrest also plays an important role.

Suggested Readings

Bristow MR. Mechanism of action of beta-blocking agents in heart failure. *Am J Cardiol* 1997;80:26L.

Cleland JGF, Swedberg K, Poole-Wilson PA. Successes and failures of current treatment of heart failure. *Lancet* 1998;352:S19.

Cohn JN. Treatment of congestive heart failure. *N Engl J Med* 1997;335:490.

Massie BM. Heart failure trials: what have we learned? *Lancet* 1998;352:S29.

Schocken DD, Arrieta M, Leaverton P, Ross E. Prevalence and mortality rate of congestive heart failure in the United States. *J Am Coll Cardiol* 1992;20:301.

Sharpe N, Doughty R. Epidemiology of heart failure and ventricular dysfunction. *Lancet* 1998;352:S3.

Essential Hypertension and Hypertensive Emergencies

1. What is the prevalence of systemic hypertension in the U.S. population?

2. What is the most common cause of systemic hypertension?

3. What is the natural history of untreated hypertension?

4. What is a hypertensive crisis?

Discussion

1. *What is the estimated prevalence of systemic hypertension in the U.S. population?*

   The overall prevalence of hypertension in the United States is approximately 25%. However, the prevalence increases with age, so that more than 60% of the population older than 70 years of age has hypertension. The incidence of hypertension and its severity is greater in blacks than whites at every age group beyond adolescence.

2. *What is the most common cause of systemic hypertension?*

   No cause is found for approximately 90% of patients with hypertension. These patients are said to have essential hypertension. Although the mechanism of essential hypertension is unknown, there are apparently both genetic and environmental factors.

3. *What is the natural history of untreated hypertension?*

   Uncomplicated hypertension often remains asymptomatic for 10 to 20 years or more. However, there is a direct relationship between the levels of both systolic and diastolic blood pressure and the incidence of stroke, coronary artery disease, and heart failure. The overall risk of premature cardiovascular disease increases substantially when additional cardiovascular risk factors are present. In fact, the likelihood of a vascular event over the next 10 years can be estimated for any patient based on their age, sex, and other risks (American Heart Association's *Coronary and Stroke Risk Handbook*). If patients with hypertension are not treated, approximately 50% die of coronary disease, 33% of stroke, and 10% to 15% of renal failure.

4. *What is a hypertensive crisis?*

   A hypertensive crisis is a situation in which hypertension requires emergent treatment. A hypertensive crisis includes hypertension with acute damage to retinal vessels (hemorrhages or exudates), which is termed *accelerated hypertension*, and hypertension with papilledema, which is called *malignant hypertension*.

   Hypertensive crises include[*]:

Accelerated or malignant hypertension
Cerebrovascular complications
Hypertensive encephalopathy
Intracerebral hemorrhage
Subarachnoid hemorrhage
Atherothrombotic cerebral infarction with severe hypertension
Cardiac
Aortic dissection
Acute pulmonary edema or left ventricular failure

---

[*]From Kaplan N. Management of hypertensive emergencies. *Lancet* 1994;344:1335.

Acute MI
Acute glomerulonephritis
Renal crisis from collagen vascular disease
Excessive circulatory catecholamines
Sympathomimetic drug use (cocaine)
Rebound hypertension due to discontinuation of antihypertensive drugs

Case   A 45-year-old African-American man is seen in the outpatient department complaining of intermittent throbbing headaches that have occurred every morning for 2 weeks. He has a history of untreated, asymptomatic, sustained high blood pressure (150 to 160/100 mm Hg) of 10 years' duration. He has no history of palpitations, sweating, tremor, or periodic paralysis. His father was also hypertensive and died from a stroke at 67 years of age. The patient has smoked cigarettes, two packs per day, for 30 years.

His physical examination reveals a blood pressure of 180/120 mm Hg and a heart rate of 90 per minute and regular. Fundal examination reveals the presence of arterial vasoconstriction. Cardiac examination reveals a laterally displaced point of maximal impulse, S_4, no S_3, and no murmur. During abdominal examination, no bruit or mass is found and the neurologic and other systems are unremarkable.

After 2 weeks of treatment, the patient is lost to follow-up. Five years later, he presents to the ER complaining of blurred vision and severe headaches. His physical examination at that time reveals a blood pressure of 270/140 mm Hg and heart rate of 100 per minute. His sensorium and orientation are normal, but fundal examination reveals retinal hemorrhages, exudates, and papilledema. Heart examination shows a left ventricular lift and an S_4. The chest radiograph shows mild to moderate cardiomegaly. His serum creatinine level is 2.4 mg/dL. The ECG shows normal sinus rhythm with increased voltage and ST segment depression and T-wave inversion.

1. What is the most likely cause of this patient's hypertension?
2. Based on initial history and physical examination findings 5 years ago, what end-organ damage was present and what was the general pathologic process?
3. What therapies and laboratory investigations would have been beneficial in this patient when he presented 5 years earlier?
4. What complications will likely develop in this patient if his hypertension is left untreated?
5. What is the appropriate diagnosis at the time of his presentation to the ER 5 years later?
6. What would be the appropriate treatment approach to adopt after the ER presentation?

Case Discussion

1. *What is the most likely cause of this patient's hypertension?*
   The most likely cause of this patient's hypertension is essential hypertension.

2. *Based on the initial history and physical examination findings 5 years ago, what end-organ damage was present and what was the general pathologic process?*

Based on the findings revealed by physical examination (left ventricular lift, S_4), this patient had left ventricular hypertrophy.

3. *What therapies and laboratory investigations would have been beneficial in this patient when he presented 5 years earlier?*

The plan of management in this patient should commence with oral antihypertensive drugs (usually at least two drugs for the control of severe hypertension), with the aim to maintain blood pressure at less than 140/90 mm Hg. Eliminating coexisting cardiovascular risk factors (especially smoking) and exercising regularly are also recommended. Moderate sodium restriction may also be beneficial.

The laboratory investigation should include chest radiography, ECG, urinalysis, and measurement of the fasting blood sugar, blood urea nitrogen, serum creatinine, electrolytes, cholesterol [total and low-density lipoprotein (LDL) and high-density lipoprotein], and triglyceride levels to yield a baseline evaluation of target organ involvement for the purposes of risk stratification and long-term follow-up.

This man already had some findings that would place him in the high-risk category for the development of cardiovascular complications. These factors are black race, younger age of onset of hypertension, male sex, hypercholesterolemia, cigarette smoking, diabetes mellitus, obesity, and evidence of end-organ damage (ventricular hypertrophy).

4. *What complications will likely develop in this patient if his hypertension is left untreated?*

Based on the preceding discussion, any or all of the complications of hypertension could evolve. These complications can be divided into two major categories:

Those caused by the hypertension itself, including left ventricular hypertrophy, CHF, renal failure, cerebral hemorrhage, retinopathy, and aortic dissection
Those caused by accelerated atherosclerosis of the coronary, cerebral, or peripheral arteries, resulting in angina pectoris, myocardial and cerebral infarction, arrhythmia, and peripheral vascular disease

5. *What is the appropriate diagnosis at the time of his presentation to the ER 5 years later?*

The appropriate diagnosis when he is seen 5 years later in the ER is hypertensive crisis and accelerated malignant hypertension. A hypertensive crisis is considered a medical emergency. Such high blood pressure can cause immediate vascular damage, as seen in this patient. The presence of severe hypertension (diastolic blood pressure of 115 mm Hg or greater) in conjunction with grade 3 (retinal hemorrhage and exudate) or grade 4 (papilledema) funduscopic changes is defined as accelerated or malignant hypertension, respectively. The term *hypertensive encephalopathy* should be reserved to refer to the presence of significant alterations in consciousness.

Table 2-1. Parenteral Agents Used to Treat Hypertensive Emergencies

Drug	Route	Onset	Duration	Dose or dosage
Vasodilators				
Sodium nitroprusside	IV infusion	Seconds–1 min	3–5 min	0.25–10 μg/kg/min
Nicardipine hydrochloride	IV	5–10 min	1–4 hr	2–10 mg/hr
Fenoldopam mesylate	IV infusion	<5 min	30 min	0.1–0.3 μg/kg/min
Nitroglycerin	IV infusion	1–2 min	3–5 min	5–100 μg/min
Diazoxide	IV bolus or infusion	1–5 min	6–12 hr	50 mg IV every 5–10 min over 30 sec, or 15–30 mg/min by IV infusion
Hydralazine	IV	10–20 min	3–8 hr	10–20 mg IV
	Intramuscular (also oral)	30 min	3–8 hr	10–50 mg IM
Enalaprilat	IV bolus	15–30 min	6 hr	1.25–5 mg
Adrenergic Inhibitors				
Labetalol	IV	5 min	3–6 hr	0.5–2 mg/min IV infusion or 20–80 mg every 10 min to a maximum cumulative dose of 300 mg
Trimethaphan	IV infusion	1–5 min	10 min	0.5–5 mg/min
Phentolamine	IV bolus	1–2 min	3–10 min	Load 5–15 mg IV every 5 min
Esmolol	IV bolus then infusion	1–2 min	10–20 min	250–500 μg/kg $\times$ 41 min, then 50–300 μg/kg/min IV

IV, intravenous.

6. *What would be the appropriate treatment approach after the ER presentation?*
    Because the papilledema is consistent with the presence of severe hypertension and represents early brain edema, which may compromise the autoregulation of cerebral blood flow, the treatment approach should be to admit the patient to the intensive care unit and start him on parenteral antihypertensive drug therapy. Sodium nitroprusside is one of the most effective and suitable drugs in this situation because of its rapid onset of action, ranging from a matter of seconds to 1 minute, and short duration of action of 3 to 5 minutes. The goal of treatment should be to maintain the diastolic blood pressure between 100 and 110 mm Hg or the mean arterial pressure at not less than 120 mm Hg, because an abrupt decrease in the blood pressure to "normal" levels may produce hypoperfusion to the brain, heart, and kidney.
    A list of parenteral agents used to treat hypertensive emergencies is given in Table 2-1. If therapy is less urgent, a number of oral antihypertensive agents are available and are described in the *JNC VI* (see Bibliography). Short-acting nifedipine should not be used because of the increased risk of MI.

Suggested Readings

Appel LJ, Moore TJ, Obarzanek E, et al. A clinical trial of the effects of dietary patterns on blood pressure. *N Engl J Med* 1997;336:1117.
Burt VL, Whelton P, Roccella EJ, et al. Prevalence of hypertension in the US adult population: results from the third national Health and Nutrition Examination Survey, 1988–1991. *Hypertension* 1995;25:305.

Hansson L, Zanchetti A, Carruthers SG, et al. Effects of intensive blood-pressure lowering and low-dose aspirin in patients with hypertension: principal results of the Hypertension Optimal Treatment (HOT) randomised trial. *Lancet* 1998;351:1755.

Joint National Committee on Detection, Evaluation, and Treatment of High Blood Pressure. The sixth report of the Joint National Committee on Detection, Evaluation, and Treatment of High Blood Pressure (JNC VI). *Arch Intern Med* 1997;157:2413.

MacMahon S, Peto R, Cutler J, et al. Blood pressure, stroke, and coronary heart disease: part 1. prolonged differences in blood pressure: prospective observational studies corrected for the regression dilution bias. *Lancet* 1990;335:765.

Pickering G. Hypertension: definitions, natural histories and consequences. *Am J Med* 1972;52:570.

Wilson PW. Established risk factors and coronary artery disease: the Framingham Study. *Am J Hypertens* 1994;7:75.

Myocardial Infarction

1. What are the major known risk factors for coronary artery disease?
2. What is the male-to-female ratio associated with ischemic heart disease deaths in the U.S. population?
3. What is the most common cause of acute MI?
4. In placebo-controlled trials, what types of treatment have been shown to improve outcome in patients with acute MI?

Discussion

1. *What are the major known risk factors for coronary artery disease?*

   Cigarette smoking, diabetes mellitus, hypertension, and dyslipidemia are the major modifiable risk factors for coronary artery disease. Advanced age, a family history of coronary artery disease, and male sex are nonmodifiable risk factors. Other modifiable risk factors include obesity and physical inactivity. Factors that appear to increase risk and are still being studied include fibrinogen, homocysteine, elevated coagulation factor VII levels, decreased fibrinolytic activity and elevated plasminogen activator inhibitor-1 levels, stress, and low levels of circulating antioxidants.

2. *What is the male-to-female ratio associated with ischemic heart disease deaths in the U.S. population?*

   The male-to-female ratio associated with ischemic heart disease deaths in the U.S. population is 1:1; coronary artery disease is the leading cause of death in both men and women. However, the onset of symptomatic coronary artery disease is 10 to 15 years later in women than in men.

3. *What is the most common cause of acute MI?*

   Atherosclerosis is the underlying cause of MI in 95% or more of patients. In most of these patients, an acute thrombus has formed at the site of rupture of an atherosclerotic plaque.

4. *In placebo-controlled trials, what types of treatments have been shown to improve outcome in patients with acute MI?*

   Aspirin, thrombolytic agents, β-adrenergic blockers, and ACE inhibitors have all been shown to reduce mortality after MI. Acute percutaneous transluminal coronary angioplasty (primary PTCA), when performed promptly, appears to improve survival more than thrombolytic drugs, at least in the short term. Chronically, lowering the LDL cholesterol with HMG-CoA reductase inhibitors decreases the risk of recurrent MI.

Case 1   A 62-year-old man with a history of hypertension is mowing his lawn at 9:00 a.m. on a Saturday morning when he experiences a heavy sensation in his chest. He stops mowing the lawn and within 10 minutes his symptoms resolve, and he resumes cutting the grass. Approximately 10 minutes later, he experiences severe, crushing chest pain associated with shortness of breath and pain radiating down his left arm. As he walks to his house, he becomes diaphoretic and nauseated, and vomits twice. At this point, he calls an ambulance and is taken to the ER. When you arrive to examine him, he is still experiencing severe pain. A 12-lead ECG reveals 3-mm of ST segment elevation in leads V_2, V_3, V_4, and V_5 with inferior ST segment depression. The pain has been present a total of approximately 45 minutes.

1. What initial actions should be taken in this patient?
2. Is this patient's hypertension a contraindication to thrombolytic therapy?
3. What are the risks associated with thrombolytic therapy, and how long after the onset of acute MI is therapy beneficial?
4. Which is the better reperfusion therapy for acute MI—thrombolytic therapy or primary PTCA?

   The patient is given a thrombolytic agent and has an uneventful course, with complete resolution of the chest pain and ECG changes within 30 minutes of the beginning of the infusion.

5. What therapies should be administered acutely with thrombolysis or primary PTCA?

   On the following morning, the patient's ECG shows small Q waves and biphasic T waves in leads V_2, V_3, and V_4, and his CPK level has peaked at 980 U/L with a 15% CPK-MB fraction, and the troponin I level is 108 ng/mL.

6. What measures should be carried out before this patient is discharged?
7. Under what circumstances should the patient undergo coronary angiography?

Case Discussion

1. *What initial actions should be taken in this patient?*

   The first actions that should be taken in this patient are to administer oxygen and sublingual NTG and establish venous access. Morphine may be given if the pain does not resolve with NTG. Arterial puncture for performing blood gas measurement should be avoided because this would only increase the likelihood of a complication in the event of thrombolytic therapy. You should also inquire about the existence of any contraindications to thrombolytic therapy. (Discussed in question 2.) If acute MI is present and there are no contraindications, thrombolytic therapy should be begun within 30 minutes of the patient's arrival in the emergency department. Alternatively, if primary PTCA is elected instead of thrombolytic therapy, the cardiac catheterization laboratory personnel should be alerted within 30 minutes of the patient's arrival.

2. *Is this patient's hypertension a contraindication to thrombolytic therapy?*

   Hypertension alone is not a contraindication to thrombolytic therapy. If the hypertension is uncontrolled and cannot be lowered quickly to a level under 180/110 mm Hg, then it would be a relative contraindication. Absolute contraindications to thrombolytic therapy include active internal bleeding, major surgery or trauma within 2 weeks, recent head trauma or intracranial neoplasm, history of hemorrhagic cerebrovascular accident, and suspected aortic dissection. Relative contraindications in addition to uncontrolled hypertension are a history of stroke, the presence of a known left heart thrombus, prolonged cardiopulmonary resuscitation, active peptic ulcer disease, a known bleeding diathesis or use of anticoagulants, diabetic retinopathy, and pregnancy.

3. *What are the risks associated with thrombolytic therapy, and how long after the onset of acute MI is therapy beneficial?*

   The major risk of thrombolytic therapy is bleeding. If vascular puncture (particularly arterial puncture) is avoided, the overall risk of major bleeding requiring transfusion is 0.1% to 0.4%. The risk of intracranial hemorrhage with thrombolytic therapy is approximately 0.75%. Factors that increase the risk of intracranial hemorrhage include age greater than 65 years, weight less than 70 kg, hypertension at presentation, and use of tissue plasminogen activator rather than streptokinase. Patients with acute MI benefit from thrombolytic drugs for up to 12 hours after the onset of the infarction. However, the earlier the patient is treated, the greater the benefit because there is more myocardial salvage with earlier therapy.

4. *Which is the better reperfusion therapy for acute MI—thrombolytic therapy or primary PTCA?*

   The best therapy is the one that can be administered most rapidly in the hospital in which the patient presents. If facilities and personnel are available for rapid primary PTCA and the operators are experienced, primary PTCA seems to be better than thrombolytic therapy.

   In the patient with cardiogenic shock, primary PTCA is the preferred therapy, although randomized trial data are not yet available.

5. *What therapies should be administered acutely with thrombolysis or primary PTCA?*

   Aspirin (162.5 mg) should be administered immediately once the diagnosis is made in all patients unless there is a contraindication to aspirin (i.e., aspirin allergy or active bleeding). β Blockade should be instituted if there are no contraindications. Contraindications to β blockers include heart failure, second- or third-degree atrioventricular block, systolic blood pressure less than 100 mm Hg, bronchospasm or a history of asthma, and a heart rate less than 50 per minute. ACE inhibitors should be begun within the first 12 hours if there are no contraindications. Contraindications to ACE inhibitors include systolic blood pressure less than 100 mm Hg, a known allergy (such as angioedema), renal insufficiency with a serum creatinine greater than 3.0 mg/dL, or hyperkalemia.

6. *What measures should be carried out before this patient is discharged?*

Appropriate lipid-lowering therapy should be started. Fasting lipids should be measured within 24 hours of admission because LDL cholesterol levels fall within the first 24 hours after an acute MI. The patient should undergo a submaximal exercise test and have a measure of left ventricular EF. If the coronary anatomy and left ventricular EF are known because the patient had primary PTCA, these tests may not be necessary. If an intracoronary stent was placed during primary PTCA, ticlid or clopidogrel usually is given for 2 weeks in addition to aspirin.

All patients should be counseled in smoking cessation and a low-fat diet. Each patient should be taught how to use NTG and should be instructed when to call for problems.

7. *Under what circumstances should the patient undergo coronary angiography?*

Patients with recurrent ischemic chest pain, a positive submaximal exercise test, or an EF less than 40% should undergo coronary angiography if it has not already been performed during primary PTCA.

Case 2   A 67-year-old woman is in town visiting her children when she presents to your office complaining of severe symptoms of shortness of breath that have worsened over the past 12 hours. She tells you that she has had (type II) diabetes mellitus for the past 20 years and hypertension that has been fairly well controlled for 15 years. Your examination reveals an S_3 gallop and rales to her mid-scapular area. She also tells you that she has experienced chest heaviness and a "cold" for approximately 2 days. When the ECG is done, there are Q waves in leads V_2, V_3, V_4, and V_5. A call to her regular physician reveals she had a normal ECG when he saw her only 1 month ago.

1. At this point, what should you do?
2. What therapeutic interventions should be instituted at the time of admission?
3. Before discharge, she has an echocardiogram performed. What findings would favor long-term anticoagulant therapy with sodium warfarin?
4. Should this patient undergo coronary angiography or should she have a submaximal exercise test?
5. Would you recommend PTCA, surgery, or medical therapy

Case Discussion

1. *At this point, what should you do?*

Your patient has had a recent anterior MI. Her symptoms are related to left ventricular failure in the setting of a recent acute MI. She needs to be hospitalized immediately for treatment of her heart failure and for monitoring for arrhythmias and recurrent ischemia. Thrombolytic therapy or primary PTCA would not be indicated because this is a completed infarction, probably nearly 48 hours old.

2. *What therapeutic interventions should be instituted at the time of admission?*

Initial treatment consists of oxygen if hypoxemia is present, diuresis, assessment of electrolytes to maintain potassium above 4.0 mmol/L, and assessment of renal function in this diabetic woman. Aspirin should be started. Telemetry monitoring is necessary to detect arrhythmias. If the patient is not hypotensive and has no contraindications, ACE inhibitors should be started. Heparin should be considered in this patient with a large anterior MI because of the likely possibility of left ventricular apical thrombus; however, there are no prospective, randomized data for heparin in this situation. If the patient's heart failure resolves, β blockers should be started, beginning with low doses because of the history of heart failure.

3. *Before discharge, she has an echocardiogram performed. What findings would favor long-term anticoagulant therapy with sodium warfarin?*

An apical thrombus, especially if mobile, suggests a high risk for embolization, and the patient should be anticoagulated. A dyskinetic or akinetic ventricular segment has a risk for formation of left ventricular thrombus, and anticoagulation with sodium warfarin is recommended and continued for 3 to 6 months or until thrombus is no longer present. A dyskinetic or akinetic segment or an EF less than 30% are probably indications for chronic anticoagulation. No randomized, prospective data are available for any of these indications.

Two clear indications for anticoagulation in this setting are the presence of atrial fibrillation or an embolic episode.

4. *Should this patient undergo coronary angiography or should she have a submaximal exercise test?*

This woman has presented with a large MI and heart failure suggesting severe coronary disease. Her mortality risk is high and an exercise test is not necessary to stratify her risk. Therefore, she should undergo coronary angiography.

Coronary angiography shows a 90% proximal right coronary artery obstruction, a 90% proximal left anterior descending (LAD) obstruction, and a 100% proximal circumflex obstruction. Her EF by left ventricular angiography is 34%, with moderate anterior hypokinesis.

5. *Would you recommend PTCA, surgery, or medical therapy?*

With severe three-vessel disease and left ventricular dysfunction, coronary artery bypass surgery is indicated in this patient.

Suggested Readings

Falk E. Plaque rupture with severe preexisting stenosis precipitating thrombosis: characteristics of coronary atherosclerotic plaque underlying fatal occlusion thrombi. *Br Heart J* 1983;50:127.

Fibrinolytic Therapy Trialists' (FTT) Collaborative Group. Indications for fibrinolytic therapy in suspected acute myocardial infarction: collaborative overview of early mortality and major morbidity results from all randomised trials of more than 1000 patients. *Lancet* 1994;343:311.

Global Use of Strategies to Open Occluded Coronary Arteries in Acute Coronary Syndromes: GUSTO IIb Angioplasty Substudy Investigators. A clinical trial comparing primary coronary angioplasty with tissue plasminogen activator for acute myocardial infarction. *N Engl J Med* 1997;236:1621.

Hennekens CH, Albert CM, Godfried SL, et al. Adjunctive drug therapy of acute myocardial infarction: evidence from clinical trials. *N Engl J Med* 1996;335:1660.

Weaver WD, Simes RJ, Betriu A, et al. Comparison of primary coronary angioplasty and intravenous thrombolytic therapy for acute myocardial infarction: a quantitative review. *JAMA* 1997;278:2093.

Unstable Angina

1. What is unstable angina?
2. What is a non–Q-wave MI?
3. What common pathophysiologic processes underlie both unstable angina and non–Q-wave MI?
4. What is the estimated incidence of silent ischemic episodes in the setting of unstable angina?
5. What measures have been shown to improve the clinical outcome in the setting of acute coronary syndromes?

Discussion

1. *What is unstable angina?*

   Unstable angina is defined as typical anginal chest pain that is new in onset, is increased in frequency or severity, or occurs at rest.

2. *What is a non–Q-wave MI?*

   A non–Q-wave MI is an MI in which no Q waves develop on the ECG. The initial ECG may show ST segment elevation or depression, T-wave changes, or no changes at all. Previously, non–Q-wave MIs were called *subendocardial* because it was thought that infarctions with Q waves were transmural and non–Q-wave infarctions were subendocardial. However, there is substantial overlap, and some patients with Q waves have subendocardial damage only, whereas some non–Q-wave infarctions are transmural. The distinction between Q-wave and non–Q-wave infarctions is valuable clinically because early (hospital) mortality rates are higher in Q-wave infarctions, but patients with non–Q-wave infarctions have higher reinfarction and mortality rates in the subsequent 6 months to 1 year.

3. *What common pathophysiologic processes underlie both unstable angina and non–Q-wave MI?*

   Almost all patients with either unstable angina or non–Q-wave MI have underlying atherosclerosis. There usually is plaque rupture or fissuring with superimposed thrombus, platelet aggregation, and coronary vasospasm. In general, the thrombus is more gray (platelet rich) than red (fibrin rich) and is less often occlusive than in patients who present with acute ST segment elevation. However, there is significant overlap in the pathophysiologic processes behind the acute coronary syndromes and ST segment elevation because patients with ST segment elevation may not have infarction, or may have positive enzymes without Q-wave development. Without reperfusion, most patients who present with acute ST segment elevation manifest Q waves in the leads with ST segment elevation. However, with reperfusion, fewer patients manifest Q waves.

4. *What is the estimated incidence of silent ischemic episodes in the setting of unstable angina?*

   The estimated incidence of silent ischemia in the setting of unstable angina ranges from 70% to 90% of patients. Silent ischemia is defined as evidence of ischemia (e.g., typical ECG changes) that is not accompanied by typical anginal chest pain.

5. *What measures have been shown to improve the clinical outcome in the setting of acute coronary syndromes?*

   Aspirin, platelet glycoprotein IIb/IIIa inhibitors, heparin, and low–molecular-weight heparin have all been shown to improve clinical outcomes in patients with acute coronary syndromes. Low–molecular-weight heparin appears to be more effective than unfractionated heparin. β-Adrenergic blockers improve symptoms and probably improve outcome. Coronary bypass surgery and PTCA probably improve outcome if patients are properly selected, although prospective, randomized data are not available.

Case 1   A 42-year-old registered nurse is seen because of pain in the chest. She describes a "pain in my heart" and points to a 1-cm^2 area above the left breast. The pain is intensified by deep breathing, coughing, recumbency, and twisting motions. It has lasted continuously for 2 days. Three days ago, she noted extreme fatigue and shortness of breath lasting for 24 hours. Findings from a complete physical examination are normal.

1. What is the most likely diagnosis in this patient, and why?

   As you are about to discharge this patient, her husband tells you he is concerned about his wife because her sister underwent coronary bypass surgery at 44 years of age and her brother at 34 years of age. Because the pain has some features of pericarditis, you decide to do an ECG. It shows normal sinus rhythm with Q waves in the inferior leads and diffuse ST segment elevation.

2. What is your diagnosis, and what do you do?

Case Discussion

1. *What is the most likely diagnosis in this patient, and why?*

   Chest wall pain or pericarditis are the most likely initial diagnoses in this patient. Angina pectoris is uncommon in women in this age group, and this pain is not anginal chest pain. Acute cholecystitis manifests clinically with right upper quadrant tenderness and occasionally a palpable gallbladder. A pneumothorax is associated with acute shortness of breath, and physical examination in this setting reveals hyperresonance to percussion and diminished breath sounds on the affected side. Pain arising from the chest wall is the most common cause of chest pain in any age group, and often has no discernible cause. A friction rub is often but not always audible in the setting of acute pericarditis. This rub has a coarse, "leathery," and close-to-the-ear sound, with accentuation during systole and early and late diastole. Inspiration intensifies the rub. Its features often include a precise localization and tenderness on palpation over the affected area. Deep breathing, position changes, and specific body movements such as twisting often accentuate the pain. Its duration varies from a few seconds to days. Therapy is nonspecific, consisting of reassurance and simple analgesics.

2. *What is your diagnosis, and what do you do?*

This patient probably had a silent inferior MI a few days ago and now has postinfarction pericarditis. There are Q waves inferiorly, suggesting an inferior infarction, and diffuse ST segment elevation suggestive of pericarditis. Additional history is that she has had type II diabetes mellitus for 20 years and had a recent cholesterol screening at a health fair. Her LDL cholesterol was 242 mg/dL, consistent with familial heterozygous hypercholesteremia.

You admit this patient for telemetry observation. Troponin I is still likely to be elevated and should be drawn. When you ask the patient to sit up, lean forward, and exhale, a two-component pericardial friction rub is noted. Aspirin should be given for her MI and indomethacin for her pericardial symptoms. The remainder of her treatment is as discussed for patients with acute MI, except that this infarction is older and acute reperfusion is not indicated. Silent ischemia is more common in diabetes. Although women younger than 50 years of age do not often have symptomatic coronary disease, diabetes erases the benefit of female sex for coronary disease risk. It is important to consider all risk factors for coronary disease when evaluating patients with chest pain.

Case 2   A 57-year-old automobile salesman who is hypertensive and a heavy cigarette smoker describes a pressure-like sensation that developed for the first time 3 weeks before. The discomfort, which begins in the retrosternal area, radiates to the left side of his lower jaw, occurs when he walks rapidly in cold air, and more recently occurs at rest. Careful history reveals that it lasts for 10 to 15 minutes, but an especially severe episode awakened him the night before and lasted nearly half an hour before resolving spontaneously. Except for a blood pressure of 150/100 mm Hg, the physical examination findings are normal. An ECG (obtained after the pain has disappeared) reveals deep and symmetric T-wave inversion in leads V_1 to V_4. The patient is admitted and given IV heparin and oral aspirin.

1. What is your diagnosis?
2. What are some common physical findings during an ischemic episode?
   Approximately 4 hours after admission, the patient again experiences transient chest pressure. You order an ECG. The T waves are now upright in leads V_1 to V_4.
3. What are these ECG changes called, and what do they represent?
4. How should the recurrent chest pain be treated?
5. What should be done next?

Case Discussion

1. *What is your diagnosis?*

   This patient has either unstable angina or a non–Q-wave infarction. The pain is both new in onset and occurs at rest. The T-wave inversions confirm the diagnosis of ischemia. The results of cardiac enzyme tests separate unstable angina (enzymes negative) from non–Q-wave MI (enzymes positive).

2. *What are some common physical findings during an ischemic attack?*

   Increases in heart rate and blood pressure are the most common findings during ischemia. Physical examination performed during an ischemic attack may reveal an S_4, a dyskinetic apical impulse on palpation, or a mitral regurgitation murmur. Because left ventricular compliance decreases (increased "stiffness") as a consequence of ischemia, left ventricular filling pressures increase, and the resultant increase in atrial pressure produces an audible filling sound at end-diastole, the S_4. However, an S_4 is a nonspecific finding and is frequently heard in older adults. Also as a consequence of ischemia, a localized contraction abnormality may appear and cause a transient outward bulge of the left ventricle. Palpation with the palm of the hand, especially with the patient in the left lateral decubitus position, may disclose a dyskinetic impulse. Ischemia of the papillary muscles leads to failure of these muscles to shorten during systole. Therefore, the mitral leaflets are not fully apposed and mitral regurgitation results. The latter findings are infrequent. Hypotension or rales developing during chest pain suggests that a large amount of myocardium is ischemic.

3. *What are these ECG changes called, and what do they represent?*

   When previously inverted T waves become upright in the presence of chest pain, it is called *pseudonormalization*. This is strongly suggestive of ischemia.

4. *How should the recurrent chest pain be treated?*

   The pseudonormalization of the T waves clearly indicates myocardial ischemia. This pain should be treated with morphine and sublingual NTG, followed by IV NTG and β blockade if there are no contraindications. The patient is already receiving aspirin and heparin. Substantial data suggest that the platelet glycoprotein IIb/IIIa inhibitors such as abciximab, eptifibatide, and integrilin are of value in the patient with unstable angina. Although it is not an acute treatment, attention should also be focused on risk factors with measurement of the lipids. If the LDL cholesterol is elevated, it should be treated appropriately, as should any other lipid abnormalities.

5. *What should be done next?*

This patient had signs of myocardial ischemia on admission and has had recurrent pain on IV heparin in the hospital. Both the recurrent pain and the diffusely inverted T waves suggest the presence of substantial ischemia, and the deeply inverted T waves in leads V_1 to V_4 mostly likely represent a high-grade proximal LAD stenosis. This patient should undergo coronary angiography. PTCA is appropriate if there is only one- or two-vessel disease and normal or near-normal left ventricular function. If there is three-vessel disease and left ventricular dysfunction, coronary artery bypass surgery with an internal mammary artery graft to the LAD and saphenous vein grafts to the other two vessels usually is indicated. The use of PTCA versus coronary surgery may depend on patient or physician preference, lesion anatomy, the presence of proximal LAD disease, or the patient's other medical problems.

Suggested Readings

Braunwald E, Jones RH, Mark DB, et al. Diagnosing and managing unstable angina: Agency for Health Care Policy and Research. *Circulation* 1994;90:613.

Calvin JE, Klein LW, VandenBerg BJ, et al. Risk stratification in unstable angina: prospective validation of the Braunwald classification. *JAMA* 1995;273:136.

Collins P, Fox KM. Pathophysiology of angina. *Lancet* 1990;1:94.

Davies MJ, Thomas AC. Plaque fissuring: the cause of acute myocardial infarction, sudden ischemic death, and crescendo angina. *Br Heart J* 1985;53:363.

Nademanee K, Intrachot V, Josephson MA, et al. Prognostic significance of silent myocardial ischemia in patients with unstable angina. *J Am Coll Cardiol* 1987;10:1.

Patel DJ, Knight CJ, Holdright DR, et al. Long-term prognosis in unstable angina: the importance of early risk stratification using continuous ST segment monitoring. *Eur Heart J* 1998;19:240.

Stone PH, Thompson B, Anderson HV, et al. Influence of race, sex, and age on management of unstable angina and non-Q-wave myocardial infarction: the TIMI III registry. *JAMA* 1996;275:1104.

Theroux P, Fuster V. Acute coronary syndromes: unstable angina and non-Q-wave myocardial infarction. *Circulation* 1998;97:1195.

Zwaan C, Bar FWHM, Gorgels AGM, et al. Unstable angina: are we able to recognize high-risk patients? *Chest* 1997;112:244.

Sudden Cardiac Death

1. What kind of heart disease is seen most commonly in adults who die suddenly? In young athletes?
2. Which types of arrhythmias are associated with cardiac arrest and sudden cardiac death (SCD)?
3. Which patients are at highest risk for SCD?
4. What is the cause of SCD in the long QT syndrome?

Discussion

1. *What kind of heart disease is seen most commonly in adults who die suddenly? In young athletes?*

Approximately 90% of cases of SCD occur in patients with preexisting organic heart disease. In adults with SCD, the most common underlying heart disease is coronary artery disease, seen in 80% of cases. In young athletes, SCD is very rare, but when it does occur it is usually due to hypertrophic cardiomyopathy.

2. *Which types of arrhythmias are associated with cardiac arrest and SCD?*

In the field, paramedics most commonly record ventricular fibrillation or ventricular tachycardia. Less frequently seen, and associated with poorer prognosis, are bradyarrhythmias, asystole, and electrical–mechanical dissociation.

3. *Which patients are at highest risk for SCD?*

Patients at highest risk for SCD are those who have previously survived an episode of SCD or have a history of rapid sustained ventricular tachycardia and reduced left ventricular function. Although most of the therapeutic interventions designed to prevent SCD are used in this patient group, this is a relatively small population of patients compared with the total population of patients at risk for SCD. One of the best measures of the risk of SCD is left ventricular function. The risk of SCD increases as left ventricular function decreases.

4. *What is the cause of SCD in the long QT syndrome?*

The long QT syndrome is a cause of syncope and SCD in patients with structurally normal hearts. Several genetic defects involving cardiac ion channels have been identified in families in which this syndrome is inherited. Several classes of drugs that affect cardiac ion channels can also cause this syndrome. Cardiac repolarization is prolonged, reflected in a long QT interval on the ECG. Syncope and SCD are caused by a polymorphic ventricular tachycardia called *torsade de pointes* ("twisting of the points").

Case   A 65-year-old man complains of chest discomfort on the golf course and within seconds collapses and is unresponsive. His companions initiate bystander cardiopulmonary resuscitation and an ambulance is called. Paramedics arrive within 10 minutes. A "quick look" at the rhythm using the defibrillator paddles reveals ventricular fibrillation. After two shocks (200 followed by 360 J), sinus rhythm is restored, and a pulse is felt. The patient is transported to the hospital. Initial ECG shows Q waves in the precordial leads, and diffuse, nonspecific ST segment and T-wave abnormalities, with a normal QT interval. Serum electrolytes are normal. Initial and subsequent cardiac enzyme determinations do not indicate evidence of an acute MI. Family members state that the patient was on no cardiac medications and had no cardiac history. The patient, initially unresponsive and requiring mechanical ventilation, recovers neurologically over the next 48 hours and is extubated. Aside from a mild short-term memory deficit, he seems to be back to his usual self and none the worse for the experience.

1. What tests should be performed on this patient now?
2. Will coronary revascularization be of benefit in preventing recurrent SCD in this patient?

3. Is there a role for electrophysiologic testing in this patient?

4. What is the best treatment to prevent recurrent SCD in this patient?

Case Discussion

1. *What tests should be performed on this patient now?*

Despite the near-miraculous recovery of this patient, his risk of recurrent SCD is high and measures should be taken to identify the cause of SCD in his case and to prevent recurrence. Although most cases of SCD in his age group are related to coronary artery disease, it can be unclear in a particular patient whether the initiating event was a primary arrhythmia or ischemia. Ischemia can be due to increased metabolic demands (e.g., exercise) in the face of a fixed coronary obstruction, or due to transient decreased coronary blood flow from atherosclerotic plaque rupture or coronary vasospasm. It is likely that many episodes of SCD are multifactorial, superimposing transient triggering events (e.g., ischemia, changes in autonomic tone, electrolyte abnormalities, or premature ventricular complexes) on an arrhythmogenic substrate such as the cell damage created by a previous MI. This patient's complaint of chest discomfort before collapse may on first consideration suggest ischemia as the initiating event, but patients with coronary disease who have ventricular tachycardia sometimes complain of chest pain because they become ischemic secondary to the rapid heart rate. The ECG evidence of an anterior infarction without the enzyme changes characteristic of acute infarction suggest that, despite his negative cardiac history, he may have had a previous "silent" MI. This old ventricular scar may be a substrate for a primary reentrant ventricular tachycardia. To define his cardiac disease better, including his left ventricular function, and to determine if he has a substrate for recurrent ischemia, cardiac catheterization should be performed. Cardiac catheterization in this patient showed a 100% proximal LAD artery occlusion as well as a 90% occlusion of the first obtuse marginal branch of the left circumflex artery. The right coronary artery was normal. The left ventricular EF was reduced at 30% (normal, ≥55%). There was an anteroapical left ventricular aneurysm. The lateral wall of the left ventricle (supplied by the left circumflex artery) had normal motion.

2. *Will coronary revascularization be of benefit in preventing recurrent SCD in this patient?*

As discussed previously, SCD may be multifactorial and it is difficult to determine the precise triggers for an SCD episode. This patient has evidence on catheterization of a previous anterior infarction, with an anteroapical left ventricular aneurysm. This aneurysm may be a substrate for reentrant sustained monomorphic ventricular tachycardia. In addition, he has a significant stenosis in an obtuse marginal artery, with normal left ventricular wall motion in the region served by this artery. This is a substrate for ischemia. In an attempt to correct possible triggering factors like ischemia, it would be reasonable to dilate the obtuse marginal stenosis with balloon angioplasty, and this was performed in this patient. Unfortunately, in patients with reduced left ventricular function who have an aborted episode of SCD, there is no evidence that antiischemia measures alone prevent recurrent SCD.

3. *Is there a role for electrophysiologic testing in this patient?*

Most patients with presentations similar to this patient's have inducible sustained monomorphic ventricular tachycardia during electrophysiologic testing. In the past, many such patients underwent electrophysiologic testing and then were treated with antiarrhythmic drug therapy guided by serial electrophysiologic testing. Patients who failed drug therapy or who did not have inducible sustained monomorphic ventricular tachycardia were treated with empiric amiodarone or an implantable defibrillator. A number of randomized, controlled clinical trials have been performed that compare the efficacy of the implantable defibrillator with antiarrhythmic drug therapy. These trials all suggest that therapy with the implantable defibrillator is superior to antiarrhythmic drug therapy guided by electrophysiologic testing or empiric amiodarone in preventing recurrent SCD. In the AVID (Antiarrhythmics Versus Implantable Defibrillators) trial, patients who were enrolled had hemodynamically significant sustained ventricular tachycardia and a left ventricular EF of 40% or less, or ventricular fibrillation. There was a 31% reduction in the total mortality rate after 3 years with implantable defibrillators compared with antiarrhythmic drug therapy. For this reason, electrophysiologic testing is usually not performed in SCD survivors, and was not performed in this patient.

4. *What is the best treatment to prevent recurrent SCD in this patient?*

This patient was a good candidate for an implantable defibrillator, and he received one. The defibrillator was implanted in the left pectoral region in the electrophysiology laboratory, using local anesthesia and conscious sedation. The patient was discharged home the day after the implant. In addition, this patient received other medical therapy that has been shown to reduce the risk of SCD. β-Blocking drugs have been shown to reduce total mortality after MI as well as improve pump function in some cases. Aspirin may help prevent reinfarction. ACE inhibitors have been shown to improve survival in patients with reduced left ventricular function. Lipid-lowering agents may prevent progression of atherosclerosis and should be used in patients with lipid abnormalities. Other risk factor modifications, such as smoking cessation, would be recommended. Amiodarone may reduce SCD after MI, but it does not clearly reduce total mortality. Its empiric use to prevent SCD remains controversial. In this patient, there would be no added value in using amiodarone because he already has an implantable defibrillator. In fact, amiodarone, by its effect of increasing the electrical defibrillation threshold, might actually interfere with the function of the defibrillator, and thus should be avoided.

Suggested Readings

The Antiarrhythmics Versus Implantable Defibrillators (AVID) Investigators. A comparison of antiarrhythmic drug therapy with implantable defibrillators in patients resuscitated from near fatal ventricular arrhythmias. *N Engl J Med* 1997;337:1576.

Maron BJ, Epstein SE, Roberts WC. Causes of sudden death in competitive athletes. *J Am Coll Cardiol* 1989;7:204.

Moss AJ, Hall WJ, Cannom DS, et al, and the Multicenter Automatic Defibrillator Implantation Trial Investigators. Improved survival with an implanted defibrillator in patients with coronary disease at high risk for ventricular arrhythmia. *N Engl J Med* 1996;335:1933.

Roden DM, Lazzara R, Rosen M, et al, for the SADS Foundation Task Force on LQTS. Multiple mechanisms in the long QT syndrome: current knowledge, gaps, and future directions. *Circulation* 1996;94:1996.

Zipes DP, Wellens HJJ. Sudden cardiac death. *Circulation* 1998;98:2334.

Valvular Heart Disease

1. What is the difference between valvular insufficiency and valvular regurgitation?
2. What types of myocardial hypertrophy can result from valvular abnormalities?
3. What is the most serious long-term consequence of either concentric or eccentric hypertrophy?
4. What is the relationship between the pressure gradient across a stenotic valve, the blood flow across the valve, and the valve area?

Discussion

1. *What is the difference between valvular insufficiency and valvular regurgitation?*

    Regurgitation and *insufficiency* are interchangeable terms to describe backward flow of blood across a valve at a time in the cardiac cycle when there would be no flow across a competent valve.

2. *What types of myocardial hypertrophy can result from valvular abnormalities?*

    When there is a pressure load on the ventricle (such as aortic stenosis), concentric hypertrophy develops. Concentric hypertrophy means that the myocardial wall thickness is increased with a normal or decreased internal ventricular diameter. A volume load (such as aortic insufficiency or mitral regurgitation) results in eccentric hypertrophy; the wall thickness is normal but the internal diameter of the ventricle is increased. Overall left ventricular mass is increased in both types of hypertrophy.

3. *What is the most serious long-term consequence of either concentric or eccentric hypertrophy?*

    With long-standing hypertrophy of either type, myocardial dysfunction and heart failure may result.

4. *What is the relationship between the pressure gradient across a stenotic valve, the blood flow across the valve, and the valve area?*

    The pressure gradient across a valve is proportional to the blood flow across the valve divided by the valve area. Therefore, if blood flow (cardiac output) decreases and the valve area is fixed, the pressure gradient decreases. Conversely, as a valve becomes more stenotic, the pressure gradient across a valve increases if cardiac output remains constant.

Case 1   A previously healthy but inactive 42-year-old man is seen in the ER after a first
episode of syncope, which occurred while he was playing full-court basketball
for the first time in 10 years. On questioning, he describes a 2-month history of
exertional chest pain. He has not seen a physician during his adult life. Physical
examination reveals the following findings. His supine blood pressure is 100/80
mm Hg without any significant orthostatic change. There is no jugular venous
distention, but there are slowly rising, small-amplitude, and somewhat sustained
carotid pulses. His lungs are clear. A sustained and slightly laterally displaced
apex beat is noted, as well as a soft S_1 and single S_2, prominent S_4, and a grade
III/VI harsh, late-peaking, crescendo-decrescendo systolic murmur heard best
at the cardiac base and radiating to the carotids with a high-frequency component
at the cardiac apex. No clubbing, cyanosis, or edema is noted.

1. What is the most likely valvular lesion in this patient?
2. What is the most likely underlying cause of aortic stenosis in this age group?
3. What is the average survival of patients with uncorrected aortic stenosis after
the onset of syncope?
4. How is the severity of aortic stenosis most accurately determined?
5. What is the best therapy for symptomatic aortic stenosis?

Case Discussion

1. *What is the most likely valvular lesion in this patient?*
    The history of angina and syncope and the classic physical examination
findings make aortic stenosis an almost certain diagnosis in this patient. The
characteristic arterial pulses described have been referred to as *pulsus parvus
et tardus*. The single S_2 indicates the absence of the aortic component of S_2,
suggesting severe immobility of the aortic valve. The murmur is also characteristic of aortic stenosis with its crescendo-decrescendo quality and the late
peaking. Do not be fooled by the high-frequency component at the cardiac
apex. Although a second murmur may be present, the murmur typically encountered in the setting of aortic stenosis commonly radiates to the apex,
where it may be mistaken for the murmur of mitral regurgitation.
2. *What is the most likely underlying cause of aortic stenosis in this age group?*
    Between 35 and 65 years of age, degenerative change in a congenitally
bicuspid aortic valve is the predominant cause of aortic stenosis. Beyond 65
years of age, aortic stenosis usually results from calcification of a previously
normal tricuspid aortic valve (senile calcific aortic stenosis). Although the exact
cause of senile aortic stenosis is not clear, it is associated with hypertension and
hyperlipidemia. Isolated aortic stenosis rarely results from rheumatic disease.
Instances of aortic stenosis stemming from rheumatic disease are invariably
associated with mitral valve disease.
3. *What is the average survival of patients with uncorrected aortic stenosis after
the onset of syncope?*

According to studies conducted before valve surgery was available, such patients could expect to survive an average of 3 years after the onset of syncope. Patients with aortic stenosis may remain asymptomatic for years, but, once symptoms develop, the course of the disease may be quite fulminant. The average survival after the onset of angina pectoris or heart failure is 5 years and 2 years, respectively.

4. *How is the severity of aortic stenosis most accurately determined?*

The severity of aortic stenosis can be precisely determined by cardiac catheterization and calculation of the aortic valve area. The normal aortic valve area is 3 cm^2. Mild aortic stenosis exists when the valve area is less than 1.5 cm^2. Aortic stenosis is said to be critical when the valve area is 0.7 cm^2 or less. Simple pressure gradient measurements fail to account for the dependency of the gradient on the volume and rate of transvalvular flow. Physical examination findings can be suggestive but are inaccurate compared with the information yielded by the aortic valve area. Doppler echocardiography is the most commonly used tool for estimating the severity of aortic stenosis. With Doppler echocardiography, the aortic pressure gradient and aortic valve area can be reliably determined. Echocardiography can also determine the EF and the presence of left ventricular hypertrophy.

5. *What is the best therapy for symptomatic aortic stenosis?*

Aortic valve replacement is the best therapy for symptomatic aortic stenosis. Long-term results of balloon aortic valvuloplasty (a catheter-based procedure) have been disappointing. Therefore, it is used primarily for palliation for patients who are not candidates for aortic valve replacement because of other medical problems.

Case 2   A 50-year-old woman who had an "innocent" murmur diagnosed in childhood presents with dyspnea on exertion, orthopnea, and paroxysmal nocturnal dyspnea of several months' duration. On questioning, she describes a 1-year history of fatigue and exhaustion that has limited her daily activities. She has not seen a physician in years.

On physical examination, her blood pressure is 110/70 mm Hg. Her jugular venous pressure is 8 cm H$_2$O and she exhibits 1+ pulses with normal arterial upstrokes and bibasilar rales. There is a laterally displaced apex but with a palpable S$_3$, a soft S$_1$, a widely split S$_2$, a loud S$_3$, and a grade III/IV blowing, high-pitched systolic murmur heard best at the apex and radiating to the axilla and left infrascapular area. There is trace edema but no clubbing or cyanosis.

1. What is the valvular lesion in this patient?
2. What is the most common underlying cause of severe mitral regurgitation in the adult U.S. population?
3. The medical therapy for mitral regurgitation with left ventricular dysfunction may include what classes of drugs?

4. When should surgery be considered for patients with severe mitral regurgitation?

5. What are the choices for mitral valve surgery?

Case Discussion

1. *What is the valvular lesion in this patient?*

Chronic mitral regurgitation, the most insidious of all left-sided valvular lesions, is the most likely diagnosis in this patient. Severe left ventricular dysfunction is not uncommon at presentation in this disorder. The holosystolic apical murmur is characteristic of chronic mitral regurgitation. The S_3 suggests that the mitral regurgitation is severe, indicating that there is a large volume of blood crossing the mitral valve in early diastole. However, it does not necessarily imply heart failure. The murmur described is typical but must be distinguished from a VSD, tricuspid regurgitation, and aortic stenosis. The murmur characteristic of aortic stenosis is distinguished by its quality (crescendo-decrescendo), location, and radiation, as described in Case 1. The tricuspid insufficiency murmur is usually well localized to the left sternal border, with little radiation, and increases in intensity with inspiration. The murmur characteristic of VSD is typically heard best at the left sternal border, often has a harsh quality, and does not change with respiration. The murmur of VSD is rarely heard in adults because most are detected in childhood and correct spontaneously or with surgery. A VSD is a rare complication of acute MI in adults.

2. *What is the most common underlying cause of severe mitral regurgitation in the adult U.S. population?*

Myxomatous valve disease usually as an isolated lesion or sometimes associated with other connective tissue disorders (e.g., Marfan's and Ehlers-Danlos syndromes) constitutes the most common cause of severe mitral regurgitation necessitating mitral valve replacement or repair in the United States, especially in younger people. A smaller number of cases are due to rheumatic heart disease, infective endocarditis, or spontaneously ruptured chordae tendineae. In older people, severe mitral regurgitation often accompanies left ventricular enlargement and dysfunction due to coronary artery disease. The mitral regurgitation is due to a combination of stretching of the entire valvular apparatus along with papillary muscle dysfunction and wall motion abnormalities.

3. *The medical therapy for mitral regurgitation with left ventricular dysfunction may include what classes of drugs?*

Medical therapy for chronic mitral regurgitation consists of vasodilators to improve forward blood flow. There are no data, however, that vasodilators prevent gradual ventricular dysfunction or delay the time to surgery.

4. *When should surgery be considered for patients with severe mitral regurgitation?*

Mitral regurgitation results in a chronic volume overload and ultimately results in left ventricular contractile dysfunction. Mitral valve surgery should be performed before ventricular dysfunction occurs, but no perfect method to determine this time exists. Serial Doppler echocardiography is recommended and surgery should be recommended if the EF falls below 60% or the left ventricular end-diastolic dimension approaches 45 mm. Despite these recommendations, the decision for mitral valve surgery is often an extremely difficult decision.

5. *What are the choices for mitral valve surgery?*

Mitral valve replacement with a mechanical or bioprosthetic valves and, more recently, mitral valve repair constitute the surgical treatments available for severe mitral regurgitation. Mitral valve repair is associated with a lower operative mortality rate and a better long-term outcome than mitral valve replacement, and is the preferred procedure when repair is possible.

Case 3   A 36-year-old man with a history of bilateral lens dislocations is seen because of progressive fatigue, dyspnea on exertion, orthopnea, and paroxysmal nocturnal dyspnea.

At physical examination, he is noted to be quite tall, with a height of 6 ft., 6 in. (195 cm). His blood pressure is 160/60 mm Hg. There is no jugular venous distention, but systolic pulsations of the uvula are noted, as is quick collapse of the arterial pulses, which is seen in the nail beds with gentle pressure. There are bibasilar rales, together with a diffuse and hyperdynamic apex beat that is displaced laterally and inferiorly, a soft S_1 and S_2, a loud S_3, and a grade III/VI, high-pitched, nearly holodiastolic murmur heard best at the cardiac base (particularly the right upper sternal border). A late diastolic rumble is heard at the apex.

1. What is the most likely valvular lesion in this patient?
2. What is the likely underlying cause of aortic regurgitation in this patient?
3. What is the appropriate medical therapy for the patient with aortic regurgitation?
4. When should aortic valve replacement be considered in a patient with chronic aortic regurgitation?
5. What clinical variables confer an increased risk of early mortality after cardiac valve replacement?

Case Discussion

1. *What is the most likely valvular lesion in this patient?*

This case represents a classic example of chronic severe aortic regurgitation. There are many physical signs to look for in the setting of aortic regurgitation, some of which are seen in this patient. These include de Musset's sign (the head bobs with each heartbeat), Corrigan's sign or waterhammer pulses, Traube's sign (booming systolic and diastolic sounds heard over the femoral arteries), Müller's sign (systolic pulsation of the uvula), Quincke's sign (capillary pulsations seen in the nail beds), and others. All of these are signs of large stroke volume and wide pulse pressure characteristic of chronic aortic regurgitation. The mid to late diastolic rumble, the Austin Flint murmur, is created by rapid retrograde flow from the aorta striking the anterior mitral leaflet. Another explanation for this murmur is that the large volume of regurgitant flow partially closes the mitral valve, creating a late diastolic mitral valve gradient.

2. *What is the likely underlying cause of aortic regurgitation in this patient?*

In this tall young man with a history of bilateral lens dislocations, Marfan's syndrome is the most likely cause of the aortic regurgitation. The proximal aortic root is severely dilated, preventing coaptation of the aortic valve leaflets. In fact, the patient's father, who also had Marfan's syndrome, died at the age of 36 years from an acute aortic dissection with acute aortic regurgitation. Other causes of aortic regurgitation can be broken down into two categories—valvular disease and aortic root disease. Rheumatic heart disease, infective endocarditis, trauma, bicuspid valve, other congenital valvular defects (e.g., a fenestrated valve), systemic lupus erythematosus, rheumatoid arthritis, ankylosing spondylitis, and Whipple's disease may cause primary valvular disease. Cystic medial necrosis of the aorta (isolated or associated with Marfan's syndrome or Ehlers-Danlos syndrome), atherosclerosis, hypertension, syphilitic aortitis, and others may cause aortic root dilatation, and result in aortic regurgitation.

3. *What is the appropriate medical therapy for the patient with aortic regurgitation?*

In asymptomatic patients, nifedipine delays the need for surgery by 2 to 3 years. It is likely, although not confirmed in clinical trials, that other vasodilators such as ACE inhibitors would also be effective.

4. *When should aortic valve replacement be considered in a patient with chronic aortic regurgitation?*

Aortic valve surgery should be considered if the patient has symptoms of heart failure. In the asymptomatic patient, the "rule of 55" is a good general rule. If EF falls below 55% or the end-diastolic dimension increases above 55 mm, aortic valve replacement should be considered.

5. *What clinical variables confer an increased risk of early mortality after cardiac valve replacement?*

In approximate order of descending importance, severe ventricular dysfunction, previous cardiac surgery, uncorrected coronary disease, emergency surgery, and advanced age (>70 years) may all increase the risk associated with valve surgery.

Case 4 A 32-year-old woman who recently moved to the United States from Mexico is seen because of the recent onset of palpitations associated with dyspnea on exertion, orthopnea, and paroxysmal nocturnal dyspnea with hemoptysis.

On physical examination, her blood pressure is 110/90 mm Hg and her heart rate is 120 per minute and irregularly irregular. She has pinkish-purple patches on her cheeks. Jugular venous distention to 10 cm H_2O with a prominent V wave and a slow Y descent is noted, as are diminished arterial pulses and bibasilar rales (up to half of the lung fields bilaterally). Additional findings include a nondisplaced apex beat, a right ventricular heave palpable in the left parasternal region, a palpable pulmonic closure sound in the second left intercostal space, an accentuated S_1, a loud pulmonic second sound (P_2), a right-sided S_4, and a grade III/IV, low-pitched, rumbling, nearly holodiastolic murmur heard best at the cardiac apex. There is 1 to 2+ pitting edema noted in the lower extremities and presacral area.

1. What is the most likely valvular lesion in this patient?
2. What is the most common cause of mitral stenosis in adult patients?
3. What is the mortality rate associated with medically treated mitral stenosis?
4. For what major complications is this patient at risk?
5. What is the best treatment for symptomatic patients with mitral stenosis?

Case Discussion

1. *What is the most likely valvular lesion in this patient?*

   The clinical picture exhibited by this patient is characteristic of severe mitral stenosis with secondary pulmonary hypertension and cor pulmonale, as evidenced by the loud P_2 and right ventricular heave, right-sided S_4, elevated neck veins, and peripheral edema. Paroxysmal nocturnal dyspnea with hemoptysis is a major clue to this diagnosis. However, this patient does not display one of the more common auscultatory findings typical of mitral stenosis, the opening snap. This sign appears to be due to a sudden tensing of the valve leaflets after the valve cusps have completed their opening excursions, and occurs shortly after (0.08 to 0.12 second) the aortic second sound (A_2). The rumbling, low-pitched diastolic murmur heard at the apex is characteristic of mitral stenosis.

2. *What is the most common cause of mitral stenosis in adult patients?*

   Mitral stenosis in adults is almost exclusively due to rheumatic heart disease. This patient described a prolonged illness consistent with acute rheumatic fever that occurred at the age of 12 years.

3. *What is the mortality rate associated with medically treated mitral stenosis?*

   From the time of the initial diagnosis, patients with medically treated mitral stenosis can expect a mortality rate of 20% at 5 years and 40% at 10 years. This patient faces a much less favorable prognosis because of her pulmonary hypertension and right heart failure. However, the risk is significantly reduced if she undergoes valve replacement, commissurotomy, or mitral balloon valvotomy.

4. *For what major complications is this patient at risk?*

   In patients with uncorrected mitral stenosis, there is a 20% lifetime risk of thromboembolism. Eighty percent of patients with systemic emboli are in atrial fibrillation. This risk is decreased by the use of anticoagulant therapy with sodium warfarin. Infective endocarditis occurs less frequently but may be a disastrous complication.

5. *What is the best treatment for symptomatic patients with mitral stenosis?*

Options for correction of mitral stenosis include percutaneous transvenous mitral valvuloplasty, surgical mitral commissurotomy, or mitral valve repair. In balloon valvuloplasty, the balloon is passed from the femoral vein to the right atrium, across the atrial septum, and across the mitral valve. The balloon is inflated, cracking open the valve. This is the preferred procedure in experienced hands if the valve anatomy is favorable and there are no contraindications. Results are also excellent with surgical commissurotomy or mitral valve replacement.

Suggested Readings

Bonow RO, Lakatos E, Maron BJ, Epstein SE. Serial long-term assessment of the natural history of asymptomatic patients with chronic aortic regurgitation and normal left ventricular systolic function. *Circulation* 1991;84:1625.

Carabello BA, Crawford FA Jr. Valvular heart disease. *N Engl J Med* 1997;337:32.

Carabello BA, Usher BW, Hendrix GH, et al. Predictors of outcome for aortic valve replacement in patients with aortic regurgitation and left ventricular dysfunction: a change in the measuring stick. *J Am Coll Cardiol* 1987;10:991.

Cheitlin MD, Douglas PS, Parmley WW, et al. Task force 2: acquired valvular heart disease. *J Am Coll Cardiol* 1994;24:874.

Lambo NJ, Dell'Italia LJ, Crawford MH, O'Rourke RA. Bedside diagnosis of systolic murmurs. *N Engl J Med* 1988;318:1572.

Lieberman EG, Bashore TM, Hermiller JB, et al. Balloon aortic valvuplasty in adults: failure of procedure to improve long-term survival. *J Am Coll Cardiol* 1995;26:1522.

Pellikka PA, Nishimura RA, Bailey KR, Tajik AJ. The natural history of adults with asymptomatic, hemodynamically significant aortic stenosis. *J Am Coll Cardiol* 1990;15:1012.

Reyes VP, Raju BS, Wynne J, et al. Percutaneous balloon valvuloplasty compared with open surgical commissurotomy for mitral stenosis. *N Engl J Med* 1994;331:961.

Rozich JD, Carabello BA, Usher BW, et al. Mitral valve replacement with and without chordal preservation in patients with chronic mitral regurgitation: mechanisms for differences in postoperative ejection performance. *Circulation* 1992;86:1718.

Vongpastanasin W, Hills LD, Lange RA. Medical progress: prosthetic heart valves. *N Engl J Med* 1996;335:407.

3 Endocrinology, Metabolism, and Diabetes

E. Chester Ridgway and Jane E. Reusch

Adrenal Insufficiency

1. What are the general categories of adrenocortical insufficiency?
2. Can you explain why thyroid function tests should be evaluated in a patient with primary adrenal failure?
3. What are the characteristic signs and symptoms of acute and chronic adrenal insufficiency?
4. What criteria are used to make the diagnosis of adrenal insufficiency?
5. What are the considerations in deciding on long-term replacement therapy for Addison's disease?
6. What other metabolic abnormalities may occur in association with adrenal insufficiency?
7. What are the events that take place in the regulation of cortisol secretion by the hypothalamic–pituitary–adrenal axis?
8. What are the specific causes of primary and secondary adrenal failure?

Discussion

1. *What are the general categories of adrenocortical insufficiency?*
   Adrenocortical insufficiency results primarily from deficient cortisol production and in some cases deficient aldosterone and androgen production by the

adrenal gland. Because the adrenal cortex is normally stimulated by pituitary adrenocorticotropic hormone (ACTH; corticotropin), cortisol deficiency may result from adrenal disease (**primary adrenal insufficiency** or Addison's disease) or from pituitary or hypothalamic disease with ACTH deficiency (**secondary adrenal insufficiency**).

2. *Can you explain why thyroid function tests should be evaluated in a patient with primary adrenal failure?*

The association between autoimmune thyroiditis and autoimmune adrenal disease is well recognized. In general, patients with Addison's disease are more frequently afflicted with Hashimoto's thyroiditis than with Graves' disease. Approximately 50% or more of affected patients have high titers of thyroid antimicrosomal antibodies, although these patients often have no thyroid-related symptoms. Graves' hyperthyroidism can occur in association with primary adrenal failure. The association of thyroid failure and adrenal failure can also reflect hypopituitarism, with a consequent deficiency of both ACTH and thyroid-stimulating hormone (TSH). Therefore, high titers of thyroid antimicrosomal antibodies have been seen in the settings of both primary and secondary hypoadrenalism, making thyroid function tests an important component of the evaluation of a patient with primary adrenal failure.

3. *What are the characteristic signs and symptoms of acute and chronic adrenal insufficiency?*

Acute adrenal insufficiency is a potentially fatal medical emergency, and the clinical features include nausea, fever, and shock, progressing to diarrhea, muscular weakness, increased and then decreased temperature, hypoglycemia, hyponatremia, and hyperkalemia.

The cardinal signs of chronic adrenal insufficiency are weakness, fatigue, and anorexia, along with gastrointestinal complaints of nausea, vomiting, diarrhea, and vague abdominal pain. Other symptoms include salt craving (20% of the patients) and muscle cramps. Physical findings may consist of weight loss, hyperpigmentation, hypotension, and vitiligo. The ear cartilage may calcify in patients with long-standing adrenal insufficiency.

4. *What criteria are used to make the diagnosis of adrenal insufficiency?*

The diagnosis of adrenocortical insufficiency is based primarily on the plasma cortisol determinations made during the rapid ACTH stimulation test (Cortrosyn test). Any screening tests for adrenal insufficiency include determination of a basal level of cortisol and ACTH, together with a rapid ACTH stimulation test. This test is performed by administering 25 units (0.25 mg) of synthetic ACTH intravenously (IV) and measuring the response of cortisol and aldosterone. It is performed to assess initially whether the adrenals can respond to exogenous ACTH. A clearly normal response excludes the possibility of both primary and secondary adrenal failure. For the cortisol response to be normal, the cortisol level after ACTH administration should be twice the baseline level and increased by at least 10 ng/dL over the basal levels. Normally, the aldosterone levels parallel the cortisol levels, with an increase of at least 14 ng/dL above the basal levels. Patients with Addison's disease exhibit very low cortisol levels and a clearly elevated ACTH level, whereas the levels of both tend to be low in patients with hypopituitarism. In the classic situation, the response of aldosterone to ACTH is absent in patients with primary adrenal failure, whereas it is preserved in patients with secondary adrenal failure.

5. *What are the considerations in deciding on long-term replacement therapy for Addison's disease?*

Long-term replacement therapy in patients with Addison's disease involves the oral administration of a cortisone preparation in physiologic replacement doses. Usually, two thirds of the total dose is given in the morning and the remainder is given in the evening to mimic the normal circadian secretion of cortisol. Cortisone acetate can be taken in a dose of 25 mg in the morning and 12.5 mg in the evening. Alternatively, hydrocortisone can be taken in a dosage of 30 to 40 mg per day. However, because cortisone must be converted to hydrocortisone in the body, hydrocortisone is considered the more closely physiologic agent. Despite this, prednisone (7.5 mg per day) is frequently prescribed for long-term replacement because it costs less than hydrocortisone. The side effects from the excessive administration of glucocorticoids include increased appetite, weight gain, insomnia, edema, and hypertension.

Mineralocorticoid replacement (fluorohydrocortisone therapy) is necessary in patients with primary Addison's disease, although the exact replacement dose must be titrated to the patient's response. Dramatic fluid retention may occur with the initial treatment, but this subsides as the dose is adjusted.

6. *What other metabolic abnormalities may occur in association with adrenal insufficiency?*

Hyperkalemia occurs frequently in patients with primary adrenal failure (approximately 64%). This is in part due to the renal tubular loss of sodium, with conservation of the potassium level stemming from the mineralocorticoid deficiency. In addition, glucocorticoids help to maintain the function of the sodium pump and the normal gradient between the intracellular and extracellular concentrations of sodium and potassium. Without cortisol, this gradient is not maintained, so that potassium moves out of the cell and sodium moves into the cell, thus resulting in hyperkalemia.

Hypoglycemia occurs infrequently, and primarily in patients with Addison's disease who have fasted for any period. It is due to defective gluconeogenesis.

A mild **acidosis** may eventuate in patients with mineralocorticoid deficiency because of the decreased secretion of ammonia and hydrogen ions.

Increased circulating levels of **antidiuretic hormone** (ADH) may occur and contribute to the hyponatremia. The excessive loss of sodium by the renal tubules leads to an increased water loss. This is counterbalanced by an increase in the ADH levels, which tends to cause water retention. The low cardiac output and hypovolemia also serve as stimuli for ADH release.

The **inability to excrete a water load** was once used as a diagnostic test for Addison's disease. This phenomenon is primarily caused by glucocorticoid deficiency, even in the presence of euvolemia. A bolus of cortisol completely reverses the effect and a "water diuresis" ensues, but this also involves the interplay of other factors, such as an improvement in cardiac output, an increase in the effective circulating volume, an increase in the glomerular filtration rate, a reduction in ADH levels, and direct effects on the renal tubule.

Peripheral **eosinophilia** is a common finding in the setting of primary adrenal insufficiency.

7. *What are the events that take place in the regulation of cortisol secretion by the hypothalamic–pituitary–adrenal axis?*

Adrenocortical cell growth and steroid secretion are primarily controlled by the pituitary hormone ACTH. The secretory regulation of the hypothalamic–pituitary–adrenal axis involves the release of corticotropin-releasing hormone (CRH) by the hypothalamus into the hypophyseal-portal system. This hormone causes the pituitary secretion of ACTH, which is transported by the peripheral circulation to the adrenal glands, where it is bound by specific receptors and triggers steroid synthesis and secretion. Hormonal and neural input from higher brain centers stimulates or inhibits CRH synthesis and secretion in a 24-hour cycle, which causes both ACTH and cortisol secretion to exhibit a circadian rhythm. Cortisol inhibits both CRH and ACTH release, whereas ACTH has a negative feedback effect on CRH release. The circadian rhythm can be overcome by stress, however, and the adrenal glands atrophy in the absence of endogenous ACTH. Cortisol circulates bound to cortisol-binding globulin (transcortin) and the free cortisol enters a cell and interacts with a specific receptor to exert its physiologic effects.

8. *What are the specific causes of primary and secondary adrenal failure?*

Primary adrenal insufficiency (Addison's disease) is most commonly caused by idiopathic adrenal atrophy stemming from autoimmune destruction (68%), tuberculosis (17%), or some other etiology (15%). Ninety percent of the gland must be destroyed before Addison's disease becomes apparent. Less common causes of adrenal insufficiency include other granulomatous diseases, such as histoplasmosis and sarcoidosis, or infiltrative diseases, such as amyloidosis, hemochromatosis, metastatic tumor, and adrenal leukodystrophy, as well as chronic anticoagulation and bilateral adrenal hemorrhage. Gram-negative septicemia, bilateral adrenalectomy, abdominal irradiation, adrenal vein thrombosis, adrenal artery embolus, and adrenolytic drugs are also rare causes of adrenal failure.

Adrenal insufficiency is found in some patients with the acquired immunodeficiency syndrome (AIDS). The main presentation of adrenal insufficiency in AIDS is fatigue; electrolyte abnormalities are uncommon. Development of adrenal insufficiency in patients with at least one AIDS-defining disease is associated with poor prognosis.

Secondary adrenal insufficiency is commonly caused by iatrogenic corticosteroid therapy, which suppresses CRH and ACTH secretion and results in adrenal atrophy. Other, less common causes include pituitary and hypothalamic tumors, irradiation, trauma, pituitary necrosis, and surgical procedures.

Case   A 60-year-old man is hospitalized because of severe nausea, vomiting, and diarrhea of 4 days' duration. He admits to having experienced mild increasing fatigue and malaise for the past 6 months, plus poor appetite, frequent abdominal cramps, and a 20-pound (9-kg) weight loss over the past 4 months. He feels dizzy in the morning and lightheaded after standing for more than an hour. He notes that he tends to take a nap in the later afternoon. Four days before, abdominal cramps, vomiting, and diarrhea developed. He denies any skin changes and prolonged sun exposure. He admits to a decline in sexual desire. He has no history of hypertension, diabetes, asthma, or tuberculosis, and takes no medications.

Physical examination reveals a very tanned man, who appears acutely ill and somewhat dehydrated. He weighs 63 kg. His supine blood pressure is 106/68 mm Hg and his supine pulse is 90 beats per minute; his standing blood pressure is 80/50 mm Hg and his standing pulse is 104 beats per minute.

His skin shows decreased turgor. His face, hands, extensor surfaces, chest, and back are notably tanned. The findings from the head, eyes, ear, nose, and throat examination are normal, except for the presence of hardened earlobes. No heart abnormalities are noted and his lungs are clear. Abdominal examination reveals the presence of diffuse tenderness, but no rebound or localized tenderness. The bowel sounds are hyperactive. There is decreased axillary hair. His testes are normal and central nervous system findings are unremarkable.

The following laboratory data are obtained: hemoglobin (Hgb), 10.6 g, normochromic normocytic anemia; white blood cell count (WBC), 6,600 cells/mm^3; sodium, 128 mEq/L; potassium, 5.9 mEq/L; creatinine, 2.0 mg/dL; bicarbonate (HCO$_3^-$), 20 mEq/L; chloride, 96 mEq/L; blood urea nitrogen (BUN), 39 mg/dL; and calcium, 11.1 mg/dL.

The chest radiographic study findings are normal and the abdominal radiographic study shows a normal gas pattern, but bilateral adrenal calcification. His electrocardiogram (ECG) is normal.

Seven months later, the patient becomes severely fatigued and weak and complains of cold intolerance, dry skin, somnolence, and constipation. Physical examination at that time reveals a pale patient, with a supine blood pressure of 110/60 mm Hg and pulse of 64 per minute. He weighs 72 kg. His skin is dry and warm and exhibits decreased turgor. Periorbital freckling and vitiligo are present, as well as mild, diffuse thyromegaly. Neurologic examination reveals generalized muscle weakness and decreased deep tendon reflexes symmetrically.

Laboratory data are as follows: WBC, 6,900 cells/mm^3 with normal differential; serum sodium, 135 mEq/L; potassium, 4.7 mEq/L; chloride, 99 mEq/L; HCO$_3^-$, 24.8 mEq/L; glucose, 78 mg/dL; creatinine, 1.0 mg/dL; and BUN, 18 mg/dL. Thyroid function tests reveal the following findings: serum thyroxine (T$_4$), 3.2 μg/dL (normal, 412 μg/dL); triiodothyronine (T$_3$) resin uptake, 20% (normal, 25% to 35%); and TSH, 16 μU/mL (normal, 0.55.0 μU/ml). The test for antimicrosomal antibodies is positive, with a value of 1:50,000.

1. What is the most likely diagnosis in this patient?
2. What would be the first step in the diagnostic evaluation of this patient?
3. Based on the findings from the diagnostic evaluation, what is the diagnosis in this patient?
4. What would you recommend as an initial therapy?
5. How would you treat this patient's hypercalcemia?
6. What additional abnormalities may be seen in association with Addison's disease?
7. Based on the findings when the patient is seen 7 months later, what kind of thyroid disease does he have?
8. What is the most important advice to give this patient?

Case Discussion

1. *What is the most likely diagnosis in this patient?*

   The most likely diagnosis in this patient is acute adrenal insufficiency resulting from either primary or secondary adrenal failure. This patient illustrates the nonspecific nature of symptoms in the setting of chronic adrenal insufficiency, even though he exhibits the classic history and findings.

   This patient's electrolyte changes suggest primary adrenal failure. The hyperkalemia and hyponatremia are due to mineralocorticoid deficiency, often seen in the setting of primary adrenal failure. Because ACTH is not the predominant regulator of aldosterone secretion, electrolyte abnormalities are less common in patients with secondary adrenal failure.

   Adrenal crisis occurs when a stressful situation brings about decompensation. The nature of the stress may range from mild (e.g., the flu) to severe (e.g., trauma or surgery). Adrenal decompensation is marked by dehydration, hypovolemia, profound hypotension, hyponatremia, hyperkalemia, hypoglycemia, and hypothermia. Classic renal failure can mimic several aspects of chronic adrenal failure, including fatigue, malaise, anorexia, hyponatremia, and hyperkalemia. In this patient, the BUN and creatinine abnormalities are more indicative of prerenal azotemia than of acute renal failure.

   Decreased libido, which is common in patients with hypopituitarism, can also be seen in patients with Addison's disease and is due to both the debilitating nature of the illness and the associated primary gonadal failure.

   Calcification of the auricular and costal cartilage is uncommon in patients with Addison's disease, but can occur incidentally. A lack of axillary hair is actually a more common finding in female patients. The amount of pubic hair may also be diminished.

2. *What would be the first step in the diagnostic evaluation of this patient?*

   The ACTH stimulation test should be performed initially to assess whether the adrenal glands can respond to exogenous ACTH by increasing the levels of cortisol and aldosterone. Simultaneously, the plasma ACTH level should be measured because patients with Addison's disease have very low cortisol levels but an elevated ACTH level. Adrenal autoantibody testing is now available and has a 70% sensitivity. In addition, because of the abdominal radiographic finding of adrenal calcification, purified protein derivative (PPD) skin tests should be performed to assess for tuberculosis.

An ACTH stimulation test reveals a basal cortisol level of 2.8 μg/dL, which is then 2.8 μg/dL at 30 minutes and 3.0 μg/dL at 60 minutes. The aldosterone level is 2.5 ng/mL at 0 minutes, 2.5 ng/mL at 30 minutes, and 3.1 ng/mL at 60 minutes (normal values—cortisol: 925 μg/dL a.m. fasting, and 216 μg/dL p.m. fasting; aldosterone, normal salt upright: men, 622 ng/dL; women, 431 ng/dL). The plasma ACTH level is found to be 779 pg/mL (normal, <580 pg/mL at 8:00 a.m. upright; 526 pg/mL at 8:00 a.m. supine; and <517 pg/mL at 4:00 p.m. supine). The PPD test result is negative.

3. *Based on the findings from the diagnostic evaluation, what is the diagnosis in this patient?*

The results of the ACTH stimulation test in this patient are clearly abnormal, showing subnormal responses to ACTH indicative of adrenal failure. This is the classic situation in patients with primary adrenal failure—that is, the response of both cortisol and aldosterone to ACTH is absent; in secondary adrenal failure, the aldosterone response is preserved.

The plasma ACTH level is markedly elevated in this patient, and such extreme elevations may be seen in the context of severe stress, such as that caused by surgery, anesthesia, and hypoglycemia. Calcification of the adrenal glands can occur in the setting of tuberculosis, histoplasmosis, and occasionally in autoimmune adrenal disease. Thus, the cause of this patient's adrenal gland failure is primary adrenal failure, most likely secondary to the autoimmune destruction of the adrenals. The negative PPD supports a nontuberculous etiology of the primary adrenal failure.

4. *What would you recommend as an initial therapy?*

Because the clinical presentation suggests adrenal crisis, therapy should be instituted immediately because adrenal crisis is a life-threatening emergency and any delay in treatment could prove fatal. Such therapy includes the immediate IV administration of a soluble corticosteroid preparation, such as hydrocortisone (100 mg), followed by rapid infusions of glucose and normal saline at a rate of 2 to 4 liters per day. The glucocorticoids and volume repletion cause the serum potassium levels to decrease. Definitive diagnostic testing should be carried out after the acute therapy has been instituted. Mineralocorticoid therapy should be deferred until the patient can take medication orally.

5. *How would you treat this patient's hypercalcemia?*

Because this patient's hypercalcemia is mild, it requires no special treatment other than hydration with normal saline. Both hypercalcemia and hypocalcemia have been reported to occur during an adrenal crisis. This may stem from dehydration, but may also be a consequence of the increased absorption of calcium from the gut due to glucocorticoid deficiency. Occasionally, mild hypercalcemia may coexist with adrenal failure caused by a pituitary tumor that compromises the function of corticotrophs [multiple endocrine neoplasia type I (MEN1)]. Hypocalcemia may occur in patients whose hypoadrenalism is a part of the autoimmune polyglandular syndrome type I (polyglandular failure).

6. *What additional abnormalities may be seen in association with Addison's disease?*

Other abnormalities that may arise in patients with Addison's disease include hypoglycemia, hyperkalemia, high ADH levels, metabolic acidosis, vitiligo, and high levels of anti-thyroid antibodies. All of these can be a frequent component of the clinical picture in patients with adrenal insufficiency.

7. *Based on the findings when the patient is seen 7 months later, what kind of thyroid disease does he have?*

The findings are consistent with those of Hashimoto's thyroiditis. Patients with idiopathic Addison's disease are prone to other autoimmune disorders, which may develop before or after adrenal failure is diagnosed. These disorders include Graves' hyperthyroidism, Hashimoto's thyroiditis, pernicious anemia, diabetes, hypoparathyroidism, primary hypogonadism, vitiligo, and moniliasis. Areas of vitiligo form in 4% to 6% of the patients with Addison's disease, especially in those whose disease has an autoimmune cause.

In this man who has a goiter, low T_4 and high TSH levels, and strongly positive anti-thyroid antibody titers, levothyroxine therapy should be started, but only when adequate steroid replacement has been achieved and after the patient has been on steroid replacement therapy for at least 2 weeks. An adrenal crisis could be precipitated if levothyroxine is given to a patient who is in a hypoadrenal state because of the resulting increased metabolic demands that levothyroxine imposes on the body.

8. *What is the most important advice to give this patient?*

In any patient with adrenal insufficiency, it is critical to emphasize the need for increasing the dosage of glucocorticoids during periods of stress or illness, such as colds, flu, diarrhea, infections, trauma, or surgery. Failure to do so might precipitate the rapid development of an acute adrenal crisis. In addition, the patient must be instructed to wear an identification bracelet or carry a card at all times indicating that he has the disease and needs supplemental steroids during stress. This is a crucial life-preserving measure and cannot be overemphasized.

Suggested Readings

Bartalena L, Marcocci C, Bogazzi F, et al. Relation between therapy for hyperthyroidism and the course of Graves' ophthalmopathy. *N Engl J Med* 1998;338:73.

Berenson JR, Lipton A. Pharmacology and clinical efficacy of bisphosphonates. *Curr Opin Oncol* 1998;10:566.

De Luca F, Baron J. Molecular biology and clinical importance of the Ca(2+)-sensing receptor. *Curr Opin Pediatr* 1998;10:435.

Fitzgerald PA. *Handbook of clinical endocrinology*, 2nd ed. Norwalk, CT: Appleton & Lange, 1992.

Fulfaro F, Casuccio A, Ticozzi C, Ripamonti C. The role of bisphosphonates in the treatment of painful metastatic bone disease: a review of phase III trials. *Pain* 1998;78:157.

Mundy GR, Guise TA. Hypercalcemia of malignancy. *Am J Med* 1997;103:134.

Schrier RW. *Current medical therapy*, 2nd ed. New York: Raven, 1989.
Wilson JD, Foster DW, eds. *Williams' textbook of endocrinology*, 8th ed. Philadelphia: WB
  Saunders, 1992.

Cushing's Syndrome

1. What is the difference between Cushing's syndrome and Cushing's disease?
2. What is the most common cause of Cushing's syndrome?
3. What are the clinical features of Cushing's syndrome?
4. What are the biologic effects of glucocorticoids?
5. What are the screening tests used to diagnose Cushing's syndrome?

Discussion

1. *What is the difference between Cushing's syndrome and Cushing's disease?*

   Cushing's syndrome refers to the phenotypic and clinical sequelae due to hypercortisolism resulting from any cause. *Cushing's disease* refers specifically to the hypercortisolism due to an ACTH-secreting pituitary corticotroph adenoma or pituitary corticotroph hyperplasia.

2. *What is the most common cause of Cushing's syndrome?*

   The widespread use of potent corticosteroids in the practice of clinical medicine, particularly in the treatment of autoimmune, allergic, and pulmonary disorders, has made iatrogenic hypercortisolism the most common cause of Cushing's syndrome. However, once iatrogenic causes are eliminated, pituitary adenoma (68%) becomes the most common cause.

3. *What are the clinical features of Cushing's syndrome?*

   Cushing's syndrome is associated with many clinical features. **Obesity**, found in 94%, is the most common manifestation and weight gain is usually the earliest symptom of Cushing's syndrome. The obesity tends to be central, but fat can also be redistributed to the face (moon facies; 75%), as well as supraclavicular (80%) and dorsocervical areas ("buffalo hump"; 80%). These latter two, particularly the supraclavicular fat pad, are more specific findings for Cushing's syndrome.

   Skin changes occur in 85% of the patients and arise because cortisol-induced atrophy of the epidermis leads to thinning and a transparent appearance of the skin, facial plethora, easy bruisability, and the formation of striae. The latter are purplish-red areas that are depressed below the skin surface, but are wider than the pinkish-white striae that appear after pregnancy or weight loss. Wounds heal slowly in these patients and may dehisce. Hyperpigmentation occurs in the setting of the ectopic ACTH syndrome, but is rare in patients with Cushing's disease and should not be found in those with primary adrenal Cushing's syndrome. Acne (40%) is also a symptom and is due to androgen excess; it may be more generalized than that which the patient experienced before.

   Hirsutism affects 80% of the patients and typically consists of a darkening and coarsening of the hair. Female patients complain of increased growth of hair over the face, upper thighs, abdomen, and breasts. Virilism occurs in approximately 20% of the cases of adrenal carcinoma. **Hypertension** is a problem in 75% of the patients. Elevated diastolic blood pressure is a classic feature of spontaneous Cushing's syndrome, and it contributes greatly to the morbidity and mortality associated with the disorder. The increased sodium retention also leads to edema (18%). Congestive heart failure (22%) can be aggravated because of the increased blood pressure and fluid load.

Gonadal dysfunction occurs in 75% of the patients. Elevated androgen levels can result in amenorrhea and infertility in 75% of affected premenopausal women. In men, the elevated cortisol level may cause a decrease in libido.

Muscle weakness arises in 60% of patients, in particular proximal weakness that most often occurs in the lower extremities. This weakness stems from the catabolic effects of glucocorticoids on muscle tissues, steroid-induced myopathy, and possibly electrolyte imbalances. Radiographically detectable **osteoporosis** is present in most patients with Cushing's syndrome (60%), and back pain is the initial complaint in 58% of the cases. Pathologic fractures are found in the ribs and vertebral bodies in severe cases. It takes some time for the hypercortisolism to decalcify bone; thus, Cushing's syndrome due to adrenal carcinoma and some ectopic ACTH cases is not present long enough to cause osteoporosis.

Psychological disturbances can arise in 40% of patients. These complaints range from mild symptoms, such as emotional lability, increased irritability, anxiety, insomnia, euphoria, poor concentration, poor memory, and mild depression, to severe symptoms, which include frank psychosis associated with delusions or hallucinations, paranoia, severe depression, and even suicide.

Renal calculi form in 15% of patients as a result of glucocorticoid-induced hypercalcemia. Renal colic may be the presenting symptom of Cushing's syndrome. **Thirst** and **polyuria** are seen in 10% of patients. The thirst is due to glucocorticoid-induced hyperglycemia (or worsening of the diabetes mellitus) that causes an osmotic (glucose) diuresis. Diabetic ketoacidosis (DKA) and diabetic microvascular complications are rare in the diabetes seen in Cushing's syndrome.

4. *What are the biologic effects of glucocorticoids?*

From a **molecular** perspective, glucocorticoid hormones enter the cell by diffusion and activate specific gene transcription by binding to the nuclear glucocorticoid receptor. The glucocorticoid receptor is thus a conditional transactivator that influences the rate of RNA polymerase II transcription initiation by binding to specific short DNA sequence elements (glucocorticoid response elements) in the promoter regulatory region of the various target genes. Although this is the best-established pathway of glucocorticoid action, other mechanisms that mediate the rapid effects of glucocorticoids, such as the fast-feedback inhibition of ACTH secretion and possibly modulation of the γ-aminobutyric acid receptor, must also exist.

In terms of their effects on **metabolism**, glucocorticoids accelerate hepatic gluconeogenesis by stimulating phosphoenolpyruvate carboxykinase and glucose-6-phosphatase activity, and induce a permissive effect in other gluconeo-genic hormones (glucagon and catecholamines). Glucocorticoids also enhance hepatic glycogen synthesis and storage and inhibit glycogen breakdown. In muscle, glucocorticoids inhibit amino acid uptake and protein synthesis and stimulate protein breakdown and the release of amino acids, lactate, free fatty acids (FFAs), and glycerol. In adipose tissue, glucocorticoids primarily accelerate lipolysis, with a resultant release in the formation of glycerol and FFAs. Although glucocorticoids are lipolytic, an increased central fat deposi-tion is a classic feature of Cushing's syndrome. The steroid-induced increase in appetite and hyperinsulinemia may account for this, but the basis for this abnormal fat deposition in the setting of hypercortisolism remains unknown.

5. *What are the screening tests used to diagnose Cushing's syndrome?*

A key aspect of the initial workup in a patient with suspected Cushing's syndrome is to distinguish true hypercortisolism from obesity, depression, or alcoholism, or a combination of these, because many clinical and laboratory features of these disorders display significant overlap. A key aid in establishing the clinical diagnosis of hypercortisolism is to examine sequential photographs of the patient that span several years. Once Cushing's syndrome is suspected on clinical grounds, the overnight 1-mg dexamethasone suppression test (DST) and the 24-hour urinary free cortisol (UFC) determination are used as screen-ing tests. If the results of the overnight 1-mg DST are normal (8 a.m. plasma cortisol <5 μg/dL after the administration of 1 mg of dexamethasone at 11 p.m. the night before), the diagnosis is very unlikely. If the results of the UFC are also normal (i.e, <90 to 100 μg/day), Cushing's syndrome is effectively excluded. Several situations can cause false-positive results to the screening DST, including acute and chronic illness, obesity, high-estrogen states, certain drugs (phenytoin and phenobarbital), alcoholism, anorexia, renal failure, and depression. However, in the setting of obesity, high-estrogen states, and drugs, the results of a 24-hour UFC are normal. In the other situations, repeated testing is necessary to exclude the diagnosis. Rarely, false-negative results can occur, such as in the event of prolonged dexamethasone clearance or episodic hypercortisolism.

Case   A 36-year-old white woman comes to you complaining of fatigue, irritability, depression, and a 30-pound (13.5-kg) weight gain over the past 2 years. She recounts that she has noticed a significant change in her energy level for at least the past 2 years. She states that she has always been a hard worker but, 6 months before, she had to quit her job as a waitress because of extreme muscle weakness and fatigue. She has also noted increased mood swings, manifested by increased irritability, spontaneous crying episodes, and depression. She reports that her face seems rounder than it was 2 years before. On further questioning, she admits that her menstrual periods have been irregular for the past 2 years. She also admits to drinking "a six-pack of beer" at least once a week, but denies smoking. She has also noted that she bruises easily. She denies any other medical problems, and states that she is not taking any medications. She specifically denies any glucocorticoid therapy. In asking about her family history, you find out that her mother has adult-onset diabetes mellitus.

Physical examination reveals an obese white woman who is crying while she sits on the examining table, but otherwise she does not appear to be acutely ill. Her weight is 193 pounds (87 kg); height, 5 ft 7 in (167.5 cm); blood pressure, 165/100 mm Hg; and heart rate, 86 per minute and regular.

Her face is very round and plethoric compared with that in old photographs. Dorsocervical (buffalo hump) and supraclavicular fat pads are noted. She has mild facial hirsutism, some acne is noted over the face and chest, and wide purple striae are present in the lower abdomen. Her extremities are thin and she has proximal muscle weakness.

The following laboratory findings are encountered: fasting blood glucose, 180 mg/dL; potassium, 3 mEq/L; HCO_3^-, 34 mEq/L; liver function tests, all normal; 8 a.m. cortisol, 38 μg/dL, which decreases to 32 μg/dL after the administration of 1 mg of dexamethasone. The 24-hour UFC level is 876 μg.

1. What is the most likely diagnosis in this patient, and why?
2. What studies would you perform to establish the anatomic cause of her hypercortisolism?
3. What is the role of magnetic resonance imaging (MRI) and computed tomographic (CT) scanning of the pituitary and adrenal glands, as well as inferior petrosal sinus sampling, in patients with Cushing's syndrome?
4. What is the optimal therapeutic approach for this patient?
5. Why is there a need for steroid therapy in the postoperative period, and sometimes beyond, in patients with Cushing's disease?

Case Discussion

1. *What is the most likely diagnosis in this patient, and why?*

Having excluded exogenous glucocorticoid medications in the history, the differential diagnosis list would include (a) pituitary corticotroph adenoma (or hyperplasia), or Cushing's disease, (b) ectopic ACTH [or corticotropin-releasing factor (CRF)] syndrome, (c) adrenal adenoma, (d) adrenal cancer, (e) obesity, (f) depression, and (g) alcoholism.

The most frequently encountered dilemma in the differential diagnosis of Cushing's syndrome is the clinical picture consisting of an obese, depressed patient who consumes excessive amounts of alcohol. These patients can display many of the phenotypic features and laboratory findings consistent with hypercortisolism, and yet not have Cushing's syndrome. Thus, the patient's history of consuming a six-pack of beer per week is of concern because this could produce alcoholic pseudo-Cushing's syndrome. In this disorder, the effects of chronic alcoholism result in central obesity (ascites), a round, plethoric face, easy bruising, and some abnormal results from the screening tests for Cushing's syndrome. However, this patient has no abnormal liver function findings and she has physical findings (a marked change in her facial appearance compared with that in old photographs, hypertension, dorsocervical and supraclavicular fat pads, purple abdominal striae, acne, and hirsutism) and laboratory data (hyperglycemia, hypokalemia, an elevated basal cortisol level that does not suppress in response to the 1-mg DST, and an elevated 24-hour UFC) that are all highly consistent with the clinical suspicion of hypercortisolism.

The lack of virilization and the relatively slow (>2 years) onset of the clinical symptoms argue against adrenal carcinoma. In addition, the lack of a smoking history and any hyperpigmentation, together with the slow onset, suggest that ectopic ACTH arising from small cell lung carcinoma is unlikely to be the cause. This leaves pituitary adenoma (or hyperplasia), ectopic ACTH or CRF (from a carcinoid, pancreatic islet cell tumor, medullary thyroid carcinoma, or pheochromocytoma), and adrenal adenoma in the differential diagnosis. Given that pituitary adenomas constitute 68% of all noniatrogenic causes of hypercortisolism, this is the most likely diagnosis. However, further workup is required to document the precise source of the elevated cortisol levels in this patient.

2. *What studies would you perform to establish the anatomic cause of her hypercortisolism?*

Once the diagnosis of hypercortisolism (Cushing's syndrome) has been confirmed by the findings yielded by the clinical evaluation and screening laboratory tests, the combined use of the following diagnostic techniques can establish the diagnosis in almost all instances: determination of a basal plasma ACTH level, a high-dose (8-mg) DST, radiographic imaging, and inferior petrosal sampling (with or without CRF stimulation). Thus, by simultaneously measuring the plasma cortisol and ACTH levels, the possibility of an adrenal adenoma can be assessed, because the autonomous production of glucocorticoids by the adrenal adenoma suppresses ACTH to levels below 20 pg/mL. To differentiate between a pituitary adenoma and the ectopic tumor production of ACTH, several studies need to be performed because many of the laboratory and radiographic results can overlap for these two distinct causes of Cushing's syndrome. For example, the ACTH level can range between 40 and 200 pg/mL in the setting of Cushing's disease and between 100 and 10,000 pg/mL in the setting of ectopic ACTH. In the classic 2-day high-dose DST (2 mg of dexamethasone is given every 6 hours for 2 days, and 24-hour UFC samples are collected the day before and on the second day of dexamethasone administration), patients with pituitary tumors (Cushing's disease) typically exhibit a suppression less than 50% of baseline values; those with ectopic ACTH or primary adrenal hypercortisolism display little or no reduction. However, some carcinoid tumors that produce ACTH ectopically maintain some degree of negative feedback through the influence of exogenous steroids, and the suppression observed may be equivalent to that seen in patients with pituitary tumors.

The abbreviated high-dose DST involves administering 8 mg of dexamethasone at 11 p.m. the night before and measuring the plasma cortisol level the next morning at 8 a.m. In this test, a suppression below 50% of basal plasma cortisol levels is seen in patients with pituitary tumor, but not in those with ectopic ACTH and primary adrenal cortisolism. This version of the high-dose DST is preferred because it appears to be more specific and does not require two 24-hour urine collections. For a more precise definition of the cause of the disorder, however, specific radiographic procedures must be performed.

3. *What is the role of MRI and CT scanning of the pituitary and adrenal glands, as well as inferior petrosal sinus sampling, in patients with Cushing's syndrome?*

The major problem with the CT and MRI evaluation of the pituitary and adrenal glands is that they can detect asymptomatic lesions in up to 15% and 8%, respectively, of the normal population. Because of this incidence of nonspecific radiographic "lesions," the clinician must be cautious about basing the diagnosis of pituitary or adrenal Cushing's syndrome on the results of these imaging studies.

Pituitary adenomas causing Cushing's disease tend to be small (1 to 5 mm; rarely >10 mm), and thus are detectable by contrast-enhanced CT scanning in as few as 30% to 35% of cases and by gadolinium–DTPA-enhanced MRI in 55% of cases. Thus, because of its better sensitivity, MRI has replaced CT in the assessment of these tumors. Patients whose imaging studies yield negative findings need to undergo inferior petrosal sampling to document further the pituitary anatomic location of the tumor. In addition, as already discussed, even if an abnormality is detected by these imaging methods, this does not constitute unequivocal evidence that the abnormality is responsible for the syndrome. As the resolution of CT and MRI improves, the ability to detect these "incidental" and clinically silent microadenomas will also increase and further confound the diagnostic workup. An ectopic CRF syndrome could also result in an enlarged pituitary due to corticotroph hyperplasia, and yet the primary disorder may actually be a carcinoid of the lung.

Computed tomography, MRI, ultrasonography, and isotope scanning with iodocholesterol can be used to define the nature of **adrenal lesions**. These procedures are not necessary in patients with ACTH hypersecretion, however. Nevertheless, some physicians use these tests to exclude the presence of a solitary adrenal adenoma or carcinoma, and thus to confirm the presence of bilateral adrenal hyperplasia or nodular adrenal hyperplasia in the setting of pituitary-based disease. These procedures are most useful for localizing adrenal tumors because these tumors usually must be larger than 1.5 cm to cause significant cortisol production and result in Cushing's syndrome. However, as noted previously, because of the 1% to 8% incidence of silent adrenal nodules, biochemical testing must be performed with localization studies to ensure that the lesion identified is biologically significant.

To distinguish between the various causes of Cushing's syndrome when conflicting or overlapping data are obtained, bilateral simultaneous **inferior petrosal venous sampling** (with or without CRF stimulation) can successfully distinguish Cushing's disease from ectopic ACTH secretion and adrenal disease with greater accuracy than any other test. Because ACTH is rapidly metabolized (half-life, 7 to 12 minutes) and is secreted episodically, advantage can be taken of the concentration gradient between the pituitary venous drainage through the inferior petrosal sinus (central) and the peripheral venous values of ACTH to determine further whether an ACTH-producing corticotroph adenoma is present in the pituitary; the inclusion of CRF stimulation makes the test more sensitive. Bilateral and simultaneous inferior petrosal sinus samples are obtained to circumvent the problem of isolated secretory bursts or timing issues if catheters have to be repositioned. Thus, ACTH samples are obtained from the inferior petrosal sinus, from the jugular bulb, and from other sites (e.g., superior or inferior vena cava), and the findings are compared with those from simultaneously obtained peripheral vein samples. In patients with Cushing's disease, the inferior petrosal sinus/peripheral ratio (IPS:P) of ACTH exceeds 2. In patients with ectopic ACTH, the ratio is less than 2 and selective venous sampling (e.g., of the pulmonary, pancreatic, or intestinal beds) may localize the ectopic tumor. The administration of CRF during bilateral inferior petrosal sinus sampling can increase the diagnostic accuracy of the test by eliciting an ACTH response in the few patients with pituitary tumors who do not exhibit a diagnostic IPS:P gradient in the basal samples. All patients with Cushing's disease have an IPS:P greater than 3 after CRF stimulation, whereas patients with ectopic ACTH or adrenal disease can have an IPS:P of ACTH less than 3 after CRF stimulation. Inferior petrosal sinus sampling (with or without CRF stimulation) has not been extensively studied in the context of normal people, however, and thus the correct interpretation of the results requires that the patient be hypercortisolemic at the time of the study so that the response of normal corticotrophs to CRF is suppressed. Thus, the importance of inferior petrosal sampling, with or without CRF stimulation, in excluding the ectopic ACTH syndrome has become increasingly clear.

4. *What is the optimal therapeutic approach for this patient?*

Once the tumor has been localized to the pituitary, the next goal is surgically to remove the corticotroph adenoma using the technique of selective transsphenoidal surgery. Because the tumors are small, it requires an experienced neurosurgeon to sucessfully identify and resect the adenoma. Thus, meticulous exploration of the intrasellar contents is mandatory and, once the tumor is found, it is selectively removed and the remaining normal pituitary is left intact. If the tumor cannot be identified, it is necessary to perform larger pituitary resections and, in some cases, a total hypophysectomy may be necessary. Transsphenoidal surgery is successful in approximately 85% of patients with microadenomas (tumor <10 mm), and surgical damage to the normal anterior pituitary is rare. The major side effects of the procedure include transient diabetes insipidus, possible cerebrospinal fluid leak, sinusitis, and, rarely, postoperative bleeding. All patients with Cushing's disease who are successfully treated by transsphenoidal surgery become adrenally insufficient for variable periods of time and must receive replacement doses of glucocorticoids (see question 5).

The success rates for transsphenoidal surgery drop drastically (15% to 25%) in the setting of large (>10 mm) tumors, locally invasive tumors, tumors not identified at operation, and corticotroph hyperplasia. In these instances, adjunctive radiation therapy is usually administered (450 to 500 Gy). However, the major problem with radiation therapy is the lag time (6 to 12 months) for it to take effect and the 10% to 20% incidence of hypopituitarism and visual field deficits, even blindness, that may eventuate.

5. *Why is there a need for steroid therapy in the postoperative period, and sometimes beyond, in patients with Cushing's disease?*

The successful surgical removal of the ACTH-producing pituitary microadenoma eliminates the drive for adrenal glucocorticoid production and renders the patient dependent on the remaining normal corticotrophs. However, because these cells have been suppressed for years by the excess cortisol, they are dormant. Thus, those patients with Cushing's disease who have been successfully treated experience transient (1 to 18 months) adrenocortical insufficiency and require exogenous glucocorticoid support; in those who are not cured by the surgical procedure, the production of excessive amounts of glucocorticoids continues and they do not depend on an exogenous source of steroids.

Suggested Readings

Frohman LA. Diseases of the anterior pituitary. In: Felig P, Baxter JD, Broadus AE, Frohman LA, eds. *Endocrinology and metabolism*, 2nd ed. New York: McGraw-Hill, 1987.

Tyrrell JB, Ron DC, Forsham PH. Glucocorticoids and adrenal androgens. In: Greenspan FS, ed. *Basic and clinical endocrinology*, 3rd ed. Norwalk, CT: Appleton & Lange, 1991.

Diabetes Mellitus

1. What are the clinical manifestations of diabetes mellitus?
2. What are the major types of diabetes mellitus and what are their distinguishing features?
3. What are the major acute and chronic complications of the disease?
4. What aspects of the medical history require special emphasis?
5. What aspects of the physical examination require special attention?
6. What laboratory tests are essential in the evaluation of the patient with suspected diabetes?
7. What are the goals of diabetes therapy and what treatment modalities are available? How should these be individualized?

Discussion

1. *What are the clinical manifestations of diabetes mellitus?*

Diabetes mellitus is a complex metabolic disorder characterized by abnormalities of carbohydrate, lipid, and protein metabolism resulting either from a deficiency of insulin or from target tissue resistance to its cellular metabolic effects. It is the most common endocrine-metabolic disorder and affects an estimated 14 million people in the United States, with the incidence of new cases increasing by more than 700,000 cases per year.

Diabetes is manifested by the finding of hyperglycemia and the time-dependent development of chronic complications (retinopathy, neuropathy, nephropathy, and accelerated atherosclerosis) resulting from the multiple metabolic derangements. Accordingly, the presenting clinical signs and symptoms can be due to either hyperglycemia or the complications of the disease, or both. In general, the major classic symptoms of polydipsia, polyuria, weight loss, and fatigue are found in the setting of new-onset diabetes in young patients whose disease is due to insulinopenia. On the other hand, older patients with diabetes may be relatively free of symptoms for a long time. In such patients, the diabetes is first detected either incidentally or because one of its chronic complications is discovered. It is estimated that approximately half of all the adult cases of diabetes in the United States remain undiagnosed.

2. *What are the major types of diabetes mellitus and what are their distinguishing features?*

The current classification (according to the National Diabetes Data Group) of diabetes mellitus and other categories of glucose intolerance consists of three clinical classes: (a) diabetes mellitus, which includes type I, or insulin-dependent diabetes mellitus (IDDM), and type II, or non–insulin-dependent diabetes mellitus (NIDDM); (b) impaired glucose tolerance test; and (c) gestational diabetes mellitus. Of these, type I and II diabetes represent the largest category and are discussed here in further detail. Impaired glucose tolerance is defined as an abnormality in glucose levels intermediate between normal and overt diabetes, whereas gestational diabetes mellitus is defined as carbohydrate intolerance with onset or first recognition during pregnancy.

Type I diabetes, or IDDM, constitutes approximately 5% to 10% of all cases of diabetes and is due to insulin deficiency resulting from the autoimmune destruction of insulin-producing pancreatic islet cells. Therefore, such patients are prone to ketoacidosis and are absolutely dependent on exogenous insulin to sustain life (hence the term *insulin-dependent diabetes*). The onset in these patients is relatively abrupt and usually occurs in youth (mean age, 12 years), although it may arise at any age.

Type II diabetes, or NIDDM, accounts for approximately 90% to 95% of all cases of diabetes and the insulin levels of affected patients may be normal, increased, or decreased, but there is not an absolute insulin deficiency. Therefore, such patients are not prone to ketoacidosis under basal conditions and are not absolutely dependent on exogenous insulin to sustain life (hence the term *non–insulin-dependent diabetes*). However, insulin may be required in patients with NIDDM for adequate control of hyperglycemia. Obesity is frequently associated with NIDDM and the disease is usually diagnosed after 40 years of age, but can also occur at a younger age. There is usually a strong family history of diabetes mellitus in these patients.

3. *What are the major acute and chronic complications of the disease?*

Diabetic ketoacidosis and hyperglycemic, hyperosmolar, nonketotic coma (HHNKC) are the major acute complications of diabetes mellitus. DKA is a complication of IDDM and is initiated by an absolute or relative insulin deficiency and an increase in catabolic hormones, leading to the hepatic overproduction of glucose and ketone bodies. HHNKC, a complication of NIDDM, is characterized by the insidious development of marked hyperglycemia, hyperosmolarity, dehydration, and prerenal azotemia in the absence of significant hyperketonemia or acidosis. Finally, hypoglycemia can occur as an acute complication of the therapy of both types I and II diabetes mellitus.

Retinopathy, nephropathy, neuropathy, and atherosclerotic cardiovascular disease represent the chronic complications of both type I and II diabetes. These complications occur as a function of the disease's duration and, in general, in proportion to the degree of poor metabolic control. Although all of these complications can arise in the setting of both type I and II diabetes, microvascular complications (retinopathy and nephropathy) tend to be more common in the former, whereas macrovascular complications (atherosclerotic cardiovascular disease) tend to be more common in the latter. The apparent reason for this is that most patients with NIDDM acquire their disease in middle age after age-dependent underlying atherosclerotic vascular changes have already set in.

4. *What aspects of the medical history require special emphasis?*

A comprehensive medical history in a patient with suspected diabetes should be directed not only toward confirming the diagnosis, but should be used to review the nature of previous treatment programs and diabetes education, the degree of glycemic control, and whether acute and chronic complications exist. Patients should be queried about their dietary, weight, and exercise history. Current medications for the management of diabetes, as well as other medications that may affect glycemic control, should be recorded. In addition, the presence, severity, and treatment of the acute and chronic complications of diabetes should be reviewed, including sexual function, as well as prior or current infections, especially of the skin, feet, teeth and gums, and genitourinary system. Finally, the history should include a review of the presence of risk factors for atherosclerosis, including family history, smoking, hypertension, obesity, and dyslipidemia.

5. *What aspects of the physical examination require special attention?*

During the complete physical examination of a patient with suspected or known diabetes, particular attention should be directed toward checking for the presence and severity of microvascular and macrovascular complications of the disease, as well as assessing for the presence of peripheral and autonomic neuropathy. Careful examination of the feet is also indicated.

6. *What laboratory tests are essential in the evaluation of the patient with suspected diabetes?*

The laboratory evaluation in a patient with suspected diabetes is used to establish the diagnosis, to determine the degree of metabolic control, and to define the associated complications and risk factors. Although the extent of such tests should be individualized, they usually should include the following: the plasma glucose concentration (fasting or random), the Hgb A_{1c}, a fasting lipid profile, the serum creatinine level, BUN, and urinalysis (to check for the presence of microalbumin, ketones, glucose, and protein, as well as a microscopic examination). A baseline ECG is indicated for adults with diabetes. Because the frequency of thyroid disease is increased in patients with type I diabetes, assessment of thyroid function is helpful in these patients.

7. *What are the goals of diabetes therapy and what treatment modalities are available? How should these be individualized?*

In general, the goals of diabetes therapy are (a) to alleviate the signs and symptoms of the disease (e.g., polydipsia, polyuria, and nocturia); (b) to prevent the acute complications (i.e., DKA and HHNKC); and (c) to attempt to prevent the long-term complications of the disease (i.e., retinopathy, nephropathy, neuropathy, and atherosclerotic cardiovascular disease). Although the first two goals are relatively easy to achieve, until recently it was not clear if the available treatment modalities ensure prevention of the long-term complications. However, the randomized, prospective trial, the Diabetes Control and Complications Trial (DCCT), has demonstrated that tight metabolic control of type I diabetes leads to definite beneficial effects on the rate of complications. This also held true for patients with type 2 diabetes in the recently completed United Kingdom Prospective Diabetes Study (UKPDS). Therefore, it is prudent to attempt to maintain blood glucose levels in patients with both type I and II diabetes as close to the normal range as possible. The limiting factor in such attempts is an increased frequency of hypoglycemic episodes.

Although insulin is the mainstay of IDDM therapy, other treatments, including diet, exercise, and sulfonylurea agents, can be used in patients with NIDDM. Diet and exercise form the cornerstone of NIDDM therapy. They should be instituted first and patient adherence encouraged and maximized. Oral sulfonylurea agents, which enhance β-cell insulin secretion, or metformin, which decreases hepatic glucose output, are added to this treatment if diet and exercise alone fail to control hyperglycemia optimally. These agents also can be used effectively in combination because they have different mechanisms and their actions are additive. Additional oral agents include acarbose, which slows postprandial carbohydrate absorption, and troglitazone, which enhances insulin action in the periphery. Combination therapy with multiple classes of drugs is effective, but cost and monitoring for toxicity can be prohibitive. With the increased duration of type II diabetes, β-cell exhaustion leads to relative insulin insufficiency, and patients then need to be switched to insulin therapy for adequate glycemic control. However, certain patients with NIDDM, particularly the lean subjects with marked hyperglycemia on presentation, may need to be started and maintained on insulin therapy beginning at the time of initial diagnosis.

DIABETES CARE FLOW SHEET

Recommended Visit Schedule:

Patients meeting treatment goals—Semi-Annually
More often if: (1) patient unstable, (2) newly diagnosed
or (3) not meeting treatment goals

Enter results or date as appropriate on flow sheet

Area	Recommended frequency	Date	Date	Date	Date
Physical Findings (multiple Algorithm annotations–see footnote #)					
History and physical [1 & 2]	Comprehensive 1× annually Focused at other visits				
Weight [1 & 2] goal is BMI < 27	Every visit				
Blood pressure [4] goal ≤ 130/85	Every visit				
Dilated eye exam referral [4]	Annually				
Foot exam— [4] • Sensation, pedal pulses, deformities, ulcers, color • Comprehensive vascular, neurological and musculoskeletal	Every visit Annually				
Laboratory Tests (Algorithm annotation #3)					
HbA1c Depends on age, physical condition of patient. Evaluate Rx plan when >8%	2× annually—more often when not meeting treatment goals				
Urinalysis	Annually				
Microalbumin (if urine negative for protein) • Urine albumin/creatinine ratio in a random spot-check 24-hour collection with creatinine clearance	Annually—if positive, repeat test within 3 months				
Blood lipids • Cholesterol <200 mg/dl • Triglycerides <200 mg/dl • LDL <130 mg/dl (<100 with CAD) • HDL >35 mg/dl	Annually				
Diabetes Management Plan (Algorithm annotation #5 and #7)					
• Self blood glucose monitoring results • Nutrition • Exercise/physical activity • Compliance	Every visit with comprehensive review annually				
Preventive Care/Lifestyle (Algorithm annotation #4)					
Pneumococcal	At least one time				
Influenza vaccine	Annually				
Smoking cessation	Every visit				
Preconception counseling (women of childbearing age)	Every visit				
Referrals (Algorithm annotation #6)					
Diabetes Education, Endocrinologist, Diabetologist, Other specialists	As indicated				

Superscript notations refer to number of Algorithm found in Guideline Document

Case 1   A 14-year-old boy with an 8-year history of diabetes mellitus has been sick since yesterday, when he began vomiting. His diabetes has been reasonably well controlled on a dosage of 35 units of Lente insulin taken daily. He has had several episodes of DKA in the past, but not for approximately 4 years. Yesterday, when he began vomiting, his urine glucose concentration was 4+ and his urine acetone was negative, so he took his usual dose of insulin. He has had intense polyuria and polydipsia for the past 24 hours. This morning, approximately 6 hours ago, his mother decided to withhold his insulin because of continued nausea and vomiting.

Physical examination reveals a drowsy young man who can respond to questioning. His blood pressure is 90/70 mm Hg; pulse, 124 per minute; respirations, 30 per minute; and temperature, 38.3°C. His mucous membranes are dry and the ocular globes are soft and sunken, but the funduscopic findings are normal. Bowel sounds are absent and he has generalized abdominal tenderness without rebound. The deep tendon reflexes are hypoactive, but there are no localizing neurologic signs. The rest of the examination findings are normal.

Laboratory data consist of the following: Hgb, 16.4 g/dL; hematocrit (Hct), 53%; WBC, 16,942/mm^3 (93% polymorphonuclear leukocytes); BUN, 40 mg/dL; creatinine, 1.8 mg/dL; glucose, 847 mg/dL; serum ketones, strongly positive at 1:4 dilution; sodium, 126 mEq/L; potassium, 4.3 mEq/L; chloride, 100 mEq/L; and bicarbonate, 6 mEq/L. Urinalysis reveals a specific gravity of 1.030; glucose of 4+; acetone, strongly positive; and trace amounts of protein. Arterial blood gas analysis reveals a pH of 7.08, partial pressure of carbon dioxide (P_{CO_2}) of 12 mm Hg, and partial pressure of oxygen (P_{O_2}) of 80 mm Hg. An ECG shows sinus tachycardia with flat T waves. A chest radiographic study is normal. Abdominal radiographs show gastric distention, but otherwise the findings are normal.

1. What is the diagnosis and pathophysiologic process of this patient's disease?
2. How is the liver involved in the genesis of DKA?
3. What is the status of the patient's fluid and electrolyte levels?
4. What are the major goals of therapy?
5. What precipitated this episode of DKA?

Case Discussion

1. *What is the diagnosis and pathophysiologic process of this patient's disease?*

This patient has IDDM and is presenting with an episode of DKA. DKA is initiated by an absolute or relative insulin deficiency and an increase in the level of counterregulatory catabolic hormones, leading to the hepatic overproduction of glucose and ketone bodies. Consistent with this, the patient's laboratory data show the presence of marked hyperglycemia, ketonemia, ketonuria, and severe metabolic acidosis. The patient's tachypnea is also consistent with his acidotic state.

The destruction of pancreatic β cells, leading to type I diabetes, is thought to be mediated by the activation of autoimmune processes in genetically predisposed people. The presence of anti-islet and anti-insulin antibodies, the existence of inflammatory cells around the islet cells, and the temporary amelioration of new-onset type I diabetes by immunosuppressive therapy, all provide strong evidence for an autoimmune basis of pancreatic β-cell destruction.

2. *How is the liver involved in the genesis of DKA?*

Hepatic ketogenesis and the development of DKA depend on both the rate of substrate (FFA) supply to the liver and the activation of the hepatic ketogenic process, the latter being modulated by the relative increase in the glucagon-to-insulin ratio that prevails during DKA. The insulin deficiency leads to the activation of lipolysis and an increased supply of circulating FFA. In the liver, these molecules undergo successive β-oxidation to acetyl coenzyme A (CoA). During DKA, the unrestrained FFA mobilization and oxidation trigger the production of excess amounts of acetyl CoA, which undergo condensation to acetoacetyl CoA, a precursor of the ketone bodies acetoacetate, acetone, and β-hydroxybutyrate.

3. *What is the status of the patient's fluid and electrolyte levels?*

The patient's physical examination reveals signs of severe dehydration and intravascular hypovolemia (note his hypotension, tachycardia, and the dry mucous membranes). DKA, if not treated early, results in a severe total-body depletion of fluid (usually several liters) and electrolytes due to the following factors:

(1). The hyperglycemia and hyperketonemia lead to osmotic diuresis and the urinary loss of fluid and electrolytes.

(2). Because of acidosis, potassium is also shifted from the intracellular to extracellular fluid space and then lost during osmotic diuresis. Thus, the serum potassium levels may not accurately reflect the total-body deficiency.

(3). Vomiting, as in this patient, causes the further loss of fluid and electrolytes.

(4). Muscle catabolism (proteolysis), which results from the insulin deficiency, leads to the loss of potassium, phosphate, magnesium, and nitrogen.

4. *What are the major goals of therapy?*

The immediate therapeutic goals are (a) to replenish the fluid (starting with isotonic saline) and electrolytes; and (b) to provide adequate insulin to inhibit lipolysis (and thus ketogenesis) and normalize carbohydrate metabolism, both in the liver (by inhibiting glucose production) and in the peripheral tissues (by enhancing disposal of glucose and ketone bodies). During the fluid and electrolyte as well as insulin therapy, which is best administered in the form of a continuous IV infusion, the patient's blood glucose and electrolyte levels (especially potassium) should be monitored frequently and appropriate adjustments made. Additional therapeutic objectives include the identification and management of possible precipitating factors (e.g., infection, stress, and medication errors) and the implementation of measures to prevent the recurrence of DKA.

5. *What precipitated this episode of DKA?*

The immediate precipitating event of this patient's DKA is the withholding of insulin. An underlying stress or infection (e.g., gastroenteritis), which may also be present in this patient, should be evaluated and managed.

Case 2   A 63-year-old man is brought to the emergency room in an unconscious state. He was apparently in good health until 1 week before admission, when he experienced an insatiable thirst that he attempted to satisfy by drinking large quantities of beer and soda drinks. He had complained of having nocturia for several days, and yesterday had several bouts of diarrhea. He took to his bed yesterday and was found unconscious this morning. He takes no drugs, has not seen a physician for several years, and works regularly as a house painter. His previous health has been good. There is no significant family medical history.

Physical examination reveals a deeply unconscious, acutely ill man who has several focal right-sided seizures during examination. His skin and mucous membranes are dry and his ocular globes are quite soft. His blood pressure is 98/60 mm Hg, pulse is 120 per minute, and rectal temperature is 38°C, and he exhibits unlabored respirations at a rate of 13 per minute. Except for the findings of minimal hepatomegaly, absent knee jerks, and bilateral Babinski reflexes, the examination findings are otherwise normal.

Laboratory data consist of the following: Hgb, 16.2 g/dL; Hct, 51%; and WBC, 21,340/mm^3 (92% polymorphonuclear leukocytes). Urinalysis reveals a specific gravity of 1.030; pH, 6.0; glucose, 4+; acetone, moderate amounts; and protein, trace amounts. Arterial blood gas analysis reveals a pH of 7.41, P_{CO_2} of 35 mm Hg, and P_{O_2} of 68 mm Hg. Both chest radiographic and head CT scan findings are normal. His ECG shows sinus tachycardia with nonspecific ST-T–wave changes. Serum findings are BUN, 68 mg/dL; creatinine, 2.3 mg/dL; glucose, 1,420 mg/dL; ketones, trace amounts; sodium, 153 mEq/L; potassium, 4.6 mEq/L; chloride, 110 mEq/L; and bicarbonate, 26 mEq/L.

1. What is the diagnosis in this patient and how do you relate it to the major physical and laboratory findings?
2. What is the nature of this patient's endogenous insulin secretion, and is this type of diabetes hereditary?
3. Why did ketoacidosis not develop in this patient?
4. How is his liver involved in the pathogenesis of his hyperglycemia?
5. What are the major hormones that are counterregulatory to insulin action? Are they playing any role in this man's illness?
6. What would you predict about the state of his intravascular volume?
7. What are the major therapeutic goals in this patient?

Case Discussion

1. *What is the diagnosis in this patient and how do you relate it to the major physical and laboratory findings?*

   This elderly patient presents in a comatose state preceded by several days of progressive symptoms consisting of polyuria, polydipsia, and nocturia. His laboratory data show the presence of marked hyperglycemia but no acidosis. In this setting, his moderate ketonemia and ketonuria are most likely secondary to starvation. Thus, the diagnosis in this patient is HHNKC. His serum osmolality can be calculated using the formula: estimated osmolality = 2([Na] + [K]) + [glucose]/18 + [BUN]/2.8. For this patient, the estimated osmolality is calculated to be 418, which is consistent with a severe hyperosmolar state.

2. *What is the nature of this patient's endogenous insulin secretion, and is this type of diabetes hereditary?*

   This patient has type II diabetes or NIDDM. When NIDDM is of short duration, such as in this patient, and when patients are obese, the endogenous insulin levels are typically normal or elevated. In thin type II diabetic patients, especially in cases of prolonged duration, relative hypoinsulinemia may develop in response to meals or glucose challenge. Nevertheless, such patients are still able to maintain sufficient endogenous insulin secretion to prevent ketoacidosis from developing under basal conditions.

   Heredity plays an important role in the acquisition of NIDDM, although the mode of inheritance is largely unknown. NIDDM is also a heterogenous disorder, and different forms of genetic influences or defects may exist. Evidences for a genetic influence in the acquisition of NIDDM include (a) a strong family history of the disease in patients with NIDDM in the general population; (b) a very high prevalence of the disease in certain population groups (e.g., the Pima Indians and Micronesians of Nauru); (c) a concordance rate of 90% to 100% for NIDDM in monozygotic twins; (d) an apparent autosomal dominant mode of transmission of maturity-onset diabetes of the young, a form of NIDDM; and (e) the demonstration of multiple types of genetic mutations of the insulin receptor gene in certain patients with hyperinsulinemic insulin-resistant diabetic states. Such patients constitute a subset of NIDDM.

3. *Why did ketoacidosis not develop in this patient?*

   This patient has sufficient endogenous insulin to (a) prevent lipolysis (FFA levels are lower in the setting of HHNKC than of DKA), and (b) prevent full activation of the hepatic ketogenic system. In the presence of a reasonable level of endogenous insulin, the glucagon-to-insulin ratio is not high enough to lead to significant ketogenesis and ketoacidosis.

4. *How is his liver involved in the pathogenesis of his hyperglycemia?*

   The hyperglycemia in this patient results from the increased hepatic production of glucose due to increased glycogenolysis and gluconeogenesis, and from the decreased uptake and utilization of glucose by the liver, muscle, and adipose tissue. All of these changes are due to the underlying insulin resistance of NIDDM and the relative, but not absolute, insulin deficiency in the presence of acute stressful conditions.

5. *What are the major hormones that are counterregulatory to insulin action? Are they playing any role in this man's illness?*

Glucagon, cortisol, catecholamines, and growth hormone (GH) are the major insulin counterregulatory hormones that are elevated in major stressful conditions like HHNKC. Through the operation of several specific mechanisms, they counteract insulin's effects, and this worsens the hyperglycemic state.

6. *What would you predict about the state of his intravascular volume?*

The intravascular volume is severely depleted in this patient (note the related findings revealed by the physical examination). The following sequence of events may take place in patients with NIDDM if they are not adequately treated: hyperglycemia→osmotic diuresis→loss of fluid and electrolytes→dehydration→worsening hyperosmolarity and osmotic diuresis→hemoconcentration and hypovolemia→prerenal azotemia→circulatory insufficiency/shock/lactic acidosis→irreversible coma→death. Thus, if this patient's condition is not rapidly treated, irreversible coma and death may ensue.

7. *What are the major therapeutic goals in this patient?*

The major immediate therapeutic goals are (a) replacement of fluid and electrolytes; (b) correction of the hyperglycemia (relatively small doses of insulin are sufficient for patients in HHNKC compared with DKA); and (c) identification and management of the precipitating factors. HHNKC is a very serious medical emergency with a high risk of mortality unless an immediate, aggressive, and comprehensive management regimen is instituted. Once the acute situation is resolved, the patient's diabetes may be managed in the long term either with diet and oral agents or with insulin.

Suggested Readings

Bayraktar M, Van Thiel DH, Adalar N. A comparison of acarbose versus metformin as an adjuvant therapy in sulfonylurea-treated NIDDM patients. *Diabetes Care* 1996;19:252.

Bretzel RG, Voigt K, Schatz H. The United Kingdom Prospective Diabetes Study (UKPDS) implications for the pharmacotherapy of type 2 diabetes mellitus. *Exp Clin Endocrinol Diabetes* 1998;106:369.

Diabetes Control and Complications Trial Research Group. The effect of intensive treatment of diabetes on the development and progression of long-term complications in insulin dependent diabetes mellitus. *N Engl J Med* 1993;329:977.

Foster DW. Diabetes mellitus. In: Wilson JD, Braunwald E, Isselbacher KJ, et al, eds. *Harrison's principles of internal medicine*. New York: McGraw-Hill, 1991.

Melmed S, Jackson I, Kleinberg D, Klibanski A. Current treatment guidelines for acromegaly. *J Clin Endocrinol Metab* 1998;83:2646.

National Diabetes Data Group. Classification and diagnosis of diabetes mellitus and other categories of glucose intolerance. *Diabetes* 1979;28:1039.

Pickup JC, Williams G, eds. *Textbook of diabetes*, Vols 1 and 2. Oxford: Blackwell, 1991.

Shimon I, Melmed S. Management of pituitary tumors. *Ann Intern Med* 1998;129:472.

Swearingen B, Barker FG II, Katznelson L, et al. Long-term mortality after transsphenoidal surgery and adjunctive therapy for acromegaly. *J Clin Endocrinol Metab* 1998;83:3419.

Turner RC. The U.K. Prospective Diabetes Study: a review. *Diabetes Care* 1998;21:35.

UK Prospective Diabetes Study (UKPDS) Group. Effect of intensive blood-glucose control with metformin on complications in overweight patients with type 2 diabetes (UKPDS 34): UK Prospective Diabetes Study (UKPDS) Group. *Lancet* 1998;352:854.

UK Prospective Diabetes Study (UKPDS) Group. Intensive blood-glucose control with sulphonylureas or insulin compared with conventional treatment and risk of complications in patients with type 2 diabetes (UKPDS 33): UK Prospective Diabetes Study (UKPDS) Group. *Lancet* 1998;352:837.

Unger RH, Foster DW. Diabetes mellitus. In: Wilson JD, Foster DW, eds. *Williams textbook of endocrinology*. Philadelphia: WB Saunders, 1992.

Disorders of the Thyroid

1. What are the key features in a patient's history that are important in assessing for a possible functional thyroid disorder?
2. What are the important physical examination findings?
3. What laboratory data are used to confirm or refute the existence of a functional thyroid abnormality?

Discussion

1. *What are the key features in a patient's history that are important in assessing for a possible functional thyroid disorder?*

   When assessing a patient's history for clues to a functional thyroid disease, it is important to keep in mind that thyroid hormones in general control metabolism. Thus, in questioning patients about their medical history, it is important to ask specifically about elements related to metabolism. For example, in the setting of hyperthyroidism, weight loss, anxiety, tremor, palpitations, heat intolerance, hyperdefecation, insomnia, restlessness, and changes in the hair or skin are important features. In contrast, in patients with suspected hypothyroidism, look for clues that indicate decreased metabolic activity. These include weight gain, cold intolerance, constipation, dry, scaly skin, thick hair, depression, increased sleeping and fatigue, and generalized lethargy.

2. *What are the important physical examination findings?*

   Like the history, the physical examination should be performed to look for signs of hypermetabolism or hypometabolism. In the setting of hyperthyroidism, a fast pulse, tremor, sweating, thin, soft, and velvety hair, very brisk reflexes, and a hyperdynamic precordium are all features of increased metabolism. In addition, a very critical finding is an enlarged thyroid gland. If this is found in conjunction with a bruit, then the clinician can assume that the thyroid gland itself is overactive and overproducing thyroid hormone. In contrast, the findings characteristic of hypothyroidism include pale, sallow skin, thick hair, puffiness in the face and ankles, cool extremities, very delayed deep tendon relaxation, bradycardia, and a very quiet precordium. Again, an enlarged thyroid is an important physical examination finding. In this event, a firm, woody, or pebbly texture would indicate the presence of lymphocytic infiltration or Hashimoto's thyroiditis.

3. *What laboratory data are used to confirm or refute the existence of a functional thyroid abnormality?*

There is now a very sensitive and specific laboratory protocol to determine whether the patient has a functional thyroid disorder. The first diagnostic test should be measurement of the serum TSH level using the sensitive TSH assays. If this assay result proves to be within the normal range, then a functional abnormality of the thyroid has virtually been excluded. In contrast, an elevated TSH level means that the thyroid gland is failing and the patient has primary thyroid gland failure, most commonly due to autoimmune thyroid disease. Conversely, if the serum TSH level is low and undetectable, this indicates hyperthyroidism due to Graves' disease, a multinodular goiter, a hot nodule, excessive thyroid hormone ingestion, subacute thyroiditis, postpartum thyroiditis, or silent thyroiditis. If the TSH value proves to be in either the high or low range, the thyroid hormone status should be assessed. This can be done either by obtaining a total T_4 with a T_3 resin uptake (to assess T_4-binding globulin), or simply ordering a free T_4. Only in special circumstances is it necessary to test for total T_3 or free T_3 levels. Finally, in evaluating a patient with suspected hyperthyroidism, if both the TSH level is low and the free T_4 level is high, the next step is to perform a radioactive iodine uptake test and scan. This test is very important for distinguishing causes of hyperthyroidism related to overproduction (i.e., Graves' disease, a multinodular goiter, or a hot nodule) from those related to excessive release but not production (i.e., subacute thyroiditis, postpartum thyroiditis, or silent thyroiditis), as well as excessive thyroid hormone ingestion.

Case

A 31-year-old mother of two is seen because of complaints of headaches and amenorrhea, which has lasted for 3 months. She delivered her second child 10 months ago. The headaches developed after she was in a motor vehicle accident 4 months before. At that time, the patient experienced a temporary loss of consciousness but has since been normal; an extensive neurologic examination in the emergency room yielded negative findings. On further questioning, the patient also admits to a 15-pound (6.75-kg) weight loss despite a normal appetite, as well as mild heat intolerance and excessive sweating during the summer months. Recently she has noted that her hands shake and that her handwriting has become uneven. Of significance in her exercise history, she had been running 5 to 6 miles a day 5 days a week, and has participated in marathon running competitions. However, over the past 3 months, her tolerance for exercise has decreased and her running times have deteriorated. In questioning about her family history, it is found that her mother takes levothyroxine for hypothyroidism, a maternal grandmother has adult-onset diabetes mellitus, and her father has hyperlipidemia and coronary artery disease.

Physical examination reveals a well developed, well nourished, thin woman who appears somewhat anxious. Her blood pressure is 130/50 mm Hg and her pulse is 120 beats per minute. Her hair is fine with streaks of gray. Her eyes exhibit no exophthalmos, but there is a stare and lid lag. The extraocular muscles are normal. The thyroid is diffusely enlarged at approximately 40 g. There is a high-intensity bruit audible over the right lobe of the thyroid. The cardiac examination reveals a normal first and second heart sound and a grade I/VI systolic ejection murmur. The lungs are clear to auscultation and percussion. Abdominal examination findings are negative. Her hands exhibit an outstretched tremor and her skin is noted to be warm, smooth, and slightly moist. Her reflexes are symmetrically brisk. There is slight proximal muscle weakness detected in the thighs and shoulder girdle muscles.

1. What is the differential diagnosis in this patient, and should it include a normal pregnancy?
2. What is the most efficient approach to the laboratory evaluation in this patient?
3. To distinguish silent thyroiditis from Graves' hyperthyroidism, what is the most important diagnostic tool?
4. If the patient has silent thyroiditis, what is the appropriate therapy?
5. If the patient has Graves' disease and is treated with radioactive iodine, what is likely to occur?
6. If the patient is treated with antithyroid drugs, what is the likely short- and long-term prognosis?

Case Discussion

1. *What is the differential diagnosis in this patient, and should it include a normal pregnancy?*

   A normal pregnancy can mimic many of the symptoms of hyperthyroidism, including increased energy, anxiety, heat intolerance, sweating, and, in areas of the world where iodine deficiency is common, a mild increase in the thyroid gland size. In addition, pregnancy can certainly decrease the tolerance for maximal exercise. Features that are not characteristic of pregnancy are the moderate (40 g) thyroid enlargement, the lid lag and stare, and, most important, the bruit over the right side of the thyroid gland. A bruit in the thyroid gland reflects the presence of increased blood flow due to hyperplasia and excessive thyroid gland function. These features are absent in pregnancy, and thus a bruit would not be heard. However, previously silent thyroid disease may become apparent during pregnancy. In addition, a 15-pound (6.75-kg) weight loss, despite a normal appetite, would be distinctly unusual in the pregnant state. Thus, a normal pregnancy is an unlikely cause of this patient's symptoms. The differential diagnosis therefore consists of hyperthyroidism due to Graves' disease, a multinodular goiter, and silent thyroiditis. A multinodular goiter is unusual in a 31-year-old patient, and is usually seen in the older population. Furthermore, multinodular goiters are not associated with a bruit, even when producing hyperthyroidism. The diffuse enlargement of the thyroid gland at 40 g is also unusual in the setting of a multinodular goiter because, in this event, multiple nodules should be appreciated on the physical examination. A stare and lid lag can be found in patients with hyperthyroidism due to a multinodular goiter because these findings reflect the hyperthyroidism, not the autoimmune process.

The important differential diagnostic exercise to perform in this case should focus on whether the hyperthyroidism is due to Graves' disease or silent thyroiditis. Graves' disease is the most common cause of hyperthyroidism and is found more frequently in women than in men, with a ratio of 4 to 1. In addition, hyperthyroidism due to Graves' disease usually afflicts younger people between 20 and 50 years of age. The 15-pound (6.75-kg) weight loss, heat intolerance, excessive sweating, tremor, decreased exercise tolerance, moderate enlargement of the thyroid with a bruit, and the warm, smooth, and slightly moist skin are all characteristic of hyperthyroidism due to Graves' disease. In addition, the patient has a family history of autoimmune disease, in that the mother is being treated for hypothyroidism and the grandmother has adult-onset diabetes mellitus. In addition, the patient appears to have premature gray hair. The absence of exophthalmos does not conflict with this diagnosis because this finding may be clinically evident in only 10% to 20% of patients with Graves' hyperthyroidism. (However, when more sophisticated techniques for evaluating eye function are used, as many as 80% to 90% of the patients with Graves' hyperthyroidism prove to have discernible eye abnormalities.)

Hyperthyroidism due to silent thyroiditis is becoming an increasingly well recognized diagnostic entity. The exact etiology of this disorder is obscure, but appears to be an autoimmune process. Silent thyroiditis is perhaps identical to postpartum thyroiditis, which arises after 5% to 8% of all pregnancies in the United States. This disorder usually appears between 2 and 6 months postpartum (10 months is slightly excessive). The patient exhibits the signs and symptoms of hyperthyroidism and an enlarged thyroid gland, but has no evidence of exophthalmos or pretibial myxedema. Unlike subacute thyroiditis, the thyroid is not painful and her condition is not temporally associated with a viral infection. In the setting of subacute thyroiditis, the erythrocyte sedimentation rate is elevated, which reflects the existence of a presumed viral infection; in the presence of silent or postpartum thyroiditis, the sedimentation rate is normal. It is critical to distinguish hyperthyroidism due to Graves' disease from hyperthyroidism due to silent thyroiditis because the treatments of the two disorders are quite different. Because amenorrhea can occur in all forms of hyperthyroidism, it is not a helpful clue for identifying the ultimate cause of the hyperthyroidism. Finally, the bruit over the right lobe of the thyroid is an important clue that points toward a diagnosis of Graves' disease in this patient. A bruit over the thyroid gland should not be present in hyperthyroidism due to a multinodular goiter, silent thyroiditis, or subacute thyroiditis. Thus, based on the patient's history, physical examination findings, and statistical considerations, the most likely diagnosis is hyperthyroidism due to Graves' disease. However, formal laboratory studies should be done first to determine whether hyperthyroidism is indeed present and then to identify the cause of the hyperthyroidism.

2. *Which is the most efficient approach to the laboratory evaluation in this patient?*

The key issue in deciding on the nature of the laboratory evaluation is which test best determines whether hyperthyroidism is indeed present. Total T_4 and T_3 resin uptake were traditionally regarded as the best tests for establishing the presence of hyperthyroidism and for distinguishing hyperthyroidism from a normal pregnancy. In all forms of hyperthyroidism, both the total T_4 and T_3 resin uptake are elevated, whereas in pregnancy, the total T_4 is elevated because of an increase in the T_4-binding globulin level, and the T_3 resin uptake is reduced, again because of the increased T_4-binding globulin level. However, these same abnormalities in thyroid function can occur in the absence of pregnancy, such as in a patient taking birth control pills, in an older woman taking replacement estrogen, or in a woman with congenital X-linked T_4-binding globulin excess. Furthermore, confusion can arise when both hyperthyroidism and excessive estrogens coexist because the T_4 concentration can be elevated and the T_3 resin uptake may be variable (low, normal, or high values) in this setting. The total T_3 is a good test for hyperthyroidism but, because T_3 is also bound to T_4-binding globulin, its levels are elevated in the context of a normal pregnancy. Thus, it cannot be used to discriminate hyperthyroidism from pregnancy. The most efficient laboratory tests in this case are determinations of the free T_4 and TSH levels. The free T_4 level is elevated in hyperthyroidism but normal in pregnancy. Likewise, the TSH level is suppressed and undetectable in the setting of hyperthyroidism but normal in pregnancy. Thus, this laboratory profile is ideal for discriminating between hyperthyroidism and pregnancy. However, the free T_4 and TSH levels cannot discriminate between hyperthyroidism due to Graves' disease, a multinodular goiter, or silent thyroiditis.

3. *To distinguish silent thyroiditis from Graves' hyperthyroidism, what is the most important diagnostic tool?*

The most important diagnostic tool for distinguishing silent thyroiditis from Graves' disease is a radioactive iodine uptake test. Graves' disease, which is a state of thyroid hormone overproduction, involves an excessive uptake of iodine into the thyroid gland and thus a high radioactive iodine uptake. In contrast, silent thyroiditis is not an overproduction state but a state in which there is an excessive release of thyroid hormone into the circulation that suppresses TSH, stemming from autoimmune damage to thyroid follicular cells. These events render the thyroid gland incapable of taking up iodine. Thus, in the setting of silent thyroiditis, the radioactive iodine uptake is very low, in striking contrast to the elevated values found in patients with Graves' hyperthyroidism.

4. *If the patient has silent thyroiditis, what is the appropriate therapy?*

Distinguishing silent thyroiditis from Graves' disease is important because the therapy for the two conditions is dramatically different. Because silent thyroiditis is a destructive process without overproduction, it does not respond to either antithyroid drugs or radioactive iodine. The low radioactive iodine uptake in silent thyroiditis renders radioactive iodine therapy ineffective, and the lack of overproduction of thyroid hormones negates the effectiveness of antithyroid drugs. Because silent thyroiditis is a self-limited process with a triphasic course, the recommended therapy is the judicious use of β blockers to control symptoms, particularly tremor and tachycardia, and observation of the patient during the spontaneous resolution of the process. Typically, the hyperthyroid phase lasts for 1 to 3 months, after which the process is dramatically reversed; in fact, hypothyroidism can occur transiently for another 1 to 3 months. During the hypothyroid phase, many patients benefit from a short course of thyroid hormone replacement. However, in most cases, both the hyperthyroidism and hypothyroidism resolve spontaneously and normal thyroid function is restored. In only 10% to 25% of cases does permanent hypothyroidism eventuate. Perhaps the most important clinical clue to the resolution of silent thyroiditis is normalization of the thyroid gland size. Because silent thyroiditis is a self-limited process that resolves spontaneously, thyroid surgery usually is unnecessary. However, this option can be reserved for particularly severe cases that have protracted or recurrent courses.

5. *If the patient has Graves' disease and is treated with radioactive iodine, what is likely to occur?*

The most common therapy for Graves' disease in the United States is radioactive iodine, which is given in the form of a small capsule containing 5 to 10 mCi of iodine-131. The radioactive iodine is quickly absorbed from the gastrointestinal tract into the bloodstream and then incorporated into the thyroid gland, where it induces radioactive damage and kills thyroid cells. Radioactive iodine, which does not enter the thyroid gland, is quickly excreted through the kidneys into the urine. Because radioactive iodine induces damage and the eventual death of thyroid follicular cells, the chance of hypothyroidism developing is very high. In general, hypothyroidism develops in the first year in 50% to 60% of the patients treated; thereafter, the rate of development of hypothyroidism is 1% to 3% per year. Thus, hypothyroidism will develop in most patients treated with radioactive iodine and they will require lifelong thyroid hormone replacement therapy.

6. *If the patient is treated with antithyroid drugs, what is the likely short- and long-term prognosis?*

Antithyroid drugs (propylthiouracil and methimazole) are derivatives of thiourea and their mechanism of action is to inhibit both thyroid hormone synthesis and, in the case of propylthiouracil, the peripheral conversion of T_4 to T_3. These drugs are an ideal choice of therapy for patients with hyperthyroidism due to Graves' disease. They are most commonly used in children and pregnant patients, and in relatively mild cases of hyperthyroidism in which the thyroid gland is only moderately enlarged. Propylthiouracil is given in a dose of approximately 100 mg three or four times a day. Methimazole (Tapazole; Eli Lilly, Indianapolis, IN) has a slightly longer half-life than propylthiouracil and may be given in a single daily dose of 10 to 30 mg each day. Both agents exhibit a similar profile of side effects, which occur in 1% to 3% of the patients. The most common side effects are skin rash, urticaria, arthralgias, fever, and transient leukopenia. Minor gastrointestinal side effects and arthritis occur occasionally. The major rare side effect is agranulocytosis, which occurs in 0.2% to 0.5% of the patients. Other rare side effects include aplastic anemia, hepatitis, thrombocytopenia, vasculitis, and cholestatic jaundice. The side effects usually arise early in the course of therapy and, in the case of methimazole, the reactions appear to be dose dependent.

The antithyroid drugs usually are given for a 1- to 2-year period in hopes of inducing permanent remission. The frequency with which permanent remission takes place has been analyzed in many studies and has been found to tend to occur in those patients who have mild disease and smaller thyroid glands. However, when all patients are considered, the chance for permanent remission is only between 20% to 40%. Thus, 60% to 80% of patients have a relapse of their hyperthyroidism, usually within 2 years of discontinuing the antithyroid drug. In cases of relapse, the antithyroid drug can either be reinstituted or a more definitive ablative form of therapy, such as radioactive iodine, can be carried out.

Growth Hormone-Secreting Pituitary Tumors

1. What are the clinical symptoms of GH excess (i.e., acromegaly)?
2. What are the physical signs of acromegaly?
3. What is the best screening test to exclude the diagnosis of acromegaly?
4. What laboratory tests can confirm the diagnosis of acromegaly and assess other pituitary hormone functions?
5. What imaging studies are necessary?
6. What is the treatment of choice and what are the alternatives?

Discussion

1. *What are the clinical symptoms of GH excess (i.e., acromegaly)?*

   Acromegaly is the clinical syndrome resulting from excessive GH production and is usually due to a pituitary tumor. The symptoms and signs are gradual in onset, which often causes diagnosis to be delayed for 6 to 8 years. The classic symptoms consist of headache, visual disturbances (due to an enlarging tumor compressing on the optic nerves), enlargement in glove and shoe size, excessive sweating, arthralgias, loss of libido, impotence in men, amenorrhea in women, muscle weakness, and problems with an underbite or spaces between the teeth.

2. *What are the physical signs of acromegaly?*

   The physical signs of acromegaly include coarsening of the physical features (which can be determined by looking at old photographs); frontal bossing; thick, coarse skin; doughy, sweaty palms; prognathism (an enlarged mandible); widely spaced teeth and underbite; severe osteoarthritis; prominent lips, tongue, and nose; acanthosis nigricans; skin tags; enlargement of all organs; entrapment of peripheral nerves (i.e., carpal tunnel); hypertension with cardiomyopathy; visual field abnormalities; glucose intolerance; and diabetes.

3. *What is the best screening test to exclude the diagnosis of acromegaly?*

   The best screening test for acromegaly is measurement of the insulin-like growth factor I (IGF-1; somatomedin C) level. This is a liver protein induced by GH and the test constitutes an integrated assessment of GH action. GH levels are pulsatile in nature: fasting levels are usually less than 10 ng/mL in adults and the GH concentration increases at night during sleep. The levels in patients with acromegaly can range from 5 to 10 ng/mL, so the GH level is helpful if very high, but less specific if not severely elevated.

4. *What laboratory tests can confirm the diagnosis of acromegaly and assess other pituitary hormone functions?*

   To confirm the diagnosis and assess the pituitary function in a patient, the GH response to an oral glucose load is tested. To perform it, 100 gm oral glucose is given to the fasting patient and blood for GH determination is obtained at 0, 30, 60, 90, and 120 minutes. In a normal response to a glucose load, the GH levels are suppressed to less than 2 ng/mL. In patients with acromegaly, the GH levels are either not suppressed or paradoxically increase (approximately 30% of patients). This test, if done in conjunction with a somatomedin C test, is the best way of assessing cure after surgery. In addition, approximately 30% of the patients show an increase in their GH levels after a thyrotropin-releasing hormone (500 μg) IV push; normal patients do not. This test is more often used in a research setting or for the purpose of assessing tumor recurrence.

   Other blood tests for determining pituitary function include measurement of the prolactin level, which can be elevated because of the interruption of dopamine tone secondary to stalk compression or the cosecretion of prolactin by the tumor. The follicle-stimulating hormone (FSH), luteinizing hormone (LH), and testosterone or estrogen levels are used to assess the status of the reproductive axis. The thyroid status is checked by a free T_4; measurement of the TSH level is not helpful because, if there is thyroid deficiency, it is secondary to thyrotropin deficiency. The adrenal axis is assessed with a morning cortisol determination; if less than 5 mg/dL, a formal Cortrosyn (cosyntropin; Organon Teknika, Durham, NC) stimulation test of the ACTH reserve should be performed. Blood is drawn at 0, 30, and 60 minutes after one ampule (0.25 mg) IV push of synthetic ACTH. In normal subjects, the cortisol levels increase to 18 or more and are often double the baseline value. An α subunit level may be helpful as a tumor marker because some GH tumors cosecrete other pituitary hormones.

5. *What imaging studies are necessary?*

   The imaging procedure of choice is an MRI scan of the pituitary. It provides the greatest detail of the tumor's extent and landmarks for the surgeon's use during surgical removal. A coronal CT scan with fine cuts can detect most large tumors, but a lateral skull film is not sensitive. Formal visual field testing should be done in all patients with macroadenomas to serve as a baseline for assessing postoperative improvement.

6. *What is the treatment of choice and what are the alternatives?*

The treatment of choice for these tumors, which are usually macroadenomas (>1 cm), is transsphenoidal resection of the tumor, although surgical cure is often difficult. If postoperative hormonal testing reveals continued abnormal GH production, radiation therapy is often necessary. Medical therapy with bromocriptine (if the tumor costains for prolactin) may also reduce the GH levels and tumor size, while the results of irradiation are awaited. Somatostatin analogues can inhibit GH production, but they are short acting, and thus frequent subcutaneous injections are required. Reports describe symptomatic responses but only modest tumor reduction in response to these drugs. In 1999, the U.S. Food and Drug Administration (FDA) has released a once-monthly somatostatin analogue that appears to have similar efficacy to the short-acting agent.

Case

A 40-year-old man is seen because of headaches, muscle aches, and chronic low back and joint pain. As he enters the office, you notice his coarse facial features, frontal bossing, and large jaw. When you shake his hand, you find he has large, doughy, sweaty palms and, when he smiles, you note his teeth are widely spaced.

He has not seen a physician in 10 years and is taking no medications. His back and joint pain have been worsening for 6 years, but his headaches started 6 months ago.

His physical examination findings are significant for a blood pressure of 150/100 mm Hg, pulse of 60 per minute, and respiratory rate of 12 per minute.

He returns in 2 weeks with old photographs that confirm a change in his physical appearance over time, and the laboratory test results confirm your clinical impression.

1. What is your initial diagnosis in this patient?
2. Besides the back and joint pain and the headaches, what other symptoms would you look for to confirm or refute your diagnosis?
3. Besides the physical features you observe initially, what other abnormalities would you look for on physical examination?
4. What laboratory tests should be performed initially?
5. What additional testing should be performed once the initial laboratory results are known?
6. What is the preferred treatment in this patient?

Case Discussion

1. *What is your initial diagnosis in this patient?*

Acromegaly should be your initial diagnosis.

2. *Besides the back and joint pain and the headaches, what other symptoms would you look for to confirm or refute your diagnosis?*

Other symptoms to look for in this patient include a change in glove and shoe sizes, spaces between the teeth and an underbite, decreased libido and impotence, sweating, polyuria, polydipsia, and a change in vision.

3. *Besides the physical features you observe initially, what other abnormalities would you look for on physical examination?*

Other physical features to look for in this patient include thick, coarse skin, skin tags, enlarged extremities and organs, entrapment neuropathies, visual field abnormalities, and decreased body hair and testicular size. Old pictures would confirm the clinical suspicion.

4. *What laboratory tests should be performed initially?*

Initial laboratory tests in this patient would consist of the measurement of somatomedin C and fasting GH levels. If the levels are elevated, this would suggest the diagnosis of acromegaly, which would be confirmed if the GH levels did not suppress to less than 2 ng/mL in response to a glucose load.

5. *What additional testing should be performed once the initial laboratory results are known?*

If the initial laboratory results indicate acromegaly, a fasting blood sugar test should be performed to rule out diabetes. Pituitary tests should include measurement of the prolactin, FSH, LH, testosterone, and α-subunit levels. An MRI scan can show the extent of the tumor, and formal visual field testing should be performed.

6. *What is the preferred treatment in this patient?*

The preferred initial treatment is surgical removal of the tumor. Bromocriptine or a somatostatin (octreotide) analogue may be useful as medical adjuncts. Radiation therapy is indicated for the destruction of residual tumor if reoperation or surgical cure is not feasible. Postoperative hormonal testing is indicated to reassess pituitary function.

Prolactin-Secreting Pituitary Tumors

1. What symptoms and signs are associated with an elevated prolactin level in women and in men?

2. What is the underlying pathophysiologic process responsible for the effects of elevated prolactin levels?

3. What are the causes of an elevated prolactin level other than a pituitary tumor?

4. What testing is necessary to confirm or refute a diagnosis of a prolactinoma?

5. What are the treatment options for a prolactinoma?

Discussion

1. *What symptoms and signs are associated with an elevated prolactin level in women and in men?*

In women, an elevated prolactin level is associated with disturbance of the menstrual cycle ranging from the occurrence of short cycles with an inadequate luteal phase, oligoovulation, and infertility, to amenorrhea. Galactorrhea, hirsutism, mood disturbances, and headaches are also frequent complaints. In men, symptoms include decreased libido, impotence, and infertility. Galactorrhea is a rare finding. Visual field defects are seen in the setting of large tumors. Osteopenia and fractures can occur in both sexes and are due to the hypogonadism involved.

2. *What is the underlying pathophysiologic process responsible for the effects of elevated prolactin levels?*

   Prolactin is under tonic inhibitory control from dopamine in the hypothalamus. Stalk compression, which causes dopamine tone to be inhibited, or prolactin secretion from a tumor inhibits the hypothalamic–pituitary–gonadal axis at all three levels. The major effect, however, is to terminate the gonadotropin-releasing hormone–induced pulsatile release of the pituitary gonadotropins, LH and FSH. This disordered gonadotropin secretion then results in inadequate gametogenesis and steroidogenesis, and hence hypogonadism with or without infertility. For galactorrhea to occur, there must be estrogen priming of the breast in addition to an elevated prolactin level, which is why milk production does not develop in most men unless their prolactin level is chronically very elevated with suppression of testosterone release, elevation of the estradiol level, and gynecomastia.

3. *What are the causes of an elevated prolactin level other than a pituitary tumor?*

   Elevated prolactin levels may be due to physiologic causes such as pregnancy, stress, sleep, exercise, or frequent breast stimulation. Systemic disorders associated with elevated prolactin levels include hypothyroidism, hypoadrenalism, chronic renal failure (elevated production and decreased clearance), and liver failure. Drugs that elevate the prolactin level include phenothiazides, tricyclic antidepressants, opiates, metoclopramide, cimetidine, methyldopa, reserpine, and amphetamines, all of which interfere with dopamine inhibitory tone.

4. *What testing is necessary to confirm or refute a diagnosis of a prolactinoma?*

   A prolactin level of over 100 ng/mL suggests the presence of a tumor, although tumors or other causes can be associated with lower elevations. No stimulation or suppression test is needed. An MRI scan of the pituitary is necessary to detect a microadenoma and exclude a large pituitary or hypothalamic mass that is causing stalk compression.

5. *What are the treatment options for a prolactinoma?*

   The treatment of choice for prolactinomas is the dopamine agonist, bromocriptine. It effectively lowers prolactin levels and reduces tumor size. Surgical removal is reserved for noncompliant or bromocriptine-intolerant patients because of the high recurrence rate of 20% to 50% at 5 years. Major side effects of bromocriptine therapy include orthostatic dizziness, dry mouth, nausea, and vomiting, although these may be minimized by slow titration of the drug along with food intake at night. Lifelong therapy is probably necessary. Lack of treatment leads to prolonged gonadal steroid deficiency and the risk of osteopenia and fracture. The premature cardiovascular risk has not been assessed.

Case   A 28-year-old woman is seen because of irregular periods and infertility. Her menarche occurred at 12 years of age and she had regular periods with moliminal symptoms (breast tenderness, bloating, and cramping) until approximately 2 years ago. After that, her periods have become lighter and irregular without moliminal symptoms. She has decreased libido, occasional headaches, and is moody and irritable. She has noted a milky discharge from both nipples. She took birth control pills for 2 years, 5 years ago.

Her examination is significant for the following findings: normal visual fields, galactorrhea, and a decreased estrogen effect on the vaginal mucosa.

1. What is the most likely diagnosis in this patient?
2. What other historical facts are important to elicit in an effort to determine the cause of her symptoms?
3. What laboratory tests or studies would you have done?
4. What is the treatment of choice in this patient?

Case Discussion

1. *What is the most likely diagnosis in this patient?*

   The most likely diagnosis in this patient is hyperprolactinemia.
2. *What other historical facts are important to elicit in an effort to determine the cause of her symptoms?*

   It is important to find out whether she might be pregnant and whether she takes drugs that would inhibit dopamine tone. In addition, a history of hypothyroidism, hypoadrenalism, excessive breast stimulation, and renal or liver disease should be sought.
3. *What laboratory tests or studies would you have done?*

   A serum prolactin level should be measured to determine the extent of the elevation. In addition, liver function studies and determination of the BUN and creatinine levels should be done to rule out liver or kidney disease. The human chorionic gonadotropin level should be measured to rule out pregnancy, as well as the TSH and cortisol levels, if there are symptoms or signs of hypothyroidism or hypoadrenalism. An MRI scan should be obtained to distinguish between a microadenoma and a macroadenoma.
4. *What is the treatment of choice in this patient?*

   The treatment of choice is the dopamine agonist bromocriptine. Treatment is begun at night with the intake of food to decrease the side effects of postural hypotension, nausea, and dry mouth. The goal is to normalize the prolactin levels. Other long-acting dopamine agonists are available if patients fail to tolerate bromocriptine, such as cabergoline, pergolide, and dihydroergotoxine.

Hypercalcemia

1. What conditions can cause hypercalcemia?
2. What two medical conditions account for most cases of hypercalcemia?
3. In the hypercalcemic patient, what are the laboratory findings seen in the setting of hyperparathyroidism?
4. What is the treatment for hypercalcemia?
5. What are the indications for parathyroidectomy?

Discussion

1. *What conditions can cause hypercalcemia?*

   The causes of hypercalcemia that need to be considered in any patient who exhibits a bona fide elevation in their serum calcium level as documented on at least three repeat determinations are listed in Table 3-1.

2. *What two medical conditions account for most cases of hypercalcemia?*

   Of the many causes of hypercalcemia listed in Table 3-1, the most common are malignancy (45%) and hyperparathyroidism (45%). The lengthy differen-

Table 3-1. Causes of Hypercalcemia

Primary Hyperparathyroidism
  Sporadic (90%–95% of all cases of hyperparathyroidism)
  Familial syndromes (MEN I and MEN II)
    MEN I (tumors of pituitary, pancreas, and parathyroid)
    MEN IIA (medullary thyroid carcinoma, hyperparathyroidism, pheochromocytoma)
    MEN IIB (medullary thyroid carcinoma, pheochromocytoma, mucosal neuromas, marfanoid habitus, and parathyroid hyperplasia)
Neoplastic Diseases
  Local osteolysis (breast and lung carcinoma metastatic to bone, and myeloma)
  Humoral hypercalcemia of malignancy
Endocrine Disorders
  Hyperthyroidism
  Adrenal insufficiency
  Benign familial hypocalciuric hypercalcemia
Medications
  Thiazide diuretics
  Vitamin D and rarely vitamin A intoxication
  Milk-alkali syndrome
  Lithium
Granulomatous Diseases
  Sarcoidosis
  Berylliosis, tuberculosis, coccidioidomycosis, histoplasmosis
Miscellaneous
  Immobilization (associated with high bone turnover rates such as in children or in patients with Paget's disease)
  Recovery phase of acute and renal failure (rare)
  Idiopathic hypercalcemia of infancy (rare)
  Dehydration (due to hemoconcentration)

MEN, multiple endocrine neoplasia.

Table 3-2. Parathyroid Hormone Action on Kidney

Action	Manifestation
Increases tubular resorption of calcium	Hypercalcemia, mild hypercalciuria
Inhibits proximal tubule bicarbonate resorption	Type II renal tubular acidosis, hyperchloremic metabolic acidosis
Increases phosphate clearance (decreases tubular resorption of PO_4)	Phosphaturia, decreased $[PO_4]$ (increased $Cl/PO_4 > 33$)
Stimulates renal cAMP	Increased nephrogenous cAMP
Increases 1α-hydroxylase activity for 1,25-dihydroxyvitamin D synthesis	Increased levels of 1,25-dihydroxyvitamin D
Aminoaciduria	Aminoaciduria
Activates renal tubular enzymes (alkaline phosphatase, glucose-6-phosphate dehydrogenase), promotes renal gluconeogenesis	Increased renal glucose production

PO_4, phosphate radical; $[PO_4]$, PO_4 concentration; cAMP, cyclic adenosine monophosphate.

tial diagnosis (see Table 3-1) includes the other 10% of the causes. Hence, from a practical standpoint, hypercalcemic disorders can be broken down into two categories: parathyroid hormone (PTH)-mediated and non–PTH-mediated hypercalcemia.

3. *In the hypercalcemic patient, what are the laboratory findings seen in the setting of hyperparathyroidism?*

    For the sake of simplicity, the many causes of hypercalcemia can be separated into two categories according to the PTH actions involved (Tables 3-2 and 3-3).

4. *What is the treatment for hypercalcemia?*

    A hypercalcemic emergency is diagnosed when the calcium level exceeds 14 mg/dL or the patient exhibits symptoms of hypercalcemia, consisting of profound weakness, impaired mental function, nausea and vomiting, and central nervous system depression leading to stupor, lethargy, or coma. Urgent treatment of the hypercalcemia is mandatory in these situations (Table 3-4).

Table 3-3. Causes of Hypercalcemia

Variables	PTH-mediated	Non–PTH-mediated
Phosphate	Low (<2.2 mg/dL)	$\downarrow$, normal, or $\uparrow$
Chloride	High (>104 mEq/dL)	Usually <100 mEq/dL
Metabolic acidosis	Mild	Not present
Cl/PO_4	>33	<33
PTH	High	Low
Hyperparathyroidism[a]	Neoplasia with or without humoral hypercalcemia of malignancy Other non–PTH-mediated causes (see Table 3-1)	

[a]Remember to exclude benign familial hypocalciuric hypercalcemia.
PTH, parathyroid hormone; PO_4, phosphate radical.

Table 3-4. Therapy of Hypercalcemia

Urgent Therapy
1. Saline
   a. Usually safe with 200–300 mL/hr but may need over 10 L/day with careful monitoring. Use NS:D$_5$W alternate in 4:1 ratio with 20 mEq KCl/bottle (can follow urinary K$^+$, Na$^+$, and volume to document losses)
   b. May need 15 mg magnesium/hr
2. Saline plus furosemide
   a. With aggressive management, 80–100 mg furosemide IV q1–2h and replace urinary electrolytes (*N Engl J Med* 1970;283:836)
   b. Less urgent management—40 mg furosemide q4–6h
   c. Before using furosemide, be sure patient is adequately hydrated
3. Calcitonin: 4–8 IU/kg subcutaneously q6–12h
4. Calcitonin plus glucocorticoids
   a. 4–8 MRC units/kg q6–12h
   b. Prednisone: 40–60 mg/d
5. IV diphosphonates
   a. IV etidronate: 7.5 mg/kg, with 3 L of saline given over 24 hr and repeat daily for 3 d
   b. IV APD (Aredia): 60–90 mg as single 24-hr infusion with adequate saline hydration; allow a minimum of 7 days to elapse before retreatment
6. Gallium nitrate (avoid use if creatinine >2.5 mg/dL): 100–200 mg/m^2 of body surface area in 1,000 mL NS over 24 hr daily for 5 d
7. IV phosphate
   a. Given as 1,000 mg of elemental phosphate (0.16 mg/kg) over 8–12 hr during each 24-hr period (caution: can cause hypotension)
   b. Avoid use if serum phosphate elevated
8. Dialysis
9. IV EDTA
   a. Avoid use because of formation of insoluble calcium compounds that damage kidney

Long-Term Therapy (Adjunct Therapy in Addition to Treatment of Primary Cause)
1. Mobilization
2. Oral phosphates
   a. 1,000–2,000 mg of elemental phosphate (K-Phos; 3 tablets three times daily)
   b. Avoid use if elevated serum phosphate
3. Mithramycin (may also be used in semiacute situations): 25 μg/kg in 50 mL D$_5$W given as infusion over 3 hr
4. Glucocorticoids—prednisone: 50–60 mg/d
5. Diphosphonates—oral etidronate: 5–20 mg/kg/d

NS, normal saline; D$_5$W, 5% dextrose in water; IV, intravenous; EDTA, ethylenediaminetetraacetate.

5. *What are the indications for parathyroidectomy?*

The following indications for parathyroidectomy in hyperparathyroid patients have been proposed by a National Institutes of Health (NIH) consensus conference:

(1). Patient younger than 50 years of age

(2). Elevated serum calcium to a concentration of 1.0 to 1.6 mg/dL above normal laboratory values

(3). History of a life-threatening hypercalcemic episode

(4). Reduced creatinine clearance

(5). Presence of kidney stones

(6). Urine calcium excretion of greater than 400 mg per 24 hours

(7). Bone mass reduced by more than 2 standard deviations below normal

Case   A 47-year-old white male computer consultant is seen in the walk-in clinic complaining of severe right hip pain and difficulty walking. He has been taking ibuprofen for pain relief. The pain in his right hip and right proximal lower extremity has been present for approximately 4 months, and has progressed to become a sharp, localized right hip joint pain during the past month. The patient has noted a 10-pound (4.5-kg) weight loss over the preceding 2 months, but ascribes this to a self-enforced diet. He has nocturia with two to five micturitions per night, and complains of excessive thirst. In addition, he is aware of a decrease in his ability to concentrate over the preceding several months.

His past medical history is significant for nephrolithiasis requiring hospitalization 10 years earlier, and an upper gastrointestinal hemorrhage 5 years ago, secondary to peptic ulcer disease. His family history is noncontributory.

Radiographic studies of the patient's pelvis and right hip show a lytic lesion in the right sacrum and femoral acetabulum. The patient is admitted for further evaluation.

Physical examination reveals a pleasant, middle-aged man who is experiencing considerable pain in his right hip. His blood pressure is 160/98 mm Hg; pulse, 96 beats per minute; respiratory rate, 20 per minute; and temperature, 97.8°F (36.8°C). No significant skin lesions are found. On examination of the oral pharynx, a white mass on the hard palate is noted. The patient has no cervical, axillary, or inguinal adenopathy. Thyroid examination reveals a fullness in the left lower lobe. Range-of-motion exercises of the right lower extremity elicit severe right hip tenderness. A neurologic examination reveals diminished strength in the right hip flexors and extenders with normal deep tendon reflexes throughout. The patient's mental status is appropriate.

Initial laboratory data reveal the following: WBC, 5,800; Hgb, 13.3 g/dL; Hct, 39.7%; and platelet count, $274 \times 10^3/mm^3$. The following electrolyte and serum chemistry values are reported: sodium, 138 mEq/L; potassium, 3.9 mEq/L; chloride, 108 mEq/L; CO_2, 21.5 mEq/L; BUN, 18 mg/dL; creatinine, 1.0 mg/dL; and fasting glucose, 94 mg/dL. Other significant laboratory values include the following: calcium, 11.5 mg/dL; phosphate, 2.0 mg/dL; total protein, 6.8 g/dL; albumin, 2.8 g/dL; and magnesium, 1.7 mEq/L. Urinalysis findings are normal. The erythrocyte sedimentation rate is 9 mm per hour and the alkaline phosphatase level is 396 IU/L.

Chest film findings are normal. In a review of the pelvis and hip radiographic studies, lytic changes with bony destruction are found in both hemipelves, but these are greater on the right. Right femoral head involvement is also noted.

A pelvic CT scan shows the existence of multiple destructive soft tissue lesions in the bone of the pelvis; the largest of the lesions measures 8 cm. A radionuclide bone scan reveals increased uptake in the pelvic lesions and in several ribs, as well. A large-bore needle biopsy specimen from the gingivopalatal mass and the right ilium shows the appearance of a giant cell tumor mixed with fibroblasts.

Special endocrine studies reveal an ionized calcium level of 2.7 mmol/L (normal, 1.15 to 1.35 mmol/L). The 24-hour urine calcium and phosphate excretions are 290 and 856 mg, respectively.

1. Given the patient's hypoalbuminemia of 2.8 g/dL, what is the corrected calcium level?
2. What is the explanation for the patient's polyuria and polydipsia?
3. Based solely on the patient's admission electrolyte levels, what is the likely diagnosis?
4. What is the most likely explanation for the multiple bone lesions in this patient?
5. What is the special laboratory test that needs to be performed in this patient?
6. What is the best localizing procedure in patients such as this one?

Case Discussion

1. *Given the patient's hypoalbuminemia of 2.8 g/dL, what is the corrected calcium level?*

   As a rule, approximately 45% of the measured serum calcium is protein bound; 55% is diffusible. The protein-bound fraction is greater for albumin than for globulin. For a serum calcium level of 10 mg/dL, approximately 0.8 mg/dL is bound to globulin and 3.7 mg/dL is bound to albumin. In the setting of a low albumin state, approximately 1 g of albumin binds 0.8 mg of calcium. For example, this patient has a serum calcium level of 11.5 mg/dL and a serum albumin level of 2.8 g/dL. The corrected calcium level is calculated as follows:

   | 4.0 Normal albumin |
   | -2.8 Patient's albumin |

   1.2 Difference
   $\times 0.8$ (amount of calcium bound per gram of albumin) = 0.96

Patient's measured calcium:	11.5
Add correction for low albumin:	+ 0.96
Corrected calcium:	12.46 mg/dL

2. *What is the explanation for the patient's polyuria and polydipsia?*

   Hypercalcemia causes a vasopressin-resistant nephrogenic diabetes insipidus. This can promote dehydration in hypercalcemic patients, thereby aggravating the symptoms and worsening the hypercalcemia.

3. *Based solely on the patient's admission electrolyte levels, what is the likely diagnosis?*

   The electrolyte levels in this patient strongly support a diagnosis of primary hyperparathyroidism. Hypophosphatemia is seen in nearly 40% to 60% of patients with hyperparathyroidism, and its presence depends on the dietary phosphate intake. In addition, the chloride concentration greater than 104 mmol/L and the serum bicarbonate value in the mildly acidotic range suggest hyperparathyroidism. A chloride-to-phosphate ratio of greater than 33 is seen in the setting of hyperparathyroidism. In this patient, this ratio is 54, which indicates PTH-mediated hypercalcemia. An elevated 1,25-dihydroxyvitamin D level may be seen in patients with primary hyperparathyroidism, but, if there is magnesium deficiency, these levels may be normal or low.

4. *What is the most likely explanation for the multiple bone lesions in this patient?*

The turnover state of bone formation and resorption is high in patients with hyperparathyroidism. The classic histologic picture found in bone biopsy specimens is an increased number of osteoclasts, together with increased tetracycline labeling and increased rates of bone formation. The marrow in these patients may show focal areas of fibrosis. In extremely advanced cases of hyperparathyroidism, osteoclastomas, or giant cell tumors of bone may be seen. This patient had multiple such tumors.

5. *What is the special laboratory test that needs to be performed in this patient?*

The special laboratory test that needs to be done in this patient is measurement of his PTH level, which proves to be markedly elevated to a value of 811 pg/mL (normal, 1,065 pg/mL).

6. *What is the best localizing procedure in patients such as this one?*

Approximately 80% to 90% of patients with primary hyperparathyroidism have a single parathyroid adenoma, 10% to 15% have parathyroid hyperplasia, and less than 1% have parathyroid carcinoma. The preoperative localizing procedures add little in terms of sensitivity and specificity to the initial information obtained in patients with hyperparathyroidism. They are also expensive. Instead, the best approach to localization is an experienced surgeon who can, in almost all cases, remove the adenoma or identify the parathyroid hyperplasia and remove three and one-half glands. This patient proved to have a large, 16-g parathyroid adenoma, which was easily identified and removed.

Suggested Readings

Bilezikian JB. Management of acute hypercalcemia. *N Engl J Med* 1992;326:1196.

Broadus AE, Mangin M, Ikeda K, et al. Humoral hypercalcemia of cancer: identification of a novel parathyroid hormone-like peptide. *N Engl J Med* 1988;319:556.

Colao A, Di Saruo A, Landi ML, et al. Long-term and low-dose treatment with cabergoline induces macroprolactin shrinkage. *J Clin Endocrinol Metab* 1997;82:3574.

Consensus Development Conference. Diagnosis and management of asymptomatic primary hyperparathyroidism. *Ann Intern Med* 1991;114:593.

Davies PH, Stewart SE, Lancranjan L, Sheppard MC, Stewart PM. Long-term therapy with long-acting octreotide (Sandostatin-LAR) for the management of acromegaly. *Clin Endocrinol* 1998;48:311.

Henderson JE, Shustik C, Kremer R, et al. Circulating concentrations of parathyroid hormone-like peptide in malignancy and in hyperparathyroidism. *J Bone Miner Res* 1990; 5:105.

Lufkin EG, Kao PC, Heath H. Parathyroid hormone radioimmunoassays in the differential diagnosis of hypercalcemia due to primary hyperparathyroidism or malignancy. *Ann Intern Med* 1987;160:559.

Muratori M, Arosio M, Gambino G, Romando C, Biella O, Faglia G. Use of cabergoline in the long-term treatment of hyperprolactinemic and acromegalic patients. *J Endocrinol Invest* 1997;20:537.

Ralston SH, Gallacher SJ, Patel U, et al. Cancer-associated hypercalcemia: morbidity and mortality. *Ann Intern Med* 1990;112:499.

Yeh PJ, Chen JW. Pituitary tumors: surgical and medical management. *Surg Oncol* 1997; 6:67.

Hypoglycemia

1. What constitutes medically significant hypoglycemia?
2. What are the common symptoms of hypoglycemia?
3. What is the best first step in classifying hypoglycemia?
4. What are the causes of medically significant hypoglycemia?
5. In people with diabetes, what factors are associated with an increased risk of hypoglycemia?
6. What is reactive hypoglycemia and how should it be evaluated?

Discussion

1. *What constitutes medically significant hypoglycemia?*

   Medically significant hypoglycemia is diagnosed on the basis of only three findings (Whipple's triad): (a) blood glucose level of less than 50 mg/dL; (b) the presence of symptoms consistent with hypoglycemia; and (c) the resolution of symptoms after the ingestion of carbohydrates. The lower limit of normal for glucose is 70 mg/dL, but this is the lower limit for "normal" people after a 12-hour fast. During a 72-hour fast, up to 40% of "normal" women may have blood glucose values below 45 mg/dL and some as low as between 20 and 30 mg/dL. These low values may also be seen in apparently normal women 3 to 4 hours after the administration of 75 g of glucose orally (the oral glucose tolerance test), but almost none has symptoms of hypoglycemia and, therefore, medically significant hypoglycemia. Conversely, many people who exhibit symptoms consistent with hypoglycemia 3 to 4 hours after eating that respond to the ingestion of carbohydrate also do not have true hypoglycemia. The blood glucose levels in these women are rarely less than 50 mg/dL at the time they experience symptoms. These people have a condition that has been called *postprandial syndrome* or *functional hypoglycemia*.

2. *What are the common symptoms of hypoglycemia?*

   The symptoms of hypoglycemia can be divided into two categories: adrenergic and neuroglycopenic (Table 3-5). A substantial reduction in the blood glucose level stimulates the release of cortisol, GH, glucagon, and catecholamines. The attendant rise in sympathetic nervous system activity is experienced as nervousness, sweating, and palpitations. Because the brain is critically dependent on glucose for normal neuronal functioning, inadequate delivery of glucose to the brain rapidly results in alterations in mentation, which can take many forms. The signs and symptoms of neuroglycopenia can even mimic those associated with structural brain lesions or psychiatric conditions.

Table 3-5. Symptoms of Hypoglycemia

Adrenergic	Neuroglycopenia
Anxiety	Headache
Nervousness	Blurred vision
Tremulousness	Paresthesias
Sweating	Weakness
Hunger	Tiredness
Palpitations	Confusion
Irritability	Dizziness
Pallor	Amnesia
Nausea	Incoordination
Flushing	Abnormal mentation
Angina	Behavioral change
	Feeling cold
	Difficulty waking in the morning
	Senile dementia
	Organic personality syndrome
	Transient hemiplegia
	Transient aphasia
	Seizures
	Coma

3. *What is the best first step in classifying hypoglycemia?*

There are a variety of methods for categorizing the conditions that cause hypoglycemia, but none of these schemes is completely satisfactory. One approach is to divide the causes into those involving increased insulin levels, those involving increased glucose consumption, or those involving decreased glucose production. In reality, however, most of the causes of hypoglycemia embrace a combination of these mechanisms. An alternative and more useful scheme is based on the history and physical examination findings. The key features of this approach are to assess whether the hypoglycemia occurs with fasting or postprandially, and whether the affected person appears healthy. In general, the hypoglycemia that occurs with fasting or that found in people who appear generally ill is a more ominous form of the disorder.

4. *What are the causes of medically significant hypoglycemia?*

The specific causes of hypoglycemia are numerous (Table 3-6). The history, physical examination, and initial laboratory tests are performed in an effort to rule out the common causes.

The most common cause of hypoglycemia overall is the administration of a hypoglycemic agent, either insulin or an oral hypoglycemic agent. These medications may have been prescribed for the control of diabetes or may be ingested in error. If this cause is not obvious from the patient's history, the diagnosis can be made by performing an oral hypoglycemic screen on a sample of plasma, or measuring an insulin and C peptide level at the time of hypoglycemia. C peptide is a by-product of endogenous insulin production. If the insulin-producing hypoglycemia is exogenous, the insulin level is high and the C peptide level is suppressed.

Table 3-6. Etiologic Classification of Hypoglycemia

Hypoglycemia Associated Predominantly with Fasting
  Hypersecretion of insulin due to islet cell adenoma, carcinoma, hyperplasia, or nesidioblas-
    tosis
  Hepatic disease
    Generalized hypofunction
    Ethanol hypoglycemia associated with prior poor nutrition and decreased glycogen stores
    Sepsis
  Endocrine deficiencies
    Anterior pituitary insufficiency—growth hormone, adrenocorticotropic hormone
  Adrenocortical insufficiency
  Hypothyroidism
  Large nonislet cell tumors
  Renal disease
  Deficient carbohydrate stores or intake
    Severe inanition
    Severe exercise
  Autoimmune with insulin antibodies or antibodies to the insulin receptor
  Drug induced
Reactive or Stimulative Hypoglycemia
  Idiopathic functional hypoglycemia
  Alimentary hyperinsulinism
  Prediabetic functional hypoglycemia
  Endocrine deficiencies
Factitious and Artifactual Hypoglycemia
  Surreptitious insulin administration
  Surreptitious sulfonylurea ingestion
  Elevated leukocyte count—leukemia or polycythemia
Hypoglycemia of Infancy
  Abnormalities in hormone secretion
  Abnormalities of production and utilization of metabolic fuels
  Abnormalities in substrate availability

In one series consisting of hospitalized patients with hypoglycemia, the second most common cause of hypoglycemia was renal failure. Renal failure causes hypoglycemia for several reasons. First, because the kidneys play an important role in insulin clearance, insulin clearance may be decreased and insulin levels inappropriately high in the presence of renal failure. Second, during prolonged fasting, the kidneys may be responsible for as much as 30% of the net gluconeogenesis that takes place, and this would be compromised in the setting of renal failure. Finally, it appears that uremic toxins may suppress hepatic glucose output. As with other forms of hypoglycemia, inadequate caloric intake during a medical illness often contributes to the development of hypoglycemia.

Hypoglycemia may occur in association with a number of tumors (Table 3-7). These are usually large tumors located in the mediastinum or retroperitoneum. The mechanism by which these tumors cause hypoglycemia remains somewhat obscure. One explanation may be high levels of glucose extraction and utilization by the tumor mass. A second contributing feature is poor nutrition in these patients. An increased activity of IGF-II has been shown in some patients with non-islet cell tumors. IGF-II can interact with the insulin receptor, although with less affinity than insulin itself. Normally, IGF-II cleaves to a smaller protein with minimal insulin-like activity. It has been shown that although the IGF-II levels are not increased in these patients with hypoglycemia associated with cancer, there are increased levels of "big IGF-II." This is the uncleaved form of the hormone that has more insulin-like activity.

Another common cause of hypoglycemia is the ingestion of a drug that stimulates peripheral glucose utilization, inhibits hepatic glucose production, or stimulates insulin release, and there is a large number of such drugs. The drugs most often implicated are in part a function of the age of the patient (Table 3-8). Alcohol may actually be the most common drug associated with hypoglycemia because it causes an increase in the ratio of nicotinamide adenine dinucleotide hydrogenase (NADH) to NAD^+, which decreases the gluconeogenic capacity of the liver. The antiparasitic drug pentamidine is now widely used in the treatment of *Pneumocystis carinii* pneumonia in patients with AIDS. It can produce hypoglycemia by injuring the pancreatic islet cells, thereby causing insulin release and inappropriate hyperinsulinemia. As with all forms of hypoglycemia, inadequate caloric intake often contributes to the development of symptomatic hypoglycemia.

Leukemia and polycythemia vera can cause pseudohypoglycemia because of the high WBC or Hct value in these settings, which can result in continued glucose consumption in the test tube after the blood sample is obtained. In this situation, the blood glucose level is extremely low but the patient is without symptoms. To determine the actual blood glucose level in such patients, blood should be drawn into a tube that contains a substance that poisons the blood elements and prevents glycolysis from occurring after collection.

Table 3-7. Nonislet Cell Tumors Associated with Hypoglycemia

Mesenchymal
  Mesothelioma
  Fibrosarcoma
  Rhabdomyosarcoma
  Leiomyosarcoma
  Liposarcoma
  Hemangiopericytoma
Carcinomas
  Hepatic: hepatoma, biliary carcinoma
  Adrenocortical carcinoma
  Genitourinary: hypernephroma, Wilms' tumor, prostate carcinoma
  Reproductive: cervical carcinoma, breast carcinoma
Neurologic and Neuroendocrine
  Pheochromocytoma
  Carcinoid tumor
  Neurofibroma
Hematologic
  Leukemias
  Lymphoma
  Myeloma

Table 3-8. Drugs Associated with Hypoglycemia in a Variety of Age Groups

Age range (yr)	No. of patients	Drugs most frequently used (no. of cases)
Newborn	47	Sulfonylurea (mother) (14); propranolol (19); ritodrine, etc. (14)
0–2	26	Salicylate (17); propranolol (9)
2–10	48	Alcohol (28); quinine (15); propranolol (3); sulfonylurea (2)
11–30	79	Sulfonylurea (34); insulin (factitious) (20); quinine (10); alcohol (8); insulin + drug[a] (3); insulin + alcohol (2); propranolol (2)
31–40	78	Alcohol (50); sulfonylurea (14); quinine (4); insulin + alcohol (3) or drug (3); insulin (factitious) (2); propranolol (2)
41–50	71	Alcohol (33); sulfonylurea (19); insulin + alcohol (5); propranolol (3); alcohol + drug (2); quinine (2); disopyramide (1)
51–60	177	Sulfonylurea (86); alcohol (72); propranolol (4); sulfonylurea + insulin (3) or alcohol (3) or drug (3); disopyramide (3); quinine (1)
61–70	242	Sulfonylurea (173); alcohol (35); sulfonylurea + drug (10) or phenylbutazone (8) or insulin (4); disopyramide (5); propranolol (3)
Over 71	273	Sulfonylurea (219); alcohol (23); sulfonylurea + drug (12) or phenformin (6); disopyramide (5); propranolol (3)
Total	1,041 (69%)[b]	

[a] An agent without intrinsic hypoglycemic activity.
[b] Percentage of 1,418 patients for whom data were available.

Postprandial (reactive) hypoglycemia can occur in as many as 20% of patients after gastric surgical procedures. This condition is also called *alimentary hypoglycemia* and can occur after a variety of procedures, including gastrectomy, gastroenterostomy, pyloroplasty, and vagotomy. Although biochemical hypoglycemia is not rare in these patients during a long oral glucose tolerance test, symptomatic hypoglycemia is uncommon.

Other causes of hypoglycemia are much less common. Fasting by itself is a rare cause. However, extremely long periods of inadequate nutrition are required for hypoglycemia to occur in the absence of other metabolic defects. This is seen in the setting of anorexia nervosa and starvation. Likewise, liver disease produces hypoglycemia only in its most severe forms or in conjunction with inadequate caloric intake. Hypoglycemia is occasionally produced by the presence of autoantibodies either to insulin itself or to the insulin receptor, but these conditions usually occur in the presence of a known autoimmune syndrome. Finally, age plays an important role in the susceptibility to hypoglycemia. Elderly people lose counterregulatory hormone responses to hypoglycemia, are frequently on multiple medications, and may have mild organ dysfunction (renal failure, liver dysfunction, or congestive heart failure), all of which can increase the likelihood of multifactorial hypoglycemia. In addition, they may have alterations in their mental status that blunt the normal behavioral responses to hypoglycemia.

5. *In people with diabetes, what factors are associated with an increased risk of hypoglycemia?*

Hypoglycemia occurs all too frequently in treated diabetic patients, and is either directly or indirectly the cause of death in 3% to 5% of all people with type I diabetes. It results from excessive insulin administration, inadequate caloric intake, or excessive exercise. In nondiabetic people, if hypoglycemia develops, a number of hormones respond to increased glucose production and maintain a normal blood sugar level. In addition, the person notices symptoms of hypoglycemia and ingests carbohydrate to counteract these. In people with long-standing diabetes, however, there may be hypoglycemic unawareness and autonomic neuropathy, both of which blunt the normal response to hypoglycemia. Another factor that plays a role in the hypoglycemia that occurs in diabetics has to do with the introduction of recombinant human insulin, such that very few patients now remain on purified pork insulin. This has raised some concerns, particularly in Europe, about the greater risk of hypoglycemia in patients treated with human insulin because of differences in the ability of human insulin to enter the brain.

During the development of type I diabetes, there may be a period when islet cells are damaged but still retain their capacity to synthesize and store insulin. During this period, insulin may be released in a dysfunctional manner in response to nonphysiologic stimuli, or in inappropriate quantities. This may result in episodes of symptomatic hypoglycemia, but, later, as the islet cells are completely destroyed, insulinopenia and hyperglycemia predominate.

Historically, there has been a strong desire to normalize the blood glucose levels in patients with diabetes in an effort to prevent long-term complications. With the advent of home glucose monitoring, multiple daily injections of short- and long-acting insulins, insulin pumps, and glycosylated Hgb determinations, tight control is attainable. What has been learned, however, is that there is a trade-off, in that tight control can be achieved only by accepting a substantial increase in the risk of symptomatic and life-threatening hypoglycemia. The DCCT has demonstrated that tight control of blood glucose in patients with type I diabetes prevents or delays the development of diabetic complications. It is prudent to strive toward tight control while avoiding frequent hypoglycemic episodes.

6. *What is reactive hypoglycemia and how should it be evaluated?*

The term *hypoglycemia* is recognized by much of the lay public as a common problem that occurs at 10:30 a.m. in women whose breakfast consisted of a cup of coffee and a strawberry Danish. Some physicians have evaluated these reactive hypoglycemic symptoms with oral glucose tolerance tests. However, this approach is problematic because most of the women with these symptoms do not have blood glucose levels that are less than 50 mg/dL at the time of their symptoms and, in fact, most of these women's symptoms resolve spontaneously without the ingestion of carbohydrate. In addition, some "normal" women can have blood glucose values that are less than 50 mg/dL 3 to 4 hours after a 100-g oral glucose load, and yet not have symptoms. In general, these people do not have a serious illness and virtually never have an insulinoma in the absence of more typical episodes that occur with fasting. Instead, they need reassurance and a practical approach to their symptoms. Diets that are low in carbohydrate, high in protein, and high in fiber have not been conclusively shown to be of benefit, and extreme diets should be avoided. The regular ingestion of a balanced diet in perhaps four to five meals over the course of the day instead of the traditional three may be of benefit in these people.

Case   A 52-year-old white woman has an 18-month history of episodic confusion and poor work performance, but neurologic evaluation, including CT scan of the head and an electroencephalogram, are unrevealing. Dilantin and then phenobarbital are prescribed but do not alter the frequency of the attacks, and are eventually discontinued. On the day of admission, she has a generalized seizure at work. The paramedics are called, find her unconscious, and administer Narcan [naloxone hydrochloride (Du Pont Merck Pharmaceutical, Wilmington, DE)] and 1 ampule of 50% dextrose IV. She then regains consciousness. Her blood glucose level before receiving the 50% dextrose is 28 mg/dL. She denies consuming alcohol or taking any prescription medications. Her family history is unremarkable and she has no history of gastric surgery. On physical examination, she is found to be a thin woman who appears to be in good health. Her examination findings are normal, as are her initial laboratory results.

1. What is the likely diagnosis in this patient?
2. If she had a family history of this problem, what other endocrine tumors would you look for?
3. What diagnostic test, or tests, are useful in making this diagnosis?
4. If the results of the biochemical studies indicate she has an insulinoma, what should the next test be?
5. What is the proper therapy for an insulinoma?

Case Discussion

1. *What is the likely diagnosis in this patient?*

The patient's history suggests the presence of an insulinoma because the hypoglycemia is severe, recurrent, progressive, symptomatic, and reversed by the administration of IV glucose. The symptomatic episodes of hypoglycemia associated with an insulinoma may occur in the postprandial state, but almost never exclusively in this state (Table 3-9). Most people with adrenal insufficiency, tumor-associated hypoglycemia, or alimentary hypoglycemia have other signs or symptoms, appear ill, or have a known surgical history.

2. *If she had a family history of this problem, what other endocrine tumors would you look for?*

Table 3-9. Association of Hypoglycemia Symptoms with Eating in People with Insulinoma

	No. of patients	Percentage of total
1. Symptoms during or after overnight fast only (before breakfast)	20	26
2. Fasting and daytime postprandial (before lunch or dinner) symptoms	21	27
3. Symptoms after missed meal only	6	8
4. Postprandial (before lunch and dinner) symptoms only	23	29
5. Uncertain about timing of symptoms	7	9
6. No symptoms experienced	1	1
	78	100
Symptoms exacerbated by exercise	24	31

There are three generally recognized syndromes of MEN [or multiple endocrine adenomatosis (MEA)]. People with MEN I can have tumors of the pituitary (e.g., prolactinomas or Cushing's disease), the pancreas (insulinoma and gastrinoma most commonly), or the parathyroid glands. Usually hypercalcemia due to hyperparathyroidism develops first. Those affected with MEN IIA are at risk for medullary carcinoma of the thyroid, pheochromocytoma, and, less commonly, hyperparathyroidism. All these features can be found in people with MEN IIB, together with mucosal neuromas. These syndromes can occur either in families or sporadically. In all patients with insulinomas, the serum calcium and prolactin levels should be checked and a complete history and physical examination performed to look for evidence of the other potentially associated conditions. Among the cases of sporadic nonfamilial insulinomas, 80% are solitary and benign, 11% are multiple and benign, and 6% are single and malignant. The remaining 3% of the patients have multiple malignant tumors or islet hyperplasia. Ten percent of the insulinomas occur in association with MEN I, and are multifocal 80% of the time.

3. *What diagnostic test, or tests, are useful in making this diagnosis?*

The traditional diagnostic approach in patients with a suspected insulinoma is a supervised 72-hour fast. If symptomatic hypoglycemia develops and the blood glucose level is less than 50 mg/dL, then insulin and C peptide levels should be determined. In one series of patients with insulinomas, hypoglycemia occurred in the first 12 hours of fasting in 29%, within 24 hours in 71%, within 48 hours in 92%, within 60 hours in 92%, and within 72 hours in 98%. In this series, the blood glucose level at the time symptoms appeared was less than 46 mg/dL in 100%, less than 39 mg/dL in 70%, less than 35 mg/dL in 50%, and less than 28 mg/dL in 25%. Because the insulin secretion from an insulinoma is often sporadic, not all insulinomas can be diagnosed on the basis of a single fast. It is important to determine the C peptide level to demonstrate that the insulin is produced endogenously. A proinsulin level can also be helpful in diagnosing insulinomas. Proinsulin is the prohormone from which insulin and C peptide are cleaved, and accounts for only 15% to 20% of the circulating immunoreactive insulin in normal people. In those with an insulinoma, however, it constitutes greater than 22% of the insulin mass in 80% to 90% of the patients. There are other specialized tests for evaluating a patient with a suspected insulinoma but, although advocated by some, they usually are not necessary. A serum drug screen to rule out a drug-induced hypoglycemia and an ACTH stimulation test to rule out adrenal insufficiency are useful in the evaluation of hypoglycemia of unknown cause, but are not helpful in establishing the diagnosis of hyperinsulinism.

4. *If the results of the biochemical studies indicate she has an insulinoma, what should the next test be?*

Once the biochemical diagnosis of insulinoma has been established, an anatomic study usually is done. Although no single study is completely satisfactory, abdominal CT scanning and ultrasonography possess a relatively high sensitivity, pose no risk to the patient, and are relatively inexpensive, making them a good first step. Abdominal ultrasound is advocated by some as the superior study, but its utility varies from institution to institution. Angiography is more sensitive but carries some risk and is quite expensive. Some groups have advocated transhepatic venous sampling. In this method, by measuring insulin levels in the venous blood draining a particular region of the pancreas, the tumor can be localized, although not visualized. The newest preoperative localizing technique is endoscopic ultrasound. In this technique, the ultrasound transducer is endoscopically placed in the duodenum. From this site, the head of the pancreas can be well visualized, yielding a sensitivity better than that of traditional abdominal ultrasound. This technology is not yet widely available, however. The main problem with all of these approaches is that most insulinomas are small (average, 1.5 cm, 2 g), and the diagnosis hinges on the clinical presentation and the results of biochemical studies. If the anatomic studies are unrevealing and the biochemical results are convincing, the patient should undergo exploratory surgery performed by a surgeon experienced in pancreatic surgery. For this reason, extensive preoperative anatomic studies are not advocated.

5. *What is the proper therapy for an insulinoma?*

Surgical removal performed by an experienced surgeon is the primary form of therapy for insulinomas. Intraoperative direct ultrasonic examination of the pancreas combined with manual palpation by an experienced surgeon successfully localizes the tumor 80% to 90% of the time. Once the tumors are resected, most patients are cured. For those who are not cured by surgical means, long-acting somatostatin analogues can be used to decrease the frequency and severity of the hypoglycemic episodes. Diazoxide, verapamil, phenytoin, and propranolol have been used successfully in a few cases. For these patients, frequent scheduled meals are an important component of therapy.

Suggested Readings

Adrogue HJ. Glucose homeostasis and the kidney. *Kidney Int* 1992;42:1266.

Field JB. Hypoglycemia: definition, clinical presentations, classification, and laboratory tests. *Endocrinol Metab Clin North Am* 1989;18:27.

Fischer KF, Lees JA, Newman JH. Hypoglycemia in hospitalized patients: causes and outcomes. *N Engl J Med* 1986;315:1245.

Kurlan R. Postprandial (reactive) hypoglycemia and restless leg syndrome: related neurologic disorders? *Mov Disord* 1998;13:619.

Leonetti F, Foniciello M, Iozzo P, et al. Increased nonoxidative glucose metabolism in idiopathic reactive hypoglycemia. *Metabolism* 1996;45:606.

Newell-Price J, Trainer P, Besser M, Grossman A. The diagnosis and differential diagnosis of Cushing's syndrome and pseudo-Cushing's states. *Endocr Rev* 1998;19:657.

Piedrola G, Cassado JL, Lopez E, Moreno A, Perez-Elias MJ, Garcia-Robles R. Clinical features of adrenal insufficiency in patients with acquired immunodeficiency syndrome. *Clin Endocrinol* 1996;45:97.

Ross RJ, Trainer PJ. Endocrine investigation: Cushing's syndrome. *Clin Endocrinol* 1998;49:153.

Seltzer HS. Drug-induced hypoglycemia: a review of 1418 cases. *Endocrinol Metab Clin North Am* 1989;18:163.

Service FJ. Hypoglycemia. *Endocrinol Metab Clin North Am* 1997;26:937.

Service FJ. Hypoglycemias. *West J Med* 1991;154:442.

Soderbergh A, Winqvist O, Norheim I, et al. Adrenal autoantibodies and organ-specific autoimmunity in patients with Addison's disease. *Clin Endocrinol* 1996;45:453.

Xiao XR, Ye LY, Shi LX, Cheng GF, Li YT, Zhou BM. Diagnosis and treatment of adrenal tumours: a review of 35 years' experience. *Br J Urol* 1998;82:199.

Metabolic Bone Disease

1. Which diseases of bone are considered to be metabolic in origin?
2. What is osteopenia?
3. What conditions may cause osteopenia?
4. What are the risk factors for osteoporosis?
5. What simple laboratory tests can help assess the patient with osteopenia?
6. When are bone density measurements indicated?

Discussion

1. *Which diseases of bone are considered to be metabolic in origin?*

   Metabolic bone diseases are those conditions in which all the metabolic bone units throughout the skeleton are equally affected by the disease process. These diseases include osteoporosis, osteomalacia, osteitis fibrosa cystica, and osteogenesis imperfecta. Diseases that affect either a single area or multiple areas in bone are considered localized bone diseases, and include Paget's disease, fibrous dysplasia, bone cysts, healing fractures, Sudeck's atrophy, and injury disuse osteoporosis.

2. *What is osteopenia?*

   Osteopenia constitutes a diagnosis based on radiographic findings, in that the mineral content of the bones is seen to be reduced on radiography. Usually, before these studies can show bone loss, however, approximately 30% to 40%

of the skeleton must have demineralized. Any of the metabolic bone conditions listed can cause osteopenia.

3. *What conditions may cause osteopenia?*

There are many disease processes to be considered in the osteopenic patient. The most often encountered condition in such patients is age-related, idiopathic osteoporosis. Type I osteoporosis is postmenopausal osteoporosis and is usually manifested clinically by vertebral fractures; type II osteoporosis has been termed *senile osteoporosis* and is characterized by hip fracture.

There are many secondary causes of osteopenia seen in the setting of nutritional deficiency; renal, liver, gastrointestinal, and endocrine and metabolic disease; drug usage; and certain lifestyles (Table 3-10). In many of these conditions, alterations in the calcium level or vitamin D metabolism, secondary hyperparathyroidism, osteomalacia, acidosis, or a combination of these conditions is the underlying mechanism responsible for the osteopenia.

4. *What are the risk factors for osteoporosis?*

Smoking, poor calcium intake, immobilization, malnutrition, a hypogonadal state, and a family history of osteoporosis are all risk factors for osteoporosis. Smoking is a risk factor because it induces hepatic enzymes to inactivate circulating sex hormones, such as estrogen. A hypogonadal state can occur in either men or women, but in women it may result from a total hysterectomy and oophorectomy or from the spontaneous menopausal state, both of which lead to lowered estrogen levels. Other factors include the ingestion of soft drinks, most of which contain phosphoric acid. This substance increases the ingested phosphate load, which in turn depresses the serum calcium level and stimulates PTH release. Coffee is a calciuretic substance, and, as such, excessive consumption contributes to osteoporosis. The fat cell can act as an endocrine organ; thus, in lean people whose fat cell mass is decreased, the conversion of adrenal androgens to estrogens is decreased, and this can lead to osteoporosis. Some of the lifestyle risk factors can be modified to prevent osteoporosis.

5. *What simple laboratory tests can help assess the patient with osteopenia?*

A complete blood count with erythrocyte sedimentation rate and a standard serum chemistry profile that includes electrolyte, calcium, phosphate, alkaline phosphatase, creatinine, BUN, calcium, and phosphate measurements plus liver function tests are the simple blood tests needed. A 24-hour urine specimen is obtained for determination of the calcium, phosphate, and creatinine content. Bone densitometry establishes the severity of bone loss. All these laboratory tests can be used quickly to assess the patient with osteopenia. If the patient has anemia and an elevated sedimentation rate, the clinician should consider the possibility of a multiple myeloma and have either a serum protein or urine protein electrophoresis, or both, performed. Abnormalities in calcium balance can be assessed by identifying hypocalcemic or hypercalcemic disorders. Abnormalities of liver and kidney function represent secondary causes of osteoporosis. The electrolyte levels help suggest the presence of renal tubular acidosis syndromes. Alkaline phosphatase is a marker of bone osteoblast function and its measurement helps identify those patients with high-

Table 3-10. Causes of Osteopenia

Idiopathic Age-Related
  Juvenile
  Young adults
  Postmenopausal (type I)
  Senile (type II)
Secondary to Disease States
  Metabolic conditions
    Calcium deficiency
    Vitamin D deficiency states
    Malnutrition
    Idiopathic hypercalciuria
    Renal tubular acidosis and other systemic acidosis
    Diabetes mellitus
    Scurvy
  Endocrine conditions
    Thyrotoxicosis
    Cushing's syndrome
    Male and female hypogonadal state
    Hypoamenorrheic female runners
    Prolactinoma
    Hyperparathyroidism
  Renal disease
  Gastrointestinal–liver disease
  Inheritable connective tissue disease
    Osteogenesis imperfecta
    Homocystinuria
    Ehlers-Danlos syndrome
    Marfan's syndrome
  Bone marrow infiltration
    Multiple myeloma
    Lymphoma
    Leukemia
  Drugs
    Dilantin
    Phenobarbital
    Thyroid hormone
    Corticosteroids
    Prolonged heparin therapy
  Lifestyle
    Nutrition
    Alcohol
    Smoking
    Inactivity
    Immobilization
    Excessive coffee and soft drinks
  Miscellaneous
    Rheumatoid arthritis
    Systemic mastocytosis

turnover osteoporosis or osteomalacia. A 24-hour urine calcium determination can identify patients who have idiopathic hypercalciuria or low urine calcium losses, suggesting a calcium-deficient state. An extremely low urine phosphate value may reflect the consumption of a vegetarian diet. Other laboratory tests, including measurement of the PTH level, serum osteocalcin level, vitamin D metabolites, and urine hydroxyproline or hydroxypyridinium, are reserved for those patients in whom these are specifically indicated. A bone density measurement establishes the presence or absence of significant osteoporosis.

6. *When are bone density measurements indicated?*

   The National Osteoporosis Foundation and the NIH have established that bone density measurements are warranted when estrogen replacement therapy is being considered, when evaluating hypoamenorrheic runners, when assessing patients who have radiographic evidence of osteopenia, when evaluating patients with hyperparathyroidism for surgery, in steroid-treated patients, and when monitoring patients undergoing therapy for osteoporosis.

Case   A thin, 55-year-old, white, postmenopausal woman is seen in her primary care clinic because of muscle aches and weakness. She has been seen by numerous physicians for evaluation of this condition, and has been referred to the psychiatry department for treatment of a "stress reaction." The patient's past medical history is significant for a gastrectomy approximately 15 years earlier for the treatment of peptic ulcer disease. She has noticed loose stools since that time. The patient admits to a poor calcium intake, but otherwise consumes a nonvegetarian diet. She suffers hot flashes and insomnia, but has never been evaluated for estrogen therapy. During her evaluation, osteopenic changes are noted on the chest film. The patient's laboratory evaluation reveals the following findings: calcium, 8.4 mg/dL (normal, 8.7 to 10.3 mg/dL); phosphate, 2.0 mg/dL (normal, 2.7 to 4.5 mg/dL); chloride, 108 mEq/L; sodium, 145 mEq/L; potassium, 4.5 mEq/L; CO_2, 23 mEq/L; and albumin, 4.1 g/dL. Her kidney and liver function test results are normal. The alkaline phosphatase level is elevated to 380 IU/L (normal, 39 to 117 IU/L). Her 24-hour urine excretion of calcium is 40 mg (normal, 100 to 300 mg); creatinine, 1.1 g; total hydroxyproline, 86 mg (normal, 25 to 77 mg); and phosphate, 780 mg (normal, 400 to 800 mg). The osteocalcin level is 7.1 ng/mL (normal, 1.8 to 6.6 ng/mL).

1. What are the risk factors for osteoporosis in this patient?
2. Based on the patient's history and laboratory findings, what is the differential diagnosis?
3. What additional laboratory tests should be obtained in this patient?
4. Based on the laboratory findings, what would you anticipate the bone biopsy specimen to show?
5. What should the treatment be in this patient?
6. What would you advise this patient regarding the advantages and disadvantages of estrogen replacement therapy?

Case Discussion

1. *What are the risk factors for osteoporosis in this patient?*

   This thin, white, postmenopausal woman with poor calcium intake is at risk for osteoporosis.

2. *Based on the patient's history and laboratory findings, what is the differential diagnosis?*

   This patient's history suggests that, at her age of 55 years, she is entering a postmenopausal state, as indicated by the hot flashes and insomnia. In addition, poor calcium balance may be likely because of her lifelong history of poor calcium intake and the gastrectomy for peptic ulcer disease, which could lead to poor vitamin D absorption. Confirming a state of negative calcium balance is the patient's hypocalcemia, low urine calcium excretion, and electrolyte levels, which all suggest the presence of secondary hyperparathyroidism with hyperchloremia and low serum phosphate levels.

3. *What additional laboratory tests should be obtained in this patient?*

   The patient may be deficient in vitamin D. Measuring the 25-vitamin D level, which is the major circulating form of vitamin D, can establish the diagnosis of simple vitamin D deficiency. Some patients may also have a deficiency of 1,25-dihydroxyvitamin D, particularly older patients and those with renal disease. A PTH value can establish the diagnosis of secondary hyperparathyroidism due to a calcium-deficient state stemming from the vitamin D deficiency. As treatment is initiated, a PTH value that returns to normal confirms that the patient is in a state of normal calcium balance.

   In this patient, the 25-vitamin D level is 10 ng/mL (normal, 16 to 74 ng/mL) and the PTH value is 120 pg/mL (normal, 10 to 65 pg/mL).

4. *Based on the laboratory findings, what would you anticipate the bone biopsy specimen to show?*

   A tetracycline-labeled bone biopsy is performed by having the patient ingest 250 mg of tetracycline four times a day for 3 days, then withhold the tetracycline for 10 days, and then take tetracycline for another 3 days. These two tetracycline labels determine the rate of bone formation. Osteoclast counts can be determined on bone histomorphologic analysis, and the amount of tetracycline that has surfaced can be measured as an indication of active bone formation. This patient proved to have a high-turnover osteoporosis with an increased tetracycline surface and an increased osteoclast count, as borne out by the high PTH level. In addition, the high osteocalcin, alkaline phosphatase, and urinary hydroxyproline or pyridinium levels indicate a state of high bone turnover. Early in vitamin D deficiency (hypovitaminosis-D I), secondary hyperparathyroidism predominates, leading to a high-turnover osteoporosis. In the setting of severe vitamin D deficiency, especially childhood rickets (hypovitaminosis-D II and III), a low–bone-turnover state exists in which there is little tetracycline uptake.

5. *What should the treatment be in this patient?*

   Because this patient has a combined disorder of both estrogen and vitamin D deficiency, she needs to receive a cyclic course of 0.625 mg of conjugated estrogens, together with 10 to 14 days of a progestin, because of her intact uterus. The patient most likely will not respond to small doses of vitamin D, but may require 50,000 units of vitamin D, given once or twice weekly, or Calderol (calcifediol; Organon Teknika), 20 to 50 μg daily, because of the poor gastrointestinal absorption of vitamin D stemming from her gastrectomy. When treating osteoporosis, the clinician should always use the FDA-recommended treatments, which consist of oral estrogens or transdermal estradiol and injectable thyrocalcitonin. Another effective means of treating osteoporosis is with bisphosphonates. The initial experience with increased bone density on these medication was with etidronate (Didronel; Procter & Gamble, Cincinnati, OH). Alendronate is a newer bisphosphonate that both increases bone mineral density and decreases fracture rate in prospective, randomized trials.

6. *What would you advise this patient regarding the advantages and disadvantages of estrogen replacement therapy?*

Estrogens are the most effective agents for treating osteoporosis by stabilizing bone density and preventing fractures. However, estrogen therapy alone in a patient with an intact uterus is associated in a dose-dependent manner with an increased incidence of endometrial cancer; with the addition of 10 to 14 days of a progestin, however, this risk is abolished.

Estrogen therapy may not be indicated in certain patients who have estrogen-related neoplasia of the breast or patients with a strong family history of breast carcinoma. Estrogen therapy is relatively contraindicated in patients with thromboembolic disease, estrogen-related headaches, or hypertension. The use of estrogen therapy may also be associated with an increased incidence of gallstones. A marked triglyceride elevation may develop in some patients when estrogen therapy is initiated; hence, lipid levels need to be checked within 4 to 8 weeks after the start of therapy. Patients in whom adverse lipid abnormalities to oral estrogens develop may respond to transdermal estradiol therapy.

Estrogens also have a cardioprotective effect by lowering serum low-density lipoprotein levels and raising high-density lipoprotein (HDL) levels. A further cardioprotective effect is that they increase the levels of calcitonin-related peptide, a potent vasorelaxer, and stabilize vasomotion in patients with established atherosclerosis or hypercholesterolemia.

Suggested Readings

Armanento-Villereal R, Villereal DT, Avioli LV, Civitelli R. Estrogen status and heredity are major determinants of premenopausal bone mass. *J Clin Invest* 1992;90:2464.

Hofeldt FD. Proximal femoral fractures. *Clin Orthop* 1987;218:12.

Jacobs HS, Loeffler FE. Postmenopausal hormone replacement therapy. *BMJ* 1992;2:1403.

McClung M, Clemmesen B, Daifotis A, et al. Alendronate prevents postmenopausal bone loss in women without osteoporosis: a double-blind, randomized, controlled trial: Alendronate Osteoporosis Prevention Study Group. *Ann Intern Med* 1998;128:253.

Miller PD, Watts NB, Licata AA, et al. Cyclical etidronate in the treatment of postmenopausal osteoporosis: efficacy and safety after seven years of treatment. *Am J Med* 1997;103:468.

Parfitt AM, Rao DS, Stanciu AR, et al. Irreversible bone loss in osteomalacia: comparison of radial photon absorptiometry with iliac bone histomorphometry during treatment. *J Clin Invest* 1985;76:2403.

Riggs BL, Melton LJ. The prevention and treatment of osteoporosis. *N Engl J Med* 1992;327:620.

Wimalawansa SJ. A four-year randomized controlled trial of hormone replacement and bis-phosphonate, alone or in combination, in women with postmenopausal osteoporosis. *Am J Med* 1998;104:219.

Erectile Dysfunction

Case 1 A 65-year-old man presented with erectile dysfunction—he had noted gradual onset of difficulty in achieving and maintaining an erection during the past 4 years. He had had hypertension for 10 years and recently had been told that his blood cholesterol level was high. His family history was positive for coronary artery disease, hypertension, and hypercholesterolemia.

The patient's medications included atenolol, 50 mg twice a day; hydrochlorothi-azide, 50 mg per day; and aspirin, 325 mg per day. He had smoked a pack of cigarettes a day for 30 years, but quit 2 years earlier. He drank three beers each night.

Physical examination showed a blood pressure of 160/90 mm Hg, the presence of arcus corneae, and an S_4 heart sound. The liver and testicular examinations were normal, as were reflexes. The pedal pulses were diminished.

Laboratory test results were testosterone, 450 ng/dL (normal, 300 to 1,000); liver enzymes, normal; total cholesterol, 350 mg/dL; triglycerides, 300 mg/dL; and HDL, 25 mg/dL.

Case Discussion

From the history alone, it would be expected that this patient's erectile dysfunction has a vascular cause and perhaps iatrogenic exacerbation. Coronary artery disease is a risk factor for erectile dysfunction, and recent studies have suggested that merely having a history of hypercholesterolemia points to an underlying vascular etiology. His long-standing hypertension also suggests vascular disease.

This patient is taking two medications that have been associated with erectile dysfunction. Among the classes of currently used antihypertensive agents, β blockers and diuretics are most often at fault. Of the diuretics, hydrochlorothi-azide is more of a problem than furosemide.

Smoking, of course, increases the risk of vascular disease. Excessive alcohol intake is directly toxic to the testicles and can result in decreased testosterone production. Alcohol is also directly toxic to the liver, and the resulting liver dysfunction can cause imbalance in testosterone and estradiol metabolism, which is often associated with gynecomastia.

The patient's blood pressure reading indicates that his hypertension is inade-quately controlled, and the S_4 heart sound indicates that the hypertension is of long standing and has affected his heart. The presence of arcus corneae signifies prolonged hypercholesterolemia. Diminished pedal pulses offer fur-ther evidence for vascular disease.

Hypogonadism cannot be reliably detected by clinical assessment alone; hence, measurement of the testosterone level was indicated. Liver function testing was performed in light of the history of significant alcohol intake. The lipid panel confirmed hypercholesterolemia.

There have been many studies on how to distinguish between psychogenic and vascular erectile dysfunction—for example, by monitoring for nocturnal erections. No controlled study has shown that the methods change the management strategy; however, the work-up can be limited to the history, physical examination, and some laboratory testing to exclude other treatable causes of erectile dysfunction.

In this patient, atenolol and hydrochlorothiazide were replaced with enalapril. The patient was counseled on dietary changes that would help to lower his cholesterol level. A vacuum pump device was prescribed for the erectile dysfunction.

Two months later, the patient's blood pressure was normal. He reported successful resumption of sexual intercourse using the vacuum pump.

Evaluation of this patient's erectile dysfunction provided the opportunity to address the underlying hypertension and hypercholesterolemia. Otherwise, he might not have presented until a stroke or heart attack occurred.

Changing antihypertensive medication is especially important if the initiation of treatment and onset of erectile dysfunction coincide. In this case, a medication change was further justified because of inadequate blood pressure control. Angiotensin-converting enzyme (ACE) inhibitors do not appear to cause erectile dysfunction and calcium channel blockers rarely do, so these are the drugs that may be prescribed if medication is interfering with sexual functioning. Unfortunately, a change in antihypertensive medication alone is unlikely to restore erectile function.

Correction of this patient's blood lipids is long overdue. If dietary changes do not sufficiently improve his lipid profile within a few months, he will be a candidate for therapy with an HMG-CoA reductase inhibitor.

The vacuum pump device can treat erectile function in a case like this man's. The vacuum pump device consists of a Lucite tube and pump; the suction pulls blood into the penis. Once an erection has been produced, a rubber ring is placed at the base of the penis to maintain the erection. The vacuum pump has no major side effects, it can be used as often as the patient wishes, it can be used in all types of erectile dysfunction, and it has the highest success rate—it is effective in 90% to 95% of cases. Obviously, it is not meant for a man who is not in a stable relationship, largely because of poor patient acceptance. There has been some speculation that vacuum pump devices might be contraindicated in patients taking warfarin because of the potential for ecchymosis from the ring, but studies have eliminated that concern.

Case 2   A 52-year-old diabetic man presented with erectile dysfunction. His pubertal development had been normal. The diabetes had been diagnosed 15 years earlier.

At the time of diagnosis, he had had problems with impotence that resolved as the hyperglycemia was brought under control. Erectile dysfunction had returned gradually during the past 2 years. He rarely had morning erections. The erectile dysfunction has created stress in his relationship with his wife.

The patient had taken an oral hypoglycemic agent for 5 years after diagnosis of diabetes and had been on insulin for the past 10 years. He had diabetic complications, including mild retinopathy, proteinuria, and mild peripheral neuropathy. Symptoms of gastroparesis had developed during the past 6 months.

His current insulin regimen consisted of 30 units of NPH (neutral protamine Hagedorn) and 15 units of regular insulin in the morning, and 10 units of NPH and 8 units of regular in the evening.

Other medications included lisinopril (15 mg per day) and simvastatin (10 mg per day). He did not smoke or drink excessive amounts of alcohol.

Noteworthy findings on the physical examination included a blood pressure reading of 120/80 mm Hg without significant orthostasis, retinopathy, absence of an S_4 heart sound, and slightly soft testes. Sensation to pinprick on the calf was decreased.

Laboratory test results were serum testosterone, 200 ng/dL; total cholesterol, 150 mg/dL; triglycerides, 250 mg/dL; and HDL, 35 mg/dL. Glycosylated Hgb was 10% (normal, <6.5%).

Case Discussion

Diabetes is one of the most common causes of erectile dysfunction. A combination of vascular and neurologic disease is usually at fault, although hormone deficiency, medications, and psychogenic aspects also may be involved. All five components may be present in a single patient.

Men with type II diabetes often have acute erectile dysfunction at the onset of the disease, simply as a result of severe hyperglycemia. The mechanism of erectile dysfunction may include hypogonadotropic hypogonadism as well as metabolic and neurologic dysfunction (caused by glucose toxicity) in the testes. Vascular factors also may be involved because the hyperglycemia is usually associated with severe hyperlipidemia. The erectile dysfunction associated with new-onset diabetes may improve when hyperglycemia is brought under control.

In a patient with long-standing diabetes, the presence of other end-organ complications makes it more likely that erectile dysfunction is due to diabetes. In this patient, clinical assessment suggests a strong neurogenic component; the diminished sensation denotes peripheral neuropathy and the gastroparesis indicates autonomic neuropathy (although the lack of orthostasis suggests that the neuropathy is not severe). The proteinuria suggests a vascular component and, even though the absence of an S_4 argues against that, it should be remembered that an S_4 is not always present in diabetic patients with coronary artery disease.

Drug-induced erectile dysfunction does not appear to be an issue in this patient because neither the ACE inhibitor nor the HMG-CoA reductase inhibitor causes erectile dysfunction.

The testicular softness suggests a minor hormonal component, and indeed the testosterone level is slightly decreased. A low-normal or slightly low testosterone level is a typical finding in diabetic patients with erectile dysfunction. Although the reading confirms that hormone deficiency is one of his problems, a testosterone level of 200 ng/dL would not by itself cause significant hypogonadism and symptoms.

In addition, this patient's blood pressure needs to be monitored; if it increases, he will need an additional antihypertensive medication because he is already taking a maximal dose of lisinopril. Increasing data suggest that tight control of blood pressure with ACE inhibitors helps to prevent both the renal and the vascular complications of diabetes. Consequently, aggressive antihypertensive therapy to lower blood pressure to less than 130/85 mm Hg is indicated.

The patient's low-density lipoprotein level is low, but the triglyceride level is not optimal. If changes in his diet do not reduce the triglyceride level, he will be a candidate for treatment with atorvastatin.

The patient was managed with intracavernosal injection of alprostadil and androgen replacement with a low-dose testosterone patch. He reported improved erectile function and increased energy and a sense of well-being. In addition, the patient received dietary counseling and the insulin regimen was adjusted. The glycosylated Hgb decreased to 8%.

In diabetic patients with erectile dysfunction, injection of alprostadil into the corpora cavernosa of the penis can be effective. The treatment is particularly suited to diabetic patients because they often have neurologic complications, making the injections less painful than in other patients. In addition, those who are taking insulin are already familiar with needles and syringes and are less likely to be squeamish about injecting the penis. Intracavernosal injection is effective in approximately 65% of cases. The vacuum pump is held in reserve as second-line treatment.

Implantable penile prostheses were commonly used to treat erectile dysfunction in the 1970s and 1980s. They are used much less frequently today because they are expensive and may have many complications. Infection and poor wound healing are particular problems in diabetic patients, often necessitating removal of the implant—at which point the option for injection therapy has been eliminated. However, some of the newer implants may be appropriate for young men with severe erectile dysfunction that does not respond to other therapy.

Intraurethral placement of vasoactive medication was introduced as an alternative to intracavernosal injections. However, several studies have shown it to be less effective, with a success rate as low as 30% in diabetic patients.

Side effects of intracavernosal injection include priapism and penile fibrosis. Patients with neurogenic or psychogenic erectile dysfunction should use a low dose of alprostadil. If the dose is too high, the risk of priapism is significant.

When priapism occurs, the patient has to go to an emergency room, where he is treated with IV epinephrine or an 18-gauge needle that is inserted into the corpora cavernosa to withdraw blood. There have been only rare reports of more severe consequences, such as loss of the penis due to infarction.

The rate of priapism as a complication varies according to the agent used. Alprostadil has a much lower risk of priapism and fibrosis than do papaverine and phentolamine. However, alprostadil is more likely to cause a burning sensation. For that reason, it used to be mixed with papaverine, but papaverine has been withdrawn as a treatment for outpatients. Because of neuropathy, diabetic patients may not experience a burning sensation with alprostadil.

It is not clear whether better control of this patient's diabetes during the previous 10 years would have prevented erectile dysfunction. It seems logical that tight control of blood glucose levels will forestall erectile dysfunction, just as it can prevent retinopathy, renal failure, and macrovascular disease. Nevertheless, there are no prospective, double-blinded, placebo-controlled studies to confirm that long-term tight blood glucose control reduces the incidence of erectile dysfunction.

Case 3

A 48-year-old man had experienced acute onset of erectile dysfunction 6 months earlier. He had no other medical problems. Pubertal development had been normal. He was the father of three children.

On further questioning, the patient said that he had lost his job 4 months ago. He was having problems in his relationship with his wife, and had increased his alcohol consumption from two beers a week to four beers a day.

The physical examination was normal. The serum testosterone level was 450 ng/dL.

The patient was advised that his drinking was probably contributing to his erectile dysfunction and that he should reduce his intake. Referral for psychological counseling was offered, but he refused because of the cost. Instead, the physician discussed the patient's circumstances with him. A 6-week trial of yohimbine, 5.4 mg three times a day, was prescribed.

The patient returned 8 weeks later and reported some improvement in erectile function.

He felt that yohimbine had been helpful; however, he had also found a job, was experiencing less psychological stress, and had reduced his alcohol consumption.

1. What was the major factor in this patient's erectile dysfunction?
2. How do you approach psychological erectile dysfunction?
3. What are the pharmacologic options for treatment?

Case Discussion

1. *What was the major factor in this patient's erectile dysfunction?*

Although the history in this case indicated that psychological stress was the major trigger for the erectile dysfunction, it was important to consider the possibility of other components. As noted, erectile dysfunction rarely results from an isolated cause. In this case, further questioning was needed to reveal that alcohol was almost certainly a major contributor.

Obtaining an accurate history of alcohol intake is notoriously difficult. Instead of asking the patient, "Do you drink?" ask, "When you drink, do you drink beer, whiskey, or wine?" After identifying the drink of choice, pick a large amount and let patients come down from there; with beer, for example, ask if they drink a six-pack at a time. Determining the true amount of alcohol intake often requires several discussions.

Also ask patients when they drink, because they may not understand that intermittent drinking can have persistent effects. Some patients who drank heavily on the weekend and nothing at all during the week may present with erectile dysfunction and painful right-sided gynecomastia (which was worse on Mondays). Their liver enzymes were not severely elevated, but the drinking had nevertheless caused a symptomatic imbalance of testosterone and estradiol.

In patients with a history of chronic alcohol abuse, liver function tests should be ordered. Their erectile function may not return even if they reduce their alcohol intake. Because this patient's increase in alcohol intake was fairly acute, his erectile function improved as soon as he began to drink less.

2. *How do you approach psychological erectile dysfunction?*

Despite the ubiquity of the psychological component in erectile dysfunction, there have been no controlled studies to show whether psychotherapy or counseling actually helps. Even assuming that such intervention would be helpful, there are no data on the best approach. Should patients receive behavioral therapy? Counseling? Is simply talking with the primary care physician sufficient?

The primary care physician should at least acknowledge psychological stress as a component of erectile dysfunction. Sometimes acknowledging the problem is enough; the patient just needs to talk about it. Sometimes further intervention is required. Whether this is provided by the primary care physician depends on his or her level of comfort with that aspect of treatment. As in this case, insurance coverage is often an important factor as well.

3. *What are the pharmacologic options for treatment?*

With a patient such as this man, whose erectile dysfunction appears largely psychogenic, occasionally a trial of **yohimbine**, an α_2-adrenergic antagonist, may increase intracavernosal blood flow. The drug often is not efficacious; however, it is inexpensive and has virtually no side effects aside from minimally lowering blood pressure in some cases. One older study showed that yohimbine was effective in 50% of men with psychogenic impotence; placebo was effective in 30% of cases. According to more recent studies, the effectiveness of yohimbine may be improved by combining it with the serotonin agonist trazodone.

The options for treatment of erectile dysfunction have radically changed with the introduction of **sildenafil**, the first truly effective oral medication for this condition.

Advances in our knowledge of the physiology of erection have facilitated understanding of the pharmacodynamics of sildenafil. Erection is initiated by dilation of the arterial bed, which increases blood flow and pressure; it is maintained by restriction of venous outflow. Previously it was believed that the parasympathetic system was critical in maintaining erection. Now, we know that the major player is the nonadrenergic, noncholinergic (NA-NC) system, which was identified 50 years ago, but never studied in detail until relatively recently. The NA-NC system uses nitric oxide as a neurotransmitter. Through its second messenger, cyclic guanine monophosphate (cGMP), nitric oxide triggers relaxation of penile endothelium and smooth muscle, allowing expansion of the lacunar spaces within the corpora and the trapping of blood by compression of peripheral draining venules.

Sildenafil, a type 5 phosphodiesterase inhibitor, prevents the breakdown of cGMP, thus prolonging erection. It has no effect on libido and it does not cause erection without stimulation, but it maintains an erection once it has been achieved. Although the NA-NC system is particularly prominent in the penis, it is also found in the heart, the brain, and other organs. Its presence in the eye explains the blue visual hue that some patients experience after taking sildenafil.

The most common side effects of sildenafil are headache, flushing, and dyspepsia. It can also decrease blood pressure. Because the decrease in blood pressure may be synergistic with the hypotensive action of nitrates, sildenafil is contraindicated in patients taking a medication that contains nitrates, such as nitroglycerin.

In addition, sildenafil alters the half-life of many other medications, and many medications change the half-life of sildenafil. The list of agents that can interact with sildenafil includes such common medications as nonselective β blockers, erythromycin, itraconazole, potassium-sparing diuretics, and cimetidine. It is not known whether those interactions affect the side effects of sildenafil, particularly the incidence or severity of hypotension. In initial clinical trials, hypotension was reported in approximately 3% of patients, but those trials included a large percentage of young men with psychogenic impotence. Obviously, patients with vascular disease or diabetes have more problems with blood pressure regulation and theoretically with orthostatic hypotension. Deaths have been reported among patients taking sildenafil since it became available. The FDA is investigating those deaths.

Evaluating sildenafil has been difficult because it is one of several drugs that have been approved since 1997 through a new FDA process. Previously, a drug was not approved until studies had been published. Now, the FDA allows pharmaceutical companies to submit unpublished studies. With this streamlined process, a drug can be approved before clinicians have the chance to read peer-reviewed data and decide whether their patients fall into the same category as patients in the initial studies. Instead, the physician has only the drug company brochure, which does not offer the detail of a peer-reviewed journal article.

The first study of data on different patient populations taking sildenafil was published several months after the drug became available for clinical use. Although the package insert indicated an overall efficacy of 82% (versus 24% for placebo), analysis showed that the efficacy was 68% in patients with hypertension, 57% in diabetes, and 61% after transurethral prostatectomy. Moreover, those results were obtained in a selected patient population, not from general clinical use.

Physicians need additional information from peer-reviewed studies so that they can assess the risk–benefit ratio of sildenafil and make rational treatment decisions in individual cases. Meanwhile, third-party payers are trying to decide whether they should reimburse the cost of the drug. Arguments against coverage include the fact that erectile dysfunction is not a life-threatening condition. Also, because many third-party payers do not pay for oral contraceptives for women, they believe that they should not reimburse for a drug that enhances sexual performance in men.

In any case, newspaper reports indicate that sales of sildenafil have slowed. The decrease has been attributed to refusals for insurance coverage and increasing reports of side effects. A human element may also be involved. For example, in several studies of penile prostheses, patient interviews confirmed that the prostheses functioned well, but interviews with the patients' wives revealed that the patients were not using it. Similar findings have been reported in studies of other treatments for erectile dysfunction; the actual frequency of use is much less than that initially described by the patient. The ability to have sex is only one element in a complicated equation that determines whether or how often a patient has sexual relations.

Future Possibilities

Other oral agents for erectile dysfunction are undergoing clinical trials and should soon be available. Apomorphine, an opiate antagonist, has shown up to 70% efficacy in patients with psychogenic impotence; it will probably be available for clinical use by late 1999. Also under FDA review is an oral preparation of phentolamine. This agent blocks norepinephrine, causing smooth muscle relaxation and vasodilation. In preliminary studies, it was effective in 60% to 80% of patients and had fewer side effects than sildenafil.

For patients using intracavernosal injection, a combination of vasoactive intestinal peptide and phentolamine is under investigation. Both agents are smooth muscle relaxants, and vasoactive intestinal peptide appears to increase production of nitric oxide.

4 Gastroenterology

William R. Brown

Chronic Inflammatory Bowel Disease

1. What is the pathogenesis responsible for chronic ulcerative colitis (CUC) and Crohn's disease?
2. Compare and contrast the principal clinical features of CUC and Crohn's disease.
3. What are the respective risks of intestinal malignancy in CUC and Crohn's disease?
4. What are the principal medical therapeutic measures used for patients with CUC and Crohn's disease?

Discussion

1. *What is the pathogenesis responsible for CUC and Crohn's disease?*

   The cause and pathogenesis of both these chronic inflammatory bowel diseases (CIBDs) are unknown. Both are characterized by a chronic inflammatory cell infiltrate of the bowel. However, whereas CUC is restricted to the colon, Crohn's disease can involve the entire alimentary tract from the mouth to the anus, although the distal ileum and colon are the portions most frequently affected. Another distinguishing feature of Crohn's disease is the involvement of all layers of the bowel, whereas the inflammation seen in CUC is mostly limited to the mucosa. In addition, focal granulomas are common in Crohn's disease but rare in CUC. However, neither disease has pathognomonic features, and Crohn's disease of the colon cannot be histologically distinguished from CUC in 15% to 25% of cases of chronic colitis.

2. *Compare and contrast the principal clinical features of CUC and Crohn's disease.*

Both CUC and Crohn's disease are widely variable in terms of the severity, clinical course, and prognosis. Onset in both occurs most often in early adulthood. The symptoms of CUC may range from slight rectal bleeding to fulminant diarrhea with colonic hemorrhage and hypotension. Most patients have intermittent attacks, although some can have continuous symptoms without remission. The clinical features of Crohn's disease depend on the severity and location of the bowel involvement; the principal features are diarrhea, abdominal pain, hematochezia, intestinal obstruction, fissures, and fistulas.

Extraintestinal manifestations are common in both Crohn's disease and CUC, but more common in CUC. The manifestations include arthritis, arthralgia, iritis, uveitis, liver disease, and skin lesions. The arthritis may present as a migratory arthritis, involving large joints, sacroiliitis, or ankylosing spondylitis. Primary sclerosing cholangitis, which is associated with an increased frequency of cholangiocarcinoma, and chronic hepatitis are common hepatobiliary abnormalities.

The principal features that differentiate Crohn's disease from CUC are listed in Table 4-1.

Table 4-1. Features that Distinguish between Crohn's Disease and Ulcerative Colitis

Factors	Crohn's disease	Ulcerative colitis
Pathologic Features	Transmural inflammation Deep ulcers Granulomas common	Mucosal inflammation Superficial ulcers Granulomas absent
Distribution	Mouth to anus (ileum and proximal colon most common)	Colon
Clinical Features		
Rectal bleeding	20%–40%	98%
Fulminating episodes	Uncommon	Common
Obstruction	Common	Rare
Fistulas	Common	Rare
Perianal disease	Common	Less common
Sigmoidoscopic and Radiographic Findings		
Rectal involvement	50%	95%–100%
Extent	Patchy	Continuous
Ulcers	Longitudinal, deep	Shallow, collar button
Pseudopolyps	Uncommon	Common
Strictures	Common	Uncommon
Ileal involvement	Narrowed lumen with thickened wall	Dilated lumen with diminished folds but histologically normal

From Schaefer J, Mallory A. Gastrointestinal disease. In: Schrier RW, ed. *Medicine: diagnosis and treatment.* Boston: Little, Brown, 1988.

3. *What are the respective risks of intestinal malignancy in CUC and Crohn's disease?*

The frequency of intestinal cancer is increased in Crohn's disease, but not to the extent it is in CUC. According to some reports, the frequency of colon cancer in adults who have CUC involving the entire colon is approximately 25 times greater than that in the general population. The risk of colon cancer developing in patients with CUC is positively correlated with the extent and duration of the disease.

4. *What are the principal medical therapeutic measures used for patients with CUC and Crohn's disease?*

The **general measures** to control the symptoms of both diseases include correction of fluid–electrolyte imbalances; iron, folate, or vitamin B_{12} supplementation as needed for the treatment of anemia; and dietary adjustments aimed at maintaining adequate nutrition. **Total parenteral nutrition** may be required for the short-term treatment of severe acute disease, but "bowel rest" and hyperalimentation are of dubious value in the long term. **Antidiarrheal agents** such as loperamide are usually contraindicated in patients with CUC because they may contribute to the development of toxic megacolon, but they may help alleviate the diarrhea and abdominal cramps in the setting of stable Crohn's disease.

In CUC, **corticosteroids** are useful for inducing remissions or improvement in an acute attack, and they may be required for long-term management. However, the possible benefits of corticosteroids in the long term are offset by their many adverse side effects. The rectal administration of steroids can be beneficial, especially when rectal involvement (proctitis) is severe. Significant absorption of rectal steroids can occur, however, so systemic effects of the agents (both beneficial and undesirable) may arise when they are given by this route. **Sulfasalazine** is metabolized by colonic bacteria, releasing sulfapyridine and 5-aminosalicylate (5-ASA); the latter is believed to be the active compound. Sulfapyridine is absorbed systemically, which accounts for the side effects of sulfasalazine (e.g., headache, occasional megaloblastic anemia, skin rash). The greatest utility of sulfasalazine in patients with CUC is in long-term management, where it has been proved to reduce the frequency of relapses. 5-ASA, given rectally by enema or suppository, is well tolerated and effective. Given orally, 5-ASA is rapidly denatured by gastric acid, so alternatives to plain 5-ASA, such as microencapsulated (Pentasa; Hoechst Marion Roussel, Kansas City, MO) or acrylic-based resin-coated (Asacol; Procter & Gamble Pharmaceutical, Norwich, NY) forms of 5-ASA, may be used. Because the relative risk for development of CUC is greater in nonsmokers than in smokers (the opposite is true in Crohn's disease), nicotine is being tried in the treatment of CUC; some benefit has been reported, but additional research is needed.

There is no uniformly effective treatment available for Crohn's disease. However, corticosteroids have documented efficacy in diminishing the activity of the disease process. Sulfasalazine has some effectiveness, especially in colonic Crohn's disease, but is less effective than corticosteroids. Metronidazole may be at least as effective as sulfasalazine. When Crohn's disease cannot be controlled by these medications, the immunosuppressive agent azathioprine and its metabolite 6-mercaptopurine are sometimes tried; their use can result in a reduction in the corticosteroid dose needed, but this advantage may be offset by their toxic effects.

Case

A 37-year-old man with documented CUC was first seen at 19 years of age because of severe bloody diarrhea and left lower quadrant abdominal pain that necessitated hospitalization. After 10 days of treatment with high-dose prednisone and sulfasalazine, his symptoms were controlled, and he has since been managed with these medicines, with the dosages adjusted depending on his disease activity. He has not required corticosteroids except for flare-ups of disease. Subsequent to his initial presentation, after his disease activity had subsided, he underwent colonoscopy for histologic confirmation of the disease and to determine the extent of intestinal involvement; this examination revealed diffuse mucosal inflammation involving the entire colon (pancolitis). The terminal ileum appeared normal. Colonic biopsy specimens revealed a diffuse mucosal inflammatory infiltrate with little involvement of the submucosa, acute and chronic inflammatory cells, and frequent crypt abscesses but no granulomas.

The patient went on to graduate from college and was then hired as a sales representative for a pharmaceutical company. Because his disease has been quiescent, and because of a busy schedule, he has not taken his medications regularly and has rarely seen his physician.

Approximately 2 months ago, he began to feel tired, and intermittent rectal bleeding developed. His physical examination findings are unremarkable, but the fecal occult blood test is positive. The hemoglobin is 11 g/dL; hematocrit, 33%; and leukocyte count, 7,700 cells/mm^3, with a normal differential count.

1. What is your differential diagnosis of his recent symptoms?
2. What tests are necessary to make the correct diagnosis?
3. How should this patient's CUC have been managed over the previous 18 years?

Case Discussion

1. *What is your differential diagnosis of his recent symptoms?*

The differential diagnosis in this patient includes three possibilities. First, this episode could be an acute flare-up or exacerbation of his ulcerative colitis. Second, he could have an acute, self-limited colitis superimposed on his ulcerative colitis; infection with *Campylobacter*, *Salmonella*, or *Shigella* species, or with parasites can cause such a colitis. Third, the rectal bleeding and anemia could be the result of adenocarcinoma.

2. *What tests are necessary to make the correct diagnosis?*

Stool cultures and the examination of stool for ova and parasites would be an important initial laboratory test in this patient. These all proved to be negative.

Flexible sigmoidoscopy with the acquisition of biopsy specimens is also an important diagnostic procedure. In contrast to CIBD, the histologic features of acute self-limited colitis consist of normal crypt architecture and an acute but not chronic inflammatory infiltrate in the lamina propria. Inflammation is more likely to be found in the upper mucosa in acute colitis, and in the crypt bases in CIBD. When an acute self-limited colitis, such as infection with *Campylobacter jejuni, Salmonella,* or *Shigella,* resolves, the mucosa is normal, whereas crypt distortion and atrophy are often seen in the setting of healed CIBD. In other acute colitides, the histologic features found in mucosal biopsy specimens may suggest a specific infection; these include viral inclusions, parasites, or pseudomembranes.

In this patient, flexible sigmoidoscopy was performed to a depth of 30 cm and revealed a very mild granularity of the mucosa without bleeding, although some blood was seen coming from above 30 cm. Active CUC almost always involves the rectum, so the finding of only mild changes in this patient's rectum suggests that the significant pathologic process was higher in the colon. A colonoscopic examination showed a sessile, fungating mass in the descending colon, which proved to be an adenocarcinoma.

3. *How should this patient's CUC have been managed over the previous 18 years?*

There is not yet agreement on the most cost-effective approach for the surveillance for colonic cancer in patients with CUC. However, after a patient has had extensive disease for 8 to 10 years, it is probably wise to perform complete colonoscopy every 1 to 2 years, with multiple biopsy specimens obtained every 10 to 12 cm from normal-appearing mucosa and targeted specimens obtained from villous areas of mucosa, areas of ulceration with a raised edge, and strictures. Colectomy is recommended if multifocal or high-grade dysplasia is seen in the biopsy specimens and confirmed by an experienced pathologist. If a mass lesion associated with any degree of dysplasia is identified, this is also a generally accepted indication for colectomy. The management of persistent low-grade dysplasia without a mass is more controversial, however (Fig. 4-1).

Cancer prevention is an important topic to consider when advising young patients with extensive colitis about the possible need for surgical treatment. The decision to recommend prophylactic proctocolectomy after many years of colitis must be based on several considerations in the individual patient. These include the intractability of symptoms, age, psychological makeup, medical compliance, and the availability of newer surgical procedures. A prophylactic colectomy should be recommended to a noncompliant patient who acquires extensive ulcerative colitis at a young age. Patients who have CUC should be fully informed of their risk for development of cancer, as well

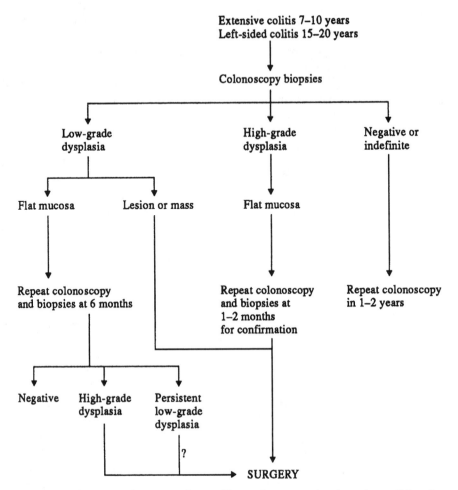

Figure 4-1. A proposed system of surveillance for cancer in ulcerative colitis using colonoscopy and biopsy. (Adapted from Lennard-Jones J, Ritchie J, Morson B, Williams C. Cancer surveillance in ulcerative colitis. *Lancet* 1983;2:149.)

as the limitations of endoscopic surveillance and the availability of surgical alternatives. If a patient is unwilling to assent to the surgical procedure, then he or she must be committed to undergoing regular surveillance.

Suggested Readings

Jewell DP. Ulcerative colitis. In: Feldman M, Scharschmidt BF, Sleisenger MH, eds. *Sleisenger and Fordtran's gastrointestinal and liver disease: pathophysiology, diagnosis, management,* 6th ed. Philadelphia: WB Saunders, 1998:1735.

Stenson WF, MacDermott RP. Inflammatory bowel disease. In: Yamada T, Alpers D, Owyang C, Powell DW, Silverstein FE, eds. *Textbook of gastroenterology,* 2nd ed. Philadelphia: JB Lippincott, 1995:1748.

Chronic Liver Disease

1. What are some specific causes of chronic liver disease?
2. What are the principal laboratory abnormalities in the setting of chronic liver disease?
3. What are the two major histologic categories of chronic hepatitis due to viral infection?

Discussion

1. *What are some specific causes of chronic liver disease?*

    Chronic liver disease may be the sequela of several kinds of toxic, metabolic, infectious, immunologic, or hereditary conditions. The following is a partial list (asterisk [*] indicates most frequently encountered):

    Drugs and chemicals
        Acetaminophen
        Alcohol*
        Amiodarone
        Arsenic and inorganic salts
        Isoniazid
        Nitrofurantoin
        Propylthiouracil
        Vinyl chloride
    Viral hepatitis
        Hepatitis B and C (non-A, non-B)*
        Cytomegalovirus
    Granulomatous infections
        Bacterial (tuberculosis), spirochetal (secondary syphilis), mycotic*
        Drugs and foreign substances
        Other
        Sarcoidosis
    Primary biliary cirrhosis
    Disorders in immunity
    Complications of ulcerative colitis and Crohn's disease (primary biliary cirrhosis and pericholangitis)*
        Primary biliary cirrhosis*
        Autoimmune chronic hepatitis*
    Inherited diseases
        Wilson's disease*
        Hemochromatosis*
        Inborn errors of metabolism (glycogen storage disease and Gaucher's disease)
        α_1-Antitrypsin deficiency

2. *What are the principal laboratory abnormalities in the setting of chronic liver disease?*

The clinically available liver function tests include those that assess, at least in part, liver synthetic function (serum albumin and bilirubin concentrations, and prothrombin time) and those that mostly evaluate the hepatocellular release of enzymes (aminotransferases and alkaline phosphatase). The aminotransferase [alanine aminotransferase (ALT), aspartate aminotransferase (AST), and alkaline phosphatase] levels often are not markedly elevated in patients with chronic liver disease, and consequently do not accurately predict prognosis. The serum albumin and bilirubin concentrations and the prothrombin time are more likely to be distinctly abnormal, and more accurately reflect the true status of the liver's functional capacity.

3. *What are the two major histologic categories of chronic hepatitis due to viral infection?*

In the past, chronic viral hepatitides were classified as chronic persistent hepatitis, which was regarded as a nonprogressive disease, and chronic active hepatitis, a disease of more severe hepatocellular necrosis and fibrosis that often progressed to cirrhosis. A newer classification of these diseases, constructed by international committees, consists of three components: the etiology of the diseases, grading of disease activity (i.e., the severity of the necroinflammatory process), and staging of the disease (i.e., the degree of fibrosis subsequent to necroinflammatory insults). The grading and staging usually are given a semiquantitative score (0 to 4) or a descriptive characterization (e.g., minimal to severe inflammation, or no fibrosis to cirrhosis).

Case

A 60-year-old man is brought to the hospital by his wife because he has not been acting his usual self. For the past 3 days, he has not been sleeping at night and has been napping during the day. There is no history of recent trauma, new medications, or suicidal ideation. He has been taking diazepam, 5 mg nightly, for insomnia. Risk factors for chronic liver disease, according to his wife, include the consumption of two beers nightly for 35 years and a blood transfusion for the treatment of a bleeding peptic ulcer 25 years ago. Past history is remarkable only for an "ulcer operation" 25 years ago.

On physical examination, he appears sleepy but arousable. The vital signs are normal. Several large spider angiomas are present on the torso. There is no scleral icterus. The parotid glands are enlarged bilaterally, and wasting of the temporal muscles is noted. The heart and lung examination findings are normal. His abdomen is slightly distended, and shifting dullness and a midline scar are present. The liver is not palpable below the right costal margin but is palpable 10 cm below the xiphoid process; it is firm and percussed to a span of 8 cm in the right mid-clavicular line. The spleen is palpable. The abdomen is not tender to palpation or percussion. The testes are small. The rectum is found to contain hard, brown stool, which is positive for occult blood. There is mild edema of the legs and moderate muscle wasting. Asterixis is present. The cranial nerves and deep tendon reflexes are intact. The patient is somewhat uncooperative but his muscular strength is not focally diminished; his plantar reflexes (Babinski) are normal.

Laboratory data are as follows: peripheral blood white cell count, 2,500 cells/mm³; hemoglobin, 10 g/dL; hematocrit, 33%; platelet count, 125,000/mm³; serum AST, 100 IU/L (normal, <30 IU/L); ALT, 80 IU/L (normal, <645 IU/L); total bilirubin, 1.2 mg/dL; alkaline phosphatase, 150 IU/L (normal, <130 IU/L); total protein, 8.0 g/dL; albumin, 3.1 g/dL; and prothrombin time, 13 seconds (control, 11 seconds).

1. What features help you to diagnose chronic, versus acute, liver disease in this patient?
2. Does any particular factor help you determine the cause of this man's liver disease?
3. What reversible factors could be contributing to this man's presumed portosystemic encephalopathy (PSE)?
4. When, if ever, should this man's ascites be sampled? If it should, how and where should it be sampled?
5. What are three possible explanations for the occult blood in his stool?
6. What is the serum–ascites albumin gradient, and of what value is it?
7. Would you start diuretic therapy now? Why or why not?
8. Why are his testes small?
9. Why are his parotid glands enlarged?
10. Is this man at increased risk for hepatocellular carcinoma?
11. How could you exclude hepatocellular carcinoma?
12. What is included in your differential diagnosis of this man's chronic liver disease?
13. Why is hepatitis A not in your differential diagnosis?

The results of additional tests are available within 4 hours of admission. The ascites is sampled from a left lower quadrant paracentesis, yielding a clear yellow fluid with a white blood cell count of 380 cells/mm³, 2% polymorphonuclear leukocytes, an albumin concentration of 0.5 g/dL, and a total protein level of 1 g/dL. No organisms are seen on Gram-stained specimens.

14. Do the findings from the additional tests on the ascitic fluid support the diagnosis of portal hypertension-associated ascites? Why or why not?
15. With these data in mind, what treatment would you offer this patient now, and why?
16. What areas of the patient's history should you examine at greater length, and why?
17. Would you offer this patient a liver biopsy and, if so, when?

Case Discussion

1. *What features help you to diagnose chronic, versus acute, liver disease in this patient?*

In this patient, there are no pathognomonic features of chronic liver disease, but several that suggest this condition. **Large spider angiomas** are common in the setting of chronic liver disease, but not acute liver disease, although small, nonpalpable spider angiomas may be present. **Muscle wasting** is common in moderately advanced chronic liver disease, but is not due to poor eating habits. Muscle wasting is not a feature of acute liver disease unless it is the result of a concomitant, unrelated problem. A **palpable, firm left lobe of the liver** (that portion palpable caudad to the xiphoid process) is usually a manifestation of chronic liver disease. It is always important to palpate and percuss for the liver in the midline, as well as in the mid-clavicular line. **Ascites**, due to portal hypertension, is much more a feature of chronic liver disease than of any other disorder. Ascites may occur in the setting of severe acute liver disease, but is usually not of significant quantity to warrant treatment. One notable exception is the Budd-Chiari syndrome, in which there may be ascites, although the abdominal distention in this syndrome is partially due to a congested and enlarged liver stemming from the hepatic vein occlusion. **Shifting dullness** is indicative of a large amount (>1.0 to 1.5 L) of ascites.

Pancytopenia is related to the splenic sequestration of blood cells and is not a prominent feature of liver disease unless the spleen is affected; when it is, it is usually enlarged. The degree of pancytopenia (or of individual cytopenias) may not correlate with spleen size. Hepatitis C may be associated with the development of aplastic anemia, but this is rare. However, the depression is usually transient and not a severe problem. Transient cytopenias may be seen in hepatitis, as in other viral infections. A **low serum albumin** level may be seen in any form of liver disease that has lasted for more than several weeks. A **high serum globulin** (total protein-albumin) level is a feature of chronic liver disease regardless of the cause. Extremely high serum globulin levels (i.e., ≥ 10 g/dL) should suggest the possibility of autoimmune or "lupoid" hepatitis; this disorder is usually seen in women and is frequently accompanied by other autoimmune features, such as thyroiditis and autoimmune hepatitis. Autoimmune hepatitis is important to recognize because it can usually be treated with corticosteroids.

2. *Does any particular factor help you determine the cause of this man's liver disease?*

There are no particular factors that point to the cause of this patient's liver disease. The major differential diagnoses here are alcoholic liver disease and chronic active hepatitis, probably in the cirrhotic stage. No feature of his history, physical examination, or routine laboratory tests helps distinguish between these two causes.

3. *What reversible factors could be contributing to this man's presumed PSE?*

Benzodiazepines, other sedative or hypnotic drugs, and opiates may precipitate PSE in a patient with severely impaired hepatic function. **Constipation** may also precipitate PSE in susceptible patients because of the colonic absorption of nitrogenous products. Both these reversible risk factors are present in this patient. Other reversible factors contributing to an episode of PSE include

electrolyte disturbances, notably hypokalemia and metabolic alkalosis; **increased intestinal absorption of nitrogenous products**, resulting from relatively excessive dietary protein intake or an upper gastrointestinal (GI) hemorrhage; and a **serious infection** of any nature. In patients with chronic liver disease who have acute PSE, thorough culture of the body fluids—ascitic fluid, blood, urine, and sputum—should be carried out. This patient's PSE indicates he has severe liver disease.

4. *When, if ever, should this man's ascites be sampled? If it should, how and where should it be sampled?*

    Diagnostic paracentesis should be performed as soon as possible to determine whether the patient has subacute bacterial peritonitis. This form of infectious peritonitis is a frequent cause of clinical deterioration in patients with chronic liver disease, and may be fatal if not recognized and treated early.

    The three safest locations for paracentesis are the left lower quadrant, right lower quadrant, and the infraumbilical midline area. A supraumbilical approach should never be used because the umbilical or paraumbilical vessels, which course just under the parietal peritoneum, are frequently recanalized in patients with portal hypertension whose portal vein is patent. It is also important always to stay clear of (medial or lateral to) the rectus muscles because the superficial epigastric vessels course under them and may be punctured. Last, skin puncture through or near an abdominal scar in a patient with suspected or known portal hypertension should always be avoided.

5. *What are three possible explanations for the occult blood in his stool?*

    The three possible explanations for the occult blood in this patient's stool are (a) portal hypertensive gastropathy or enteropathy, (b) rectal varices, and (c) esophageal variceal hemorrhage due to portal hypertension, which is usually a sudden event of large volume, although uncommonly varices "ooze."

6. *What is the serum–ascites albumin gradient, and of what value is it?*

    The serum–ascites albumin gradient is the numeric difference (not ratio) between the serum albumin concentration and the ascites albumin concentration. Studies have shown that when the gradient is 1.1 or greater, portal hypertension is contributing to or entirely causing the ascites. The two main causes of ascites to consider in this patient are portal hypertension and peritoneal malignancy. Determination of the serum–ascites albumin difference is a simple, minimally invasive, and fairly accurate way to diagnose portal hypertension.

7. *Would you start diuretic therapy now? Why or why not?*

    No. Diuretics are not essential now, and they may only worsen the PSE and increase the risk of hepatorenal syndrome.

8. *Why are his testes small?*

    In the setting of hepatic disease, the production of estrone from circulating androstenedione may be increased. The exact cause of this conversion is unknown but may be related to the decreased clearance of androstenedione by the liver. The consumption of excessive amounts of ethanol also may have contributed to the testicular atrophy in this patient.

9. *Why are his parotid glands enlarged?*

Parotid enlargement is seen in people who ingest excessive amounts of ethanol, and is associated with fatty infiltration of the glands. A similar situation may be seen in diabetic patients.

10. *Is this man at increased risk for hepatocellular carcinoma?*

Yes. There is a risk for the development of hepatocellular carcinoma in the setting of any form of cirrhotic liver, which this man most likely has. Certain conditions are associated with higher risks than others. Those associated with highest risk are genetic hemochromatosis, chronic hepatitis B, chronic hepatitis C, and alcoholic liver disease.

11. *How could you exclude hepatocellular carcinoma?*

The tests for excluding the existence of hepatocellular carcinoma are an imaging test [ultrasound or computed tomography (CT)] and a serum α-fetoprotein level. The preferred imaging test (to exclude a focal lesion) depends on the expertise at the institution. The serum α-fetoprotein level is very high in 60% of patients with alcoholic liver disease who have a superimposed hepatocellular carcinoma and in approximately 80% to 90% of patients with chronic hepatitis B who have this complication.

12. *What is included in your differential diagnosis of this man's chronic liver disease?*

The differential diagnosis in this patient includes alcoholic liver disease and chronic active hepatitis with cirrhosis, due to either hepatitis B or C, although hepatitis should be regarded as the more likely diagnosis. The hepatitis viruses may have been transmitted to him by the blood he received many years ago, or they may have been "sporadically" acquired.

13. *Why is hepatitis A not in your differential diagnosis?*

Hepatitis A has never been reported to cause chronic liver disease.

14. *Do the findings from the additional tests on the ascitic fluid support the diagnosis of portal hypertension-associated ascites? Why or why not?*

Yes, the findings from the tests on the ascitic fluid do support the diagnosis of portal hypertension-associated ascites because the serum–ascites albumin gradient (2.6) exceeds 1.1. There are two caveats to remember when using the serum–ascites albumin gradient in the diagnosis of ascites. First, if massive hepatic metastases cause enough liver disease to result in portal hypertension and ascites, the gradient resembles that seen in portal hypertension. Second, in ascites of mixed etiology (e.g., portal hypertension plus tuberculous peritonitis), the gradient usually resembles that seen in the setting of portal hypertension.

15. *With these data in mind, what treatment would you offer this patient now, and why?*

Hospital admission is required. Strict bed rest (for fear of self-harm) seems prudent. No benzodiazepines should be administered, although the patient should be monitored for the signs of ethanol withdrawal—agitation, tachycardia, fever, and hallucinosis. The patient should receive an enema if he is constipated. Lactulose should also be administered (by mouth or nasogastric tube) if the patient becomes too disoriented and uncooperative. The oral or nasogastric lactulose dose is variable, but the goal of therapy is to produce two to three soft stools per day. Alternatively, a nonabsorbable antibiotic could be used, such as neomycin at a dosage of 500 to 1,000 mg given orally or by nasogastric tube every 6 hours. There is no evidence that giving both medications together (lactulose and neomycin) is more effective than administering either alone. Lactulose is probably beneficial in the treatment of PSE by virtue of its ability to decrease the amount of nitrogen available for absorption (as urea) from the colon. Lactulose may accomplish this by altering the colonic flora to more urease-negative forms and by inducing an osmotic diarrhea.

16. *What areas of the patient's history should you examine at greater length, and why?*

One area of the patient's history that should be examined at greater length is his **ethanol consumption history**. This involves interviewing more of his family and friends. The alleged amount of ethanol ingested (per the patient's wife) is too low to cause liver disease in men because the alcohol content of two cans of beer is approximately 12 g. However, the parotid gland enlargement and testicular atrophy are findings that suggest his ethanol ingestion has been more than he has admitted. The amount and duration of alcohol ingestion necessary to cause chronic liver disease is highly variable among individuals, although the incidence of biopsy-proved cirrhosis, alcoholic hepatitis, or both, increases as consumption is increased. It is usually believed that the threshold amount of alcohol consumption that leads to these serious forms of chronic liver disease is on the order of 100 to 150 g per day for several years in men, but less in women. However, a large proportion of heavy drinkers do not contract serious liver diseases. It is advisable to record alcohol consumption in terms of grams per day times the number of years of consumption. A quart of 80 proof whiskey contains approximately 300 g of ethanol, a six-pack of 4% beer approximately 75 g, and 750 mL of wine approximately 90 g (150 g for "fortified" wine).

A second area of inquiry should be the patient's **family history**. In this patient, you should also ask whether anyone in the family has had liver disease, including genetic hemochromatosis. You might phrase the question in this way: "Do you have any family members who have conditions that require blood to be removed as treatment?" The manifestations of hemochromatosis may differ in various family members, and may consist of cardiomyopathy, diabetes, arthritis, or pituitary insufficiency. In this patient, the small liver is inconsistent with a diagnosis of hemochromatosis, although all else is. Moreover, he is an older man—the typical age and sex of patients who have severe chronic liver disease caused by hemochromatosis.

17. *Would you offer this patient a liver biopsy, and, if so, when?*

A liver biopsy would be of no help in the initial management of his decompensated liver disease. However, when conclusive documentation of the diagnosis would help determine management, liver biopsy might be important.

This might be the case in a patient with suspected Budd-Chiari syndrome because this is often treatable by hepatic decompression (as, for example, with a side-to-side portacaval anastomosis), or it might be the case in a patient with hemochromatosis. Once the patient's condition has stabilized, a liver biopsy might be offered, for three reasons. First, he may be a candidate for specific therapy. However, it is unlikely that there is any therapy for this patient because there is no effective treatment for alcoholic liver disease other than abstinence. In addition, interferon treatment may be dangerous in patients with advanced chronic hepatitis because of the hepatocytolysis brought about by therapy. Second, some authorities believe that liver biopsy is indicated in patients with suspected alcoholic liver disease because confirmation of that diagnosis might help persuade the patient to abstain from further ethanol ingestion. Third, if the patient becomes a candidate for hepatic transplantation, most centers require a definitive preoperative diagnosis before proceeding with the procedure.

Suggested Readings

Bacon BR, Tavill AS. Hemachromatosis and the iron overload syndromes. In: Zakim D, Boyer TD, eds. *Hepatology: a textbook of liver disease*, 3rd ed. Philadelphia: WB Saunders, 1996:1439.

Batts KP, Ludwig J. Chronic hepatitis: an update on terminology and reporting. *Am J Pathol* 1995;19:1409.

Bisceglie AM, Hoofnagle JH. Chronic viral hepatitis. In: Zakim D, Boyer TD, eds. *Hepatology: a textbook of liver disease*, 3rd ed. Philadelphia: WB Saunders, 1996:1299.

Diehl AM. Liver disease in the alcoholic: clinical aspects. In: Zakim D, Boyer TD, eds. *Hepatology: a textbook of liver disease*, 3rd ed. Philadelphia: WB Saunders, 1996:1050.

Diarrhea

1. What is the diagnostic importance of nocturnal diarrhea in a patient with chronic diarrhea?
2. What is the difference between a secretory and an osmotic diarrhea?
3. What happens to diarrheal stool volume after fasting in the following settings: a vasoactive intestinal peptide (VIP) tumor, the abrupt onset of watery diarrhea after traveling outside of the United States, and diarrhea only when drinking large amounts of carbonated beverages?
4. What is the most likely cause of diarrhea in a patient who has recently taken ampicillin and who then has low-grade fever and watery diarrhea? What is the most cost-effective way to diagnose this disease, and how would you treat this patient?
5. Why do patients with giardiasis often complain of increased stool volume and abdominal cramping when they consume milk products?
6. What are the organisms most commonly associated with diarrhea of less than 2 to 3 weeks' duration, and what are their clinical characteristics? How are such cases evaluated, and what are the various approaches to treatment?
7. What is the utility of staining stool specimens for leukocytes?

8. What would the clinician look for if surreptitious laxative abuse is suspected as a cause of chronic diarrhea?

9. A 24-year-old woman who has had a recurring rectovaginal fistula for 2 years complains of frequent small-volume stools, which occasionally contain blood and mucus. Stool cultures yield negative findings. What is the likely disease in this woman with a rectovaginal fistula, and what would be the next step in evaluating this patient?

Discussion

1. *What is the diagnostic importance of nocturnal diarrhea in a patient with chronic diarrhea?*

   Nocturnal diarrhea suggests an organic cause of the diarrhea. Patients with irritable bowel syndrome or other "functional" diarrheas rarely have diarrhea that awakens them from sleep.

2. *What is the difference between a secretory and an osmotic diarrhea?*

   Secretory diarrhea is due to the active secretion of water and electrolytes into the intestinal lumen. The mechanism of action responsible for the release of the secretagogues is variable. For instance, the diarrhea of cholera, the classic example of a secretory diarrhea, is caused by the stimulation of adenylate cyclase activity by cholera toxin; this, in turn, causes an increase in the intracellular concentration of cyclic adenosine monophosphate, which both stimulates electrogenic chloride secretion and inhibits electroneutral sodium chloride absorption. Increases in intracellular concentrations of Ca^{2+} as well as cyclic guanosine monophosphate have been proposed as the abnormalities at work in various other forms of secretory diarrhea.

   In **osmotic diarrhea**, an unabsorbable solute (often a carbohydrate or divalent mineral) increases the osmolality of the intestinal contents. This increased osmolality passively "drags" water into the intestinal lumen. Patients with osmotic diarrhea usually have a measured stool osmolality that is much greater than that yielded by the equation: $2 \times$ serum Na^+ + serum K^+; this condition constitutes an osmotic gap. A common osmotic diarrhea is that which occurs after the ingestion of milk or milk products in people who are deficient in the intestinal enzyme lactase.

3. *What happens to diarrheal stool volume after fasting in the following settings: a VIP tumor, the abrupt onset of watery diarrhea after traveling outside of the United States, or diarrhea only when drinking large amounts of carbonated beverages?*

   Vasoactive intestinal peptide is produced by the intestinal mucosa in increased amounts in the WDHA (*w*atery *d*iarrhea, *h*ypokalemia, and *a*chlorhydria) syndrome. VIP causes diarrhea by stimulating mucosal adenylate cyclase activity, and therefore would be expected to cause a secretory diarrhea. In such a condition, fasting would not change the stool volume until the patient becomes severely dehydrated.

   Travelers' diarrhea is watery and usually occurs within 3 to 6 days after arriving in another country, or on return. Symptoms typically last for 2 to 3 days. Hospitalization is rarely required, and treatment is largely supportive. The most common pathogens responsible are the enterotoxigenic strains of *Escherichia coli*, which can elaborate heat-labile and heat-stable enterotoxins. The heat-labile toxin acts similarly to cholera toxin, whereas the heat-stable toxin stimulates mucosal guanylate cyclase activity. Other types of diarrhea-producing *E. coli* and their associated symptoms are the enteropathogenic type, which causes watery diarrhea, predominantly in children and newborns; the enteroinvasive type, which causes bloody diarrhea (dysentery) in children and adults, usually after the ingestion of contaminated food and water; and the enterohemorrhagic type, which causes bloody diarrhea in people of all ages and is transmitted in contaminated food (often poorly cooked hamburger). Serotype 0157:H7 of the enterohemorrhagic type has been identified in several outbreaks of infection characterized by particularly severe disease (hemolytic uremic syndrome).

Other pathogens associated with travelers' diarrhea include *Shigella* and *Salmonella* species, *C. jejuni*, and *Vibrio parahaemolyticus*. Because of the numerous causes of traveler's diarrhea, the effect of fasting is usually unpredictable.

The osmotic diarrhea that occurs only after drinking large amounts of carbonated beverages is due to the ingestion of large amounts of fructose, which is the sugar used to sweeten these beverages (although not diet drinks) and comes in the form of corn syrup. Fructose is poorly absorbed by the proximal small intestinal mucosa. Cessation of fructose intake should cause the diarrhea to stop.

4. *What is the most likely cause of diarrhea in a patient who has recently taken ampicillin and who then has low-grade fever and watery diarrhea? What is the most cost-effective way to diagnose this disease, and how would you treat this patient?*

Pseudomembranous colitis (PMC) caused by *Clostridium difficile* is a likely diagnosis in this instance, given the patient's recent antibiotic use. The disease is usually self-limited, with the diarrhea dissipating 5 to 10 days after discontinuation of the offending antibiotic. Clindamycin was the first drug proved to cause PMC; later, ampicillin, because of its widespread use, was the drug most commonly implicated, but virtually any antibiotic can be responsible. In healthy adults, *C. difficile* colonization rates of 2% to 3% have been reported, whereas the rates in adults receiving antimicrobials but without diarrheal symptoms are as high as 10% to 15%.

The most commonly used method for diagnosing PMC is the cytotoxicity assay, which involves observation of the cytopathic effect produced by the toxin on a cell culture; it has a sensitivity of 95% to 97%. Although the latex agglutination test for the presence of toxin is both cheaper and faster to perform, it has a sensitivity of only approximately 85%. Gross colonic abnormalities in patients with PMC, which can be seen endoscopically, typically occur in the descending and sigmoid colon, making flexible sigmoidoscopy an adequate examination in most cases; however, cases with only right-sided involvement have been reported. The endoscopic findings in patients with PMC include erythematous, friable mucosa with characteristic pseudomembranes. Care must be taken to rule out bacterial or parasitic infections (especially *C. jejuni* and *Entamoeba histolytica*) and inflammatory bowel disease.

The recommended treatment for less severe cases of PMC consists of either oral metronidazole (250 mg four times a day) or vancomycin (125 to 500 mg four times a day). Parenteral doses of metronidazole [500 mg intravenously (IV) every 6 hours] should be given only when oral medication cannot be tolerated. The IV administration of vancomycin is not effective. The rates of relapse are similar for both metronidazole and vancomycin and range from 10% to 15%. Cholestyramine has been reported to be effective in the treatment of mild PMC or as an adjunctive measure, presumably by binding the toxin intraluminally. Cholestyramine may be used in conjunction with metronidazole but not with vancomycin, because it can bind and inactivate vancomycin.

5. *Why do patients with giardiasis often complain of increased stool volume and abdominal cramping when they consume milk products?*

Giardia lamblia infection causes a deficiency in the intestinal disaccharidases, including lactase. The disaccharidase deficiency can cause cramping and flatulence after the ingestion of carbohydrates, especially milk products.

6. *What are the organisms most commonly associated with diarrhea of less than 2 to 3 weeks' duration, and what are their clinical characteristics? How are such cases evaluated, and what are the various approaches to treatment?*

The evaluation of a case of acute diarrhea involves routine culture of the stools, examination of the stools for the presence of ova and parasites, and, in some instances, flexible sigmoidoscopy.

One of the **viral causes** of acute diarrhea is the Norwalk agent, which is seen in family and community epidemics, usually in older children and adults. It has an incubation period of 1 to 2 days. Vomiting and low-grade fever are common. Rotavirus infection is seen in infants and young children, primarily in winter; the incubation period is 1 to 3 days. Vomiting (occurring in 80%), upper respiratory symptoms, and fever (found in 30%) are common. Enteric adenovirus is a sporadic disease of infants and young children, and is often associated with fever and upper respiratory symptoms.

There are many **bacterial causes** of acute diarrhea. In *Shigella* infection, the major site of mucosal invasion is the colon. Penetration of the mucosa and invasion of the bloodstream are rare. Crampy abdominal pain and tenesmus are hallmarks of the disease. The organism elaborates an enterotoxin (Shiga toxin) that activates adenylate cyclase and causes a watery diarrhea in the early stages of the disease. Bloody diarrhea soon follows. The mainstay of therapy is supportive, with rehydration most important. Narcotics and anticholinergic medications should be avoided. Antibiotic treatment is reserved for those cases that do not resolve spontaneously in several days; ampicillin (500 mg four times a day, orally, for 5 days) is usually effective, but trimethoprim–sulfamethoxazole (one double-strength tablet twice daily) can be used for resistant strains. Chronic carriers, although uncommon, are prone to intermittent attacks of the disease.

The major site of *Salmonella* invasion is the ileal and sometimes the colonic mucosa. Bacteremia, with or without associated GI symptoms, occurs in approximately 10% of the cases. Carriers are usually asymptomatic, with the organism harbored in the gallbladder. Periumbilical pain and bloody diarrhea last approximately 5 days. Because antimicrobial treatment significantly increases the carrier rate, it is reserved for those cases that do not resolve spontaneously or for those patients who have an underlying predisposing condition.

C. jejuni is a common bacterial pathogen isolated from patients with acute bacillary diarrhea. Invasion of the mucosa occurs predominantly in the colon. Two features that may distinguish *C. jejuni* infection from other causes of bacterial diarrhea are (a) a prodrome of constitutional symptoms, and (b) a biphasic course, with initial improvement followed by worsening. No antibiotic regimen has been shown to lessen the symptoms or the time course of the disease.

Yersinia enterocolitica can cause enterocolitis, with a clinical picture consisting of fever, abdominal cramping, and bloody diarrhea lasting 1 to 3 weeks. Watery diarrhea is seen, possibly due to enterotoxin production. Invasive ileitis is also a feature of these infections.

Other diarrhea-producing enteric pathogens include *E. histolytica, G. lamblia,* and *Strongyloides stercoralis.*

7. *What is the utility of staining stool specimens for leukocytes?*

The presence of numerous leukocytes in stool specimens implies the existence of active inflammation of the intestinal mucosa. In cases of acute diarrhea, the presence of pus implies invasion (*Shigella, Salmonella, C. jejuni,* and *E. histolytica*), although *Shigella, E. histolytica,* and *C. jejuni* infections are usually associated with the most pus. Patients with PMC also often have large numbers of fecal leukocytes. In cases of chronic diarrhea, the presence of pus most often implies tuberculosis, amebic colitis, ischemic colitis, or inflammatory bowel disease (ulcerative colitis more so than Crohn's disease, unless the latter involves the colon).

8. *What would the clinician look for if surreptitious laxative abuse is suspected as a cause of chronic diarrhea?*

There are several tell-tale clues to surreptitious laxative abuse. Melanosis coli, a dark pigmentation of the colorectal mucosa, may exist if the diarrhea is due to long-standing use of anthracene laxatives (aloe and cascara). The pigmentation usually disappears within 12 months after discontinuation of the laxative. If the ingestion of phenolphthalein-containing laxatives is the cause of the diarrhea, alkalization of a stool specimen, by adding sodium hydroxide to it, turns it pink. (However, raising the pH too high results in loss of the color and hence a false-negative result.) An osmotic gap of the stool may be present if the ingestion of magnesium sulfate is the cause of the diarrhea. Sodium sulfate and phosphate, however, which cause an osmotic diarrhea due to the formation of the anions sulfate and phosphate, do not cause an osmotic gap, and should be suspected in someone who is thought to abuse laxatives but has an apparent secretory diarrhea.

9. *What is the likely disease in this woman with a rectovaginal fistula, and what would be the next step in evaluating this patient?*

Crohn's disease is the most common cause of rectovaginal fistulas in young women and must be considered in the evaluation of such fistulas. Small-volume, bloody diarrhea is suggestive of anorectal involvement. After routine stool culture and examination for ova and parasites, flexible sigmoidoscopy should be performed. In cases of Crohn's disease in which small bowel involvement is considered likely, a small bowel radiographic study might be next in order. In any event, cultures and tissue for histologic analysis should be obtained before empiric treatment with corticosteroids is instituted, to ensure that infectious colitis is not the cause.

Case A 32-year-old woman with a history of Crohn's disease since childhood complains of having 10 to 12 loose, frothy, burning bowel movements. Blood is occasionally intermixed in the stool. The increased stool frequency has been a problem ever since her most recent hospitalization for the treatment of small bowel obstruction, 5 weeks previously. At that time, the remaining 120 cm of her ileum and 100 cm of her jejunum were resected because of fistulization and the formation of adhesions. She denies having fever, chills, and night sweats. Her appetite has been good, and she denies having abdominal pain associated with food ingestion; however, she has lost 15 pounds (6.75 kg) since her last operation. Her medications have not been changed since her discharge from the hospital, and consist of metronidazole (250 mg four times daily), prednisone (20 mg daily), calcium, and monthly vitamin B_{12} injections. She has had a long-standing history of watery diarrhea, which had been controlled before the most recent operation with the use of cholestyramine. Her weight had been stable for many years.

The patient is pale but in no acute distress and without fever. No orthostatic changes in her vital signs are noted. Her abdomen is soft with active bowel sounds. A healing midline incision and multiple scars from previous operations are present. The liver span is 7 cm in the mid-clavicular line. No abdominal or rectal masses are found. Her legs are slightly edematous. Her stool is dark brown and positive for occult blood.

The following laboratory results are obtained: hematocrit, 32%; mean corpuscular volume, 98 μm^3; serum sodium, 136 mEq/L; potassium, 3.0 mEq/L; chloride, 91 mEq/L; bicarbonate, 19 mEq/L; and creatinine, 0.6 mg/dL. The white blood cell count, platelet count, prothrombin time, and liver test results are all normal.

1. What is the first set of tests you would order in this patient to help explain the diarrhea?

2. Is this likely to be a flare-up of the patient's Crohn's disease?

3. If the cholestyramine treatment is resumed, how will this affect the volume of her diarrhea, and why?
4. What other treatment might be prescribed in an attempt to control her diarrhea and aid her nutrition?

Case Discussion

1. *What is the first set of tests you would order in this patient to help explain the diarrhea?*

   The first step in evaluating the patient with postoperative diarrhea whose condition is stable is to rule out enteric infection, with cultures and examination of the stools for ova and parasites. Because this patient is taking metronidazole, the possibility of PMC should also be considered, and a stool cytotoxicity assay carried out. (Although metronidazole is commonly used to treat PMC, the drug also has been implicated in several cases as the causative antibiotic.) Flexible sigmoidoscopy could probably be safely performed this soon after the resection, but as long as the patient's condition is stable, the procedure can be postponed pending the culture results.

2. *Is this likely to be a flare-up of the patient's Crohn's disease?*

   No, because constitutional symptoms have not appeared or changed, and also because the character of the stool is more suggestive of a malabsorptive disorder than of an active flare-up of Crohn's disease.

3. *If the cholestyramine treatment is resumed, how will this affect the volume of her diarrhea, and why?*

   Most likely the patient's diarrhea will worsen if she takes cholestyramine, even though it was effective before her recent operation. The explanation for this difference in effect is as follows. Because bile acids are normally absorbed actively in the distal ileum and resecreted by the liver into bile, when the distal ileum is either severely diseased or resected, unabsorbed bile acids enter the colon and stimulate water and electrolyte secretion, resulting in diarrhea. If the amount of ileum involved or resected is less than approximately 100 cm, the liver can compensate for the loss of bile acids by increasing bile acid synthesis, and fat malabsorption and weight loss are thereby largely prevented. Cholestyramine is effective in controlling diarrhea in this situation by binding bile acids in the small bowel and preventing their secretory effects in the colon. Such a set of circumstances apparently existed in this patient before her recent operation. However, her last operation resulted in the loss of her remaining ileum as well as part of the jejunum. Such a large loss of bowel would most likely result in depletion of her bile acid pool beyond the liver's ability to compensate for it by increasing bile acid synthesis, with consequent malabsorption of fat. The administration of cholestyramine would further deplete the bile acid pool and aggravate the fat malabsorption, which in turn would worsen the diarrhea. The mechanism responsible for this latter event is the stimulatory effect of unabsorbed fatty acids or their hydroxy derivatives on colonic water and electrolyte secretion.

4. *What other treatment might be prescribed in an attempt to control her diarrhea and aid her nutrition?*

Medium-chain triglycerides given orally should be tried to control her diarrhea and enhance nutrition. They do not require solubilization by bile acids for efficient absorption. At the same time, the patient should observe a low-fat diet.

Suggested Readings

Bartlett JG. Antibiotic-associated diarrhea. In: Blaser MJ, Smith PD, Ravdin JI, Greenberg HB, Guerrant RL, eds. *Infections of the gastrointestinal tract.* New York: Raven Press, 1995:893.

DuPont HL. Traveler's diarrhea. In: Blaser MJ, Smith, PD, Ravdin JI, Greenberg HB, Guerrant RL, eds. *Infections of the gastrointestinal tract.* New York: Raven Press, 1995:299.

DuPont HL, Hornick RB, Dawkins AT, et al. The response of man to virulent *Shigella flexneri* 2a. *J Infect Dis* 1969;119:296.

Hoffman AF, Poley JR. Cholestyramine treatment of diarrhea associated with ileal resection. *N Engl J Med* 1969;281:397.

Kapikian AZ, Chanock RM. Norwalk group of viruses. In: Fields BN, ed. *Virology*, 2d ed. New York: Raven Press, 1990:671.

Malabsorption

1. What are the major steps in the digestion and absorption of dietary lipids, carbohydrates, and proteins?
2. What are the principal sites of intestinal absorption of various nutrients?
3. Of what does the enterohepatic circulation of bile acids consist?
4. What are some of the major disorders of maldigestion or malabsorption?

Discussion

1. *What are the major steps in the digestion and absorption of dietary lipids, carbohydrates, and proteins?*

The process of digestion can be divided into three major steps: (a) intraluminal digestion, including the action of bile acids and pancreatic enzymes; (b) digestion by the intestinal epithelium; and (c) the transport of nutrients across the epithelium to the circulation.

The major events in the **digestion and absorption of dietary lipid** include (a) the lipolysis of dietary triglycerides by pancreatic lipase; (b) micellar solubilization of the resulting long-chain fatty acids and β-monoglycerides by bile acids; (c) the absorption of fatty acids and β-monoglycerides into enterocytes; (d) the reesterification and incorporation (along with cholesterol, cholesterol esters, phospholipid, and β-lipoproteins) into chylomicrons and very–low-density lipoproteins; and (e) the transport of chylomicrons from the mucosal cell into the intestinal lymphatics.

In the **digestion and absorption of dietary carbohydrates**, starch, which accounts for most of the carbohydrate intake, is initially hydrolyzed mostly by pancreatic amylase, yielding smaller sugars (maltose, maltotriose, and dextrins). These products, as well as ingested disaccharides such as lactose (milk sugar) and sucrose, are hydrolyzed further into their component monosaccharides by glucosidases (maltase, sucrase α-dextrinase, and lactase), which are present in the brush border of epithelial cells in the proximal intestine. The monosaccharides are then absorbed by the epithelial cells and enter the portal circulation.

For the **digestion and absorption of dietary protein** to take place, proteins are first hydrolyzed by pancreatic enzymes in the intestinal lumen. These enzymes include endopeptidases (trypsin, chymotrypsin, and elastase) and exopeptidases (carboxypeptidases A and B). Oligopeptides produced by the pancreatic enzymes are further hydrolyzed by aminopeptidases located on the brush border as well as in the cytoplasm of intestinal epithelial cells. The resultant amino acids, and certain dipeptides and tripeptides, then enter the portal circulation.

2. *What are the principal sites of intestinal absorption of various nutrients?*

All dietary nutrients, with the exception of vitamin B_{12} (cobalamin), are absorbed preferentially in the proximal small intestine; most absorption of the components of a meal occurs within the first 150 cm, although absorption (especially of sugars and amino acids) can occur more distally (as in the event of disease or surgical bypass of the proximal intestine). Vitamin B_{12} is absorbed by the distal ileum, where there is a specific receptor for the cobalamin–intrinsic factor complex.

3. *Of what does the enterohepatic circulation of bile acids consist?*

Bile acids are synthesized by the liver from cholesterol and are conjugated to either taurine or glycine before secretion into bile. During fasting, the bile acids are stored in the gallbladder. After a meal, they are secreted into the duodenum. The bile acids are very efficiently absorbed from the distal ileum, carried back to the liver by the portal vein, efficiently extracted and reconjugated by the liver, and then secreted again into bile. During each cycle, more than 95% of the bile acids are absorbed, but only small amounts are absorbed in the proximal small intestine.

4. *What are some of the major disorders of maldigestion or malabsorption?*

The following are representative disorders:

Intraluminal disorders
   Pancreatic exocrine (enzyme) insufficiency
      Chronic pancreatitis
      Pancreatic resection
      Cystic fibrosis
   Bile acid deficiency
      Pancreatic or bile duct carcinoma
      Extensive distal ileal resection or disease

Bacterial overgrowth in the proximal intestine
Surgical disruption of the continuity of the upper bowel (a Billroth II gastrojejunostomy)
Disorders of enterocytes
Primary defects (epithelium histologically normal)
Primary lactase deficiency
Sucrase–isomaltase deficiency
Secondary defects (epithelium histologically abnormal)
Nontropical sprue (celiac disease and gluten-sensitive enteropathy)
Tropical sprue
Acquired immunodeficiency syndrome (AIDS) enteropathy
Whipple's disease
Disturbed transfer of metabolites from enterocytes into lymph or portal blood
Infiltrative processes of the mucosa (amyloidosis and lymphoma)
Intestinal lymphangiectasia

Case   A 27-year-old woman complains of 11 months of diarrhea, gas, and abdominal cramps. She has five or six loose bowel movements a day, and diarrhea often awakens her from sleep. She also complains of abdominal cramps that are most severe just before a bowel movement, and are then temporarily relieved with the bowel movement. In addition, she feels tired and has lost approximately 8 pounds (3.6 kg) without dieting. She has noted a tendency to bruise easily. She drinks four glasses of milk a day.

Her past medical history is positive only for fatigue, for which she saw another physician 11 months ago, before the diarrhea developed. The physician told her that she had an iron-deficiency anemia. Since then, she has taken ferrous sulfate (300 mg four times daily), but still feels fatigued. She takes no other medication.

Physical examination reveals a young woman who appears mildly underweight but is otherwise normal.

Laboratory test results are as follows: white blood cell count, normal; hematocrit, 34%; mean corpuscular volume, 74 μm^3; serum iron, 50 mg/dL; total iron-binding capacity, 435 mg/dL; stool leukocyte test, negative; stool examination for ova and parasites, negative; serum albumin, 3.2 mg/dL; serum electrolytes, normal; and prothrombin time, 2 seconds greater than control.

While awaiting these laboratory results, you advise the patient to stop ingesting all milk products. The patient reports that this reduces but does not eliminate the diarrhea or gas.

1. What additional history should you obtain from the patient?
2. What might lead you to suspect that malabsorption is the cause of this patient's diarrhea, and why? What test should be performed to confirm this, and why?

This patient's fecal fat excretion is measured and found elevated, which proves she has maldigestion or malabsorption.

3. Considering that the patient has either maldigestion or malabsorption, what are two disorders that may decrease the bile acid pool, two disorders that decrease pancreatic lipase activity, and two disorders that may decrease absorption by small bowel enterocytes?

4. How does the D-xylose test differentiate problems with digestion (e.g, bile salt depletion and pancreatic lipase deficiency) from problems with absorption? Name one disorder that may produce a false-positive result.

   The D-xylose test in this patient reveals poor absorption of this sugar, which indicates that the small bowel absorption probably is abnormal.

5. Based on the results of the D-xylose test, what test should be performed now?

   A small bowel biopsy specimen in this patient reveals mucosal villous atrophy and crypt hyperplasia, accompanied by an increased number of plasma cells and lymphocytes in the lamina propria.

6. Although the biopsy findings indicate celiac sprue, what other disorders could produce such a "flat" mucosa?

7. How can the diagnosis of celiac sprue be confirmed?

8. If the D-xylose test result was abnormal, but the small bowel biopsy findings were normal, bacterial overgrowth in the proximal small intestine might be suspected. How should this possibility be evaluated?

9. If this patient's D-xylose absorption test result had been normal, what disorder might you suspect and how should you evaluate this possibility?

10. Why did the symptoms in this patient, who had celiac sprue, abate when she stopped drinking milk?

Case Discussion

1. *What additional history should you obtain from the patient?*

   This patient has chronic diarrhea, which is arbitrarily defined as diarrhea that lasts longer than 3 weeks. Chronic diarrhea is a fairly common complaint, with a lengthy differential diagnosis. The clinical history remains the mainstay of the initial approach to diagnosis, and the history taking must include questions concerning the following factors:

   - Food: Milk consumption, sorbitol (added to diet foods and fruit), fructose (found in soft drinks, candy, and fruit), and unpasteurized milk (*Yersinia* infection).
   - Travel: To areas where giardiasis, amebiasis, or schistosomiasis might be contracted.
   - Iatrogenic factors: Operations on the GI tract. A partial gastrectomy can result in dumping (rapid emptying of the gastric contents into the small intestine) and, if a stagnant area of bowel is created, bacterial overgrowth can result (the blind loop syndrome). Medications also are a common cause of diarrhea. The administration of antibiotics can result in *C. difficile* colitis, and antacid use can produce an osmotic diarrhea. β-Adrenergic antagonists, colchicine, laxatives, and innumerable other drugs can also cause diarrhea.

- Risk factors for AIDS.
- Review of systems: This may reveal arthritis, which can accompany inflammatory bowel disease or Whipple's disease; peptic ulcer disease, which can be associated with the Zollinger-Ellison syndrome; symptoms or a history of diabetes; or hyperthyroidism.
- Past medical problems, with an emphasis on childhood diarrhea or malnutrition and operations.
- Further characterization of the diarrhea: Does it awaken the patient at night? Is it constant or does it alternate with constipation? The most common cause of chronic diarrhea in the U.S. population is the irritable bowel syndrome, which is a poorly understood motility disorder. It rarely results in diarrhea that awakens the patient at night, rarely produces weight loss, and consists of diarrhea alternating with constipation.

2. *What might lead you to suspect that malabsorption is the cause of this patient's diarrhea, and why? What test should be performed to confirm this, and why?*

   Malabsorption is suspected as the cause of the diarrhea because of the iron deficiency that does not respond to oral iron treatment and because the prothrombin time is elevated without signs of liver disease. The 2- or 3-day stool collection for quantitative fat analysis is the single most useful test to document malabsorption. Because fat absorption is such a complex process, requiring the digestion of triglycerides by pancreatic lipase, solubilization of these products by bile salts, and absorption of the subsequent products by enterocytes of the small intestine, abnormalities in any of these steps result in fat malabsorption and an increase in fecal fat excretion. Thus, measurement of the fecal fat content is a test of many steps in the digestion and absorption pathways. One of the few kinds of malabsorption that does not cause increased fecal fat loss is that due to the lack of an intestinal enzyme needed in the digestion of a particular carbohydrate, despite a histologically normal intestine. The most common example of this is primary lactase deficiency, in which lactose is not absorbed normally but fat is.

3. *Considering that the patient has either maldigestion or malabsorption, what are two disorders that may decrease the bile acid pool, two disorders that decrease pancreatic lipase activity, and two disorders that may decrease absorption by small bowel enterocytes?*

   Resection or disease of the distal small bowel can cause a decreased reabsorption of bile acids, resulting in insufficient bile salt concentrations in the proximal intestine to allow the normal solubilization and absorption of fat. Complete blockage of the bile duct prevents bile acids from entering the duodenum.

   Chronic pancreatitis or pancreatic cancer can block the pancreatic duct, resulting in decreased secretion of lipase. Increased acid content in the duodenum, such as occurs in the Zollinger-Ellison syndrome, can inactivate pancreatic lipase in the intestinal lumen.

Decreased absorption by small bowel enterocytes may be caused by celiac sprue, tropical sprue, Whipple's disease, small intestinal lymphoma, AIDS enteropathy, and several other diseases.

4. *How does the* D-*xylose test differentiate problems with digestion (e.g., bile salt depletion and pancreatic lipase deficiency) from problems with absorption? Name one disorder that may produce a false-positive result.*

D-Xylose is a five-carbon sugar that can be absorbed without the aid of bile salts, pancreatic enzymes, or intestinal enzymes. It should be absorbed normally if the small bowel is intact. Thus, the test is useful in distinguishing pancreatic enzyme insufficiency from enterocyte abnormalities. However, bacterial overgrowth in the proximal intestine is a condition that can cause malabsorption of D-xylose without affecting the enterocyte (the bacteria will consume the D-xylose before it can be absorbed), thus producing a false-positive result.

5. *Based on the results of the* D-*xylose test, what test should be performed now?*

The small bowel should now be examined, and there are two appropriate ways to do this: small bowel biopsy and a small bowel barium radiograph. A biopsy specimen gives more information about the mucosa, whereas the radiograph may permit better evaluation of diverticula, regional ileitis, or blind loops.

6. *Although the biopsy findings indicate celiac sprue, what other disorders could produce such a "flat" mucosa?*

Tropical sprue, soy and milk protein allergy (primarily in children), diffuse intestinal lymphoma, giardiasis, the Zollinger-Ellison syndrome, prolonged total parenteral nutrition, and viral gastroenteritis can produce a flat mucosal lesion that looks almost exactly like celiac sprue.

7. *How can the diagnosis of celiac sprue be confirmed?*

The diagnosis of celiac sprue can be confirmed by observing the patient's response to a gluten-free diet. Adherence to a gluten-free diet should bring about a cessation or marked reduction in the diarrhea and other intestinal symptoms, weight gain, and histologic improvement in the intestinal mucosa. Gluten is found in wheat, rye, barley, and oats, but not in rice and corn.

8. *If the* D-*xylose test result was abnormal, but the small bowel biopsy findings were normal, a bacterial overgrowth in the proximal small intestine might be suspected. How should this possibility be evaluated?*

This would be more likely to occur in patients who have had an operation that resulted in a blind loop of small intestine, or in elderly patients, who are more likely to have multiple small bowel diverticula. A small bowel barium radiographic examination should reveal these abnormalities. The bile acid breath test could be used to document bacterial deconjugation of bile acids. In this test, a radiolabeled conjugated bile acid, such as $[^{14}C]$-glycocholic acid, is given orally, and the amount and the time course of the $[^{14}C]$-O_2 exhaled is measured. Normally, most of the labeled bile acid is absorbed intact in the distal ileum; a minor amount reaches the colon, where anaerobic bacteria cleave the glycine moiety from the cholic acid moiety. The $[^{14}C]$-O_2 released in the colon is absorbed and exhaled. If the upper intestine is populated by excessive numbers of anaerobic bacteria, the deconjugation of [^{14}C]-glycocholic acid occurs earlier and to a greater degree than normal, resulting in an early and high rise in the exhaled [^{14}C]-O$_2$ level.

9. *If this patient's D-xylose absorption test result had been normal, what disorder might you suspect and how should you evaluate this possibility?*

Pancreatic insufficiency should be suspected in patients who have a history of chronic pancreatitis or, less commonly, in middle-aged or elderly people who may present with a pancreatic cancer obstructing the pancreatic duct. A patient who has malabsorption and a history of pancreatitis should undergo a trial of pancreatic enzyme treatment. If this alleviates the diarrhea, the trial can be both diagnostic and therapeutic. The secretin test can be used to evaluate pancreatic function, but it is expensive and difficult to perform, so it is rarely used. If a pancreatic cancer is suspected, an imaging study such as CT scanning or endoscopic retrograde cholangiopancreatography (ERCP) should be performed.

10. *Why did the symptoms in this patient who had celiac sprue abate when she stopped drinking milk?*

Celiac sprue damages the intestinal epithelium, thereby decreasing the amounts of digestive enzymes, such as lactase, that are normally present in the villus cells.

Suggested Readings

Mann J, Brown WR, Kern F Jr. The subtle and variable clinical expression of gluten-induced enteropathy (adult celiac disease, nontropical sprue): an analysis of 21 consecutive cases. *Am J Med* 1970;48:357.

Riley SA, Turnbrg LA. Maldigestion and malabsorption. In: Feldman M, Scharschmidt BF, Sleisenger MH, eds. *Sleisenger and Fordtran's gastrointestinal and liver disease: pathophysiology, diagnosis, management*, 6th ed. Philadelphia: WB Saunders, 1998:1501.

Trier JS. Celiac sprue and refractory sprue. In: Feldman M, Scharschmidt BF, Sleisenger MH, eds. *Sleisenger and Fordtran's gastrointestinal and liver disease: pathophysiology, diagnosis, management*, 6th ed. Philadelphia: WB Saunders, 1998:1557.

Pancreatitis

1. What are the common and uncommon causes of acute pancreatitis?
2. What pathogenetic mechanism is hypothesized to be common to these causes of acute pancreatitis, and how does it explain the clinical features of the disease?
3. What symptoms and signs typify acute pancreatitis?
4. What difficulties may be encountered in confirming the diagnosis of acute pancreatitis through the measurement of amylase levels, and how might the diagnostic accuracy be improved?
5. What clinical and laboratory indices can be used to assess the prognosis in a case of acute pancreatitis?

6. What events signal the development of local complications of acute pancreatitis, and how are they best evaluated?

7. What are the mainstays of treatment for acute pancreatitis, and what is the rationale for their use?

8. What cardinal feature distinguishes chronic pancreatitis from acute pancreatitis?

9. How does the etiology of chronic pancreatitis differ from that of acute pancreatitis?

10. What are the mainstays of treatment for chronic pancreatitis?

Discussion

1. *What are the common and uncommon causes of acute pancreatitis?*

   The common causes of acute pancreatitis are alcohol (60%), gallstones (25% to 30%), and idiopathic causes. The uncommon causes include the following:

   Postoperative
   After ERCP
   Trauma
   Metabolic (hypertriglyceridemia, hyperparathyroidism, renal failure, and acute fatty liver of pregnancy)
   Hereditary
   Infections (mumps, *Mycoplasma*, coxsackie virus, and echovirus)
   Vasculitides (systemic lupus erythematosus, thrombotic thrombocytopenic purpura, Henoch-Schönlein purpura, necrotizing angiitis)
   Ampulla of Vater obstruction (Crohn's disease, duodenal diverticula, penetrating duodenal ulcer, pancreas divisum, and scorpion venom)
   Drugs
      Azathioprine/6-mercaptopurine
      Thiazide diuretics
      Estrogens
      Furosemide
      Sulfonamides (sulfasalazine, trimethoprim–sulfamethoxazole)
      Tetracycline
      Methyldopa
      Sulindac
      Valproate
      Pentamidine
      Didanosine
      Oral 5-ASA (olsalzine and mesalamine)
      Octreotide

2. *What pathogenetic mechanism is hypothesized to be common to these causes of acute pancreatitis, and how does it explain the clinical features of the disease?*

   Autodigestion is the pathogenetic mechanism common to all the causes of acute pancreatitis. Etiologic factors are believed to lead to the premature activation of pancreatic proenzymes within the gland. Destruction of the pancreas by the activated enzymes leads to local injury (edema, necrosis, and hemorrhage). In addition, the activation and release of vasoactive peptides and enzymes compounds the systemic effects of pancreatic injury (shock, disseminated intravascular coagulation, adult respiratory distress syndrome, renal failure, hyperglycemia, and hypocalcemia).

3. *What symptoms and signs typify acute pancreatitis?*

Pain is a characteristic symptom of acute pancreatitis and is located in the mid-epigastric and periumbilical regions. Commonly, it radiates to the back and is more constant and sustained than the pain associated with other abdominal processes. It is often more intense in the supine position and ameliorated by sitting forward. Patients may exhibit marked abdominal tenderness and guarding.

Nausea and vomiting are other symptoms. In this setting, the abdomen may be distended from the accumulation of intraabdominal and retroperitoneal fluid, paralytic ileus, and chemical peritonitis. The bowel sounds may be diminished.

Hypotension may be present in as many as half of the patients; it results from the loss of plasma and blood into the retroperitoneum, vasodilation, and myocardial depressant factor.

Less common, but important, findings include periumbilical (Cullen's sign) or flank ecchymoses (Grey Turner's sign).

4. *What difficulties may be encountered in confirming the diagnosis of acute pancreatitis through the measurement of amylase levels, and how might the diagnostic accuracy be improved?*

Although the serum amylase level usually rises within 12 hours of the onset of pain and remains elevated for 3 to 5 days, a normal serum amylase value does not exclude pancreatitis. Spuriously normal serum amylase levels may result from the rapid clearance of amylase into the urine, and may be seen with hypertriglyceridemia and in late-stage ("burned out") chronic pancreatitis. The magnitude of the amylase elevation in serum or urine does not correlate with the severity of pancreatitis. In addition, hyperamylasemia is not a specific finding for pancreatitis because it may occur in a great variety of pancreatic and nonpancreatic diseases. There are salivary as well as pancreatic-type isoamylases, and salivary amylase accounts for 60% to 65% of the total amylase content. Salivary hyperamylasemia can occur in the settings of diabetic ketoacidosis, alcoholism, and malignancy (especially with hepatic metastasis). Macroamylasemia occurs without any relationship to pancreatitis and results in elevated serum (but not urine) amylase levels.

Attempts at improving the sensitivity, and especially the specificity, of the laboratory-based diagnosis of pancreatitis have included measurement of the renal amylase clearance and the ratio of renal amylase clearance to creatinine clearance (C_{am}/C_{cr}). However, the specificity of the C_{am}/C_{cr} is questionable because it may be elevated in the settings of diabetic ketoacidosis, burns, renal failure, chronic hemodialysis, pancreatic neoplasms, and alcoholic liver disease. Measurement of the pancreatic isoamylase levels has also been tried. This may provide information that changes the clinical diagnosis in 20% to 40% of patients with hyperamylasemia. Measurement of the serum lipase level is slightly less sensitive for the diagnosis of pancreatitis than is measurement of the serum amylase level, but the lipase concentration remains elevated longer and is more specific than the amylase value.

5. *What clinical and laboratory indices can be used to assess the prognosis in a case of acute pancreatitis?*

A set of the early risk factors, known as *Ranson's criteria*, has been used to predict the potential complications and mortality in a patient with acute pancreatitis:

At admission
    Age, older than 55 years
    White blood cell count, >16,000/mm^3
    Blood glucose, >200 mg/dL
    Serum lactate dehydrogenase, >350 IU/L
    AST, >250 IU/L
During initial 48 hours
    Hematocrit decrease, >10%
    Blood urea nitrogen rise, >5 mg/dL
    Serum calcium, <8 mg/dL
    Arterial partial pressure of oxygen (Po$_2$), <60 mm Hg
    Base deficit, >4 mEq/L
    Estimated fluid sequestration, >6 L

The mortality rate associated with these signs has been determined as follows: two or fewer signs, 1%; three or four signs, 16%; five or six signs, 40%; and more than six signs, 100%.

Measurement of **trypsinogen activation peptide** in urine may distinguish mild from severe pancreatitis, but the test is not generally available.

6. *What events signal the development of local complications of acute pancreatitis, and how are they best evaluated?*

Local and infectious complications of acute pancreatitis account for 80% of the mortality associated with the disease; thus, detection of these complications is crucial in minimizing the likelihood of a fatal outcome. A **pancreatic pseudocyst** should be suspected in the setting of persistent pain and hyperamylasemia and may be manifested as a palpable mass in the upper abdomen. **Pancreatic necrosis**, or phlegmon, and **pancreatic abscess** are often difficult to distinguish because they both commonly cause prolonged abdominal pain and tenderness, fever, leukocytosis, and a palpable mass.

A CT scan with oral and IV contrast enhancement is the best method for imaging these complications. Extraluminal gas may be seen on the studies and can be used to distinguish pancreatic necrosis from pancreatic abscess. However, it is CT-guided percutaneous needle aspiration that usually allows for the early diagnosis of pancreatic infection and abscess, which require either percutaneous or surgical drainage.

7. *What are the mainstays of treatment for acute pancreatitis, and what is the rationale for their use?*

By eliminating oral intake (NPO), the neural and hormonal stimuli to pancreatic exocrine secretion are minimized, thus limiting the cycle of pancreatic autodigestion and inflammation. Eliminating food intake reduces the vagal stimulation of pancreatic secretion and reduces the delivery of acid, fatty acids, and amino acids to the duodenum, which would elicit release of secretin and cholecystokinin. Nasogastric suction is useful for those patients experiencing nausea and vomiting resulting from paralytic ileus. IV fluid hydration and electrolyte (especially calcium) administration replace the losses stemming from retroperitoneal inflammation and exudation. Hypocalcemia is believed to result from a combination of factors: hypoalbuminemia, the sequestration of calcium in areas of fat necrosis, and an inadequate parathormone response. Analgesic administration is usually required to control the pain, which is often intense and prolonged.

8. *What cardinal feature distinguishes chronic pancreatitis from acute pancreatitis?*

The permanent destruction of the pancreatic gland is a cardinal feature of chronic pancreatitis. Pathologically, there is atrophy of the acini, a loss of islet cells, fibrosis, and plugging of irregular pancreatic ducts by protein. The protein plugs may be calcified and, on radiographic studies, 30% of patients exhibit pancreatic calcification. The clinical sequelae of glandular destruction include exocrine and endocrine insufficiency, manifested by steatorrhea and diabetes mellitus, respectively (the former occurring only when there is a more than 90% reduction in exocrine function). Abdominal pain is not uniformly seen and may be intermittent, constant, or absent. Because of the acinar destruction, the serum amylase levels may be only mildly elevated or normal.

9. *How does the etiology of chronic pancreatitis differ from that of acute pancreatitis?*

In western countries, most (approximately 90%) cases of chronic pancreatitis are attributable to alcoholism. Other possible causes include metabolic disorders such as hypercalcemia of any cause (perhaps hyperparathyroidism), hyperlipidemia, and congenital or hereditary conditions (pancreas divisum, cystic fibrosis, and hereditary pancreatitis).

10. *What are the mainstays of treatment for chronic pancreatitis?*

Acute relapses of chronic pancreatitis may require management identical to that for acute pancreatitis, and may be accompanied by pseudocyst formation and pancreatic ascites. Exocrine insufficiency resulting in steatorrhea and weight loss is treated with oral pancreatic enzyme replacement, whereas endocrine insufficiency (diabetes mellitus) requires insulin therapy. The management of the chronic pain has been problematic, and patients frequently become addicted to narcotic analgesics. The oral administration of high doses of pancreatic enzymes may reduce the pain. Surgical intervention (ganglionectomy, partial and total pancreatectomy, and pancreatic duct drainage operations) confers inconsistent benefits and is fraught with long-term morbidity.

Case 1   A 66-year-old man is admitted with complaints of progressively severe, constant upper abdominal pain, nausea, and vomiting of 48 hours' duration. Recently, he has consumed large quantities of vodka, but has no history of biliary tract disease and is taking no medications.

He is a thin man, wincing and clutching his abdomen. His temperature is 38°C; blood pressure, 100/60 mm Hg; pulse, 90 beats per minute; and respirations, 18 per minute. His abdomen is flat and the bowel sounds are hypoactive. There is marked direct tenderness with guarding in the mid-epigastrium, but no peritoneal signs.

The following laboratory data are gathered: white blood cell count, 10,000 cells/mm³; hematocrit, 50%; serum creatinine, 1.3 mg/dL; total serum bilirubin, 3.4 mg/dL; alkaline phosphatase, 246 IU/L; AST, 209 IU/L; and serum amylase, 741 U/L.

Plain abdominal radiographs reveal the presence of scattered air–fluid levels, predominantly in the small bowel, but no calcification or subdiaphragmatic free air. An abdominal ultrasound examination reveals a dilated, fluid-filled gallbladder, a dilated common bile duct without definite calculi, and a poorly visualized pancreas due to overlying bowel gas.

A nasogastric tube is inserted and placed at low suction, and the patient remains NPO, receiving only IV fluids. Over the ensuing 48 hours, he requires regular doses of meperidine for the control of persistent, severe pain and is noted to have a rise in his bilirubin (8.0 mg/dL), alkaline phosphatase (450 IU/L), and AST (375 IU/L) levels. ERCP, performed on the third hospital day, demonstrates a dilated common bile duct that tapers smoothly in its intrapancreatic portion and contains no stones. The gallbladder is dilated and also contains no stones. No pancreatogram is obtained.

The aforementioned management is continued, and total parenteral nutrition is started. The patient's pain, abdominal tenderness, and liver test abnormalities gradually abate over the subsequent 10 days.

1. Why was an ERCP obtained?
2. What was the cause of the patient's biliary obstruction?

Case Discussion

1. *Why was an ERCP obtained?*

The patient's laboratory data included abnormal liver test results consistent with cholestasis, and common bile duct dilation was seen on the ultrasound examination. These findings and the failure of his symptoms to subside during the early hospital course raised concern about a gallstone at the ampulla of Vater and "gallstone pancreatitis." Performance of emergency ERCP, with papillotomy when ampullary or common bile duct stones are found, has been advocated within 24 hours in patients who have acute biliary pancreatitis.

2. *What was the cause of the patient's biliary obstruction?*

The absence of gallstones on the ERCP study and the patient's gradual improvement with conservative management of acute pancreatitis support the presence of biliary obstruction due to compression of the intrapancreatic common bile duct by an inflamed pancreas.

Case 2

A 40-year-old, alcoholic man complains of chronic abdominal pain and weight loss. He had consumed 2 pints of bourbon daily for the past 10 years, until 4 years ago, when he had his first episode of abdominal pain, which was characterized as a sharp, continuous epigastric pain radiating to the back, and associated with nausea and vomiting. He was admitted to the hospital, where his symptoms gradually abated with treatment, consisting of bowel rest and IV fluids for 1 week. His abdominal radiographs at that time revealed calcification in the area of the pancreas. He subsequently reduced his alcohol intake, but required readmission to the hospital on several occasions after the consumption of relatively small quantities of alcohol.

In recent months, the patient has lost 25 pounds (11.25 kg), coincident with the passing of persistently loose and occasionally greasy stools. His abdominal pain has become constant, and a macrocytic anemia has developed.

The patient is found to be cachectic, weighing 125 pounds (56.25 kg). He has a scaphoid abdomen with normal bowel sounds and mild direct tenderness in the mid-epigastrium in response to palpation. There is moderate pedal edema.

Relevant laboratory data are: white blood cell count, 4,900 cells/mm³, with 65% segmented cells, 20% lymphocytes, and 10% monocytes; hematocrit, 37%; mean corpuscular volume, 106 μm³; prothrombin time, 14 seconds (control, 12 seconds); serum albumin, 2.7 g/dL; serum glucose, normal; serum and electrolytes and liver function tests are otherwise normal; serum vitamin B_{12}, 96 pg/mL (normal, >200 pg/mL); serum folate, normal; and 72-hour fecal fat excretion, 42 g (normal, <15 g).

The patient is started on a regimen of monthly vitamin B_{12} injections and oral pancreatic enzymes, three capsules with each meal and one capsule with snacks. At first, he fails to gain weight and observes no reduction in the frequency of his bowel movements; his abdominal pain persists at a moderate severity. The dose of enzymes is increased to six capsules with each meal, and he also begins taking cimetidine (300 mg orally four times a day). Over a period of 1 month, his pain subsides considerably and he gains 15 pounds (6.75 kg).

1. Is it unusual that the patient had his first attack of pancreatitis pain after 10 years of heavy alcohol consumption, and at that time he already had signs of chronic pancreatitis (pancreatic calcification)?

2. What is the pathophysiologic basis for vitamin B_{12} deficiency in the setting of chronic pancreatitis?

3. Why did the patient begin to gain weight only once his pancreatic enzyme dose was increased and cimetidine added?

4. Why might the patient's pain have subsided toward the end of the described course?

Case Discussion

1. *Is it unusual that the patient had his first attack of pancreatitis pain after 10 years of heavy alcohol consumption, and at that time he already had signs of chronic pancreatitis (pancreatic calcification)?*

No. It is believed that most people must consume at least 50 g of alcohol daily on a prolonged basis before chronic pancreatitis develops, and most have been drinking excessively for 5 to 20 years before their first attack. Alcohol-induced pancreatitis probably is chronic, even at the time of the first attack. Pancreatic calcifications are seen in 25% to 50% of the patients and are particularly common in alcoholics who have chronic pancreatitis.

2. *What is the pathophysiologic basis for vitamin B_{12} deficiency in the setting of chronic pancreatitis?*

The vitamin B_{12} deficiency stems from the exocrine insufficiency. Pancreatic proteases are necessary to cleave R protein from vitamin B_{12} in the proximal intestine, so that the latter may be absorbed as a complex with intrinsic factor (in the terminal ileum). Approximately 50% of patients with advanced pancreatitis have vitamin B_{12} deficiency due to exocrine insufficiency.

3. *Why did the patient begin to gain weight only once his pancreatic enzyme dose was increased and cimetidine added?*

Pancreatic enzymes can be inactivated by gastric acid, and this inactivation can be reduced by the administration of antacids or H_2 receptor antagonists. In addition, evidence suggests that certain enzyme capsules are more effective at delivering active enzyme to the small intestine than are others.

4. *Why might the patient's pain have subsided toward the end of the described course?*

Sustained pain relief in patients with chronic pancreatitis often occurs after several years and only with marked progression of the pancreatic exocrine insufficiency, rather than being a result of therapeutic intervention. However, this patient's pain seemed to subside rather quickly with the institution of high doses of pancreatic enzyme therapy. The suppression of pancreatic exocrine secretion has been accomplished in patients given intraduodenal perfusions of pancreatic extract, and the pain of chronic pancreatitis has been shown to respond in some patients to treatment with pancreatic enzymes.

Suggested Readings

Balhazar EJ, Robinson DL, Megibow AJ, Ranson JH. Acute pancreatitis: value of CT in establishing prognosis. *Radiology* 1990;174:331.

Gorelick FS. Acute pancreatitis. In: Yamada T, et al, eds. *Textbook of gastroenterology*, 2nd ed. Philadelphia: JB Lippincott, 1995:2065.

Isaksson G, Ihse I. Pain reduction by an oral pancreatic enzyme preparation in chronic pancreatitis. *Dig Dis Sci* 1983;28:97.

Owyang C, Levitt MD. Chronic pancreatitis. In: Yamada T, et al, eds. *Textbook of gastroenterology*, 2nd ed. Philadelphia: JB Lippincott, 1995:2091.

Acute Lower Gastrointestinal Hemorrhage

1. What is one of the most important diagnoses to rule out in a patient with large-volume hematochezia?

2. Which method of imaging the GI tract has no role in the evaluation of a patient with acute lower GI bleeding?

3. What are the two most common causes of acute major lower GI bleeding?

Discussion

1. *What is one of the most important diagnoses to rule out in a patient with large-volume hematochezia?*

An upper GI bleeding source must be ruled out in every patient with large-volume hematochezia. Lower GI bleeding is defined as bleeding from a source distal to the ligament of Treitz, the structure that divides the duodenum from the jejunum. Approximately 10% of patients with upper GI bleeding have hematochezia because of a rapid rate of blood loss and the subsequent rapid transit of blood through the GI tract. Because the strategy for treatment of an upper GI hemorrhage may differ drastically from that for a lower GI hemorrhage, first ruling out an upper GI tract bleeding source is mandatory in patients presenting with hematochezia.

The easiest way to exclude a significant upper GI hemorrhage with substantial reliability is through nasogastric lavage and aspiration. The aspiration of bilious contents from a nasogastric tube makes it very likely that the bleeding originates from a lower source, but this is not an infallible finding. If the source of bleeding remains in doubt after nasogastric lavage, upper GI endoscopy should be performed.

2. *Which method of imaging the GI tract has no role in the evaluation of a patient with acute lower GI bleeding?*

A barium enema examination should not be performed in the setting of acute lower GI bleeding because it has no therapeutic potential, and the barium interferes with the performance of more appropriate tests, namely ^{99m}Tc-labeled erythrocyte scanning, angiography, and colonoscopy.

At most hospitals, the ^{99m}Tc-labeled erythrocyte scan is the preferred nuclear medicine test for localizing the source of acute lower GI bleeding. To perform it, the patient's red blood cells are labeled with radioactive technetium. A scintillation camera then tracks where the labeled red blood cells collect in the patient. The ^{99m}Tc-labeled erythrocyte scan may help localize a bleeding source to the general region of the small bowel, right colon, or left colon, thereby directing the course of therapy. Under the correct circumstances, this scan may localize a source bleeding at rates as low as 0.5 mL per minute.

If arterial bleeding is occurring at a rate of approximately 1 mL per minute, angiography is useful for both diagnosis and therapy. Once catheterized, the bleeding artery may then be selectively infused with vasopressin, or embolized with metal coils, ethanol, or Gelfoam. Angiography usually is not useful if the bleeding has stopped.

Colonoscopy, because it may yield a diagnosis and provide a means for delivering therapy, regardless of whether the patient is actively bleeding, should be performed before nuclear medicine scans or angiography in most patients with acute lower GI bleeding. If possible, the lower bowel should be rapidly flushed with a polyethylene glycol electrolyte solution before colonoscopy is performed. With modern techniques, the diagnostic accuracy of colonoscopy is at least as good as that of angiography, unless the rate of bleeding is so brisk as to obscure colonoscopic visualization completely.

3. *What are the two most common causes of acute major lower GI bleeding?*

The most common cause of major lower GI bleeding is diverticulosis, accounting for approximately 40% of all cases. Diverticula are herniations in the colon wall that are believed to be acquired with age. Causal associations between low dietary fiber intake and diverticulosis have not been universally accepted, and the true etiology is probably multifactorial. In diverticulosis, as the colon wall herniates, the intramural arteries (vasa recta) may rupture, thus producing a brisk but painless hemorrhage. Although the hemorrhage stops spontaneously in approximately 80% of patients, diverticular bleeding may lead to life-threatening blood loss, particularly in the elderly. Diverticula are more common in the left colon, yet diverticular bleeding most often originates from the right colon. Diagnosis usually is based on the findings revealed by urgent colonoscopy or by angiography. Therapy by selective angiographic catheterization is successful in most cases.

Arteriovenous malformations (AVMs) or angiodysplasias in the colon are the second most common cause of major lower GI bleeding, accounting for approximately 20% of all cases. These vascular ectasias are located just beneath the columnar epithelium, and most are due to the degenerative changes of aging. A causal association between aortic stenosis and colonic AVMs has not been definitely established. AVMs are usually located in the right colon and may present as either an acute lower GI hemorrhage or as chronic low-volume bleeding manifested by iron-deficiency anemia. If the bleeding is brisk and persistent, angiography is usually the preferred method for making the diagnosis and carrying out therapy. If the bleeding has slowed or stopped, urgent colonoscopic therapy by thermal cauterization or injection is often useful.

Less common causes of acute lower GI bleeding are colonic neoplasms, inflammatory bowel disease, infectious colitis, and ischemic colitis. Ischemic colitis usually presents with acute, crampy lower abdominal pain, the urge to defecate, and passage of bloody diarrhea. "Watershed" areas of the colon, such as the splenic flexure and sigmoid colon, are most commonly involved because of their poor blood flow.

Hemorrhoids and colonic neoplasms are the most common causes of chronic lower GI bleeding.

Case   A 70-year-old woman is seen in the emergency room complaining of rectal bleeding. Her first episode occurred approximately 6 hours ago, when she passed red blood and clots. At first she attributed the bleeding to her hemorrhoids, but she has had five more episodes since, the last of which was accompanied by a sensation of dizziness. She does not smoke or drink alcoholic beverages. She takes several aspirin a day for the treatment of arthritis. Physical examination reveals a woman who is pale and anxious. Her blood pressure and pulse in the supine position are 110/70 mm Hg and 100 beats per minute, respectively. When she stands, her blood pressure and pulse are 85/50 mm Hg and 130 beats per minute, respectively. The abdominal examination reveals benign findings. Rectal examination reveals red blood in the vault and no masses.

1. What are the three most likely causes of this woman's hematochezia?
2. What diagnostic and therapeutic maneuvers must you do within the first hour?
3. What diagnostic and therapeutic tests should you consider having done over the next 24 to 48 hours?

Case Discussion

1. *What are the three most likely causes of this woman's hematochezia?*

    Diverticulosis, colonic AVMs, and upper GI bleeding are the most likely causes of this woman's bleeding, which is associated with hemodynamic instability. Hemorrhoids, inflammatory bowel disease, and colonic neoplasms only rarely cause bleeding of this degree.

2. *What diagnostic and therapeutic maneuvers must you do within the first hour?*

    This woman exhibits significant hemodynamic instability, as demonstrated by the orthostatic changes in her blood pressure and pulse. You must place at least two large-bore (18-gauge) IV catheters and start IV volume expansion using crystalloid fluid (usually 0.9N sodium chloride or an equivalent of lactated Ringer's solution). At the same time, you should draw blood for typing and crossmatch studies, hemogram, coagulation studies, and serum chemistry profile. Next, you should place a nasogastric tube to obtain gastric contents and determine whether there is an upper GI bleeding source. The aspiration of blood should prompt strong consideration for performing emergency upper GI endoscopy.

3. *What diagnostic and therapeutic tests should you consider having done over the next 24 to 48 hours?*

    If the bleeding slows or stops, rapid GI lavage with polyethylene glycol electrolyte solution followed by colonoscopy is usually the best test for diagnosis and therapy, with a diagnostic yield of 40% to 50% in this setting. Colonoscopy can still be useful if the bleeding is persistently brisk; however, in this situation, angiography is the preferred test in many hospitals. If colonoscopy and angiography fail to identify the source of the bleeding, a ^{99m}Tc-labeled erythrocyte scan may help localize the source.

Suggested Readings

Elta GH. Approach to the patient with gross gastrointestinal bleeding. In: Yamada T, Alpers D, Owyang C, Powell DW, Silverstein FE, eds. *Textbook of gastroenterology*, 2nd ed. Philadelphia: JB Lippincott, 1995:671.

Marshall JB. Acute gastrointestinal bleeding. *Postgrad Med* 1990;87:63.

Acute Upper Gastrointestinal Hemorrhage

1. Is measurement of the hemoglobin concentration and the hematocrit the best way to determine the severity of GI bleeding? Why or why not?
2. Is esophagitis a common cause of severe upper GI bleeding?
3. Is β-adrenoreceptor blockade a treatment option for acute variceal bleeding? If so, why? If not, what are some treatment options?

Discussion

1. *Is measurement of the hemoglobin concentration and the hematocrit the best way to determine the severity of GI bleeding? Why or why not?*

No. The best way to determine the severity of GI bleeding is to measure the vital signs with the patient in the supine and standing positions. If orthostatic changes in the vital signs (postural hypotension) occur in the setting of GI bleeding, this usually indicates at least a 20% loss in the total blood volume. This finding mandates immediate IV volume expansion and preparation for blood transfusion. Other physical findings associated with severe blood loss are resting tachycardia and hypotension, pallor, and agitation.

The initial blood count (hemogram) obtained from an acutely bleeding patient is a very poor reflection of the amount of blood lost. To be accurate, the blood count must be obtained when the patient's intravascular volume is normal. After an acute loss of blood, reequilibration may take up to 72 hours. The IV administration of crystalloid hastens this process (often known as *hemodilution*).

Placement of a nasogastric tube is very helpful in the initial assessment of a patient with GI bleeding, but the findings yielded can be misleading. The absence of bloody aspirate may mean the bleeding has stopped for the moment, yet the amount of blood already lost may be life threatening. Conversely, up to 15% of patients with an actively bleeding upper GI source may have a nonbloody gastric aspirate. The presence of bile in the gastric aspirate offers some reassurance that an upper GI bleed has stopped; however, up to 50% of physicians misjudge the presence or absence of a bilious aspirate. The persistence of bloody gastric aspirate indicates significant ongoing bleeding.

Melena is produced when hemoglobin is degraded by bacteria in the GI tract, and may originate from either an upper or lower GI source. The ingestion of approximately 100 to 200 mL of blood is enough to cause melena; hence, the presence of melena alone does not necessarily mean the patient has had a substantial loss of blood. On the other hand, frequent episodes of melena indicate significant bleeding. Hematochezia resulting from an upper GI bleeding source indicates massive bleeding.

2. *Is esophagitis a common cause of severe upper GI bleeding?*

No. Esophagitis accounts only for approximately 8% of all cases of upper GI bleeding. It is usually caused by gastroesophageal reflux of acid, but may also be caused by infectious agents such as *Candida albicans*, herpes simplex virus, and cytomegalovirus. Severe bleeding resulting from esophagitis is rare and usually occurs in the setting of an already hospitalized and critically ill patient, especially during mechanical respiration.

Peptic ulcer disease accounts for 40% to 50% of all the cases of upper GI bleeding, and is discussed in the next section.

Depending on the institution, **variceal bleeding** accounts for 10% to 30% of all cases of upper GI bleeding. Varices are a complication of portal hypertension, the cause of which may be classified as prehepatic (portal vein obstruction), hepatic (cirrhosis), or posthepatic (inferior vena cava thrombosis). The most common cause of portal hypertension in the United States population is ethanol-induced cirrhosis. The 6-week mortality rate associated with bleeding varices is approximately 40%, and patients with variceal bleeding should be managed in an intensive care unit. These patients often have concurrent medical problems, such as a coagulopathy and hepatic encephalopathy.

Mallory-Weiss tears are partial-thickness mucosal lacerations near the gastroesophageal junction, usually caused by forceful retching in the setting of ethanol ingestion. These tears account for approximately 10% of upper GI hemorrhages. Most Mallory-Weiss tears stop bleeding spontaneously. Persistent bleeding can be treated by either endoscopic hemostasis or angiographic embolization.

Significant acute and chronic blood loss, sometimes leading to iron-deficiency anemia, can occur from gastric erosions or ulcers within a sliding hiatal hernia. These lesions, sometimes called Cameron lesions, seem to result from the riding motion of the herniated stomach in and out of the chest during respiration.

3. *Is β-adrenoreceptor blockade a treatment option for acute variceal bleeding? If so, why? If not, what are some treatment options?*

No. β-Adrenoreceptor blockers, such as propranolol, produce a negative chronotropic and inotropic effect. The use of such drugs in an acutely bleeding patient, who is depending on an adrenergic response to maintain an adequate blood pressure, is therefore contraindicated. Some evidence supports the use of β-adrenoreceptor blockers in selected patients to reduce the risk of recurrent variceal bleeding after the acute hemorrhage has been well controlled. Although the complete mechanism of action of these drugs has yet to be delineated, they are thought to exert their beneficial effect in part by lowering the portal pressure.

Other pharmacologic approaches to the control of acute variceal bleeding are the use of parenteral vasopressin or somatostatin. Although vasopressin has been commonly used, its efficacy has not been firmly established and it has associated cardiovascular side effects. The drug's mechanism of action is thought to be splanchnic arteriolar vasoconstriction, resulting in decreased portal pressure. Increasingly, somatostatin has become popular for the control of variceal bleeding, also because of its purported lowering of portal pressure. Somatostatin has been shown to be as effective as vasopressin in controlling acute variceal hemorrhage.

Endoscopic hemostasis achieved by **endoscopic injection sclerotherapy**, which has an acute hemostasis rate of approximately 90%, had been the treatment of choice for bleeding esophageal varices. More recently, however, **endoscopic variceal ligation** has become an increasingly popular hemostasis technique because it is as effective as sclerotherapy and considerably safer.

If endoscopic techniques are either unavailable or unsuccessful, acute hemostasis may be achieved with balloon tamponade devices. Although the tamponade accomplished with devices such as the Sengstaken-Blakemore tube or the Minnesota tube is effective in approximately 40% to 90% of patients, the rebleeding rate associated with their use is approximately 50%. There is approximately a 30% rate of serious complications, such as aspiration pneumonia or esophageal rupture, resulting from the use of these tubes; therefore, their use is considered a temporary measure only.

Interventional radiologic techniques, such as the angiographic embolization of varices or the placement of a transjugular intrahepatic portosystemic stent shunt, may also be useful if endoscopic hemostasis fails or is unavailable. The surgical creation of a portosystemic shunt in an acutely bleeding patient is associated with mortality rates of 50% to 80%, and has fallen out of favor. Furthermore, such shunts make liver transplantation technically more difficult.

Case   A 42-year-old man is brought to the emergency room by ambulance after an episode of hematemesis and syncope at a local bar. He has never had prior GI bleeding, and regularly takes aspirin for the relief of chronic back pain. During your interview, he passes several liquid, maroon stools. Your physical examination reveals a supine blood pressure and pulse of 120/75 mm Hg and 110 beats per minute, respectively. When you sit him upright he complains of feeling faint and his systolic pressure drops to 90 mm Hg by palpation. His abdomen is nontender and distended. Shifting dullness is elicited and the spleen tip is palpable. The initial hemoglobin is 15 g/dL and the hematocrit is 45%.

1. How do you know this man has lost a significant amount of blood?
2. What are the most likely causes of this man's upper GI bleeding, and what should the next diagnostic step be?

Case Discussion

1. *How do you know this man has lost a significant amount of blood?*

He has significant orthostatic changes in his vital signs, indicating at least a 20% loss of total blood volume. The hemoglobin concentration or the hematocrit may be falsely reassuring in the setting of acute GI bleeding.

2. *What are the most likely causes of this man's upper GI bleeding, and what should the next diagnostic step be?*

The most likely causes of such severe upper GI bleeding are peptic ulcer disease and varices, the latter resulting from portal hypertension. This man has risk factors for both conditions. There is no way to distinguish one from the other based on the history and examination findings. After hemodynamic stabilization, emergency esophagogastroduodenoscopy should be performed for diagnosis and to carry out acute hemostasis.

Suggested Readings

Elta GH. Approach to the patient with gross gastrointestinal bleeding. In: Yamada T, Alpers DH, Owyang C, Powell DW, Silverstein FE, eds. *Textbook of gastroenterology*, 2nd ed. Philadelphia: JB Lippincott, 1995:671.

Jensen D, ed. Severe nonvariceal upper GI hemorrhage. *Gastrointest Endosc Clin North Am* 1991;1.

Stiegmann GV, Goff JS, Michaletz-Onody PA, et al. Endoscopic sclerotherapy as compared with endoscopic ligation for bleeding esophageal varices. *N Engl J Med* 1992;316:1527.

Peptic Ulcer Disease

1. What are the major risk factors for the development of peptic ulcers?
2. Is dietary adherence to bland meals and milk an accepted treatment for peptic ulcer disease? If not, what should the treatment be?

Discussion

1. *What are the major risk factors for the development of peptic ulcers?*

The major risk factors for the development of peptic ulcer disease are cigarette smoking, the ingestion of nonsteroidal antiinflammatory drugs (NSAIDs), and a family history of peptic ulcer. Peptic ulcers are thought to form when the effects of gastric acid and pepsin overwhelm the protective mucosal barrier. Diseases such as the Zollinger-Ellison syndrome increase the secretion of gastric acid. Other factors promote the breakdown of the mucosal barrier.

Ulcers are twice as likely to develop in cigarette smokers than in nonsmokers. In addition, ulcers heal more slowly and are more likely to recur in smokers. The mechanism responsible for cigarette smoke's ulcerogenic effect is not completely understood. NSAIDs disrupt the mucus–bicarbonate barrier, allowing acid to damage the underlying mucosa. The GI complications of NSAIDs are a major cause of upper GI bleeding and perforation, particularly in elderly women, and are responsible for a two- to threefold increased mortality risk in long-term users of NSAIDs. The combined use of NSAIDs and corticosteroids appears to increase the risk even further.

People who have first-degree relatives with peptic ulcers have three times the risk of acquiring ulcers, compared with the general population. The risk is even higher for the identical twin of a patient with ulcer disease.

Infection of the gastric mucosa by *Helicobacter pylori* is strongly associated with lower rates of duodenal ulcer healing and with higher rates of ulcer recurrence. The exact way in which *H. pylori* promotes ulcers is not known.

No conclusive evidence links dietary substances, including ethanol, caffeine, and spicy foods, with the development of peptic ulcers. Similarly, although a critically ill hospitalized patient may have stress ulcers, environmental stressors at home or at work have not been conclusively linked with the development of peptic ulcers. There is also no defined ulcerogenic personality.

2. *Is dietary adherence to bland meals and milk an accepted treatment for peptic ulcer disease? If not, what should the treatment be?*

No. Before the advent of modern pharmacologic therapy, the treatment of ulcer disease with frequent bland meals and milk was widely accepted. Unfortunately, such treatment actually increases the production of gastric acid and does not accelerate ulcer healing.

Histamine-2 receptor antagonists, of which cimetidine was the first agent released for use, are widely accepted as safe and effective for the treatment of peptic ulcers. These agents directly inhibit histamine-stimulated gastric acid secretion, and indirectly inhibit the histamine-potentiated, gastrin-stimulated acid secretion. When given in sufficient doses, the various H_2 receptor antagonists act equally well, with duodenal ulcer healing rates of 75% after 4 weeks, and 85% to 95% after 8 weeks of therapy. The selection of a particular agent should be determined by the patient's ability to comply with the dosing regimen, as well as the cost per dose.

Proton pump inhibitors, such as omeprazole and lansoprazole, are concentrated in the highly acidic environment of the parietal cell secretory canaliculi. When activated by protonation, these agents covalently bind to H^+/K^+ ATPase, thus causing irreversible inhibition of the enzyme and a 90% to 99% suppression of gastric acid production within 24 hours. At doses of 20 to 40 mg per day, omeprazole achieves more rapid pain relief and faster healing of peptic ulcers than do standard doses of H_2 receptor antagonists. Proton pump inhibitors are the treatment of choice for patients with nonsurgically correctable Zollinger-Ellison syndrome. These agents have displayed an excellent short-term safety profile, and, with increasing use, their long-term risk seems less than initially feared.

Sucralfate is an aluminum salt of sulfated sucrose. When placed in an acidic environment, it binds tenaciously to ulcers and promotes healing. It has no effect on acid secretion and has minimal acid-neutralizing effects. The entire mechanism of sucralfate's beneficial actions has not been determined. Sucralfate appears to be as effective as H_2 receptor antagonists in promoting the healing of acute peptic ulcers. Its systemic absorption is minimal, although its long-term effects on aluminum deposition are unknown. Its primary side effect is dose-related constipation.

Antacids are also effective in promoting the healing of gastric and duodenal ulcers. Frequent dosing is usually required to achieve an effectiveness equal to that of H_2 receptor antagonists. Such a dosing schedule often results in poor patient compliance, not to mention the side effect of diarrhea associated with the use of magnesium-containing antacids.

There is no evidence to support the use of these agents in various combinations for the primary treatment of peptic ulcers. Combination therapy with antibiotics, acid-suppresive medications, and bismuth compounds is effective in healing duodenal ulcers associated with *H. pylori* infection, and in preventing the recurrence of such ulcers.

Case A 50-year-old man has had recurrent and at times severe epigastric abdominal pain for the past several years. Antacids have given him symptomatic relief. The most recent episode began 1 week ago and has not responded completely to antacids. The pain now wakes him up at night. He smokes one pack of cigarettes per day, and he takes aspirin several times a week. His family history is unremarkable. Your examination reveals moderate epigastric tenderness without evidence of a mass. The stool is brown and positive for occult blood.

1. What are this man's risk factors for peptic ulcer disease?
2. What diagnostic tests should you consider?
3. When would you consider treatment for *H. pylori*?

Case Discussion

1. *What are this man's risk factors for peptic ulcer disease?*
   His smoking and NSAID ingestion are both risk factors for peptic ulcer disease.
2. *What diagnostic tests should you consider?*
   If the patient were younger than 40 years of age, had only mild and intermittent symptoms, and had no evidence of systemic disease or risk factors for malignancy, a trial of empiric antiulcer therapy without prior diagnostic tests would be acceptable. Otherwise, either esophagogastroduodenoscopy (EGD) or a double-contrast upper GI radiographic series is recommended. When there is a possibility of malignancy and biopsy specimens may be needed, EGD is considered superior to radiography for the purpose of diagnosis. Because the man described is older than 40 years of age, smokes cigarettes, has occult blood in the stool, and is having increasingly severe pain, a diagnostic workup (preferably EGD) rather than empiric therapy is recommended.
3. *When would you consider treatment for* H. pylori?
   Eradication of *H. pylori* when associated with duodenal ulcer usually is advocated, and eradication results in a dramatic reduction in ulcer recurrence.

Infection can be demonstrated by endoscopic biopsy, serology, or radioisotope breath test findings. A multiple-drug regimen is required for reliable eradication of the organisms. A commonly used combination has been that of a bismuth-containing compound, tetracycline, metronidazole, and either a proton pump inhibitor or an H_2 receptor antagonist. Better patient compliance and equal efficacy have been reported with combinations of clarithromycin, amoxicillin, bismuth, and a proton pump inhibitor or H_2 receptor antagonist.

Suggested Readings

Graham DY. Treatment of peptic ulcers caused by *Helicobacter pylori. N Engl J Med* 1993;328:349.

Isenberg J, McQuaid K, Laine L, et al. Acid-peptic disorders. In: Yamada T, Alpers, DH, Owyang C, Powell DW, Silverstein, FE, eds. *Textbook of gastroenterology*, 2nd ed. Philadelphia: Lippincott, 1995.

Salcedo JA, Al-Kawas F. Treatment of *Helicobacter pylori* infection. *Arch Intern Med* 1998;158:842.

Soll AH. Peptic ulcer and its complications. In: Feldman M, Scharschmidt BF, Sleisenger MH, eds. *Sleisenger and Fordtran's gastrointestinal and liver disease: pathophysiology, diagnosis, management*, 6th ed. Philadelphia: WB Saunders, 1998:620.

Gallstone Disease

1. Which group of people has the highest known prevalence of gallstones?
2. What are the different types of gallstones, and how do they form?
3. Should all patients with gallstones undergo cholecystectomy?
4. What are the common symptoms of gallstone disease, and what percentage of patients with asymptomatic gallstones eventually exhibit symptoms?
5. What is the best imaging technique to demonstrate cholelithiasis?
6. What treatment for symptomatic cholelithiasis is the standard against which other treatments are compared?

Discussion

1. *Which group of people has the highest known prevalence of gallstones?*

Studies that have examined autopsy findings with regard to gallstones have revealed that the highest known prevalence of gallstones is in the North American Pima Indians: approximately 60% for women and 25% for men. The population of Thailand has one of the lowest known prevalences: approximately 5% for women and 3% for men. The rate for whites in the United States and in north-central Europe is approximately 30% for women and 15% for men.

The composition of gallstones varies widely from population to population. The white population of the United States tends to have gallstones consisting largely of cholesterol, whereas the population of Asia tends to have brown, calcium bilirubinate stones.

The widespread variation in gallstone prevalence rates, the variation in gallstone composition among ethnic populations, and the general female-to-male ratio of approximately 2:1 all strongly implicate both hereditary and environmental factors in the etiology of gallstone disease.

2. *What are the different types of gallstones, and how do they form?*

There are three types of gallstones: cholesterol, brown pigment, and black pigment. Cholesterol gallstones are composed primarily of cholesterol monohydrate crystals mixed with mucin glycoprotein. Brown pigment gallstones are composed primarily of calcium bilirubinate. Black pigment gallstones are composed primarily of an insoluble bilirubin pigment polymer.

The formation of gallstones depends on the interplay of three factors: the production of lithogenic bile, gallbladder motility, and the nucleation of gallstones. Conditions that foster increased biliary cholesterol secretion, such as obesity, reduced bile acid secretion (as in terminal ileal Crohn's disease), and increased bilirubin production (as in sickle cell hemoglobinopathy), may all cause the production of lithogenic bile. Biliary stasis, such as that associated with prolonged total parenteral nutrition, also promotes gallstone formation. Decreased biliary immunoglobulin A (IgA) secretion, such as that found in many Asians, may allow the growth of bacteria that produce β-glucuronidase; the resulting hydrolysis of conjugated bilirubin promotes the precipitation of calcium bilirubinate. These calcium salts may then form the nuclei for gallstones.

3. *Should all patients with gallstones undergo cholecystectomy?*

No. Most patients with gallstones remain asymptomatic, and those who do become symptomatic are not at increased risk of death from either the disease or the operation. This is also true for patients with concurrent diabetes mellitus. Therefore, prophylactic cholecystectomy is not recommended for most asymptomatic patients, including those with diabetes mellitus. However, prophylactic cholecystectomy for asymptomatic gallstones is recommended for certain groups who face a high risk of morbidity. The risk of gallbladder cancer is high in Native Americans with cholelithiasis. Symptoms develop in nearly all children who have cholelithiasis. The likelihood of complications after emergency cholecystectomy is increased in patients with sickle cell hemoglobinopathy.

Patients with asymptomatic stones in the common bile duct (choledocholithiasis) experience a more morbid course; in 50% of patients with choledocholithiasis found postmortem, these ductal stones contributed to their death. Therefore, such stones should be removed either surgically or by ERCP.

4. *What are the common symptoms of gallstone disease, and what percentage of patients with asymptomatic gallstones eventually exhibit symptoms?*

Only 10% to 20% of the people with asymptomatic gallstones eventually exhibit symptoms. The onset of symptoms most commonly consists of recurrent biliary pain due to a stone in the cystic duct. This pain usually starts in the right upper quadrant or epigastrium and may radiate to the back or right shoulder. Biliary pain typically is gradual in onset and lasts several hours. Contrary to common belief, there is no particular temporal relationship to food intake or diet.

Persistent blockage of the cystic duct results in acute inflammation of the gallbladder, or acute cholecystitis. Patients with acute cholecystitis usually experience nausea, vomiting, and fever, and they complain of severe right upper quadrant pain. Elicitation of right upper quadrant abdominal tenderness in combination with leukocytosis is also highly suggestive of acute cholecystitis. The definitive treatment is cholecystectomy.

Obstruction of the common bile duct by a gallstone may result in cholangitis. Charcot's triad of symptoms (fever, chills, and jaundice) is exhibited by only 50% to 75% of patients with acute cholangitis. Most patients respond rapidly to proper antibiotic therapy; however, definitive treatment consists of decompression of the bile duct by ERCP, percutaneous cholangiography, or biliary surgery.

Acute biliary pancreatitis may result from a common bile duct stone that is transiently blocking the pancreatic duct within the ampulla of Vater. Urgent ERCP with endoscopic sphincterotomy should be considered for these patients.

5. *What is the best imaging technique to demonstrate cholelithiasis?*

Ultrasonography is the best initial method for demonstrating cholelithiasis because it has a 90% to 95% sensitivity and a 95% specificity. In addition, it is noninvasive and is encumbered by few technical limitations. Its main utility is in the demonstration of gallstones, although it is capable of detecting some additional findings, such as pericholecystic fluid, thickening of the gallbladder wall, and distention of the gallbladder, which suggest active inflammation. Ultrasonography can often reveal ductal dilatation or common bile duct stones, but failure to do so does not rule out choledocholithiasis.

Before ultrasonography became available, oral cholecystography was the test of choice for identifying gallstones. However, this procedure takes several hours to perform, is not effective when the bilirubin level exceeds 2.0 mg/dL, and the results are made unreliable by vomiting and diarrhea. This technique may be useful if there is a strong clinical suspicion of cholelithiasis but the ultrasonographic findings are equivocal.

Hepatobiliary scintigraphy is primarily used to assist in establishing the diagnosis of acute cholecystitis. If the radioactive tracer does not image the gallbladder, this strongly suggests obstruction of the cystic duct; however, this technique cannot identify stones within the gallbladder.

Endoscopic retrograde cholangiopancreatography is the best technique for diagnosing common bile duct stones, but it is far less sensitive in detecting stones in the gallbladder than is ultrasonography or oral cholecystography. Magnetic resonance cholangiopancreatography shows promise of being an accurate, noninvasive means of visualizing the bile ducts and pancreatic ducts.

In general, CT scanning visualizes gallstones poorly and adds little information in the overall effort to diagnose gallstone disease.

6. *What treatment for symptomatic cholelithiasis is the standard against which other treatments are compared?*

Open cholecystectomy has been the standard treatment of symptomatic gallstone disease. In a patient younger than 50 years of age who is free of complicating factors, the mortality rate associated with elective open cholecystectomy is less than 1%. The patient is usually hospitalized for approximately 5 days and remains on medical disability leave for an additional 4 to 6 weeks.

More recently, laparoscopic cholecystectomy has become the preferred treatment for symptomatic gallstone disease in most patients. Although this method is attended by a slightly higher rate of common bile duct injury, patients who undergo it usually require a shorter hospital stay and less time off from work than do those who undergo open cholecystectomy.

The dissolution of gallstones through the oral administration of bile acids such as ursodeoxycholic acid (ursodiol) is reserved for those patients who are either unable or unwilling to undergo surgery. This therapy is most effective for that 15% of patients with cholelithiasis who have small cholesterol gallstones floating in a functional gallbladder. After the 6 to 12 months of therapy is completed, the recurrence rate of gallstones is approximately 50% at 5 years.

Case   A 54-year-old Hispanic woman presents to the emergency room complaining of constant, severe right upper quadrant pain radiating to her right scapula that has lasted for approximately 6 hours. She has vomited twice without relief of the pain. She has experienced two similar, but less severe, episodes of such pain several weeks ago, for which she did not seek medical care. She does not have any chronic illness. Examination reveals a moderately obese woman with a temperature of 38°C. Her sclerae are slightly icteric. She exhibits abdominal guarding with moderate right upper quadrant tenderness on palpation, halting of inspiration during palpation, and normal bowel sounds. The white blood cell count is 14,000 cells/mm^3 and the alkaline phosphatase level is elevated at 200 IU/L. The total bilirubin level is 4 mg/dL. The serum aminotransferase values are normal.

1. What is the most likely diagnosis in this patient?
2. What imaging study should be performed?
3. How should you manage this patient's condition?

Case Discussion

1. *What is the most likely diagnosis in this patient?*

The most likely diagnosis is acute cholecystitis associated with choledocholithiasis and obstruction of the common bile duct by a gallstone. This woman's previous symptoms, which are consistent with recurrent biliary pain, suggest gallstone disease. The more severe symptoms she now has, which are associated with a leukocytosis, right upper quadrant abdominal tenderness, and inspiratory arrest with palpation in the right upper quadrant (Murphy's sign), suggest acute cholecystitis. The elevated alkaline phosphatase and total bilirubin levels are evidence that the common bile duct is obstructed. (The total bilirubin level rarely rises above 3 mg/dL in cholecystitis alone.)

2. *What imaging study should be performed?*

Abdominal ultrasonography should be performed routinely in patients suspected of having gallstone disease. In this patient, the typical presentation, which points toward acute cholecystitis and cholelithiasis, makes additional imaging studies unnecessary. If the ultrasonogram fails to demonstrate stones, a hepatobiliary scintigram could assist in making the diagnosis.

3. *How should you manage this patient's condition?*

Initial management should consist of the IV administration of fluids and antibiotic coverage for gram-negative organisms, together with nasogastric suction. Cholecystectomy should be performed soon after the patient's condition has stabilized because a delay in surgery is associated with higher morbidity rates. If open cholecystectomy is performed, an exploration of the common bile duct should be strongly considered. If the laparoscopic method is chosen, preoperative ERCP should be performed to remove the stone in the common bile duct. If the patient's condition does not improve rapidly and she still has obstructive jaundice, an urgent ERCP should be performed to decompress the biliary system.

Suggested Readings

Bilhartz LE, Horton JD. Gallstone disease and its complications. In: Feldman M, Scharschmidt BF, Sleisenger MH, eds. *Sleisenger and Fordtran's gastrointestinal and liver disease: pathophysiology, diagnosis, management*, 6th ed. Philadelphia: WB Saunders, 1998:948.

Lee SP, Kuver R. Gallstones. In: Yamada T, Alpers DH, Owyang C, Powell DW, Silverstein FE, eds. *Textbook of gastroenterology*, 2nd ed. Philadelphia: JB Lippincott, 1995:2187.

NIH Consensus Development Panel on Gallstones and Laparoscopic Cholecystectomy. NIH Consensus Conference: gallstones and laparoscopic cholecystectomy. *JAMA* 1993;269:1018.

Acute Hepatocellular Disease

1. What are the major signs and symptoms of acute hepatocellular injury, and which are specific to a particular process?
2. At what serum bilirubin level is jaundice detectable, and what are the main determinants of the serum bilirubin concentration?
3. What are four general causes of acute liver injury?
4. What are the features of viral hepatitis A, B, C, D, and E?
5. Match the following serologic results with the most likely clinical state.

a. HBsAg−, anti-HBs+, anti-HBc+	**1.** Acute hepatitis B
b. HBsAg−, anti-HBs+, anti-HBc−	**2.** Acute hepatitis A
c. HBsAg+, IgM anti-HBc+	**3.** Prior HBV infection, now immune
d. HBsAg+, IgM anti-HBc−	**4.** Prior HAV infection, now immune

    e. Anti-HAV(total)+, IgM anti-HAV−   **5.** Hepatitis B chronic carrier
    f. Anti-HAV(total)+, IgM anti-HAV+   **6.** Received hepatitis B vaccine

HBsAg, hepatitis B surface antigen; anti-HBs, antibody to hepatitis B surface antigen; anti-HBc, antibody to hepatitis B core antigen; anti-HAV, antibodies to hepatitis A antigens [total and immunoglobulin M (IgM) class]; −, negative; +, positive; HBV, hepatitis B virus; HAV, hepatitis A virus.

6. What hepatic enzyme pattern suggests the presence of alcoholic liver disease?
7. What are the clinical and laboratory findings characteristic of ischemic liver injury?
8. What is fulminant hepatic failure?

Discussion

1. *What are the major signs and symptoms of acute hepatocellular injury, and which are specific to a particular process?*

    The typical symptoms of hepatitis include malaise, fatigue, anorexia, nausea, scleral icterus, dark urine, abdominal pain, headache, fever, myalgia, and arthralgia. Signs include jaundice, hepatomegaly, tender liver, splenomegaly, and rash. In general, these features are nonspecific and do not help to identify the cause of liver injury.

2. *At what serum bilirubin level is jaundice detectable, and what are the main determinants of the serum bilirubin concentration?*

    A serum bilirubin level in the range of 2.5 to 3.0 mg/dL usually produces detectable scleral icterus. The serum bilirubin concentration is determined by the rates of bilirubin production (resulting from the catabolism of hemoglobin and other heme-containing enzymes) and elimination (including excretion into bile and the renal excretion of conjugated bilirubin). As a result, hemolysis and changes in renal function can considerably alter the serum bilirubin concentration.

3. *What are four general causes of acute liver injury?*

    Exposure to toxins is a common cause of acute liver injury. Such toxins include acetaminophen, halogenated hydrocarbons, and the toxin from the mushroom *Amanita phalloides*. **Infections** can also cause acute liver injury. The most common infections are those caused by hepatitis viruses A, B, C, D, and E. Parasites, bacteria, and fungi can also cause infectious hepatitis. Hepatic injury can also stem from **ischemia**. This is usually a result of severe systemic hypotension or congestive heart failure. Other sources of acute liver injury are the various **metabolic disorders** such as Wilson's disease and Reye's syndrome.

4. *What are the features of viral hepatitis A, B, C, D, and E?*

    Hepatitis A is caused by an RNA enterovirus that is usually transmitted by fecal-oral contamination. The hepatitis A virus is present in the stool only 2 weeks after infection, although symptoms do not appear until approximately 4 weeks after infection. This period of asymptomatic infectivity is partially responsible for the occasional outbreaks of hepatitis A spread by an unsuspecting food handler at a restaurant, or by children at a day-care center. Symptoms usually consist of nausea, vomiting, jaundice, and malaise, although the entire course of the disease may be subclinical, especially in children. Progression to fulminant hepatic failure is very rare, and full recovery is expected after 3 weeks of symptoms. The best serologic test for confirming *acute* viral hepatitis A is the IgM anti-HAV determination, which should be positive at the onset of symptoms. The presence of IgG anti-HAV implies the person had hepatitis A in the past and is immune. Susceptible people should be passively immunized with human immune serum globulin within 2 weeks of exposure to the hepatitis A virus. Active prophylaxis against hepatitis A for certain high-risk populations and patients with chronic liver disease is now available in the form of hepatitis A vaccine.

Hepatitis B is caused by a DNA virus that is transmitted by parenteral exposure to infected blood, usually through skin punctures by contaminated needles. Because this virus can also be transmitted across minute breaks in mucous membranes, risk factors for hepatitis B infection include sexual contact and the sharing of razors and toothbrushes with an infected person; transmission at birth from mother to child is also common. The hepatitis B virus is present in the blood approximately 2 months after infection, with symptoms appearing at approximately 3 months. IgM anti-HBc appears early in the disease and its measurement is the best single serologic test to confirm acute viral hepatitis B. The clinical course may progress to fulminant hepatic failure and death in up to 2% of the patients, or the infection may smolder in a chronic carrier state in up to 10% of the patients. Those who become chronic carriers are at high risk for early death from cirrhosis or hepatocellular carcinoma and should be considered candidates for α-interferon therapy. Immunization with vaccine made from recombinant HBsAg is highly effective and confers long-lasting protection against infection.

Hepatitis C is caused by an RNA virus that, like the hepatitis B virus, is believed to be transmitted primarily by parenteral exposure to infected blood, although a substantial percentage of patients have no identifiable risk factors. Symptoms of the acute infection are often mild. More than 50% of infected people become chronic carriers who are then at high risk for chronic hepatitis, cirrhosis, and hepatocellular carcinoma. Patients with chronic hepatitis C should be considered candidates for treatment with α-interferon or the combination of interferon and ribavirin. Serologic tests for hepatitis C continue to be improved as our knowledge of the virus increases. There is no known protective antibody and no known vaccine.

Hepatitis D is caused by a defective RNA virus that requires the presence of HBsAg for expression. Hence, infection by the hepatitis D virus occurs only as a coinfection with hepatitis B virus, or as a superinfection in those who are chronic hepatitis B virus carriers. The symptoms of hepatitis D are usually more severe than those seen with acute hepatitis B, with progression to fulminant hepatic failure and death in up to 20% of the patients. The specific serologic test for hepatitis D, anti-HD, should be carried out only if the HBsAg serology is positive. There is no vaccine specific to the hepatitis D virus, although immunization against hepatitis B confers protection against hepatitis D.

Hepatitis E is caused by an RNA virus that, like the hepatitis A virus, is transmitted primarily by fecal-oral contamination. Outbreaks of the disease can reach epidemic proportions in areas of the world where flooding and poor sanitation are prevalent. Although symptoms are mild in most patients, hepatitis E has a 20% mortality rate if it is acquired during pregnancy. Specific serologic tests are under development. There is no known vaccine for it.

5. *Match the following serologic results with the most likely clinical state.*

Following is the correct pairing of the serologic results with the most likely clinical state: a with 3, b with 6, c with 1, d with 5, e with 4, and f with 2. HBsAg is present in the settings of acute infection, chronic infection, and the carrier state. Anti-HBs and anti-HBc appear and the HBsAg level declines as the acute infection resolves. IgM anti-HBc or IgM anti-HAV is usually present only during acute infection, whereas the IgG classes of anti-HBc and anti-HAV persist, indicating a state of immunity after resolution of the acute infection. Anti-HBs appears alone, without anti-HBc, in response to hepatitis B vaccine.

6. *What hepatic enzyme pattern suggests the presence of alcoholic liver disease?*

In the setting of alcoholic hepatitis, the serum AST level is usually higher than the serum ALT level. In addition, the serum level of γ-glutamyltranspeptidase is often elevated because of induction of this enzyme by chronic ethanol ingestion.

7. *What are the clinical and laboratory findings characteristic of ischemic liver injury?*

Ischemic liver injury, or "shock liver," usually occurs in the setting of a recognized circulatory disturbance, such as hypotension or acute myocardial infarction. A rapid and dramatic rise in the AST and ALT levels is seen, with an equally rapid decline. The aminotransferase levels can rise into the thousands, approaching levels seen with acute viral hepatitis. A slow, steady increase in the serum bilirubin concentration subsequently occurs and peaks several days later. A liver biopsy is not needed for diagnosis, but, when specimens are obtained, they show centrilobular necrosis.

8. *What is fulminant hepatic failure?*

Fulminant hepatic failure is defined as progression to signs of liver failure, including hepatic encephalopathy, within 8 weeks of the onset of symptoms. Such a picture occurring 8 to 24 weeks from the onset of symptoms is considered subfulminant hepatic failure. Fulminant hepatic failure may be caused by viral, toxic, ischemic, or other causes of hepatocellular injury. The mortality rate for these entities is extremely high. Intensive support is indicated in affected patients, and liver transplantation should be considered if spontaneous recovery does not occur.

Case   A 37-year-old housewife reports 3 weeks of general fatigue, several days of dark urine, and 1 day of scleral icterus. She denies vomiting, but complains of mild, continuous pain in the right upper quadrant and intermittent nausea.

Physical examination reveals the patient to be jaundiced but comfortable. She shows no signs of malnutrition and has no spider angiomas or palmar erythema. The liver is tender and measures 15 cm by percussion in the mid-clavicular line. It is palpable 4 cm below the costal margin on inspiration. The spleen is not palpable and the examination findings are otherwise unremarkable.

1. What is your first diagnostic impression, and why? Match the laboratory findings with the various diagnostic possibilities.

	AST (IU/L)	ALT (IU/L)	Total bilirubin (mg/dL)	Alkaline phospha-tase (IU/L)	Diagnosis
A.	235	90	5.5	190	**1.** Acute viral hepatitis
B.	1,100	1,320	5.5	190	**2.** Chronic viral hepatitis
C.	235	325	5.5	190	**3.** Alcoholic hepatitis
D.	235	325	10.5	990	**4.** Bile duct obstruction

2. What other historical information is needed pertaining to risk factors?
3. What tests would you order if you suspected acute viral hepatitis?
4. If the patient has acute hepatitis A or hepatitis B, what should you tell her about the risk to her family, and what is the appropriate follow-up after she recovers?
5. What if all initial viral hepatitis serology results are nonreactive?
6. If the patient has a strong family history of liver disease, what tests are available to screen for inherited disorders?
7. Is a liver biopsy indicated in this patient?
8. Should this patient be admitted to the hospital?

Case Discussion

1. *What is your first diagnostic impression, and why? Match the laboratory findings with the various diagnostic possibilities.*

   The symptoms and examination findings are nonspecific and the laboratory findings and the various diagnostic possibilities are paired, as follows: A with 3, B with 1, C with 2, and D with 4. Very high aminotransferase levels (>1,000 IU/L) usually indicate an acute hepatocellular injury. Lower levels (two to five times normal) can be seen, however, early or late in the course of an acute injury, or in the settings of chronic hepatitis or alcoholic liver disease. An AST/ALT ratio that exceeds 1 suggests the presence of alcoholic liver disease. Alkaline phosphatase and bilirubin levels that are elevated out of proportion to the aminotransferase concentrations suggest a biliary obstructive process, but these are not specific with regard to the level of obstruction (extrahepatic obstruction versus intrahepatic cholestasis).

2. *What other historical information is needed pertaining to risk factors?*

A patient presenting with liver disease should be asked about the following: travel and hepatitis exposure (hepatitis A); parenteral risk factors, including transfusions, IV drug use, sexual contacts, and professional exposure (health care workers—hepatitis B and C); medications; environmental exposure; alcohol intake; childhood liver disease; and family history. Although prolonged excessive alcohol intake is often easily recognized, sometimes it is covert.

3. *What tests would you order if you suspected acute viral hepatitis?*

The selection of tests should be guided by the nature of the clinical history. The following tests should be done in a person suspected of having acute viral hepatitis: (a) IgM anti-HAV to check for acute hepatitis A; (b) IgM anti-HBc to check for acute hepatitis B; (c) HBsAg to determine if the patient could have acute hepatitis D; and (d) antibodies to hepatitis C antigens (anti-HCV) to check for acute hepatitis C. No other serologic tests are appropriate in the initial workup of patients with possible acute viral hepatitis.

4. *If the patient has acute hepatitis A or hepatitis B, what should you tell her about the risk to her family, and what is the appropriate follow-up after she recovers?*

The household and sexual contacts of people with acute hepatitis A should be passively immunized with immune globulin, and they should exercise careful standard precautions to avoid fecal-oral transmission. The household contacts of people with acute hepatitis B should avoid parenteral contact (the sharing of razors and toothbrushes and the like). Sexual contact should be minimized during the acute stage of the illness. After clinical recovery, it is important to determine whether the HBsAg has disappeared and anti-HBs has appeared. Failure to clear HBsAg suggests development of a chronic hepatitis B carrier state. Sexual or household contacts of hepatitis B carriers should be immunized with hepatitis B vaccine.

5. *What if all initial viral hepatitis serology results are nonreactive?*

Repeat testing for anti-HCV in 6 months is appropriate because this test may not be positive in the acute setting.

6 *If the patient has a strong family history of liver disease, what tests are available to screen for inherited disorders?*

A low serum ceruloplasmin level and a high urinary copper excretion are highly suggestive of Wilson's disease. A high serum ferritin level and high transferrin saturation are highly suggestive of hemachromatosis. The definitive test for both of these disorders is a liver biopsy.

7. *Is a liver biopsy indicated in this patient?*

Liver biopsy is not usually needed for diagnosis or prognosis in patients with acute liver diseases. Exceptions might include establishing the diagnosis of drug-induced or toxic hepatitis, ischemic liver injury, granulomatous disease, and, rarely, alcoholic hepatitis.

8. *Should this patient be admitted to the hospital?*

Most patients with acute hepatitis do not require hospital admission. However, those who exhibit evidence of severe liver injury, such as hepatic encephalopathy, a bilirubin level rising above 15 mg/dL, or an increasing prothrombin time, and those with severe anorexia or nausea, should be hospitalized.

Suggested Readings

Dolan SA. Vaccines for hepatitis A and B: the latest recommendations on safe and extended protection. *Postgrad Med* 1997;102:74.

Nanji AA, Zakim D. Alcoholic liver disease. In: Zakim D, Boyer TD, eds. *Hepatology: a textbook of liver disease*, 3rd ed. Philadelphia: WB Saunders, 1996:891.

Seeff LB. Diagnosis, therapy and prognosis of viral hepatitis. In: Zakim D, Boyer TD, eds. *Hepatology: a textbook of liver disease*, 3rd ed. Philadelphia: WB Saunders, 1996:1067.

5　Geriatrics

Laurence Robbins

Dementia

1. What is the most common cause of primary dementia in the U.S. population?
2. What are the pathognomonic postmortem findings of Alzheimer's disease?
3. Can the children of patients with Alzheimer's disease be genetically tested and told with assurance whether they will inherit the disease?
4. How can cognitive function be tested quickly and reliably?
5. Can the intellectual decline seen in patients with Alzheimer's disease be halted or reversed with medications?

Discussion

1. *What is the most common cause of primary dementia in the U.S. population?*

Alzheimer's disease is the most common cause of primary dementia in the U.S. population. Dementia affects approximately 4 million people in the United States. Primarily a disease of old age, it afflicts approximately 2% of the population between 65 and 70 years of age, and between 20% and 50% of the population older than 80 years of age. It is a clinical syndrome characterized by an acquired and global decline in intellectual functioning. Deficits in three or more of the following five areas are needed to confirm diagnosis: memory, language, visuospatial skills, cognition, and emotions.

Alzheimer's disease is more properly called *dementia of the Alzheimer's type.* This distinction in nomenclature is made because the diagnosis of Alzheimer's disease cannot actually be confirmed without the microscopic examination of brain tissue. This disease accounts for 70% or more of irreversible dementia in primary care populations older than 65 years of age. Multiinfarct dementia (caused by cerebrovascular disease), late-stage Parkinson's disease, and chronic alcoholism account for most other cases of irreversible dementia. Postmortem autopsy series suggest that at least 10% of dementias represent a combination of Alzheimer's disease and some other cause, most often multiinfarct dementia. Rare causes of dementia include diffuse Lewy body disease, Jakob-Creutzfeldt disease, Pick's disease, Huntington's chorea, and anoxic brain damage.

Although thyroid disease, vitamin B_{12} deficiency, depression, and drug toxicity may result in decreased cognition, these problems are usually distinguished from the irreversible dementing diseases already listed because their treatment may halt or reverse the memory impairment.

2. *What are the pathognomonic postmortem findings of Alzheimer's disease?*

Neurofibrillary tangles and neuritic plaques are postmortem findings pathognomonic for Alzheimer's disease, and the diagnosis is certain only if the pathologist identifies a significant number of these lesions in the typical distribution (i.e., heavy concentrations in the hippocampus and surrounding areas of the temporal lobes). Ninety percent or more of patients with clinically diagnosed dementia of the Alzheimer's type have the diagnosis confirmed at postmortem examination. Plaques and neurofibrillary tangles are also found in the brains of normal elderly subjects, but in much smaller numbers than in the elderly patients with Alzheimer's disease.

Other conditions that may be clinically confused with Alzheimer's disease are associated with different pathologic findings. A multifocal loss of brain tissue secondary to ischemia is seen in the setting of multiinfarct dementia. Degeneration of the dopaminergic cells in the substantia nigra and Lewy bodies are found in patients with Parkinson's disease. Sometimes pathologists find cortical and subcortical neuronal loss associated with Lewy bodies outside the traditional distribution of these lesions in Parkinson's disease. This entity is now identified as diffuse Lewy body disease and may represent the second most common cause of neurodegenerative dementia behind Alzheimer's disease.

3. *Can the children of patients with Alzheimer's disease be genetically tested and told with assurance whether they will inherit the disease?*

The evidence for the genetic inheritance of Alzheimer's disease has dramatically increased. Familial Alzheimer's disease rarely occurs in an autosomal dominant pattern. Representing less than 5% of all cases of Alzheimer's disease, nearly all the families with autosomal dominant disease have been found to carry one of three defective genes in chromosomes 1, 14, or 21. In general, the dementia becomes evident in the affected family members between 35 and 65 years of age, much earlier than the usual patient with Alzheimer's disease, whose dementia often does not become clinically evident until the eighth decade. Differences in apolipoprotein E (ApoE) synthesis linked to chromosome 19 may increase a person's risk for the more common form of late-onset Alzheimer's disease. Three ApoE alleles have been described, ApoE2, ApoE3, and ApoE4. ApoE4 appears to increase the risk for development of late-onset Alzheimer's disease, whereas ApoE2 reduces this risk. ApoE3 is the most commonly inherited allele and confers a risk that is intermediate between that of ApoE2 and ApoE4. However, not all people with an ApoE4 allele will acquire Alzheimer's disease and, conversely, many cases of Alzheimer's disease occur among people who are homozygous for ApoE3.

Therefore, genetic testing in the absence of an autosomal dominant pattern inheritance of the disease does not definitively tell a person whether he or she will acquire the disease. There are no treatments that clearly delay or prevent the onset of Alzheimer's disease, and this further limits any clinical benefit of genetic testing.

4. *How can cognitive function be tested quickly and reliably?*

   The Folstein Mini-Mental Status Examination (MMSE) and similar brief mental status tests (e.g., the Pfeiffer and the Blessed Dementia Scale) are quick, standardized tools to assess cognitive function and may reliably estimate the severity of mental status impairment. The MMSE measures orientation, memory, and attention as well as the status of written and spoken language and visuospatial skills. With a sensitivity of 87% and specificity of 82%, the MMSE results are reproducible when the test is administered either by a professional or by someone trained to do so. One of the best single-item screening tests is clock drawing. The inability to draw familiar, relatively simple objects may reflect apraxia, often an early sign of dementia. The examiner asks the patient to draw a clock face, fill in the numbers, and then draw the hour and minute hands indicating a time, such as 2:45. Studies suggest that this simple test has a sensitivity and specificity similar to more elaborate screening tools like the MMSE.

5. *Can the intellectual decline seen in patients with Alzheimer's disease be halted or reversed with medications?*

   Research aimed at finding medications that retard or even reverse the progression of Alzheimer's disease has increased dramatically. A single, placebo-controlled, double-blinded, randomized, 52-week trial showed that patients with Alzheimer's disease who took extract of *Gingko biloba* had slightly better scores on some mental status tests. The clinical significance of this study is unclear. Unfortunately, this substance is available only in unstandardized formulations, so that patients who wish to purchase gingko will be unable to compare the potency and efficacy of various brands. A single randomized trial of two antioxidants, vitamin E and selegiline, suggested that 1,000 IU of vitamin E twice daily may have some modest benefit in slowing the progression of Alzheimer's disease. Similar results were noted for the monoamine oxidase inhibitor, selegiline, but the combination of vitamin E and selegiline was less effective than either taken alone. Because the benefit of the individual agents was apparent only when four different outcome measures were combined into a single measure, the validity of this study remains questionable. Epidemiologic, retrospective evidence suggests that nonsteroidal antiinflammatory agents (e.g., ibuprofen) and postmenopausal estrogen replacement therapy may prevent the onset or progression of Alzheimer's disease, but prospective studies have not yet confirmed these preliminary observations.

   Recognizing that cholinergic neuronal loss is a predominant pathologic finding in Alzheimer's disease, investigators have focused on finding ways to enhance cerebral cholinergic activity. This observation led to the development of new cholinesterase inhibitors that block the breakdown of acetylcholine in the brains of patients with Alzheimer's disease. The first U.S. Food and Drug Administration–approved cholinesterase inhibitor, tacrine (Cognex; Parke-Davis, Morris Plains, NJ), had significant hepatotoxicity and gastrointestinal side effects that limited dosing and effectiveness. Donepezil (Aricept; Pfizer, New York, NY) was released in early 1997 and appears to have an efficacy similar to tacrine's while producing less toxicity. In all studies of these drugs, benefits have been studied only in trials lasting 6 months to 1 year. Most patients with early Alzheimer's disease live 10 to 12 years. Long-term studies are needed to determine whether cholinesterase inhibitors will significantly delay the clinical progression of this disease. Unfortunately, even the short-term studies to date suggest that any benefit of the available cholinesterase inhibitors disappears a few weeks after patients discontinue these drugs. This observation suggests that cholinesterase inhibitors mask the clinical appearance of symptoms for approximately 6 months but do not change the rate of deterioration of the progression disease. Former President Ronald Reagan, one of the most famous people with Alzheimer's disease, purportedly had no benefit from a trial of cholinesterase inhibitors.

Physicians can do much to reduce the functional decline of patients with Alzheimer's disease, even if they cannot stop the progression of dementia. The physician must consider nearly any medication as a potential contributor to deterioration in mental status. Medications ranging from psychoactive medications to digoxin may reversibly accelerate cognitive decline. Depression is a common complication of Alzheimer's disease and may also make patients appear to have further decline in intellectual function. Appropriate treatment of depression may lead to a dramatic improvement in cognition and functional status. Finally, physicians must support the caregivers of patients with Alzheimer's disease. Demented patients' quality of life is frequently related to the level of stress their caregivers experience in caring for them. Caregiver comfort and satisfaction will, in turn, help to maintain the demented patient's physical health and function.

Case   An 88-year-old black man is seen whose only medical problem is mild hypertension, treated with hydrochlorothiazide (12.5 mg daily). During the initial outpatient interview, his wife confides that approximately 2 years ago she began to notice he was becoming forgetful and exhibiting outbursts of anger, which were very atypical for him. She describes him as having been a very kind and gentle man, who was a teacher before his retirement. Gradually his interests and involvement in activities have declined. He began to nap throughout the day and then stay up at night. Sometimes she would find him in the kitchen "cooking dinner" at 3:00 a.m. She has become afraid to leave him home alone. Six months ago, he was involved in a motor vehicle accident and charged with failure to yield the right-of-way, but has refused to stop driving despite several near-collisions since then. Finally, during the past few weeks, he has become physically abusive toward her.

You find the patient to be a tall, well dressed man with a friendly manner. His blood pressure is 165/80 mm Hg; pulse, 75 beats per minute and regular; and respirations, 18 per minute. His temperature is 37°C. Findings during the physical examination, including a thorough neurologic examination, are normal except for a positive palmomental response. He exhibits difficulty following simple commands. His Folstein MMSE score is 16/30 (normal, >23) and he is unaware of his errors. His score of 3/30 on the Geriatric Depression Scale suggests that he is not depressed. When asked how things are at home, he is slow to respond and says, "fine." On further questioning about his relationship with his wife, all he says is that his wife is a "good woman." His self-assessment is that he is doing well "for an old man." Laboratory evaluation reveals normal hematocrit and serum creatinine values. Liver function test results are normal. His vitamin B_{12} level is 480 pg/mL (normal, 225 to 800 pg/mL); folate, at 10 ng/mL, and thyroid-stimulating hormone, at 3 IU/mL, were also normal. A rapid plasma reagin test is nonreactive. A head computed tomography (CT) scan obtained at the time of his automobile accident 6 months ago was interpreted to show "cerebral atrophy, consistent with age."

1. Which aspect of this patient's presentation is most valuable in formulating a differential diagnosis?
2. On a CT scan or magnetic resonance imaging (MRI), what findings are most characteristic of Alzheimer's disease or other causes of dementia?
3. For what potentially treatable cause of memory loss should this patient be screened?
4. Can anything be done to help his wife manage the behavior of her husband?

Case Discussion

1. *Which aspect of this patient's presentation is most valuable in formulating a differential diagnosis?*

The history provided by the patient's wife is the most informative aspect of this patient's condition. When dementia is advanced, its diagnosis is obvious. Early on, however, the patient may hide or rationalize his deficits and his cognitive changes may be so subtle that they are more apparent at home than in the clinician's office. This is where the family history becomes of utmost importance. In this case, the patient's wife supplied many clues to her husband's dementia. This information could never be obtained directly from a patient who is unaware of the problem.

A normal physical examination is common in a patient with early Alzheimer's disease. The first pathologic changes in Alzheimer's disease occur mostly in the temporal and parietal lobes of the brain and spare the motor strip. Thus, the first signs of disease are frequently limited to memory impairment, subtle personality changes (e.g., increased irritability or flattening of affect), aphasia, and apraxia. Gait disorder and motor findings are unusual.

The only significant finding during this patient's examination was a palmomental response. This response, consisting of the contraction of the mentalis and orbicularis oris muscles with brisk scratching of the palm of the ipsilateral hand, is a primitive reflex that may appear with bilateral frontal lobe lesions, which may occur in Alzheimer's disease as well as other dementias.

2. *On a CT scan or MRI, what findings are most characteristic of Alzheimer's disease or other causes of dementia?*

Computed tomography scanning or MRI may show evidence of temporal lobe atrophy in early Alzheimer's disease. However, neuroimaging evidence of cerebral atrophy correlates more with advancing age than it does with mental status decline. CT or MRI findings of white matter disease consistent with multiinfarct dementia have been reported in patients with normal cognition. Conversely, MRI and CT scans fail to show abnormalities in 20% of patients who have clinically diagnosed Alzheimer's disease. Therefore, it is not surprising that the patient's CT scan findings were normal for his age. If the dementia has gradually progressed for 2 or more years, the mental status examination shows severe impairment, and the patient has no focal neurologic findings or gait disorder, neuroimaging is extremely unlikely to reveal findings that will alter management.

3. *For what potentially treatable cause of memory loss should this patient be screened?*

The goal of the evaluation is to identify diseases that can be diagnosed confidently, or for which there is treatment that might reverse the cognitive deficits. Therefore, the physician should routinely take a careful history, complete a careful physical examination, and order a basic laboratory evaluation including a complete blood count, serum electrolytes, calcium, creatinine, thyroid-stimulating hormone, and vitamin B_{12} level. The physician orders other tests, such as CT scan or MRI, based on the results of the history and physical examination. For example, a history of recent or sudden onset of cognitive impairment after head trauma suggests the possibility of subdural hematoma and indicates the need for brain imaging. This is particularly true if the physical examination reveals a gait disorder or focal neurologic signs. The triad of dementia of recent onset, gait disorder, and urinary incontinence may suggest the diagnosis of normal-pressure hydrocephalus, another potentially reversible cause of cognitive decline. This disorder is extremely rare, and, although some patients may experience improvement with ventricular shunting, postoperative complications (e.g., subdural hematoma, infection, and shunt obstruction) are very common.

Hypothyroidism and vitamin B_{12} deficiency sufficient to affect neuronal function usually cause disturbances in attention and consciousness, and are diagnosed and treated long before dementia appears. Occasionally, however, a patient delays getting medical care until dementia is present, so all patients should be evaluated for these conditions.

Neurosyphilis is no longer a common cause of cognitive impairment. These patients usually have other neurologic findings, such as dorsal column disease manifest by loss of position and vibratory sensation, in addition to mental status decline.

A severely depressed patient may seem disoriented and perform poorly on tests of cognitive function. These deficits may be due to reversible changes that mimic the irreversible changes of dementia. Because the diagnosis of depression can be difficult and based on subtle findings in an elderly patient, many tools, such as the Geriatric Depression Scale, have been developed to aid in its diagnosis.

Unfortunately, the patient described here did not exhibit any of these potentially treatable abnormalities.

4. *Can anything be done to help his wife manage the behavior of her husband?*

Yes. There are ways to help the patient's wife manage her husband's behavior. Caring for a demented patient is a physically and emotionally exhausting job. As recommendations are made, the physician must consider not only the patient, but the caregiver. Allowing caregivers to vent emotions, acknowledging the difficulty of their task, telling them what to expect as the disease progresses, offering respite care, and referring them to support groups are small things that may help them cope better with the patient and his or her needs.

The treatment of behavioral problems is difficult, but can be effective. Regular exercise and limiting the number and duration of late afternoon or evening naps may help reduce the nocturnal insomnia that often complicates the management of demented elderly patients. Most sedatives and hypnotics, particularly the long-acting ones, should not be used because they may cause oversedation or a paradoxical increase in agitation, and may only worsen cognitive and behavioral deficits.

Delusions are common in dementia syndromes. In fact, approximately 50% of the patients with Alzheimer's disease or multiinfarct dementia experience delusions. Agitation and combative behaviors can accompany these symptoms. The cautious use of low doses of haloperidol, or other antipsychotics, may be helpful in ameliorating these behaviors.

Suggested Readings

Jagust WJ. Functional imaging in dementia: an overview. *J Clin Psychiatry* 1994;55[Suppl]:5.

Small CW, Rabins PV, Barry PP, et al. Diagnosis and treatment of Alzheimer disease and related disorders. *JAMA* 1997;278:1363.

Weytingh MD, Bossuyt PMMM, van Crevel H. Reversible dementia: more than 10% or less than 1%? A quantitative review. *J Neurol* 1995;242:466.

Falls in the Elderly

1. How commonly do falls occur in the elderly?

2. How often does injury or death result from a fall?

3. What factors make the elderly more likely to fall?

4. What should the history and physical examination focus on in a patient who is having problems with falling?

Discussion

1. *How commonly do falls occur in the elderly?*

Thirty percent of the elderly older than 65 years of age who live out in the community experience falls annually. Most patients are reluctant to tell their physician or family members of these falls, so this figure is probably an underestimate. Because a history of falls increases the risk of future falls and serious injury, physicians must elicit a history of falling and then intervene to reduce the future risk.

2. *How often does injury or death result from a fall?*

Accidental injury is the sixth leading cause of death in people older than 65 years of age, and two thirds of these deaths are related to falls. Fractures occur in 5% of falls, and the most common fracture sites are the hip, humerus, wrist, and pelvis. Another 5% of falls cause soft tissue injuries, such as sprains, joint dislocations, and hematomas, that require the patient's hospitalization. Even in those cases in which no injury is incurred, there are still consequences; a person who has fallen may become emotionally paralyzed by a "fear of falling" and begin to limit activities and thus become socially isolated. In this way, a fall may have a negative impact on a person's quality of life and independence. In nursing homes, 50% or more of the ambulatory residents fall each year, despite the presence of trained staff and careful observation of safety measures. Approximately 4% of all patients in nursing homes have traumatic bone fractures annually, particularly hip fracture.

Once elderly people become bed bound, the risk of falling obviously decreases. The risk of fracture is greater in the ambulatory patients, particularly if the patient's gait is unsteady. Falls do not occur only in frail elderly patients; many serious injuries actually occur in active elderly people who fall.

3. *What factors make the elderly more likely to fall?*

Falls may be the first sign of an acute medical illness, a so-called *sentinel fall*. Frequently, multiple factors, rather than a single problem, contribute to an elderly patient's risk of falling. It is often best to divide these factors into two categories: intrinsic and extrinsic. **Intrinsic factors** are those related to aging and disease processes. These include changes in balance and gait, pain and stiffness due to arthritis, decreased muscle strength, dizziness, postural hypotension, sensory losses (hearing, vision, and proprioception), cognitive impairment, stroke, and syncope. Other intrinsic causes to consider are vertebrobasilar insufficiency, depression, hypothyroidism, mechanical foot problems, or cardiac arrhythmias.

Patients tend to attribute their falls to **extrinsic factors**, such as tripping over obstacles, but, with advancing age, it becomes less likely that extrinsic factors alone are at fault. Indeed, most falls in frail elderly occur during routine activities of daily living. However, certain extrinsic factors such as medication side effects (e.g., orthostasis and dizziness) are common. Similarly, falling may be the first clue that leads the physician to the eventual diagnosis of alcoholism as the cause for poor balance and subsequent falls. Other extrinsic factors that may contribute to falls include inadequate lighting, slippery floors, loose throw rugs, exposed electrical cords, items out of reach (so that patients stand on unstable chairs or other supports and lose their balance more easily), lack of assistive devices such as bathroom rails to steady themselves, bed height too high (so that falls from bed more likely result in significant injury), unsafe stairs, and poorly fitting footwear. Eliminating or reducing extrinsic factors may help to reduce the risk of subsequent falls.

4. *What should the history and physical examination focus on in a patient who is having problems with falling?*

A careful history of the falling episodes should be obtained. This includes the frequency, the patient's activity at the time of the fall, where they occur, and associated symptoms such as loss of consciousness. It is important to get information from anyone who may have witnessed the fall and can provide a more detailed description of the circumstances. Ask carefully about drug usage, including over-the-counter medications. Vital signs, including pulse and blood pressure, taken lying and standing, can identify orthostatic hypotension, which often contributes to a fall risk. Physical examination must include a careful cardiac examination that looks for irregular rhythm and murmurs. On neurologic examination, visual acuity and peripheral vision, strength, and cerebellar, sensory, and mental status must be assessed, looking for impaired vision, weakness, ataxia, neuropathy, or dementia. A useful screening test for balance, strength, mobility, and endurance is the "get-up-and-go" test. To perform it, ask the patient to get up from a chair (without using his or her hands to push away from the chair), walk across the room, turn around, walk back to the chair, and sit down. It takes very little time and reveals much about the patient's gait. Beyond screening laboratory tests such as a complete blood count or chemistry panel, vitamin B_{12} and thyroid-stimulating hormone levels should be measured if there is evidence of a peripheral neuropathy or treatable causes of muscular weakness. Other tests such as visual testing, assessment of vestibular function (e.g., electronystagmography), ambulatory cardiac monitoring, or CT scanning should be done only if there are clinical clues to specific disorders that may cause falls (i.e., vertigo, syncope, or focal neurologic findings).

Case   An 86-year-old man is seen because of a history of frequent falls, reported by his wife. Other than the falls, she is able to care for him in their home. She reports that he falls at least three times per week, usually without injury. However, he has required evaluation in the emergency room and the suturing of superficial lacerations received in the falls. These falls are not accompanied by loss of consciousness, palpitations, or seizure activity. His medical history is remarkable for probable Alzheimer's dementia, severe degenerative joint disease with chronic low back pain, decreased hearing and vision, benign familial tremor, and urinary incontinence (related to his dementia). His current medications consist of calcium supplementation, propranolol (40 mg three times a day), diphenhydramine (50 mg taken at night) for insomnia, and acetaminophen as needed. His wife reports that he has a cane and a walker but rarely uses them.

Physical examination reveals a pleasant, thin, demented man. Vital signs are as follows: temperature, 37°C; respirations, 20 per minute; pulse, 55 beats per minute; and blood pressure, 105/70 mm Hg supine. On standing, his pulse rate remains at 55 beats per minute but his blood pressure drops to 90/65 mm Hg and, when asked, he says he feels "woozy." Cardiac examination findings are unremarkable; the rhythm is regular and there are no murmurs or gallops. His neurologic findings are nonfocal. His cranial nerves are intact and there is no nystagmus. He has a fine tremor in both hands, but normal tone and strength in all extremities. Sensory examination is intact. Cerebellar function is slow, but finger-to-nose and heel-to-shin testing shows accurate responses. His posture is stooped and his wide-based gait is unsteady. He walks by holding on to the office furniture. Laboratory tests consisting of complete blood count and electrolyte and creatinine measurements yield unremarkable findings.

1. What problems are contributing to this patient's falls?
2. What diagnostic tests may be the most helpful in this patient?
3. What intervention, or interventions, would you institute to decrease this patient's risk of falling?

Case Discussion

1. *What problems are contributing to this patient's falls?*

The history and physical examination findings suggest a number of factors contributing to this patient's falls. Degenerative joint disease increases the risk of falls in a number of ways. First, stiffness and change in posture affect balance and, second, joint pain experienced while walking may discourage activity and exercise, which, in turn, contributes to decreased muscle tone and an increased risk of falling. This vicious cycle may foster a fear of falling and the eventual cessation of walking. Dementia may be associated with poor judgment, which also adds to the risk of falling. For example, without supervision, a demented patient may try to maintain his balance by grasping an unstable chair or other object that cannot support his or her weight. Even if a demented patient has a cane or a walker, he or she may not remember to use it. The patient's caregiver needs to be educated about the need for the frequent verbal "cueing" of demented patients (e.g., reminding them to use assistive devices or not to grasp unstable objects for balance). The physician must always review the nature of the patient's medication to determine if side effects may be contributing to fall risk. In this case, the patient is taking a β-adrenergic blocker (propranolol) for the treatment of tremor, which may be causing bradycardia, and this, in turn, may contribute to the patient's weakness and risk of falling. Orthostatic hypotension caused by various medications is a frequent source of fall risk. Antihypertensive medications or anticholinergic medications (e.g., his diphenhydramine or tricyclic antidepressants, such as amitriptyline) are two classes of medications that frequently cause orthostatic hypotension. Sedative medications not only alter the level of consciousness, but may blunt postural reflexes. Cardiac dysrhythmias are responsible for 25% to 35% of all syncopal episodes, and they account for 2% to 10% of falls. However, in this patient, who has no history of cardiac disease or loss of consciousness, a dysrhythmia is an unlikely contributor to his falls.

2. *What diagnostic tests may be the most helpful in this patient?*

Any sensory deficits that can be alleviated may reduce the risk of falling. Ophthalmologic evaluation of his poor vision may identify a reversible problem such as cataracts. With better vision, the patient may be able to navigate more safely and thus reduce his fall risk even if his other deficits are less reversible. In addition, the patient's urinary incontinence may contribute to his falls. If urinary urgency leads the patient to rush to the bathroom and lose his balance, attention to reversible causes of his urge incontinence may reduce the risk of falling (see the discussion of urinary incontinence that follows).

More sophisticated and expensive tests, such as electroencephalography, Holter monitoring, and CT scanning of the head, may be performed in patients who are falling but should be done selectively, based on the patient's history and physical examination findings. Because this patient has no evidence of seizure activity, an electroencephalogram is unlikely to be revealing. Likewise, the diagnostic yield of 24-hour ambulatory cardiac monitoring would probably be very low, given the lack of cardiac symptoms, and is unnecessary for this patient. If he had any focal neurologic deficits or recent changes in cognition, a CT scan might be called for to rule out a subdural hematoma or a stroke but, again, there is no suggestion of such a problem in this patient.

3. *What intervention, or interventions, would you institute to decrease this patient's risk of falling?*

A patient who is elderly and has many medical problems is often expected to be frail and weak. However, even the frail elderly may improve their strength and balance by participating in a regular exercise program. Evidence is emerging that modest weight training, in addition to aerobic conditioning, may further help to increase muscle mass and balance and reduce the risk of falls. If this patient were stronger and in less discomfort, his gait and balance would likely improve with exercise.

The propranolol this patient is taking is a concern. He is likely taking it to control his tremor, which is not a dangerous condition. This β blocker is lowering his blood pressure too much and preventing his heart rate from increasing to compensate, and this is especially a problem considering that the patient has no history of hypertension. It should be reduced and perhaps eventually discontinued.

Restraints are not a safe treatment option because patients may only become weaker and despondent when "tied down." Even in nursing home settings, no evidence has been found that placing patients in restraints significantly reduces the risk of serious injuries due to falls. Families concerned about repeated falls in a loved one sometimes believe that he or she will be safer in a nursing home. However, doing this may only add to the patient's agitation, which then leads to a desire to escape. This actually increases the risk of falls, particularly because supervision cannot be constant and the intrinsic risk factors for falling still exist. As for sedation, psychoactive medications such as the longer-acting benzodiazepines (e.g., flurazepam) have been shown to be associated with an increased risk of falls, and should not be prescribed. Medications that increase the risk of falls are also likely concomitantly to worsen any underlying mental status impairment. This patient is on diphenhydramine, which may be sedating him and impairing his balance. This should be discontinued.

Suggested Readings

Hindmarch JJ, Estes EH Jr. Falls in older persons. *Arch Intern Med* 1989;149:2217.
King MD, Tinetti ME. Falls in community-dwelling older persons. *J Am Geriatr Soc* 1995;43:1146.
Rubenstein LZ, Josephson KR, Robbins AS. Falls in the nursing home. *Ann Intern Med* 1994;121:442.

Urinary Incontinence

1. How common is urinary incontinence in the elderly?
2. What are the normal changes in bladder physiology that occur with aging?
3. How is incontinence classified, and what are the characteristics of the different types?
4. Of what does the differential diagnosis of transient urinary incontinence consist?

Discussion

1. *How common is urinary incontinence in the elderly?*

   Urinary incontinence, the involuntary loss of urine, affects 10 million Americans. Of people older than 65 years of age, 5% of men and 25% of women have problems with incontinence. In 1987 alone, the direct cost of the problem was over $10 billion. Incontinence adds $3 to $12 per day to the cost of nursing home care, and 50% to 90% of all nursing home residents experience some incontinence.

   Besides the significant expense of incontinence, it is a source of many medical complications, such as rashes, pressure ulcers, catheterization, urinary tract infections, falls, and fractures. There are also social consequences, such as embarrassment, isolation, and depression. It also adds to caregiver stress.

2. *What are the normal changes in bladder physiology that occur with aging?*

   Bladder capacity and compliance decline with aging, as does the ability to postpone voiding. There are also more frequent uninhibited bladder contractions and an increase in the residual volume of urine. Because of an age-related decrease in the glomerular filtration rate and a delay in the excretion of a water load, approximately two thirds of fluid is excreted in the evening rather than during the day. This leads to nocturnal urinary frequency and the risk of nocturnal urinary incontinence.

There are also sex-specific changes. Estrogen deficiency in women leads to weakened sphincter tone and changes in the position of the bladder neck. The urethral length shortens and the maximal urethral closure pressures decline. In men, prostatic enlargement can potentially block urine outflow. All of these changes predispose elderly patients to incontinence. The encouraging news is that 50% of the cases are transient and two thirds of the remaining cases can be either cured or markedly alleviated with therapy.

3. *How is incontinence classified, and what are the characteristics of the different types?*

Urge incontinence is the most common type of incontinence in the elderly, accounting for approximately 80% of cases. Afflicted patients often describe a sudden uncontrollable urge to void that may not allow them time to reach the bathroom. The urge is caused by contraction of the bladder's detrusor muscle, which forces moderate to large volumes of urine out through the urethra. Central nervous system diseases (e.g., stroke, Alzheimer's and Parkinson's diseases, a primary brain tumor, or metastatic disease) and primary disease of the bladder (e.g., carcinoma, the effects of radiation treatment, or bladder outlet obstruction) may be associated with urge incontinence.

Stress incontinence is particularly common in elderly women. In pure stress incontinence, leakage occurs with increases in pressure caused by coughing, sneezing, laughing, or lifting. In it, only a small amount of urine leaks out after a delay of 5 to 15 seconds. The source of the problem in women is usually urethral hypermobility due to laxity of the pelvic floor musculature caused by childbearing. In men, stress incontinence is less common but may occur if the urethral sphincter is damaged during transurethral or radical prostatectomy.

Overflow incontinence is caused either by outlet obstruction or an atonic bladder (i.e., ineffective detrusor contraction due to myogenic or neurologic causes). Leakage of small amounts of urine may occur throughout the day and night. Patients may also describe urinary hesitancy and a feeling of incomplete emptying. On abdominal examination, a distended bladder may be palpated even after the patient has attempted to void.

Reflex incontinence is usually due to a suprasacral spinal cord lesion. As the bladder distends, contraction occurs. Leakage is not associated with stress and there is no warning before the onset of urination. Incontinence episodes are of moderate volume and occur frequently.

Functional incontinence is due to a problem unrelated to the urinary tract. Examples are impaired mobility or metabolic problems such as hyperglycemia or mild renal insufficiency. This diagnosis can be made only by taking a very careful history and after excluding the previously listed causes. Functional incontinence may result from the use of iatrogenic drugs that impair cognition or from imposed limitations on mobility, such as restraints.

Because urinary incontinence in the elderly is often multifactorial, all potentially contributing risk factors should be carefully reviewed to determine its cause.

4. *Of what does the differential diagnosis of transient urinary incontinence consist?*

An acute change in a patient's mental status (delirium) or a mood disorder (depression) may contribute to functional incontinence, such as the patient who is too confused to find a bathroom or too despondent to care about personal hygiene. End-stage dementia may render a patient incapable of recognizing the urge to void.

Urinary tract infection may lead to irritation of the detrusor muscle and thus urinary frequency and urgency. Similarly, inflammation caused by atrophic urethritis or vaginitis may contribute to increased urge.

Medications may foster urinary incontinence in a variety of ways. Sedatives depress the level of consciousness, leading to a functional incontinence. Diuretics increase the urine volume, which then increases urinary frequency. A larger urine volume may then trigger more frequent episodes of bladder spasm and augment the risk of urge incontinence. Anticholinergic medications, such as antihistamines, tricyclic antidepressants, and antipsychotics, inhibit detrusor contractions and lead to overflow incontinence. Calcium channel blockers (e.g., nifedipine, verapamil, and diltiazem) may similarly decrease detrusor contractility and worsen overflow incontinence.

Endocrine conditions such as hyperglycemia and hypercalcemia cause urinary frequency and, like diuretics, increase urine volumes, and hence the risk of incontinence. Restricted mobility due to severe arthritis, stroke, cardiac disease, or any other debilitating condition may simply prevent a patient from reaching the bathroom in time (i.e., functional incontinence). Finally, stool impaction may contribute to pelvic nerve compression, leading to an atonic bladder and overflow incontinence.

Case   A 73-year-old mother of six is brought to your office by her daughter to establish her mother's primary care in town. The patient has come to live with her daughter after her husband died 6 months ago. The patient's children are concerned that she is depressed and report she is not getting out of her house except when she has a doctor's appointment. Her past medical history is remarkable for hypertension (for which she takes hydrochlorothiazide daily) and some arthritis in her knees. She has undergone no surgical procedures. She denies any other problems, but, when specifically asked, she admits to having urinary incontinence for several years, which has been worse during the past few weeks. She describes getting the urge to void almost every hour and, if she does not get to the bathroom in a matter of minutes, she has started to lose enough urine such that she now needs to wear adult pads. When asked if she loses urine when she coughs or laughs, she confirms that this has occurred for many years. She says that she has not reported this embarrassing problem to her previous physicians because they never asked, and has attributed it to "just getting old." She and her husband had stopped having sex because she was afraid that it would make her incontinence worse.

Physical examination reveals a healthy-appearing elderly woman whose vital signs are normal, including her blood pressure, which is 130/76 mm Hg. Her examination findings are unremarkable except for her pelvis, which exhibits atrophic mucosa and a grade III cystocele (bladder and urethra protruding). She is asked to cough and a small amount of urine leaks from the urethra. The rectal findings are normal and there is good rectal tone. Neurologic findings are normal, including a normal anal wink (suggesting intact sphincter), and there are no lumbosacral neurologic findings. Laboratory evaluation reveals normal electrolyte and creatinine values and a random blood glucose level of 240 mg/dL. Urinalysis, with urine obtained by catheterization, reveals 5 to 10 white blood cells per high-power field, no epithelial cells, 2+ bacteria, and 3+ glucose.

1. Of what does the differential diagnosis of this patient's incontinence consist?
2. What conservative treatments could you try in this patient?
3. If these measures help but do not eliminate her incontinence completely, what would be the next step in treatment?
4. How would the emphasis of your evaluation differ for a male patient?

Case Discussion

1. *Of what does the differential diagnosis of this patient's incontinence consist?*

This patient describes symptoms of the most common type of incontinence in the elderly, namely, urge incontinence. She has a history of six vaginal deliveries and also has corresponding symptoms of stress incontinence, with suggestive findings discovered on examination (i.e., urine leaks when she laughs). The urinalysis findings are abnormal, indicating a possible urinary tract infection that could be exacerbating her symptoms of urgency and frequency. It may explain the worsening of symptoms in the past few weeks. An elevated blood glucose level may foster an osmotic diuresis that increases urine volumes and thus adds to the risk of incontinence.

A fear of leaving her home and the consequent social isolation may have been precipitated by her incontinence because patients prone to urge incontinence often limit their activities to avoid embarrassing accidents. On visual inspection, she was found to have an atrophic mucosa, which may suggest estrogen deficiency. Similar atrophy may occur in the urethral mucosa, which in turn reduces urethral sphincter competence.

She is on a diuretic, which may also exacerbate her incontinence. Her blood pressure may respond either to another agent or to diet alone, with weight reduction and sodium restriction. She also has arthritis in her knees, which limits her ability to get to the bathroom in time. It may be that the bathroom is farther from the bedroom in her daughter's home, and this could contribute to the recent worsening of symptoms. A simple rearrangement of her bedroom furniture may put her bed closer to the toilet and reduce the risk of nocturnal incontinence by shortening the distance she needs to travel to the bathroom.

2. *What conservative treatments could you try in this patient?*

First, the easily reversible causes need to be eliminated. A careful evaluation, including a pelvic examination, must precede any treatment. It would be reasonable to have her urine cultured and to treat her for a urinary tract infection to see if the urgency dissipates. If she has no contraindications to estrogen replacement, such treatment could be given orally or topically to alleviate the atrophic urethritis. Her diuretic medication could be discontinued and replaced with a different agent if weight loss and sodium reduction fail to control her blood pressure. If the distance from the bedroom to the bathroom is a source of nocturnal incontinence, this problem could be alleviated by getting the patient a bedside commode. Treatment of her diabetes, either with diet, oral agents, or insulin, will help decrease the urine volume. In general, it is reasonable to counsel all patients complaining of incontinence to refrain from drinking too much fluid before going out or near bedtime.

3. *If these measures help but do not eliminate her incontinence completely, what would be the next step in treatment?*

The patient has symptoms of both urge and stress incontinence. However, the possibility of overflow incontinence should also be assessed. This is done by catheterizing the patient after she has voided to see if there is urinary retention (>100 mL), which would indicate possible overflow incontinence. Neither stress nor urge incontinence alone should cause a high postvoid residual volume. Behavioral techniques are very effective in alleviating both urge and stress incontinence. Because the uninhibited bladder spasms associated with urge incontinence are brief, the patient should be instructed to sit calmly and allow the urge to pass. Jumping up to go to the bathroom only accentuates abdominal pressure during the contraction and makes the leakage of urine more likely. Behavior modification alone can considerably ease the patient's urge incontinence. Women with stress incontinence may reduce loss of urine by performing exercises that strengthen the pelvic floor muscles. To teach patients these exercises (Kegel exercises), ask the patient to feel the muscles she uses to stop her stream of urine or a bowel movement. She must contract these muscles without also contracting the abdominal muscles 10 to 15 times, three times a day. This practice must be continued to remain effective. If the incontinence persists even after diligent exercising for several weeks or months, the patient should be referred to a gynecologist for consideration of surgical correction of pelvic floor laxity.

4. *How would the emphasis of your evaluation differ for a male patient?*

Overflow incontinence associated with bladder outlet obstruction resulting from benign prostatic hypertrophy is an important cause of incontinence unique to men. Therefore, men should be asked carefully about urinary frequency and hesitancy, a decrease in the force of the urine stream, and if they experience a sensation of incomplete emptying. It is more important to evaluate the postvoid residual volume early in the workup of a man. A low residual volume does not absolutely rule out obstruction because of the intermittent nature of such an obstruction. However, if the volume is greater than approximately 250 mL, the diagnosis of bladder outlet obstruction is very likely. Most urologists perform cystoscopy before prostatic surgery to confirm the diagnosis and rule out detrusor flaccidity in men with large postvoid residual urine volumes. If the patient has a flaccid bladder, the urologist may be reluctant to perform prostate surgery because such patients are likely to continue to require either permanent or intermittent postoperative catheterization.

Urge incontinence is also an important diagnosis in male patients. It often coexists with obstruction because a distended bladder is more prone to contractions. Therefore, men treated for symptoms of outlet obstruction must also be asked about symptoms of urgency that may require additional treatment to prevent continued urinary incontinence after surgical correction of urinary tract obstruction.

Suggested Readings

Consensus Conference. Urinary incontinence in adults. *JAMA* 1989;261:2685.

Fantl JA, Newman DK, Colling J, et al. *Urinary incontinence in adults: acute and chronic management.* U.S. Department of Health and Human Services, Agency for Health Care Policy and Research. Rockville, MD, U.S. Government Printing Office, 1996.

McDowell BJ, Burgio KL, Dombrowski M, et al. An interdisciplinary approach to the assessment and behavioral treatment of urinary incontinence in geriatric outpatients. *J Am Geriatr Soc* 1991;40:370.

Medication Use in the Elderly

1. What is polypharmacy, and is it a significant problem in the elderly? If so, why?
2. Why do elderly patients experience an increased incidence of adverse drug reactions (ADRs)?
3. Name several ways in which ADRs might be associated with each of the following in elderly patients: new medications, the long-term use of drugs, and the sudden cessation of medications.

Discussion

1. *What is polypharmacy, and is it a significant problem in the elderly? If so, why?*

   Polypharmacy is the concurrent use of many medications. Although this term is most often used to refer to the use of "too many medications," some patients with multiple medical problems may be appropriately receiving several prescription medications. Because medications are a common cause of reversible problems in the elderly (e.g., drug-induced confusion and orthostatic hypotension), each medication prescribed for an elderly person must be carefully scrutinized to determine whether the benefits outweigh the adverse effects of the drug. Because the adverse effects frequently outweigh the benefits, it has been said of good geriatricians that they "stop more medications than they start."

Polypharmacy is a serious problem in the elderly. An average elderly person takes two to five prescription medications as well as three to four over-the-counter drugs. Although aged Americans (>65 years old) constitute 12% of the U.S. population, they consume approximately 25% of all prescription medications. They are therefore not only exposed to more drugs but also to more potential adverse drug effects. Indeed, older people have three to seven times more ADRs than do younger patients, and the frequency of ADRs correlates with the number of medications used.

2. *Why do elderly patients experience an increased incidence of ADRs?*

The management of drug therapy in the elderly differs from that in younger patients, and the resulting higher incidence of polypharmacy in the elderly population increases the risk of drug–drug interactions. These interactions may result from the altered absorption, excretion, or protein binding of the drugs involved. In addition, unanticipated drug effects may occur if one drug enhances or interferes with the hepatic metabolism of another. Such interactions may result in either toxic or subtherapeutic drug levels.

Comorbidity adds to the incidence of ADRs because the signs and symptoms of a preexisting disease may be worsened by the effects of medications given to treat another disorder. This can result either from the worsening of an underlying disease process by the offending drug (e.g., the use of β_2 blockers in patients with chronic obstructive pulmonary disease or congestive heart failure) or because the signs and symptoms of the drug's side effects mirror and therefore intensify those of the underlying disease process. An example of this includes the urinary retention caused by anticholinergic medications (e.g., tricyclic antidepressants and diphenhydramine) in a patient with an enlarged prostate. The retention occurs because the enlarged prostate obstructs the urine flow and the anticholinergic medication weakens detrusor contraction.

Elderly patients often have less physiologic reserve and therefore handle physiologic stress less successfully than do younger patients. The amount of physiologic reserve varies among elderly patients and even among different organ systems within the same individual. Sometimes physicians obtain baseline measurements to assess a patient's reserve. For example, the creatinine clearance may suggest how much kidney reserve is left. Thus, the risk of ADRs may be minimized by the careful evaluation of an individual elderly patient's function before prescribing potentially toxic medications. Sometimes simply reducing the dosage may confer an adequate therapeutic effect without producing toxicity. Those elderly patients with better reserve who are capable of the more normal metabolism of medications may need the same dosage as younger patients to obtain a therapeutic effect. In summary, therapy must be individualized to obtain the optimum effect from medication while avoiding toxicity.

Age-related physiologic changes in the elderly include a decline in lean muscle mass and total body water content, with an increased proportion of total body fat. These changes affect drug disposition in the following manner: less total body water translates into a smaller volume of distribution for water-soluble medications, resulting in higher-than-anticipated serum concentrations. Because adipose tissue is often proportionately greater in older patients, the volume of distribution for fat-soluble medications increases, prolonging the elimination period. Another physiologic change of great importance is a decline in renal function with age, occurring in approximately 65% of elderly people. For the elderly, the serum creatinine concentration alone is an unreliable indicator of kidney function because it depends on the amount of muscle mass, which decreases with advancing age. Instead, creatinine clearance is a more accurate estimate of renal function in the elderly. Age-related physiologic changes in hepatic metabolism and protein binding usually have less impact on drug metabolism than does the decline in renal function.

3. *Name several ways in which ADRs might be associated with each of the following in elderly patients: new medications, the long-term use of drugs, and the sudden cessation of medications.*

New medications may elicit ADRs by producing predictable side effects, especially if the side effects exacerbate preexisting disease-related symptoms. For example, preexisting postural hypotension can be worsened by tricyclic antidepressants. New medications can also cause adverse effects if the dosages prescribed are not those appropriate for the elderly, leading to drug intoxication. For example, digoxin toxicity may occur if the physician fails to adjust the dosage to accommodate renal impairment. When new medications are added to an already complicated medical regimen, this may also foster noncompliance, either because of patient frustration about having to take so many pills or because of confusion over complicated dosing schedules. New medications can precipitate ADRs when they become involved in drug–drug interactions, as previously discussed. Finally, patients may not tolerate new medications for idiosyncratic reasons, thus emphasizing the need for physicians to maintain vigilance in detecting an ADR. Contributing to this is the fact that drug side effects may not be recognized as such by patients because they ascribe their symptoms to old age.

The long-term use of medications may be associated with an ADR when a patient's renal, hepatic, or nutritional status changes without a concomitant dose adjustment. For instance, a drug dose tolerated for many years may become toxic as renal clearance declines. In addition, ADRs result when new medications adversely affect the pharmacokinetics of medications elderly patients have otherwise tolerated for years. An example of such interactions is the digoxin toxicity that occurs secondary to decreased clearance after the addition of verapamil to a medical regimen.

Changes in compliance can result in ADRs. Noncompliance is a common geriatric problem, with estimates of noncompliance ranging from 26% to 59% for the geriatric population, and polypharmacy increases the incidence of noncompliance. Compliance can be improved when physicians regularly ask their patients in a nonjudgmental fashion about their medication use, simplify the medical regimen, and remind elderly patients about the need for each medication. Other factors that influence compliance include cognitive, financial, and functional changes.

Adverse drug reactions can also occur when a patient is hospitalized and started on a medical regimen that the physician incorrectly assumed was being followed at home. If the patient has been taking fewer pills than actually prescribed, this "enforced" compliance may precipitate toxicity even though the dosing schedule may seem correct.

Finally, many drugs commonly used in the elderly are associated with **withdrawal syndromes**. Of particular importance are the psychotropic drugs, such as the benzodiazepines, antipsychotics, and antidepressants. Drug withdrawal syndromes may occur if these medications are discontinued abruptly or tapered too quickly, and should be considered as a potential source of a marked change in an elderly patient's behavior. Drug withdrawal may occur even when therapeutic, and not necessarily high doses are abruptly discontinued. Unfortunately, drug withdrawal frequently goes unrecognized, leading to potentially preventable adverse complications. Agitation and delirium are among the more common symptoms associated with withdrawal from some psychotropic drugs. For this reason, it is important to consider drug withdrawal as a possible cause of any unexplained delirium.

Case   An 81-year-old man who was admitted to the hospital 2 days ago for the evaluation of epigastric burning in conjunction with hemoccult-positive stools and anemia suddenly exhibits confusion. He has undergone endoscopy and was found to have gastritis. His hematocrit reading has remained stable and discharge planning is in progress. His abdominal symptoms have been alleviated with the addition of the H_2 blocker, cimetidine.

His past medical history is limited, and he is vague when answering questions about it. His daughter has reported that he has dementia. No other medical problems have been identified. The patient denied alcohol or tobacco use on admission. The medications he was taking before admission are unknown, but he is currently being given cimetidine (400 mg orally twice daily) and diphenhydramine (25 mg orally at night, as needed) for insomnia. He has no known drug allergies.

The patient is a widowed, retired plumber who lives alone. His family history is noncontributory and a review of systems is significant for insomnia.

The nurses relate that the patient was well during the day, but became progressively confused during the evening. He is found to be disoriented and irritable, with his mental status fluctuating between agitation, with perceptual distortions and visual hallucinations, and hypersomnolence.

Physical examination reveals the following findings: blood pressure, 140/80 mm Hg; temperature, 98.6°F (37.0°C); pulse, 80 beats per minute; and respirations, 16 per minute. There are no orthostatic changes.

The patient is unable to cooperate fully with mental status testing but is noted to be disoriented to time and place and appears anxious. He is flushed. Head, eye, ear, nose, and throat findings, as well as the cardiac, pulmonary, and abdominal findings are unremarkable. Neurologic examination reveals nonfocal findings.

His cranial nerves are intact and there is no asterixis. His reflexes are 2+ and symmetric. His motor ability is scored as 5/5 and symmetric. His sensation is intact to light touch, although other sensory modalities cannot be tested. His toes are downgoing bilaterally and he has no cerebellar abnormalities.

You correctly ascertain that the patient's current behavior cannot simply be due to worsening of his underlying dementia but is consistent with delirium. To exclude metabolic, infectious, traumatic, or neurologic causes, the following data are obtained: white blood cell count, 6,000 cells/mm^3 with a normal differential; hematocrit, 35% and stable compared with admission; platelets, 350 × 10^3/mm^3; sodium, 140 mEq/L; chloride, 105 mEq/L; creatinine, 0.9 mg/dL; potassium, 4.0 mEq/L; CO_2, 27 mEq/L; blood urea nitrogen, 12 mg/dL; glucose, 125 mg/dL; calcium, 9.0 mg/dL; arterial blood gases, normal; aspartate aminotransferase, 20 U/L (normal range, 14 to 30 IU/L); alkaline phosphatase, 175 IU/L (normal range, 30 to 110 IU/L); total bilirubin, 0.4 mg/dL; thyroid-stimulating hormone, 4 U/mL (normal range, 0.5 to 5 μU/mL); vitamin B$_{12}$, 600 pg/mL (normal range, 225 to 800 pg/mL); and rapid plasma reagin, nonreactive.

No pyuria is found on urinalysis and blood specimens are sent for culture.

A chest radiograph and electrocardiogram are normal, as is a CT scan of the head, which shows no evidence of hemorrhage.

The diphenhydramine is discontinued and the patient's daughter is called and told of her father's condition. She reports that on entering her father's apartment that evening, she discovered a half-empty bottle of lorazepam (a benzodiazepine) that she had not known he was taking.

1. Which of the patient's symptoms are consistent with delirium?
2. Is the presentation of benzodiazepine withdrawal in elderly patients different from that in younger patients?
3. How could this withdrawal syndrome have been prevented?
4. Are there other drugs cited in the case that can cause confusion? If so, how?

Case Discussion

1. *Which of the patient's symptoms are consistent with delirium?*

The symptoms in this patient that are consistent with delirium, which may reflect benzodiazepine withdrawal, include fluctuations in consciousness, anxiety, confusion, irritability, perceptual disturbances, and hallucinations. Because drug withdrawal is frequently unrecognized, physicians should consider the possibility of withdrawal in any geriatric patient who exhibits an abrupt alteration in behavior and cognition, particularly when other systemic causes have been excluded. Physicians must also maintain a high index of suspicion for alcohol withdrawal in both elderly men and women. Finally, as exemplified in this patient, communication with family, friends, and caregivers may provide valuable information about otherwise unreported psychoactive drug use or abuse.

Lorazepam is an intermediate-acting benzodiazepine, with an onset of withdrawal symptoms typically occurring in the first 24 to 72 hours after discontinuation, which is consistent with this patient's clinical picture. Rarely, withdrawal symptoms may be delayed for up to 2 weeks in patients taking longer-acting benzodiazepines, such as diazepam and flurazepam. The age-related increase in the proportion of total body fat of geriatric patients may provide a larger volume of distribution for fat-soluble benzodiazepines, thereby lengthening the elimination period and postponing the onset of withdrawal symptoms.

2. *Is the presentation of benzodiazepine withdrawal in elderly patients different from that in younger patients?*

The clinical manifestations of benzodiazepine withdrawal in the elderly frequently differ from those seen in younger patients. The difference in the clinical manifestations of withdrawal in elderly patients is in general due to comorbidity stemming from other diseases and impaired homeostatic reserve. In some cases, these factors result in more severe and even life-threatening withdrawal symptoms. Benzodiazepine withdrawal is associated with increased autonomic nervous system activity. In younger patients, this manifests as tachycardia, mild hypertension, and diaphoresis. In elderly patients with limited physiologic reserve, the increased autonomic nervous system activity may precipitate severe cardiovascular complications. In other situations, comorbidity or impaired homeostatic reserve, or both, may result in more subtle withdrawal symptoms in elderly patients. Health care professionals may mistakenly attribute changes in mental status to worsening dementia. In geriatric patients, abrupt and isolated confusion is sometimes the only clue to benzodiazepine withdrawal.

3. *How could this withdrawal syndrome have been prevented?*

This patient's benzodiazepine withdrawal might have been prevented, first, by finding out whether he is taking a medication associated with a withdrawal syndrome. When admitting elderly patients with cognitive impairment, it is important to communicate with the primary caregiver because this frequently provides such vitally important information. Second, if benzodiazepines are to be discontinued, the dose should be gradually tapered by 10% to 20% per week.

4. *Are there other drugs cited in the case that can cause confusion? If so, how?*

The patient was started on two new medications during his hospitalization—cimetidine and diphenhydramine. Both of these drugs can cause confusion in elderly patients, and drug-induced delirium is more common in patients with preexisting dementia (an example of a drug–disease interaction).

Cimetidine, an H_2 blocker, can produce a host of systemic effects and may participate in drug–drug interactions because of its ability to decrease the metabolism of medications that are eliminated by the liver. Cimetidine also rarely causes central nervous system symptoms such as confusion and hallucinations. The mechanism responsible for cimetidine-mediated mental status changes is unknown.

Diphenhydramine is frequently used to promote sleep, but actually is a poor choice for frail, elderly patients. Of particular concern are its potential anticholinergic side effects, which include dry mouth, urinary retention, constipation, blurred vision, and confusion. Geriatric patients may be more sensitive to anticholinergic side effects than younger people because of age-related changes in acetylcholine neurotransmission.

Suggested Readings

Ahronheim JC. *Handbook of prescribing medications for geriatric patients*. Boston: Little, Brown, 1992:1–12, 96–100, 347–348.

Beers MH. Polypharmacy and appropriate prescribing. In: Beck JC, ed. *Geriatric review syllabus*, 1991–1992 ed. New York: American Geriatric Society, 1991, p. 218.

Gerber JG, Brass EP. Drug use in the elderly. In: Jahnigen DW, Schrier RW, eds. *Geriatric medicine*, 2nd ed. Cambridge, MA: Blackwell Science, 1996.

6 Infectious Diseases

Robert T. Schooley

Urinary Tract Infection

1. What host factors lead to the development of urinary tract infections (UTIs), and how are these factors different for men and women?
2. What organisms commonly cause lower UTIs?
3. What are the signs and symptoms of lower UTI, and how do these differ from those of pyelonephritis?

Discussion

1. *What host factors lead to the development of UTIs, and how are these factors different for men and women?*

   Improper hygiene, sexual activity, incontinence, urinary tract instrumentation, diabetes mellitus, a genetic predisposition, and dehydration are all factors that can increase the likelihood of a UTI. Most UTIs are caused by endogenous flora originating from the gastrointestinal tract. These organisms have been shown to colonize the vaginal introitus and periurethral area before UTI occurs. Women who wipe their perineal area from the posterior to anterior direction after defecation, rather than vice versa, or those who are incontinent of stool, may be subject to more frequent colonization of the short female urethra with Enterobacteriaceae. The longer urethra in men makes access to the bladder more difficult for enteric flora; however, this flora may be introduced to the normally sterile bladder area as the result of Foley catheterization or cystoscopy. One of the natural defenses against cystitis after urethral colonization is the mechanical flushing of the urinary bladder that takes place during urination. Obviously, anyone who is dehydrated cannot benefit as frequently from this natural defense mechanism.Sexual activity can predispose women to acquiring UTI. In addition, as the result of a poorly understood mechanism, women who use a diaphragm for contraception seem to be more susceptible to urethral colonization and UTI, perhaps because it inflicts indirect mechanical trauma on the urethra. Diabetes mellitus may predispose to UTI through a variety of mechanisms, including the defective chemotaxis of leukocytes, phagocytic defects, and enhanced growth conditions for bacteria. Genetically determined factors, such as the type and number of receptors on uroepithelial cells to which bacteria may attach, also appear to heighten susceptibility to UTIs.

2. *What organisms commonly cause lower UTIs?*

Escherichia coli causes most (up to 80%) of the cases of community-acquired uncomplicated UTIs, with *Klebsiella, Enterobacter*, and *Proteus* organisms more likely to cause complicated or hospital-acquired UTIs. These are all gram-negative organisms that usually originate from the patient's own gastrointestinal flora. There are, however, several gram-positive organisms that occur as urinary pathogens. *Staphylococcus saprophyticus*, a coagulase-negative *Staphylococcus* organism, causes 20% or more of the UTIs in women 16 to 35 years of age. *Streptococcus faecalis* causes 2% to 3% of the UTIs in otherwise healthy young women. When *Staphylococcus aureus* is found in the urine, a bacteremic infection of the kidney should be suspected.

Chlamydia, Ureaplasma, Mycoplasma, and *Neisseria gonorrhoeae* are sexually transmitted pathogens that usually cause vaginal or cervical infections; however, they may be implicated in cases of acute urethral syndrome in which Gram's-stained urine samples exhibit pyuria without bacteriuria.

Pseudomonas and *Serratia* are more commonly nosocomial gram-negative pathogens that are not usually seen in community-acquired, uncomplicated UTIs.

3. *What are the signs and symptoms of lower UTI, and how do these differ from those of pyelonephritis?*

The term *lower urinary tract infection* actually encompasses cystitis and urethritis as well as prostatitis. Symptoms classically include urinary frequency, urgency, dysuria, and suprapubic discomfort. Signs may include fever, cloudy or foul-smelling urine, and hematuria. Because upper UTIs (i.e., pyelonephritis, acute lobar nephritis, and a perinephric abscess) often start as cystitis, the same signs and symptoms may exist; however, the fever is usually more severe, and may be accompanied by shaking chills. An upper UTI is often accompanied by costovertebral angle tenderness on the involved side. Elderly people and those with diabetes may exhibit fewer signs and symptoms than otherwise normal hosts.

Case A 19-year-old, sexually active woman presents to the emergency room complaining of a 2-day history of urinary frequency, burning, and urgency. She denies vaginal discharge or itching, fever, chills, nausea, vomiting, back pain, abdominal pain, or hematuria. She has no history of UTI or a sexually transmitted disease. She recently began using a diaphragm for birth control, and reports that her last menstrual period occurred 3 weeks ago. She has only one sexual partner, who denies penile discharge or burning on urination. On physical examination, she is noted to be afebrile with a normal blood pressure and pulse. There is no costovertebral angle tenderness. Her abdomen is soft and there is mild suprapubic tenderness in response to palpation. A urinalysis reveals 1+ protein, 2+ leukocytes, and 1+ blood. The urine pH is 5.6. Gram's staining of an unspun urine specimen reveals abundant polymorphonuclear leukocytes and moderate gram-negative rods. A clean-catch urine specimen is sent to the microbiology laboratory for culture.

The emergency room physician diagnoses an uncomplicated UTI and prescribes trimethoprim-sulfamethoxazole (TMP-SMX), one double-strength tablet twice a day for 5 days.

1. What other therapeutic options would have been appropriate in this patient?
2. What can this woman do to help prevent recurrent UTIs?
3. Should this woman's sexual partner be evaluated for UTI?
4. Was the Gram's staining an important diagnostic test, and in what way did the findings alter the management of this case?
5. What is the value of knowing the urine pH in this setting?
6. What other diagnostic or laboratory tests should have been performed?
7. What would be an appropriate analgesic for a patient with UTI who is experiencing severe urethral discomfort?
8. What side effects of therapy should this woman know about?
9. What possible consequences could arise if this woman does not comply with therapy?

Case Discussion

1. *What other therapeutic options would have been appropriate in this patient?*

Trimethoprim-sulfamethoxazole remains the drug of choice for the empirically based treatment of uncomplicated UTIs. For sulfa-allergic patients, ampicillin, amoxicillin, a first-generation cephalosporin, a quinolone, or nitrofurantoin are appropriate alternatives. Therapy may then be modified based on the results of the urine culture and the sensitivities of the infecting organism. Enterococci are not susceptible to either TMP-SMX or cephalosporins, which points up the utility of performing urine Gram's staining when deciding on antibiotic therapy. The prevalence of ampicillin-resistant *E. coli* may be as high as 30% in some communities, and this needs to be considered when selecting an appropriate antibiotic. *S. saprophyticus* responds to ampicillin, TMP-SMX, the quinolones, and nitrofurantoin.

The required duration of therapy for uncomplicated lower UTIs remains controversial. Single-dose therapy consisting of amoxicillin or TMP-SMX has been shown in large, randomized studies to be reasonably effective, and has the advantages of improved patient compliance, less expense, and a decreased incidence of subsequent vaginal candidiasis. The disadvantages of single-dose therapy with high-dose amoxicillin include a slightly higher incidence of gastro-intestinal upset and slightly decreased efficacy compared with traditional 7- to 10-day therapeutic regimens. Some reviewers have concluded that 3 days of therapy may be superior to single-dose therapy, but both single-dose and 3-day regimens continue to be recommended for the various reasons given. In general, single-dose therapy is contraindicated in patients with known anatomic or functional abnormalities, or with immunocompromising diseases such as diabetes mellitus. After single-dose therapy, urine cultures should be performed 1 to 2 weeks later to document cure. In the event of treatment failure, a longer course of the appropriate antibiotic should be administered.

Regardless of the pathogen and the choice of antibiotics, aggressive oral hydration is a reasonable recommendation in the management of an uncompli-cated UTI. Although there is no evidence that hydration improves the results of appropriate antimicrobial therapy, it does dilute the bacteria and removes infected urine by frequent bladder emptying. In addition, hippuric acid, the precursors of which are found in large quantities in cranberry juice, acidifies the urine pH and has a mild bacteriostatic effect on most urinary pathogens.

2. *What can this woman do to help prevent recurrent UTIs?*

Some women find that switching to another method of birth control consid-erably reduces the frequency of recurrent bacterial UTIs. Thorough cleansing of the perineal area of UTI-prone people before sexual relations may decrease the incidence of postcoital UTI; however, most patients find this to be an impractical and not completely effective preventive measure.

Choosing another method of birth control may not be necessary for most women if they remember to drink a large glass of water before and void after intercourse; however, studies have shown that diaphragm usage is an independent risk factor for UTI. Regular antibiotic prophylaxis should be reserved for those patients with a history of multiple recurrent UTIs, or complicated UTI or upper tract infections, or for immunocompromised hosts. The disadvantages of ongoing prophylaxis include the development of drug-related side effects and colonization with multidrug-resistant organisms.

3. *Should this woman's sexual partner be evaluated for UTI?*

No. Although lower UTIs in women are associated with sexual activity, this is not a sexually transmitted disease. The infecting organisms are usually endogenous flora. Healthy men without predisposing factors such as urinary tract instrumentation or diabetes mellitus rarely get lower UTIs. Bacterial prostatitis does not put his sexual partner at risk for cystitis.

4. *Was the Gram's staining an important diagnostic test, and in what way did the findings alter the management of this case?*

When bacteriuria is found in Gram's-stained, uncentrifuged urine, this is a very specific finding for the diagnosis of UTI. The finding of microscopic bacteriuria corresponds to urine culture colony counts of 10^5/mL in over 90% of such specimens. Distinguishing between gram-positive and gram-negative infections can be quite useful in making therapeutic decisions.

5. *What is the value of knowing the urine pH in this setting?*

Alkaline urine may be caused by infection with *Proteus* species, which produce urease. The presence of nonalkaline urine in this patient makes infection with a urea-splitting organism unlikely.

6. *What other diagnostic or laboratory tests should have been performed?*

The physical examination and diagnostic studies performed in an emergency room setting should be directed toward elucidating the nature of the patient's chief complaint and history. A pelvic examination would be appropriate if the patient had reported symptoms of increased vaginal discharge, dyspareunia, or exposure to a known sexually transmitted disease in the partner. The indications for performing cultures for sexually transmitted pathogens are similar to those for a pelvic examination. *Chlamydia, Ureaplasma, N. gonorrhoeae,* or *Mycoplasma* infection should have been considered in this patient if no organisms were seen on the Gram's-stained urine specimens, or if subsequent routine bacterial cultures grew no organisms.

Intravenous pyelography and a renal ultrasound examination should be reserved for when a complicated UTI or upper UTI such as pyelonephritis is suspected. A pregnancy test should be performed in any woman of childbearing age before prescribing an antibiotic that may be contraindicated in pregnancy.

7. *What would be an appropriate analgesic for a patient with UTI who is experiencing severe urethral discomfort?*

Phenazopyridine hydrochloride is a urinary tract analgesic agent that exerts a topical analgesic effect on the mucosa of the urinary tract through an unknown mechanism of action. The side effects are minimal, and include the urine acquiring a red or orange color that may stain fabric. It usually is not necessary to prescribe more than a 2-day supply to patients with uncomplicated UTIs who are receiving appropriate antibiotic therapy. Opioid analgesics are relatively contraindicated in UTI because they may cause acute urinary retention.

8. *What side effects of therapy should this woman know about?*

Vaginal candidiasis commonly develops after antimicrobial therapy because antibiotics eliminate much of the normal vaginal flora and create an ideal environment for the overgrowth of *Candida albicans*. Hypersensitivity reactions may occur with any antibiotic; however, TMP-SMX may rarely also be associated with interstitial nephritis, aseptic meningitis, Stevens-Johnson syndrome, or erythema multiforme. A careful history to rule out known drug allergy is important.

9. *What possible consequences could arise if this woman does not comply with therapy?*

  The consequences of noncompliance with therapy include continuing symptoms, the induction of antibiotic-resistant strains of microorganisms, and, most important, ascending infection leading to acute pyelonephritis or even a perinephric abscess.

Suggested Readings

Bailey RR, Abbott GD. Treatment of urinary tract infections with a single dose of trimethoprim-sulfamethoxazole. *CMAJ* 1978;118:551.

Dunagan WC, Ridner ML. *Manual of medical therapeutics*, 26th ed. Boston: Little Brown, 1995, p. 257.

Fihn SD, Latham RH, Roberts P, et al. Association between diaphragm use and urinary tract infection. *JAMA* 1985;254:240.

Hovelius B, Mardh P. *Staphylococcus saprophyticus* as a common cause of urinary tract infections. *Rev Infect Dis* 1984;6:328.

Latham RH, Running K, Stamm WE. Urinary tract infection in young adult women caused by *Staphylococcus saprophyticus. JAMA* 1983;250:3063.

Leibovici L, Alpert G, Laor L, et al. Urinary tract infections and sexual activity in young women. *Arch Intern Med* 1987;147:345.

Mandell GL, Douglas RG, Bennett JE. *Principles and practice of infectious diseases*, 4th ed. New York: Churchill Livingston, 1995, p. 662.

Rubin RH, Fang LST, Jones SR, et al. Single-dose amoxicillin therapy for urinary tract infection. *JAMA* 1980;244:561.

Stamey TA. *Pathogenesis and treatment of urinary tract infections*. Baltimore: Williams & Wilkins, 1980.

The Acquired Immunodeficiency Syndrome

1. What are the principles of antiretroviral chemotherapy?

2. When should antiretroviral chemotherapy be started?

3. What are the most important HIV-1-associated opportunistic infections, and the treatments used, in the HIV-1-infected individuals who live in developed countries?

Discussion

1. *What are the principles of antiretroviral chemotherapy?*

  HIV-1-associated morbidity and mortality is the direct result of immunosuppression mediated by viral replication. The goal of antiretroviral chemotherapy is to drive plasma HIV-1 levels to below the limits of detection with the most sensitive available assay. This approach affords two major benefits: A) Successful suppression of viral replication arrests destruction of the immune response and allows for immune reconstitution. This, in turn, results in a dramatic decline in HIV-1 associated morbidity and mortality; B) The emergence of drug resistance can be eliminated or greatly reduced by driving viral replication rates to extremely low levels.

  Suppression of plasma HIV-1 RNA to levels of 20 copies/ml is best achieved through the use of a combination regimen containing at least three agents. The inclusion of multiple agents is required both for potency and to interpose a significant genetic barrier to the virus with respect to the emergence of resistance. HIV-1 replication occurs at the rate of approximately 10 billion viral particles per day in each infected person. With the replicative infidelity of HIV-1's reverse transcription mechanism, this high level of replication rapidly results in the creation of a diverse quasispecies of virus. Thus, it is likely that at the institution of therapy, viral variants exist that are resistant to each currently available agent. The use of multiple agents with non-overlapping resistance mechanisms requires the virus to make multiple genetic changes in each virion in order to persist in the presence of all agents in the regimen.

At the present time, reduction of HIV-1 RNA to 20 copies/ml is best achieved with the selection of two nucleoside analogs (AZT, ddI, D4T, or 3TC) and a potent protease inhibitor (indinavir, ritonavir, amprenavir, or nelfinavir) or a potent non-nucleoside reverse transcriptase inhibitor (efavirenz or nevirapine). The selection of an individual regimen for a specific patient requires a full understanding of each of the agents on the part of the physician and a strong commitment to strict adherence to the regimen chosen by the patient. There is no single regimen that is appropriate for all patients. AZT and 3TC, D4T and 3TC, or D4T and ddI are the most commonly prescribed nucleoside analog components of the regimen. Selection of the third drug in the regimen requires a detailed discussion with the patient centered on the toxicities of each of the available alternatives. If a protease inhibitor is chosen, ritonavir and nelfinavir have the advantage of being twice daily agents with no need to avoid concomitant meals. Ritonavir is associated with circumoral paraesthesias and nausea in a significant fraction of patients. Nelfinavir is often associated with diarrhea. These toxicities are infrequently seen with indinavir, but this agent is associated with nephrolithiasis and must be given in a thrice-daily regimen with dosing intervals avoiding meals. Efavirenz is an excellent alternative agent that can be given as a single nightly dose but it may be associated with CNS side effects. Recently abacavir, a potent nucleoside analog, has been introduced as a possibly third drug in combination regimens. Although there are factors that might prompt choice of one regimen or another in an individual patient, the most important message for patients is that these regimens are flexible and if side effects are complicating adherence, it is almost always possible to make adjustments in the regimen that retain potency but which allow the patient to tolerate the regimen. Appropriate management of antiretroviral chemotherapy is both an art and a science that is best accomplished by physicians with substantial experience in management of patients with HIV-1 infection.

2. *When should antiretroviral chemotherapy be started?*

There is no single answer that is appropriate for every patient. Ongoing viral replication is always damaging to the immune response of the host. On the other hand, current antiretroviral regimens are complex, associated with side effects in many patients, and require significant discipline in order to achieve the level of viral suppression associated with durable success. As CD4 cell counts decline, patients become at greater risk for HIV-1 associated opportunistic infections. Rising plasma HIV-1 RNA levels are associated with more rapid immunological and clinical disease progression. Adequate suppression of HIV-1 is best achieved in patients with high CD4 cell counts and low plasma HIV-1 RNA levels. Thus, all things being equal, it could be argued that early institution of therapy is associated with the best chance of long-term success. The desire to start therapy early must be balanced by a consideration of long-term toxicities and the commitment of the patient to strict adherence of the regimen chosen. In general, the urgency to start therapy increases as CD4 cells fall and the plasma HIV-1 RNA level rises. Most experts recommend treatment for any symptomatic patient and for any patient with fewer than 500 CD4 cells. However, it is sometimes reasonable to follow patients with lower CD4 (but stable) cell counts and low plasma HIV-1 RNA levels.

3. *What are the most important HIV-1-associated opportunistic infections, and the treatments used, in the HIV-1-infected individuals who live in developed countries?*

In general, the risk of various HIV-1-related infections increases with disease progression and declining CD4 cell counts. Two notable exceptions to this rule, however, are pneumococcal pneumonia and tuberculosis. All HIV-1-infected patients are at increased risk for acquiring pneumococcal pneumonia and sepsis. Whether the administration of pneumococcal vaccine can prevent or lessen the severity of pneumococcal disease in these patients has not been proved, but the current practice is to administer pneumococcal vaccine to all HIV-1-infected patients whose CD4 lymphocyte counts exceed 500/mm^3. The response to vaccination of patients with counts of less than 500/mm^3 is likely to be enhanced if patients are on effective antiretroviral therapy at the time of vaccination.

Tuberculosis is one of the few HIV-1-related infections that is transmissible to immunocompetent persons. HIV-infected persons are at increased risk for acquiring tuberculosis regardless of the stage of their HIV-1-infection. Because the tuberculin skin test result may be falsely negative in HIV-1-infected patients, patients who have been exposed to tuberculosis should undergo isoniazid treatment regardless of their tuberculin skin test results.

Oral candidiasis (thrush) most frequently occurs when the CD4 lymphocyte count falls below 300/mm^3. Thrush can usually be treated with topical antifungal agents (nystatin swish and swallow, or clotrimazole troches), but more severe cases, especially when esophageal lesions are present, may require systemic antifungal agents such as ketoconazole or fluconazole.

Early in the AIDS epidemic, *P. carinii* pneumonia was the most common AIDS-defining illness. With the advent of effective prophylactic regimens, this illness has become much less frequent. Pneumocystis pneumonia is usually treated with TMP-SMX. Alternatively, intravenous pentamidine, oral trimethoprim/dapsone, or oral atovaquone can be used in sulfa-allergic patients.

HIV-1-infected persons with less than 200 CD4 lymphocytes/mm^3 are at risk for suffering several types of central nervous system (CNS) infections. One of the most common causes of intracranial masses in HIV-1-infected patients, *Toxoplasma gondi*, is treated with pyrimethamine and sulfadiazine. *Cryptococcus neoformans*, *Histoplasma capsulatum*, and *Coccidioides immitis* can cause CNS or disseminated disease in HIV-1-infected patients; infection with these pathogens is usually treated with amphotericin B.

Patients with less than 50 CD4 lymphocytes/mm^3 are at risk for suffering disseminated infection with mycobacterium avium (MAC) or ocular or systemic cytomegalovirus infections. Disseminated MAC is commonly manifested clinically by the appearance of systemic symptoms (fever, weight loss, night sweats, and anemia). Treatment with a combination consisting of rifabutin, ethambutol, and clarithromycin is the treatment of choice for MAC infection. Cytomegalovirus retinitis presents with painless loss of vision and may be accompanied by systemic evidence of infection manifest by fever, weight loss, or gastrointestinal symptoms. Treatment with ganciclovir, foscarnet, or cidofavir is usually effective.

Case

A 32-year-old woman in her first trimester of pregnancy is found to be HIV-1 seropositive in routine screening undertaken during the course of her pregnancy. The patient has no prior medical illness. Her physical examination is normal except for slight breast engorgement. Her social history reveals that she has been married to the same man for the prior three years. He is also healthy. Upon detailed questioning, he admitted to having visited a prostitute during a trip to the Far East in his early twenties. He is subsequently found to be HIV-1 seropositive with a CD4 cell count of 860 cells/mms and a plasma HIV-1 RNA level of 1300 copies/ml.

The laboratory evaluation reveals that she has a positive ELISA for antibodies to HIV-1. HIV-1 seropositivity was confirmed by a Western blot assay. Her PPD is negative, as is her serology for Toxoplasma gondii. Her RPR is negative. Her hematocrit is 43. Her white blood cell count is 5200. Her CD4 cell count is 347 cells/mm^3. Her plasma HIV-1 RNA level is 143,000 copies/ml.

1. What would you recommend to her with respect to antiretroviral chemotherapy?
2. What is the likelihood that her child will be infected?
3. What would you recommend to her husband with respect to antiretroviral chemotherapy?

Case Discussion

1. *What would you recommend to her with respect to antiretroviral chemotherapy?*

The general approach to antiretroviral chemotherapy in pregnancy should be the same as it is in a non-pregnant woman. The dual goals of therapy in this setting are to suppress viral replication to benefit the mother and to decrease the risk of transmission of HIV-1 to her baby. With her CD4 cell count and plasma HIV-1 RNA level, she is at a significant risk for disease progression over the next several years and most experts would strongly recommend antiretroviral chemotherapy to her. With the exception of efavirenz for which primate teratogenicity studies have raised concerns about the induction of severe CNS anomalies, there is little evidence that current antiretroviral chemotherapeutic agents pose any significant risk to either the mother or the fetus. Since rigorous studies have not been completed, however, and since the occurrence of morning sickness in many women is in the first trimester of pregnancy, it would be preferable to delay the initiation of therapy until the second or third trimester of pregnancy. This would also offer an opportunity to work through some of the complex psychosocial issues facing the couple in confronting the information regarding their HIV-1 infections at this unexpected point in their lives.

When therapy is initiated, the goal of therapy is to suppress plasma HIV-1 RNA levels to less than 20 copies/ml. It would be reasonable to initiate therapy with two nucleoside analogs such as AZT and 3TC or D4T and 3TC and a potent protease inhibitor or non-nucleoside reverse transcriptase inhibitor. The choice of the third drug in the regimen should balance issues related to potency and tolerability. Although many experts might recommend nevirapine as the third drug in the regimen in view of concerns that were raised in 1998 regarding the possibility that the use of protease inhibitors during pregnancy might be associated with an increased risk of premature delivery, subsequent studies revealed these concerns to be groundless. In view of her high plasma-HIV-1 RNA level, concerns might be raised about the potency of nevirapine and it would probably be most reasonable to use a protease inhibitor in this setting. In view of the Gilbert-like effects of indinavir, it would be preferable not to transplacentally expose the neonate to the drug. Since ritonavir is difficult to tolerate for many patients from the gastrointestinal standpoint, nelfinavir would be preferable in this setting.

2. *What is the likelihood that her child will be infected?*

Prior to the advent of antiretroviral chemotherapy, the likelihood of transmitting HIV-1 from mother to child was in the range of 25%. Zidovudine monotherapy administered during the third trimester of pregnancy coupled with intravenous zidovudine during delivery and six weeks of zidovudine for the child, reduced the risk of perinatal transmission to 8%. More potent contemporary antiretroviral chemotherapeutic regimens have reduced this risk to below 2%. The goal of therapy in the mother should be to reduce plasma HIV-1 RNA levels to <20 copies/ml by delivery. The baby should also receive antiretroviral chemotherapy as part of the perinatal transmission prevention strategy. Most consultants would recommend zidovudine with or without lamivudine for approximately 6 weeks following delivery. The child should not be breast fed, regardless of the mother's plasma HIV-1 level, in view of the risk of transmission of HIV-1 to the neonate by this route.

3. *What would you recommend to her husband with respect to antiretroviral chemotherapy?*

The father has been infected for more than 5 years and has maintained a low plasma HIV-1 RNA level and a near normal CD4 cell count. Although he is technically not a long-term nonprogressor since he has not been documented to be infected for more than 10 years, his plasma HIV-1 RNA level and CD4 cell count predict that his disease progression risk is very low. Most experts would not recommend antiretroviral chemotherapy to him at this point. Although antiretroviral chemotherapy is not indicated, he should undergo a full initial evaluation for HIV-1 including a PPD, an RPR, Toxoplasma gondii and cytomegalovirus serology and should be followed at 3-6 month intervals for evidence of a rising plasma HIV-1 RNA level and/or a falling CD4 cell count. He should also be vaccinated against pneumococcal disease.

Suggested Readings

Barnes PF, Bloch AP, Davidson PT, Snider DE. Tuberculosis in patients with human immuno-deficiency virus infection. *N Engl J Med* 1991;324:1644.

Carpenter CJ, Fischl MA, Hammer SM, et al. Antiretroviral therapy for HIV Infection in 1998. *JAMA* 1998; 280:78-86.

Connor EM, Sperling RS, Gelber R, et al. for the Pediatric ACTG Protocol 076 Study Group. Reduction of maternal-infant transmission of human immunodeficiency virus type 1 with zidovudine treatment. *N Engl J Med* 1994;331:1173-1180.

Gulick RM, Mellors JW, Havlir D, et al. Treatment with indinavir, zidovudine and lamivudine in adult with human immunodeficiency virus infection and prior antiretroviral therapy. *N Engl J Med* 1997;337:734-740.

Ho DD, Neumann AU, Perelson AS. Rapid turnover of plasma virions and CD4 lymphocytes in HIV-1 infection. *Nature* 1995;373:123-126.

Masur H, Ognibene FP, Yarchoan R, et al. CD4 counts as predictors of opportunistic pneumonias in human immunodeficiency virus (HIV) infection. *Ann Intern Med* 1989;111:223.

Palella FJ, Delaney KM, Moorman AC, et al. Declining morbidity and mortality among patients with advanced human immunodeficiency virus infection. HIV outpatient study investigators. *N Engl J Med* 1998;338:853-860.

Sperling RS, Shapiro DE, Coombs RW, et al. (The Pediatric AIDS Clinical Trials Group Protocol 076 Study Group). Maternal viral load, zidovudine treatment, and the risk of transmission of human immunodeficiency virus type 1 from mother to infant. *N Engl J Med* 1996;335:1621-1629.

Wei X, Ghosh SK, Taylor ME, et al. Viral dynamics in human immunodeficiency virus type 1 infection. *Nature* 1995;373:117-122.

Cellulitis

1. What factors predispose to the development of cellulitis?
2. What are the signs and symptoms of cellulitis?
3. What organisms most frequently cause cellulitis?

Discussion

1. *What factors predispose to the development of cellulitis?*

Although any person can acquire cellulitis, there are several factors that heighten the risk of this infection. Any compromise of skin integrity can introduce organisms into the skin and subcutaneous tissues. Thus, surgical procedures, trauma, the placement of intravenous catheters, burns, and bite wounds are all factors that predispose to the development of cellulitis. The risk for development of cellulitis is also increased in hosts whose sensation is impaired, such as patients with diabetes with peripheral neuropathy whose ability to perceive and appropriately react to trauma is diminished.

Impaired arterial circulation also predisposes to the development of cellulitis. Host immune mechanisms, such as polymorphonuclear leukocytes and complement, are delivered through the circulation. Therefore, if the host circulation is impaired, normal immune mechanisms, which might easily eradicate an organism, cannot be mounted. This is why cellulitis is more frequent in patients with impaired arterial circulation, such as those with diabetes and smokers with peripheral vascular disease.

Patients whose venous and lymphatic drainage is compromised are also less able to clear bacteria from their bodies, and consequently predisposed to cellulitis. Patients with chronic edema of the lower extremities are particularly vulnerable to cellulitis, which may spread very rapidly. A distinctive form of cellulitis has been found in patients whose saphenous veins have been removed for coronary artery bypass grafting. These patients, who most likely have both venous insufficiency and impaired lymphatic drainage, have been found to acquire cellulitis at the site of the saphenous venectomy. Frequently, the portal of entry for the infection is associated with tinea pedis. Besides the treatment of the cellulitis, the tinea pedis should be treated with a topical antifungal agent.

Immunocompromised patients, such as those undergoing chemotherapy or transplantation procedures, are also vulnerable to cellulitis. The infection in these patients may be more difficult to diagnose because the characteristic symptoms and signs may be more subtle owing to the antiinflammatory properties of the immunosuppression.

2. *What are the signs and symptoms of cellulitis?*

The classic appearance exhibited by cellulitis is a hot, swollen, red, and tender skin lesion. The patient may be febrile, and regional lymphadenopathy is common. Acute lymphangitis, indicated by red streaks coursing up the patient's limb from the site of the cellulitis, signifies the spread of infection along subcutaneous lymphatic channels. Not all cases of cellulitis are associated with lymphangitis, but it may be the harbinger of serious systemic illness with bacteremia.

3. *What organisms most frequently cause cellulitis?*

The most common causes of cellulitis in general are group A streptococci and *S. aureus*. These gram-positive cocci are normal constituents of human skin flora and are easily introduced into wounds by trauma. Other streptococci may also occasionally cause cellulitis.

Less common pathogens may also be introduced into a wound by trauma. For example, soil-contaminated wounds may become infected with fungi or *Clostridium* species. Animal bite wounds may become infected with bacteria from the animal's mouth. Erysipeloid, caused by *Erysipelothrix rhusiopathiae*, is a cellulitis affecting people who handle salt-water fish, shellfish, poultry, meat, or animal hides. Various *Vibrio* species may cause cellulitis in people with wounds exposed to salt water or raw seafood.

Less frequently, cellulitis may be acquired through bacteremia. Rare cases of pneumococcal cellulitis have been reported. Immunocompromised patients may also acquire cellulitis by means of a bacteremia caused by organisms, such as *C. neoformans* or *E. coli*, that are not usual causes of cellulitis in normal hosts.

Case   A 27-year-old man presents to the emergency room complaining of pain in his right hand. He was well until the previous day, when he sustained a deep scratch at the base of his right thumb while playing with his cat. He washed the wound and bandaged it tightly to stop the bleeding. Overnight, however, his palm began to swell, turned red, and became increasingly painful.

His blood pressure is 120/70 mm Hg, his heart rate is 90 beats per minute, his respiratory rate is 12 per minute, and his temperature is 38.5°C. Physical examination findings are notable for a laceration on the right thenar eminence that is 2 cm long and 0.5 cm deep. The wound is partially crusted over with blood, with a small amount of serosanguineous discharge. The surrounding tissue is erythematous, hot, and exquisitely tender. There are two red streaks ascending the lower half of his anterior forearm. He has a tender, mobile, 1-cm lymph node in the right axilla. There is full range of motion without discomfort in any of the digits or the wrist of his right upper extremity. Neurologic examination of the hand reveals normal findings, and Allen's test is normal.

The following laboratory data are found: white blood cell count, 15,000/mm³, with a differential count of 75% polymorphonuclear leukocytes, 5% band forms, 17% lymphocytes, 2% monocytes, and 1% eosinophils. His serum chemistry values are normal. A radiographic study of the hand reveals no evidence of a foreign body or subcutaneous emphysema. Gram's staining of the serosanguineous discharge from the wound reveals large numbers of small gram-negative rods and a few gram-positive cocci in chains. Samples of the discharge and blood are sent for culture.

The patient was born and raised in the United States. He has been in good health before this illness and has no history of hospitalizations. He recalls having had a tetanus booster shot 7 years ago. He has no history of allergic reactions to medications. His 7-year-old cat was also born and raised in the United States, has received all appropriate vaccinations, and is apparently healthy.

1. What infectious agents should be considered as possible causes of this patient's cellulitis?
2. What would be the most appropriate antibiotic treatment for this patient?
3. In addition to antibiotics, what other measures should be taken to treat this cellulitis?

Case Discussion

1. *What infectious agents should be considered as possible causes of this patient's cellulitis?*

Group A streptococci and *S. aureus* must always be considered as potential causes of cellulitis because they are the most common etiologic agents. In the event of animal bites or scratches, the oral flora of the animal may be an important source of infection as well. *Pasteurella multocida* is found in the oropharynx of 50% to 70% of normal cats and 12% to 60% of normal dogs. This gram-negative rod is frequently implicated in infections resulting from cat bites or scratches, and is found less often in wounds inflicted by dogs. Other important animal oral flora to consider in patients with bites and scratch wounds include aerobic and anaerobic streptococcal organisms, as well as gram-negative anaerobes, such as *Bacteroides* species and *Fusobacterium*. Organisms found in soil, such as *Clostridia* species, may also be transmitted by scratches or bites.

The rapid tempo of this patient's illness, with the development of an exqui-sitely painful cellulitis within 24 hours of a cat scratch is characteristic of *P. multocida* infection, although such a rapid course may also be seen in the setting of streptococcal infections. It would be unusual, however, for a staphylococcal infection to progress this rapidly. Moreover, the discharge from a staphylococcal infection would more likely be purulent than serosanguineous. The finding of many gram-negative rods on the Gram's-stained specimen of the wound dis-charge also suggests a *P. multocida* infection, or else a gram-negative anaerobic infection. However, a few gram-positive cocci in chains were also found, making streptococcal infection a part of the differential diagnosis.

2. *What would be the most appropriate antibiotic treatment for this patient?*

This patient has a serious hand infection, along with an impending systemic illness. Anyone with such a serious hand infection should be hospitalized and receive intravenous antibiotics to prevent advancing infection, as well as to avert the potentially devastating consequences of suboptimal therapy. Penicil-lin is the drug of choice for *P. multocida* infections, and would also be effective for the management of both streptococcal and anaerobic infections. Thus, intravenous penicillin would be the best antibiotic in this case. For patients who are allergic to penicillin, tetracycline is the best alternative drug for the treatment of *P. multocida* infections.

3. *In addition to antibiotics, what other measures should be taken to treat this cellu-litis?*

Overestimating the efficacy of antibiotics, and underestimating the critical roles played by débridement, drainage, wound elevation, and immobilization, are probably the most frequent mistakes made in the treatment of cellulitis. Drainage of a closed-space infection and removal of necrotic tissue are essen-tial to curing any infection. Even when the proper antibiotics are administered, an infection can worsen if abscesses or necrotic tissue are not drained or removed. The reason for this is that abscesses and necrotic tissue are not well vascularized, making them inaccessible to both the antibiotics and the host immune mechanisms, such as polymorphonuclear leukocytes and complement, that are normally conveyed through the bloodstream. Thus, in these inaccessi-ble regions, bacteria can freely multiply, and, in some instances, such infection can result in sepsis and death despite an appropriate antibiotic regimen.

Abscesses tend to develop in the setting of *P. multocida* infection. In addi-tion, the hand contains several physiologic spaces, such as the thenar eminence, that can serve as pockets of infection. Thus, a *P. multocida* cellulitis of the hand may require surgical débridement and drainage. Incision of a hand wound should not be performed by a novice, because there is a great potential for damaging internal structures or creating wounds that would result in serious contractures. A hand surgeon should be consulted for this purpose.

The object of elevation and immobilization in the treatment of cellulitis is to diminish the edema, which impedes the blood flow to an infected region. Elevation of the affected limb above the level of the heart is necessary to achieve optimal results. In the event of a lower extremity cellulitis, merely placing the affected limb on a chair while seated is not adequate because the abdominal contents still exert pressure on the lymphatic vessels in this position, thus perpetuating the edema. In addition to the measures just described, this patient should receive a tetanus booster shot. Any patient with a bite or deep scratch wound who has not had a tetanus booster shot within the preceding 5 years should receive one.

Suggested Readings

Centers for Disease Control: Diphtheria, tetanus, and pertussis: guidelines for vaccine prophylaxis and other preventive measures. *Ann Intern Med* 1985;103:896.

Elliot DL, Tolle SW, Goldberg L, Miller JB. Pet-associated illness. *N Engl J Med* 1985;313:985.

Francis DP, Holmes MA, Brandon G. *Pasteurella multocida*: infections after domestic animal bites and scratches. *JAMA* 1975;233:42.

Goldstein EJC. Bites. In: Mandell GL, Douglas RG, Bennett JE, eds. *Principles and practice of infectious diseases*. New York: Churchill Livingstone, 1995, p. 2765.

Swartz MN. Cellulitis and subcutaneous tissue. In: Mandell GL, Douglas RG, Bennett JE, eds. *Principles and practices of infectious diseases*. New York: Churchill Livingstone, 1995, p. 909.

A Late Complication of Tuberculosis

1. What are the goals of the modern drug treatment of active pulmonary tuberculosis?
2. What factors are likely to promote relapse?
3. What factors are likely to foster the acquisition of drug-resistant disease?

Discussion

1. *What are the goals of the modern drug treatment of active pulmonary tuberculosis?*

Fundamental to the modern drug treatment of tuberculosis is the use of multiple-drug regimens. There are two goals to this approach.

The first object of multiple-drug treatment is to prevent the emergence of resistant organisms. The findings from early studies of the use of streptomycin dramatically demonstrated the futility of monotherapy, in that patients with severe disease showed an initial gratifying response to treatment, but, after some weeks, their condition began to deteriorate. Their sputum smears became positive for organisms once again, and drug-resistant disease developed. It is believed that monotherapy selects for, rather than induces the mutation of, resistant organisms. Therefore, the larger the population of organisms, the higher the likelihood that resistant organisms are present. Thus, in the setting of an asymptomatic primary infection that involves few organisms, monotherapy (usually consisting of isoniazid) can be used safely as prophylaxis. In patients with active disease (especially cavitating pulmonary disease in which the burden of infection is immense), the probability of resistant organisms is high. Mutations leading to drug resistance are unlinked, however, so the use of two drugs (e.g., isoniazid plus rifampin) effectively prevents the emergence of secondary drug resistance (i.e., drug resistance acquired during treatment).

The second goal of therapy is to shorten the duration of treatment. To achieve a lasting cure in a high proportion of cases, regimens that comprise only rifampin plus isoniazid must be continued for 9 months. However, this can be reduced to 6 months by the addition of pyrazinamide for the first 2 months. Pyrazinamide is a powerful sterilizing drug that may exert its effect by acting on special subpopulations of organisms, such as those in a more acid environment. It has been shown that no additional benefit accrues to continuing this expensive drug beyond the first 2 months.

A factor to be considered when planning multidrug treatment is that initial drug resistance exists when the disease is caused by organisms that are resistant to at least one drug before any treatment is given. When this is suspected on epidemiologic grounds, an additional drug (usually streptomycin or ethambutol) is added to the regimen during the first 2 months, while the results of drug susceptibility studies are awaited. This approach reduces the risk of only one effective drug being given.

2. *What factors are likely to promote relapse?*

Relapse (i.e., the endogenous reactivation of previously treated tuberculosis) is most likely to occur during the first year after the end of treatment and in those patients who initially had more extensive disease. Patients who discontinue their treatment early are most likely to have a relapse. Therefore, ensuring compliance with treatment is central to preventing relapse.

3. *What factors are likely to foster the acquisition of drug-resistant disease?*

For the reasons already outlined, drug-resistant organisms emerge when a patient effectively receives only monotherapy. This may occur for a variety of reasons, and the following illustrates how it can happen. A patient on rifampin plus isoniazid may sell his powerful red rifampin capsules to his friends (or the witch doctor) for use in the treatment of gonorrhea and then take only the isoniazid himself, resulting in isoniazid monotherapy! This man acquires isoniazid resistance, cough recurs, and ethambutol is added by a kindly physician, which effectively now constitutes ethambutol monotherapy. Soon, resistance to ethambutol emerges and the man's health continues to decline. Perhaps he will start taking his rifampin, which means he is receiving rifampin monotherapy!

Such patients first need to know that they must either take both medications and get better, or neither and get worse, but at least, in this latter instance, the disease remains drug susceptible. However, it is also a mistake to add one drug at a time to a failing regimen. Instead, two new drugs should be added to protect against the emergence of resistance to each other. Fully supervised therapy prevents scenarios such as these from happening, but, unfortunately, at present it is not feasible on a global scale.

Case A 73-year-old man is admitted because of a 3-month history of intermittent hemoptysis. Approximately once a week he has been coughing up small amounts of blood-streaked sputum, but, on the day before admission, he started to cough frequently and produced approximately half a cupful of red and clotted blood over a 24-hour period. The patient had emigrated to America in the 1940s after having been interned in a labor camp in Europe during World War II. A medical examination at the time of his liberation revealed he had tuberculosis. He was then admitted to a sanatorium, where he stayed for 18 months, with treatment consisting of artificial pneumothorax. In the 1950s, he had a relapse and was treated for 18 months with isoniazid, paraaminosalicylic acid, and streptomycin. He continued to smoke a pack of cigarettes per day until an attack of pneumonia 5 years before, which caused him to stop smoking. For the past year, he has been increasingly disabled by exertional dyspnea, such that he is now unable to climb a flight of stairs without stopping. He has also had recurrent exacerbations of breathlessness with productive cough, but no previous hemoptysis. He has recently noted increasing ankle edema. He has no history of weight loss or fever.

On examination, he is found to be thin and anxious, afebrile, and normotensive, with a regular pulse of 110 beats per minute. He is slightly tachypneic and has both central and peripheral cyanosis. The jugular venous pulse is visible approximately 3 cm above the clavicle when he is at an angle of 45 degrees. He has a discrete, firm, nontender lymph node that is enlarged to approximately 2 cm in the right supraclavicular fossa. The trachea is deviated to the right, and the right upper chest is noted to be indrawn below the clavicle; it is dull to percussion and bronchial breath sounds are heard. The apex of the heart is not palpable and auscultation of the heart reveals a loud pulmonary second sound. He has bilateral ankle edema.

The chest radiographic study on admission depicts bilateral, severe fibrotic lung disease, which is most marked in the upper lobes, with elevation of the hila; the abnormalities are more pronounced on the right. The horizontal fissure is elevated on the right and projects upward. Deviation of the trachea to the right is confirmed. There are thin-walled cavities bilaterally, and a cavity on the right is found to contain an opacity that is outlined by a crescent-shaped rim of air.

1. What is the most likely diagnosis in this patient?
2. If massive hemoptysis supervenes, how should this be managed?
3. What is the most useful investigation to confirm the diagnosis?
4. Should the patient receive intravenous amphotericin B?
5. What additional late complication of tuberculosis does this patient exhibit, and how can this be relieved?

Case Discussion

1. *What is the most likely diagnosis in this patient?*

Diagnoses that should be considered in this patient include aspergilloma, reactivation of the tuberculosis, carcinoma of the bronchus, and bronchiectasis. However, this patient exhibits the classic clinical picture of aspergilloma. *Aspergillus* colonizes and grows saprophytically in cavities created by preexisting lung disease (typically those caused by tuberculosis, although occasionally other diseases such as sarcoidosis, bronchiectasis, or pulmonary fibrosis can cause the formation of cavities hospitable to such infection). A fungus ball develops in the preexisting cavity, which is lined with bronchial epithelium or granulation tissue. Chest radiographic studies, tomograms, or computed tomographic (CT) scans can show the rounded opacity within the cavity, together with a crescent-shaped rim of air between it and the cavity wall. The ball may lie free within the cavity (in which case it can be seen to change position on decubitus chest radiographs) or it may be attached by granulation tissue. Often the patient is asymptomatic, but hemoptysis is the most important complication of aspergilloma.

In this patient, reactivation of the tuberculosis is less likely than aspergilloma because, despite a 3-month history, the patient has not lost weight or had a fever. In addition, the cavities seen on the chest radiographs have thin walls, suggesting the presence of inactive disease. However, radiologically, it is impossible to distinguish with certainty between active and inactive tuberculosis.

Carcinoma of the bronchus would also be expected to cause weight loss, but it is an important consideration in patients with a history of tuberculosis because they are at higher risk than the general population because of the carcinoma (usually adenocarcinoma or alveolar cell carcinoma) that can form in scarred tissue as an aftermath of infection. This patient is also at risk for bronchial carcinoma because of his long history of smoking.

Tuberculosis commonly leads to bronchiectasis, which would undoubtedly coexist in a patient like this who has severe destructive lung disease. However, this patient's episode is dominated by hemoptysis, rather than by the expectoration of copious, purulent sputum, suggestive of an exacerbation of bronchiectasis.

2. *If massive hemoptysis supervenes, how should this be managed?*

Surgical removal is the preferred treatment in the setting of life-threatening hemoptysis due to aspergilloma, although in this patient (as in many with aspergilloma), severe underlying lung disease indicates the likelihood of a poor outcome from pulmonary surgery. There has been some success with the intracavitary instillation of *N*-acetylcysteine and amphotericin B (and, in one case, aminocaproic acid) in the control of severe hemoptysis in such patients.

Embolization of the bronchial artery has been used successfully to control severe hemoptysis due to tuberculosis, among other causes, but has not been successful in the management of severe hemoptysis caused by aspergilloma, probably because of the large collateral circulation involved.

While arrangements are made for definitive management, a patient with severe hemoptysis should be positioned on the side of the suspected source (in this case, the right side) to minimize flooding of the unaffected lung with blood. Sedation of the patient is likely to be required. An intravenous line should be established and blood crossmatched and administered when needed.

3. *What is the most useful investigation to confirm the diagnosis?*

No investigation (other than pathologic analysis of the surgical specimen) is specific in confirming the diagnosis of aspergilloma, but *Aspergillus* precipitins are present in a high proportion of cases of aspergilloma and can serve to confirm the diagnosis in a patient with the characteristic clinical and radiologic presentation, such as that described here. Sputum culture for *Aspergillus* organisms is less helpful because it may yield no organisms if the cavity does not communicate with the bronchus. Skin tests with *Aspergillus* antigens are also less reliable.

Microscopic examination of the sputum for acid-alcohol–fast bacilli should be done in a case such as this to exclude coexisting active tuberculosis, although, both clinically and radiologically, this is a less likely diagnosis. A reasonable precaution would be to place the patient in respiratory isolation until negative smear results have been obtained.

4. *Should the patient receive intravenous amphotericin B?*

There have been no prospective studies comparing the outcome in patients with aspergilloma treated with intravenous amphotericin B versus the outcome in untreated patients. The findings from retrospective studies suggest, however, that this treatment confers no beneficial effect, and this is not surprising, given that the fungal ball is isolated from the bloodstream. Asymptomatic patients may simply be monitored and resolution may occur spontaneously. Prophylactic surgical removal may be considered in patients who are fit for the procedure because of the potential for aspergilloma to cause fatal hemoptysis, and because it may effect a lasting cure. However, the poor exercise tolerance and the clinical findings indicating respiratory failure in this case suggest that the patient would be unlikely to tolerate the procedure. This could be confirmed by formal pulmonary function tests. Poor prognostic indicators would be an arterial blood gas analysis showing an elevated partial pressure of carbon dioxide (Pco_2) and a forced expiratory volume in 1 second of less than 1 L.

5. *What additional late complication of tuberculosis does this patient exhibit, and how can this be relieved?*

The patient has central cyanosis, indicating that he has hypoxia at rest. This is an additional late complication of pulmonary tuberculosis, probably exacerbated in his case by chronic obstructive pulmonary disease due to smoking. The hypoxia has resulted in pulmonary vasoconstriction and, hence, in pulmonary hypertension (indicated by the loud pulmonary second sound heard on auscultation of the heart). This, in turn, has resulted in right ventricular failure (indicated by the raised jugular venous pressure and edema), or cor pulmonale. The continuous administration of oxygen is indicated for the relief of this syndrome.

Suggested Readings

Fox W. Whither short-course chemotherapy? *British Journal of Diseases of the Chest* 1981;75:331.

Glimp RA, Bayer AS. Pulmonary aspergilloma: diagnostic and therapeutic considerations. *Arch Intern Med* 1983;143:303.

Hammerman KJ, Sarosi GA, Tosh FE. Amphotericin B in the treatment of saprophytic forms of pulmonary aspergillosis. *American Review of Respiratory Disease* 1974;109:57.

Mitchison DA. Basic mechanisms of chemotherapy. *Chest* 1979;76[Suppl]:771.

Shapiro MJ, Albelda SM, Mayock RL, McLean GK. Severe hemoptysis associated with pulmonary aspergilloma: percutaneous intracavitary treatment. *Chest* 1988;94:1225.

Sepsis

1. Is there a clinical distinction between bacteremia and sepsis?
2. What is the distinction between chills and rigors?
3. What factors are associated with a poor prognosis in the setting of gram-negative sepsis?

Discussion

1. *Is there a clinical distinction between bacteremia and sepsis?*

   It is important to differentiate among bacteremia, sepsis, and septic shock. Bacteremia is defined as the presence of viable bacteria in the blood, as demonstrated by a positive blood culture. Bacteremias may be further classified as transient, sustained, or intermittent, depending on the length of time blood cultures are positive. Transient bacteremias are common and last for only several minutes. When multiple blood cultures are positive over the course of several hours to several days, this indicates a sustained bacteremia. Intermittent bacteremias are those in which the blood cultures are intermittently positive. *Sepsis* is a clinical term that refers to a physiologic state that is associated with severe infection. In septic shock, there is hypotension (systolic blood pressure <90 mm Hg or a one-third reduction from the prior systolic blood pressure) and evidence of end-organ damage secondary to reduced blood flow.

2. *What is the distinction between chills and rigors?*

   It is very important to know the difference between chills and rigors. Rigor (a true shaking chill) is very often associated with bacteremia. The patient may experience teeth chattering and body tremors that usually last for 15 to 30 minutes. A chill is more appropriately described as a chilly sensation, not a clinical presentation. Rigors may be seen in the setting of viral infections as well as bacteremias.

3. *What factors are associated with a poor prognosis in the setting of gram-negative sepsis?*

   Despite advances in supportive therapy, the mortality rate associated with gram-negative septic shock approaches 40%. Factors that contribute to this poor prognosis are increased age, poor nutritional status, steroid use, cirrhosis, diabetes, congestive heart failure, and granulocytopenia. Outcome is also adversely affected by volume depletion, inappropriate antibiotic use, and delay in therapy.

Case   A 74-year-old white man with Alzheimer's disease is brought to the emergency room by ambulance after a 1-day history of fever and mental status changes. On arrival in the emergency room, his blood pressure is found to be 100/60 mm Hg, his heart rate is 100 beats per minute, his temperature is 38.5°C, and his respiratory rate is 24 per minute. The patient is unable to give any history; however, his wife states that he had been in his usual health until the evening before admission, when he began to complain of generalized abdominal pain and had become more confused than usual.

Physical examination reveals an agitated elderly man who is in no acute distress. His oral mucosa is dry and the lung examination reveals decreased breath sounds at the bases bilaterally. Cardiac examination reveals sinus tachycardia. Abdominal examination reveals normal bowel sounds and a palpable mass in the lower abdomen extending from 2 cm below the umbilicus down to the pelvis. Rectal examination reveals an enlarged, firm prostate, and the stool is heme negative. His extremities are cool and clammy and there is decreased skin turgor.

Admission laboratory results are as follows: white blood cell count, 16,000/mm³ with a differential count of 85% polymorphonuclear leukocytes, 10% band forms, and 5% lymphocytes; hematocrit, 47%; creatinine, 2.3 mg/dL; blood urea nitrogen, 40 mg/dL; sodium, 141 mEq/L; potassium, 4.5 mEq/L; chloride, 107 mEq/L; and carbon dioxide, 17 mEq/L. Arterial blood gas measurement performed on room air reveals a pH of 7.29, a P_{O_2} of 68 mm Hg, and a P_{CO_2} of 30 mm Hg. His chest radiographic findings are unremarkable. The patient is asked for a urine specimen but is able to void only 5 mL of cloudy, dark yellow urine, which is sent to the laboratory for urinalysis and culture.

A Foley catheter was subsequently placed and 500 mL of foul-smelling urine was obtained. On repeat examination, his abdomen was found to be soft and the mass had disappeared.

1. What system is the likely source of infection in this patient, and how could infection at this site explain his other signs and symptoms?
2. What group of organisms is most likely associated with the sepsis syndrome in this patient, and how does this group differ from the other major groups of bacteria and fungi?
3. How does endotoxin affect macrophages, and what chemical signals are produced by macrophages to contribute to the sepsis syndrome?
4. Of what should the initial management of a patient with the sepsis syndrome consist?

Case Discussion

1. *What system is the likely source of infection in this patient, and how could infection at this site explain his other signs and symptoms?*
   The most likely diagnosis that fits with this patient's constellation of symptoms is urosepsis. As brought to light by the physical examination, the patient

has the signs of septic shock—impaired tissue perfusion, hypotension, and lactic acidosis in association with positive blood cultures. Tachycardia, tachypnea, and oliguria are also usually seen in the setting of genitourinary, gastrointestinal, biliary, and gynecologic infections, and thus are not specific to urosepsis. Abnormalities in mental status may also be a feature of the initial presentation, even without infection in the CNS. In elderly patients, the symptoms of mental obtundation may be subtle and consist only of withdrawal or agitation, and they may constitute the sole indication of severe infection. The chest radiographic study in this patient was negative with no evidence of an infiltrate, making pneumonia unlikely. However, the clinician must always keep in mind that with hydration an infiltrate may blossom, so the patient's respiratory status should be monitored closely. Because the mental status changes may be one of the only early manifestations of sepsis in the elderly, more often than not a lumbar puncture yields normal fluid. This patient's physical examination findings were also remarkable for an abdominal mass, and indeed he had complained of diffuse abdominal pain for at least 1 day before admission. Certainly, elderly patients may have appendicitis, diverticulitis with an abscess, or a colon carcinoma with subsequent bacteremia, and these processes must all be included in the differential diagnosis. He was noted to have an enlarged prostate and also had difficulty voiding.

2. *What group of organisms is most likely associated with the sepsis syndrome in this patient, and how does this group differ from the other major groups of bacteria and fungi?*

The organisms most frequently isolated in the blood of patients with the sepsis syndrome are gram-negative bacilli. Shock occurs less frequently in the setting of bacteremia due to gram-positive organisms. This difference may stem from variations in the host response to different bacterial cell wall constituents. The lipopolysaccharide portion of the cell wall of gram-negative bacilli (called *endotoxin*) elicits a vigorous inflammatory response when injected intravenously into animals. The inflammatory response to lipoteichoic acid, a cell wall constituent of gram-positive organisms, is much less pronounced. This patient had not been hospitalized, nor had he undergone any kind of instrumentation. Therefore, the most likely organism to cause a UTI with subsequent bacteremia and the sepsis syndrome in this patient is *E. coli*. Other potential gram-negative organisms that may precipitate septic shock include *Klebsiella pneumoniae, Pseudomonas aeruginosa, Enterobacter aerogenes*, and *Serratia marcescens*. The primary portal of entry is the genitourinary tract, but the gastrointestinal tract, respiratory tract, and skin are also important sources of bacteremia. Enterococcus must also be considered as a potential cause of this patient's illness because it can frequently cause prostatitis. Other gram-positive organisms, such as coagulase-positive and coagulase-negative *Staphylococcus* species, can certainly cause bacteremia and sepsis syndrome; however, this occurs most commonly in hospitalized patients who have had some type of intravascular device installed.

3. *How does endotoxin affect macrophages, and what chemical signals are produced by macrophages to contribute to the sepsis syndrome?*

   Several bacterial factors are powerful mediators of sepsis, and one of the most potent is endotoxin. As stated, endotoxin is the lipopolysaccharide component of the cell wall in gram-negative bacteria. It appears that when cell injury occurs with the activation of immune defenses or the initiation of antimicrobial therapy, bacterial cell lysis takes place and the titer of detectable endotoxin in the patient's blood rises dramatically. Macrophages are then activated by endotoxin and their phagocytic functions and lysosomal enzyme production are accelerated. Once the actions of the macrophages and monocytes have been triggered, they begin to synthesize and release many mediators, including tumor necrosis factor-α (TNF-α); interleukin (IL)-1, IL-2, and IL-6; and platelet-activating factor. After the release of TNF-α, IL-1, and platelet-activating factor, arachidonic acid is metabolized to form leukotrienes, thromboxane A_2, and prostaglandin E_2. IL-1 and IL-6 activate T cells to produce interferon-γ, IL-2, IL-4, and granulocyte–macrophage colony-stimulating factor. The coagulation cascade and complement system are also activated (Fig. 6-1). Clinically, this phenomenon results in a low central venous or pulmonary capillary wedge pressure, as well as a marked drop in total systemic vascular resistance. In addition, there is a compensatory increase in cardiac output in an attempt to maintain perfusion. The end result of this process is an increase in cardiac output, a marked fall in peripheral vascular resistance, and hypotension. If uncontrolled, progressive lactic acidosis ensues, ultimately leading to death.

4. *Of what should the initial management of a patient with the sepsis syndrome consist?*

   Although antibiotic therapy is the mainstay of treatment for sepsis caused by gram-negative organisms, the amelioration of underlying conditions, elimination of predisposing factors, drainage of abscesses, removal of infected foreign bodies, and adequate supportive care are also of paramount importance for curing the infection. It is critical to remember that the immediate therapeutic intervention should be directed at increasing cardiac output and oxygen delivery to prevent or minimize hypoperfusion and reduce tissue hypoxia. An optimal intravascular volume *must* be restored and maintained. Fluid requirements are very unpredictable because of capillary leak, and, at the very least, central venous pressures should be monitored so that these requirements can be appropriately met. It may be necessary to install a Swan-Ganz catheter for monitoring cardiac function and left ventricular filling pressures in patients with left ventricular dysfunction. Respiratory status and acid–base disturbances can be observed with serial arterial blood gas measurements, which are also helpful in determining a patient's prognosis. The chance for survival in patients who are alkalemic is excellent, but this is not the case for acidemic patients. The next step is to obtain appropriate cultures and administer appropriate bactericidal agents. The antibiotic should be chosen on the basis of the presumed source of the bacteria and the susceptibility pattern of

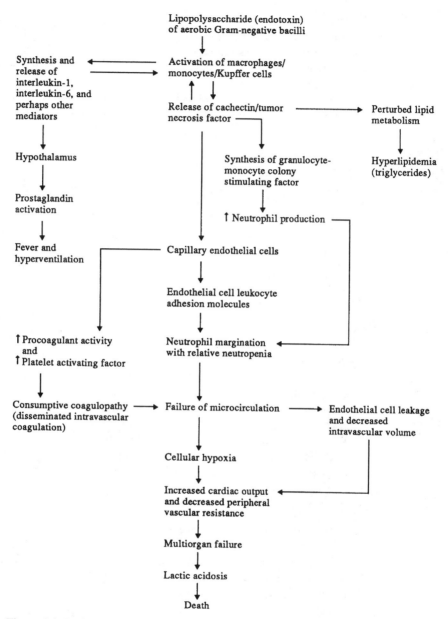

Figure 6-1. Pathogenesis of the microvascular injury and death due to endotoxin shock. (From Karchmer AW, Barza M, Drew WL, et al. *Infectious disease medicine (MKSAP IX).* Philadelphia: American College of Physicians, 1991.)

organisms from that source. In general, if bacteremia with a sepsis syndrome is suspected, combination therapy that includes two antibiotics should be instituted, such as an extended-spectrum penicillin or a third-generation cephalosporin plus an aminoglycoside. Additional therapies that are under investigation are based on the emerging knowledge of the pathophysiologic sequence of bacteremic shock. These include immunoglobulin M monoclonal antibody aimed at neutralizing endotoxin, endotoxin receptor antibodies, monoclonal antibody to TNF, and cytokine receptor antibodies or antagonists, or both.

Suggested Readings

Foltzer MA, Reese RE. Bacteremia and sepsis. In: Reese RE, Betts RF, eds. *A practical approach to infectious diseases*, 3rd ed. Boston: Little, Brown, 1991, p. 19.

Karchmer AW, Barza M, Drew WL, et al. *Infectious disease medicine (MKSAP IX)*, Part B, Book 1. Philadelphia: American College of Physicians, 1991:321–322.

Mostow SR. Management of gram-negative septic shock. *Hosp Pract* 1990;25(10):121.

Parillo JE, Parker MM, Natanson C, et al. Septic shock in humans. *Ann Intern Med* 1990;113:227.

Young LS, Glauser MP, eds. Gram-negative septicemia and septic shock. *Infect Dis Clin North Am* 1991;5(4).

Endocarditis

1. What types of organisms can cause infective endocarditis?
2. What are some important factors that increase the risk for the development of endocarditis?
3. What are the two types of bacterial endocarditis and their clinical characteristics?
4. What conditions call for surgical intervention?
5. Are there any differences in the characteristics of endocarditis between the intravenous drug abuse population and non-drug abusers?

Discussion

1. *What types of organisms can cause infective endocarditis?*

   There are many organisms that can infect the heart and cause endocarditis. The most common ones are "traditional" bacteria, but fungi, *Rickettsia* organisms, *Chlamydia* organisms, and viruses may all invade myocardial tissues and produce disease.

2. *What are some important factors that increase the risk for the development of endocarditis?*

   Many factors increase the risk for the development of endocarditis. Underlying heart diseases such as rheumatic valvular damage, a bicuspid aortic valve, patent ductus arteriosus, and small ventricular septal defects cause damaged tissue or abnormal blood flow, conditions under which bacteria can adhere to the surface and cause infection. Also implicated for the same reasons are prosthetic valves. Intravenous drug abusers are at risk for endocarditis because their valves are being constantly bombarded with impurities such as talc, which causes scarring of the valves, and also because they mix their drug of choice with contaminated water. Nosocomial infections may result from the placement of intravenous catheters or pacemaker wires, or from wound infections or genitourinary manipulation. The elderly are also at increased risk for endocarditis.

3. *What are the two types of bacterial endocarditis and their clinical characteristics?*

The two types of bacterial endocarditis are acute and subacute. Acute bacterial endocarditis is most commonly associated with intravenous drug abuse, intravenous catheter infection, and prosthetic valve infections. These infections may be rapidly fatal if left untreated, and surgical repair or replacement of the damaged valve may be necessary. Subacute endocarditis develops most often in the setting of structural heart disease (e.g., mitral valve prolapse), a history of rheumatic heart disease, or prosthetic valves. It also affects elderly patients, or it may occur in the setting of no known valvular disease. Its onset tends to be more indolent. Symptoms such as weakness, fatigue, night sweats, and weight loss may have existed for weeks to months before diagnosis. Its onset may be related to antecedent events such as dental work, although no definite predisposing event is apparent in most cases. Because some patients may have multiple risk factors and exhibit a variable clinical picture, their disease cannot be easily classified. It is always important to keep in mind the maxim that "if you don't think about endocarditis, you won't diagnose it!"

4. *What conditions call for surgical intervention?*

Surgical intervention is indicated if (a) the bacteremia persists after 2 to 3 weeks of adequate antibiotic therapy; (b) there is progressive congestive heart failure; (c) valve dysfunction results in moderate to severe congestive heart failure; (d) invasive perivalvular infection arises, as reflected by the appearance of new, persistent electrocardiographic conduction disturbances, echocardiographic evidence of a paravalvular abscess or fistula, purulent pericarditis, or persistent unexplained fever despite appropriate antibiotic therapy; (e) fungal endocarditis occurs; or (f) appropriately treated prosthetic valve endocarditis recurs.

5. *Are there any differences in the characteristics of endocarditis between the intravenous drug abuse population and non-drug abusers?*

There are several characteristics of endocarditis relatively unique to intravenous drug abusers, although these are generalizations only. A history of documented prior heart disease is unusual, and the incidence of tricuspid valve involvement is approximately 50% in this population, which is much higher than that in the nonaddict population. In addition, a murmur is frequently undetectable and there is isolated tricuspid valve involvement, unlike the murmurs of aortic or mitral valve insufficiency seen most commonly in the nonaddict population.

Case   A 27-year-old white man presents to the emergency room with a chief complaint of fevers, shaking chills, cough, and headache of 2 days' duration. He denies nausea, vomiting, diarrhea, or dysuria. History reveals that the patient smokes one pack of cigarettes per day, drinks a six-pack of beer per day, and has recently started using "skin-popping" cocaine. He has had no previous hospitalizations or undergone any surgical procedures.

Physical examination reveals a temperature of 39.0°C, blood pressure of 120/80 mm Hg, pulse of 114 beats per minute, and respiratory rate of 18 per minute. His conjunctivae are normal. His oral mucosa is moist and his dentition is good. Lung examination reveals some coarse rhonchi bilaterally. Cardiac examination reveals a grade II/VI systolic murmur that is heard best at the left sternal border but does not radiate. Abdominal and extremity findings are unremarkable. Neurologic examination reveals nonfocal findings, although the patient does complain of a global headache. There is no meningismus.

Laboratory values are as follows: white blood cell count, 18,000/mm^3 (85% polymorphonuclear cells, 10% bands, and 5% lymphocytes); hematocrit, 38%; and platelets, 170,000/mm^3. A chest radiographic study reveals bilateral nodular infiltrates. The patient is admitted to the medicine service for further evaluation and treatment.

1. What type of endocarditis does this patient likely have?
2. What is the likely cause of his pulmonary infiltrates?
3. What are the most common offending pathogens in this setting?
4. What would you prescribe as an initial antibiotic regimen?

Case Discussion

1. *What type of endocarditis does this patient likely have?*

This patient's clinical presentation illustrates a case of acute endocarditis. Tricuspid valve (right-sided) endocarditis is most likely because it is commonly associated with intravenous drug abuse, although the mitral and aortic valves could also be involved.

2. *What is the likely cause of his pulmonary infiltrates?*

The cause of this patient's pulmonary infiltrates is septic emboli that have traveled to the lung. In both acute and subacute bacterial endocarditis, signs and symptoms of embolic phenomena may appear. These episodes of vascular occlusion cause pain in the chest (pulmonary or coronary), abdomen (mesenteric or splenic), or the extremities. Bone pain (particularly vertebral and sacroiliac) is also common because of the hematogenous spread of infection to these sites. Other embolic phenomena that may occur include hematuria (emboli to the kidneys), blindness resulting from retinal artery occlusion, and acute neurologic symptoms (stroke, meningitis, seizures, and headache). Certainly, cardiac involvement such as congestive heart failure may occur in this setting as the result of progressive valvular insufficiency or myocarditis; however, this would be evidenced by the finding of Kerley's B lines or fluffy pulmonary infiltrates on chest radiographic studies.

3. *What are the most common offending pathogens in this setting?*

The organism that would most likely be the source of this patient's infection is *S. aureus*. This organism accounts for approximately 20% of the cases of endocarditis in the general population, but for 55% of the cases associated with intravenous drug abuse. It should therefore be suspected as the etiologic agent in infections associated with a history of intravenous drug abuse, as well as in the context of acute embolic phenomena and acute bacterial endocarditis. Coagulase-negative staphylococci are common in the setting of prosthetic valve endocarditis, but not in the setting of non-prosthetic valve–associated infection. Streptococci account for approximately 70% of all cases of native valvular bacterial endocarditis in the nonaddict population, and infection due to the various species is broken down as follows: 40% due to viridans streptococci; 10% due to enterococci (group E streptococci); and 20% due to other nonhemolytic, microaerophilic, anaerobic, or nonenterococcal group D streptococci. Approximately 10% of the cases are caused by other fastidious organisms, such as fungi and gram-negative bacilli.

4. *What would you prescribe as an initial antibiotic regimen?*

The initial treatment of suspected acute bacterial endocarditis should be directed toward *S. aureus* because it is the most common organism in patients with acute bacterial endocarditis. The clinician should always draw three to four blood specimens for culture before initiating antibiotic therapy. After this is done, nafcillin (2 g intravenously every 4 hours) plus gentamicin (1 mg/ kg intravenously every 8 hours) are appropriate as an initial combination until the culture results are known. This combination covers both *S. aureus* (methicillin sensitive) and enterococci infections, and, with few exceptions, any other likely bacteria. Although there are a variety of recommendations in the literature, it is generally agreed that the prolonged administration of relatively high doses of bactericidal agents is indicated. With the exception of infection caused by highly resistant organisms, it is usually fairly easy to obtain a good symptomatic response (e.g., decline in fever and decreased myalgias) and sterilization of blood cultures within a few days of the start of therapy. A bacteriologic cure with sterilization of the lesions is much more difficult, however, because although valvular lesions are bathed in blood, the valves themselves are relatively avascular. Bacteria in vegetations are surrounded by fibrin. This, in combination with the high flow rates in the cardiac chambers, makes it difficult for phagocytic cells to adhere to the site of infection. Thus, prolonged treatment with high doses of bactericidal antibiotics is essential for cure. There is *in vitro* and *in vivo* evidence that low-dose gentamicin in combination with a semisynthetic penicillin produces more rapid killing of staphylococci and sterilization of valves than does penicillin alone. This suggests that the addition of gentamicin (1 mg/kg every 8 hours for 3 to 5 days) is a reasonable regimen (if the patient has no contraindications to aminoglycoside use, such as renal failure) in an attempt to clear the bacteremia rapidly and minimize damage to the heart valves. There are, however, no data from randomized, blinded studies showing that this approach has an impact on the clinical outcome.

Suggested Readings

Brandriss MW, Lambert JS. Cardiac infections. In Reese RE, Betts RF, eds. *A practical approach to infectious diseases*, 3rd ed. Boston: Little, Brown, 1991, p. 278.

Chambers HF, Miller RT, Newman MD. Right-sided *Staphylococcus aureus* endocarditis in intravenous drug abusers: two-week combination therapy. *Ann Intern Med* 1988;109:619.

Chambers HF, Korzeniowski OM, Sande MA, et al. *Staphylococcus aureus* endocarditis: clinical manifestations in addicts and nonaddicts. *Medicine (Baltimore)* 1983;62:170.

Sullam PM, Drake TA, Sande MA. Pathogenesis of endocarditis. *Am J Med* 1985;78:110.

Fever and Abdominal Pain

1. What is the single best test to evaluate the febrile patient with abdominal pain?
2. What are the most important pathogens in the bowel flora?
3. Besides obstruction, ischemia, and injury involving the gut (and its outpouchings), what are other causes of peritonitis?
4. What are several examples of extraperitoneal diseases that can present with abdominal pain as a prominent symptom?

Discussion

1. *What is the single best test to evaluate the febrile patient with abdominal pain?*

   The febrile patient with abdominal pain can be a daunting prospect. The differential diagnosis in this setting ranges from benign, self-limited infections such as viral enteritis to severe, life-threatening infections such as peritonitis resulting from an ischemic bowel. However, despite the availability of a tremendous variety of imaging procedures and tests of bodily fluids, the single best approach to diagnosis in a patient with fever and abdominal pain remains a careful history and physical examination. Sometimes the information yielded is sufficient to make a diagnosis. More often, tests are necessary, but a careful clinical evaluation narrows the list of questions that need to be answered by tests. Fishing with a long series of tests without well-considered clinical questions occasionally hooks the true culprit, but more often nets a catch of red herrings.

2. *What are the most important pathogens in the bowel flora?*

   A common concern in the febrile patient with abdominal pain is the possible contamination of the peritoneal space from the bowel. Although a great variety of organisms live in the gut, the number of important pathogens is, fortunately, small. The Enterobacteriaceae are perhaps the best known such pathogens. Anaerobes are the dominant organisms in the colon and, of this class, *Bacteroides* species are the important pathogens. Finally, streptococci, especially enterococci, can be prominent pathogens (they are also important because of their resistance to a number of commonly used antibiotics, such as the cephalosporins).

3. *Besides obstruction, ischemia, and injury involving the gut (and its outpouchings), what are other causes of peritonitis?*

   Preexisting ascitic fluid, especially that due to hepatic cirrhosis, can become infected and cause peritonitis. Salpingitis and endometritis can lead to peritonitis through direct extension of the infection out the open abdominal ostium of the tube. Primary peritonitis is an unusual form of bacterial peritonitis that has no clear predisposing factors; it most often affects children. Finally, there are noninfectious causes of peritonitis, including bleeding into the peritoneum, which can cause pain and low-grade fevers, plus the rare familial Mediterranean fever.

4. *What are several examples of extraperitoneal diseases that can present with abdominal pain as a prominent symptom?*

Lower lobe pneumonia can be a source of considerable abdominal pain and tenderness. Neuritic pain resulting from a variety of causes (infectious causes include herpes zoster, Lyme disease, and tabes dorsalis) can produce severe abdominal pain, which is convincing enough at times to prompt performance of an exploratory laparotomy.

Case A 24-year-old woman comes to the emergency room because of a 4-day history of abdominal pain, which she describes as a sharp, progressively severe pain in the right lower chest and upper abdomen that is exacerbated by taking a deep breath, walking, or sitting erect. She feels nauseated, but has not vomited. At home she has had fevers as high as 38°C, but no rigors. She has had no previous similar episodes and has never undergone abdominal surgery. She denies cough or dyspnea, fatty food intolerance, jaundice or dark urine, dysuria, or urinary frequency. She has never been pregnant; her last menstrual period began 1 week ago and is now ending. Her past medical history is unremarkable; her only medication is an oral contraceptive. She drinks socially on weekends, but does not use tobacco. Her family history is notable in that her mother had a cholecystectomy at 34 years of age.

On physical examination, she is found to be a mildly obese young woman who is in moderate distress and lying curled up on her right side. Her temperature is 37.8°C, her blood pressure is 96/60 mm Hg, and her pulse is 110 beats per minute. Examination of her head and neck yield unremarkable findings; specifically, there is no scleral icterus or cervical adenopathy. Her chest is clear to auscultation and percussion, although she is unable to take a deep breath because of the pain in her right lower chest. She has hypoactive bowel sounds and exhibits substantial tenderness in the right upper quadrant associated with a positive Murphy's sign (an inability to take a deep breath during deep palpation of the right upper quadrant). The edge of her liver is not palpable and the span, by percussion, is normal. No masses or tenderness are found elsewhere in the abdomen, and the spleen is not palpable. Rectal examination reveals no tenderness and the stool is guaiac negative. Her skin and extremities appear normal.

She has a white blood cell count of 10,500/mm^3 with 85% segmented neutrophils and 7% band forms, a hematocrit of 39%, and a platelet count of 216,000/mm^3. Serum electrolyte and creatinine values are normal. The aspartate aminotransferase (AST) level is elevated at 56 U/mL (normal, <30 IU/mL), but her serum bilirubin, alkaline phosphatase, and amylase levels are normal. Urinalysis is notable for 20 to 50 white blood cells, 20 to 50 red blood cells, many bacteria, and many epithelial cells per high-power field. She is thought to have acute cholecystitis, but an ultrasound scan of the liver, biliary ducts, and pancreas is negative.

1. What are the various ways for you to proceed at this point?
2. What is the most likely diagnosis based on the findings from your further investigations?
3. What pathogens can cause salpingitis with perihepatitis?
4. What noninvasive tests are helpful for confirming a specific cause of salpingitis with perihepatitis?

Case Discussion

1. *What are the various ways for you to proceed at this point?*

    To elucidate the nature of this patient's disorder, you decide to proceed with the following: radionuclide biliary (lidofenin) scanning, a chest radiographic study, repeat urinalysis and culture, serologic tests for hepatitis A, B, and C, serum β-human chorionic gonadotropin (hCG) measurement, and sexual history and pelvic examination.

    During this second round of testing, you encounter the following. Because it is 6:00 p.m., the nuclear medicine facilities are not available until tomorrow morning, and therefore it is not possible to have a radionuclide biliary scan performed. The chest radiographic study is negative. Repeat urinalysis on a catheterized specimen yields normal findings, but the culture results are pending, as are the results of serologic tests for hepatitis A, B, and C. The serum β-hCG level shows she is not pregnant. Sexual history and pelvic examination reveal she is sexually active with a new partner in the past month. Because she uses an oral contraceptive, her partner does not use condoms. She has had genital warts and yeast infections in the past, but has no known history of other sexually transmitted diseases. She does not use intravenous drugs, has never received a blood transfusion, and has had no occupational exposure to blood. On pelvic examination, her external genitalia are found to be normal. There is a small amount of dark blood from the cervical os and mild tenderness with cervical motion and palpation of the right adnexa. The size of the uterus is normal and there are no adnexal masses.

2. *What is the most likely diagnosis based on the findings from your further investigations?*

    All these tests investigate important causes of acute abdominal pain and fever. Interpretation of the results allows a fairly confident diagnosis to be made. The initial concern was acute cholecystitis, but the normal ultrasound findings make this diagnosis unlikely, although they do not completely rule it out because a single stone may lodge in the distal common duct and be missed on ultrasound. Arguing against cholecystitis are her age and lack of previous pregnancies. Another possibility is right lower lobe pneumonia. In most cases of pneumonia, respiratory symptoms are the chief complaint, but lower lobe pneumonia, by irritating the parietal pleura overlying the diaphragm, can assume the characteristics of an abdominal presentation. In this case, the normal chest radiographic findings and lack of pulmonary symptoms make this diagnosis very unlikely.

Patients with pyelonephritis can experience pain anteriorly (in the upper and mid-abdomen) as well as the classic costovertebral angle tenderness in the back. However, the lack of lower urinary tract symptoms (dysuria, urinary frequency, and suprapubic pain) in this patient is not conclusive evidence against this diagnosis because these symptoms are frequently mild or even absent in patients with upper UTIs. The initial urinalysis revealed many white blood cells, a finding that on first blush seems to confirm the diagnosis of pyelonephritis. However, there are many epithelial cells as well, which makes it impossible to tell whether the white blood cells came from the urinary or the reproductive tract. A catheterized urine specimen answers this question, and the subsequent normal urinalysis findings almost rule out the possibility of pyelonephritis. Rarely, if there is infection behind an obstruction of the ureter, the urinalysis results can be normal. Such patients are usually severely ill, however, rendering this diagnosis very unlikely in this case.

Although acute viral hepatitis can cause pronounced right upper quadrant pain and tenderness, it is a very unlikely diagnosis in this patient. At the onset of symptoms, the transaminase levels in the setting of viral hepatitis are markedly elevated—usually exceeding 10 times normal. The minor elevation in the AST level in this patient would be very atypical of acute viral hepatitis.

The possibility of a ruptured ectopic pregnancy should always be considered in a young woman with abdominal pain and vaginal bleeding, but the serum β-hCG measurement rules this possibility out.

Acute salpingitis (infection of the fallopian tubes or pelvic inflammatory disease) can be manifested by right upper quadrant pain. This symptom is thought to arise as a result of secretions from the infected tube leaking into the peritoneum and traveling up the right pericolic gutter to the right upper quadrant. This can produce infection of the hepatic capsule, termed *perihepatitis* (or Fitz-Hugh–Curtis syndrome). Surprisingly, the symptoms of the perihepatitis are frequently much more prominent than the symptoms stemming from the original focus of infection in the tube. Therefore, these patients are frequently admitted and sometimes taken to surgery for treatment of a presumed cholecystitis. There are no pathognomonic laboratory or imaging findings that can confirm this diagnosis; this requires laparoscopy. However, acute salpingitis should be seriously considered in this patient—a sexually active woman with right upper quadrant pain, fevers, and no signs of cholecystitis. With the additional factor that she has a new sexual partner coupled with the finding of right adnexal tenderness, salpingitis with perihepatitis becomes the most likely diagnosis.

3. *What pathogens can cause salpingitis with perihepatitis?*

Gonorrhea is the classic cause of this syndrome. In Fitz-Hugh's original description, Gram's staining of the fluid from the hepatic capsule showed gram-negative diplococci. Since then, as in the case of acute urethritis, it has become clear that *C. trachomatis* is a common cause of acute salpingitis with perihepatitis.

4. *What noninvasive tests are helpful for confirming a specific cause of salpingitis with perihepatitis?*

Gram's staining of a cervical smear, although relatively insensitive (50%) for detecting gonococci, is specific enough (95%) to be used as the basis for presumptive therapy if results are positive. A cervical culture for gonorrhea allows the detection of smear-negative cases. It is possible to culture *Chlamydia*, but this is a relatively expensive procedure and the means of doing so are not available in many clinics and small hospitals. However, a number of antigen detection systems (using, for example, an enzyme-linked immunosorbent assay) have been developed and marketed. These have an acceptable sensitivity and specificity, with results available in 24 hours or less.

Suggested Readings

Bolton JP. Perihepatitis. *Br Med Bull* 1983;39:159.

Fitz-Hugh T. Acute gonococcic peritonitis of the right upper quadrant in women. *JAMA* 1934;102:2094.

Katzman DK, Friedman IM, McDonald CA, Litt IF. *Chlamydia trachomatis* Fitz-Hugh–Curtis syndrome without salpingitis in female adolescents. *American Journal of Diseases of Children* 1988;142:996.

Muller-Schoop JW, Wang SP, Munzinger J, et al. *Chlamydia trachomatis* as possible cause of peritonitis and perihepatitis in young women. *BMJ* 1978;1:1022.

Wood JJ, Bolton JP, et al. Biliary-type pain as a manifestation of genital tract infection: the Curtis–Fitz-Hugh syndrome. *Br J Surg* 1982;69:251.

Central Nervous System Infection

1. What principles are important in selecting an antimicrobial regimen to treat a CNS infection?

2. How do cerebrospinal fluid (CSF) findings such as the protein and glucose levels, the white blood cell count, and differential help determine the differential diagnosis of a CNS infection?

3. What are the most common pathogens causing bacterial meningitis, and how does the prevalence of the bacterial pathogens that cause meningitis vary, depending on the age of the host?

Discussion

1. *What principles are important in selecting an antimicrobial regimen to treat a CNS infection?*

The blood–brain barrier functions to help prevent the entry of circulating pathogens into the CNS. Unfortunately, however, it also has the effect of decreasing antibiotic penetration into the CSF. The cephalosporins, penicillins, chloramphenicol, and TMP-SMX are commonly used antibiotics that all demonstrate good CSF penetration. In contrast, the aminoglycosides have extremely poor CSF penetration, and an infection requiring aminoglycoside therapy must usually be managed with the intrathecal administration of these antibiotics. Other drugs, such as vancomycin, exhibit intermediate CSF penetration, and their efficacy depends on the presence of inflamed meninges to permit a therapeutic level of antibiotic to be reached.

Another important principle is to choose an empiric antibiotic regimen that covers the most likely pathogens. This choice therefore depends on the epidemiologic background of the patient and on his or her recent exposure history. After the pathogen has been identified and the drug susceptibility determined, therapy can be more specifically tailored. Finally, as with any new drug regimen, the patient's history of drug allergy should be carefully reviewed.

2. *How do CSF findings such as the protein and glucose levels, the white blood cell count, and differential help determine the differential diagnosis of a CNS infection?*

In adults, the normal range of the CSF glucose level is 45 to 80 mg/dL. A glucose level of less than 30 mg/dL suggests bacterial, fungal, or tuberculous meningitis. An elevated level may be seen in the setting of diabetes mellitus. A CSF protein level greater than 150 mg/dL suggests bacterial meningitis, and an extremely high protein level (>350 mg/dL) suggests a complete block of the spinal canal, as seen in certain cases of epidural abscess or tumors. The normal range for the lumbar CSF protein level in adults is 9 to 58 mg/dL. A white blood cell count greater than 1,200/mm^3 suggests bacterial meningitis. However, a count of less than this does not necessarily imply viral infection because bacterial meningitis is also frequently associated with this finding. Neutrophil predominance (>50%) also suggests bacterial meningitis, although there is considerable overlap with other types of meningitis in this regard. Lymphocyte predominance may be seen in the context of tuberculous, viral, fungal, partially treated bacterial, or aseptic meningitis.

3. *What are the most common pathogens causing bacterial meningitis, and how does the prevalence of the bacterial pathogens that cause meningitis vary, depending on the age of the host?*

The four most common pathogens causing meningitis for all age groups are *Streptococcus pneumoniae, Haemophilus influenzae, Neisseria meningitidis,* and *E. coli.* However, there is considerable variation in the prevalence of these various pathogens among the different age groups. The highest attack rate of bacterial meningitis occurs in the very young and very old. Lower attack rates are seen in young to middle-aged adults. In the United States, 0- to 1-month-old infants most commonly get group B streptococcus, *E. coli,* and *Listeria* meningitis; children 1 month to 5 years of age predominantly get *H. influenzae* meningitis (up to 70% of the cases). Forty percent of the patients with meningitis 5 to 29 years of age acquire *N. meningitidis* infection, and *S. pneumoniae* is the most common meningitis pathogen in patients 29 years of age and older. Elderly patients are more vulnerable to *Listeria monocytogenes*, gram-negative bacilli, and pneumococcus.

Case

A 79-year-old man who is a resident of a nursing home is brought to the emergency room by the nursing home staff. He had been in his usual state of health until that morning, when headache, fever, and chills developed. He slept through breakfast, after which his caretakers found him to be lethargic, and this prompted them to bring him to the hospital. On initial examination he is found to be stuporous. His temperature is 102.6°F (39°C), and he has prominent nuchal rigidity. Funduscopic examination reveals no evidence of papilledema. A grade II/VI systolic ejection murmur is found on cardiac examination. Pulmonary auscultation reveals the presence of bibasilar fine crackles. An indwelling Foley catheter is in place, which the nursing home staff explains he has required for the past 18 months because of urinary incontinence. A past medical history is notable for two episodes of UTIs, both occurring after the insertion of the Foley catheter, and mild chronic interstitial lung disease.

A CT scan of the head reveals no evidence of increased intracranial pressure, no shift or mass effect, and no intracranial bleeding, but atrophic changes consistent with age. A lumbar puncture is performed, blood and urine cultures are obtained, and appropriate therapy is begun.

1. What is the most likely pathogenesis of this man's meningitis?
2. What aspects of the emergency room management should have been different in this case?
3. What empiric intravenous antibiotic therapy would be most appropriate to treat the bacterial meningitis in a patient of this age, and how long should he be treated?
4. What physical findings could point to an anatomic source of bacterial meningitis?
5. What CSF findings would be expected if this patient has bacterial meningitis?
6. If the Gram's staining of the CSF and the cultures had yielded no organisms in this patient, what should you suspect?
7. If this patient had experienced the gradual onset of fevers, headache, and nuchal rigidity, what other possible diagnoses might you have entertained?

Case Discussion

1. *What is the most likely pathogenesis of this man's meningitis?*

Several possible scenarios could explain the presence of bacteria in normally sterile CSF, despite an intact blood–brain barrier. These include any of a number of processes leading to the development of bacteremia and meningeal seeding. One of the more common sources of infection is nasopharyngeal colonization by bacteria, which is then followed by sinusitis, local invasion, bacteremia, and meningeal seeding. Another pathogenic mechanism is trauma (such as an occult skull fracture), leading to a breach in the blood–brain barrier and the entry of skin flora.

The most likely scenario in this patient is that a plugged Foley catheter led to the reflux of bladder contents into the ureters up to the kidneys, with consequent seeding of the bloodstream by urinary pathogens. Bacteremia can then lead to meningitis, especially in the immunocompromised or elderly host. Although the mechanism of bacterial transport across a presumably intact blood–brain barrier is largely unknown, the findings from some studies have suggested that a high concentration of bacteria in the bloodstream, and the presence of bacterial virulence factors such as antiphagocytic polysaccharide capsules, the S fimbriae of *E. coli*, or other components of bacterial cell walls, may facilitate this process.

2. *What aspects of the emergency room management should have been different in this case?*

The head CT scan was unnecessary because the funduscopic and nonfocal neurologic findings were sufficient to rule out a significant intracranial mass effect. Otherwise, the management of this patient was correct, and it illustrated a number of important concepts. It is important to attempt to identify the pathogen in a patient with meningitis before the initiation of antibiotic therapy. Lumbar puncture should be delayed or deferred only in the following two instances. First, lumbar puncture should not be performed if a minor delay in therapy could be hazardous, as in patients in bacterial shock or those who face a high risk of bacterial shock because of the rapid onset of purpura or because of low blood pressure. It also should not be performed when there is a possible danger of uncal herniation, as in the event of rapidly developing coma, focal neurologic signs, convulsions, or papilledema. Otherwise, appropriate management consists of quickly excluding papilledema, focal neurologic signs, shock, and purpura, followed by prompt lumbar puncture and the subsequent administration of appropriate antibiotics.

The respiratory isolation of patients with suspected meningitis is appropriate only when there is a strong suspicion of *N. meningitidis*, tuberculous meningitis, or *H. influenzae* type B (in pediatric patients). The close contacts of patients with *N. meningitidis* (such as the person performing an intubation) should receive prophylactic rifampin treatment (10 mg/kg orally twice a day for 2 days, to a maximum of 600 mg twice a day).

3. *What empiric intravenous antibiotic therapy would be most appropriate to treat the bacterial meningitis in a patient of this age, and how long should he be treated?*

The approaches to age-specific empiric antibiotic therapy for bacterial meningitis are based on knowledge of the most common pathogens that affect each group, as already outlined. The combination of ampicillin plus a third-generation cephalosporin is appropriate for infants 0 to 12 weeks of age as well as for the elderly (older than 50 years of age). The ampicillin is added mainly to ensure coverage for *L. monocytogenes*. Once the pathogen and its susceptibility pattern are known, therapy can be individualized. Children and adolescents 3 months to 18 years of age are most appropriately treated with either a third-generation cephalosporin or with ampicillin plus chloramphenicol. For nonimmunocompromised young adults and the middle-aged (18 to 50 years of age), either penicillin G or ampicillin alone is appropriate because of the overwhelming predominance of *S. pneumoniae* and *N. meningitidis* in this age group. The duration of antibiotic therapy for bacterial meningitis is still largely based on tradition: 10 to 14 days for acute bacterial meningitis caused by any of the three major meningeal pathogens, and approximately 3 weeks for gram-negative bacillary meningitis. The dosages of the antibiotics for the treatment of meningitis are usually higher than those used for other infections to ensure adequate bactericidal activity in the CSF. For example, intravenous penicillin G should be given every 4 hours to a total daily dose of 20 to 24 million units, and 2 g of ceftriaxone should be given every 12 hours. The aminoglycosides, which do not adequately traverse the blood–brain barrier, must be administered intrathecally as well as intravenously when indicated, as in the event of meningitis due to a highly resistant gram-negative organism.

4. *What physical findings could point to an anatomic source of bacterial meningitis?*

   Important physical findings that are clues to an anatomic source of bacterial meningitis include otitis media, sinusitis, skull fracture or other evidence of cranial trauma such as CSF leaking from the external auditory meatus, neurosurgical scars, or the presence of a ventriculostomy shunt.

   Most cases of meningitis result from the attachment of bacteria to epithelial cells of the nasopharyngeal and oropharyngeal mucosa, followed by transgression of the mucosal barrier. These events are also associated with the development of otitis media and sinusitis. Any anatomic breach of the blood–brain barrier, either through trauma or neurosurgery, can introduce bacteria into the CNS. Meningitis develops in up to 30% of patients who have a ventriculoatrial or ventriculoperitoneal shunt. Other pertinent physical findings in a patient with meningitis include a dermal sinus or mastoiditis.

5. *What CSF findings would be expected if this patient has bacterial meningitis?*

   The clinician would expect to see the following constellation of findings: a low glucose level, a high protein content, and an elevated white blood cell count, with a neutrophil predominance (see earlier discussion).

6. *If the Gram's staining of the CSF and the cultures had yielded no organisms in this patient, what should you suspect?*

   The lack of organisms on Gram's-stained CSF specimens does not rule out bacterial meningitis; however, this test should be performed on a centrifuged sediment of CSF. Negative findings are encountered in 10% to 20% of the patients with bacterial meningitis whose CSF cultures are positive for organisms. In cases of partially treated bacterial meningitis, Gram's staining of the CSF more often yields negative findings. An acid-fast smear of spun CSF is only rarely positive in cases of tuberculous meningitis.

7. *If this patient had experienced the gradual onset of fevers, headache, and nuchal rigidity, what other possible diagnoses might you have entertained?*

Fungal meningitis, a brain abscess, tuberculous meningitis, and carcinomatous meningitis all tend to be rather insidious in onset and assume a more chronic course than that seen with acute bacterial meningitis. The onset of tuberculous meningitis may occasionally be rapid in an immunocompromised host, but this would usually occur only in the course of miliary tuberculosis or with the rupture of a subependymal tubercle. More commonly, however, patients with tuberculous meningitis have symptoms for more than 2 weeks. One of the hallmarks of tuberculous meningitis is the development of ocular palsies, seen in 30% to 70% of the cases.

An epidemiologic history is useful in diagnosing chronic meningitis. Prior exposure to tuberculosis, a history of skin test positivity, or recent travel to or residence in areas endemic for *Histoplasma* or *Coccidioides* is important information to elicit. Carcinomatous meningitis usually occurs in the setting of a known underlying malignancy.

Suggested Readings

Quagliarello V, Scheld WM. Bacterial meningitis: pathogenesis, pathophysiology and progress. *N Engl J Med* 1992;327:864.

Scheld WM, Whitley RJ, Durak DT. Cerebrospinal fluid in central nervous system infections. In: Gillin BG, Weingarten K, Gamache PW, Hartman B, eds. *Infections of the central nervous system*. New York: Raven, 1991, p. 861.

Scheld WM, Whitley RJ, Durak DT. Epidural abscess. In: Gillin BG, Weingarten K, Gamache PW, Hartman B, eds. *Infections of the central nervous system*. New York: Raven, 1991, p. 499.

Schoenbaum SC, Gardner P, Shillito J. Infections of cerebrospinal fluid shunts: epidemiology, clinical manifestations and therapy. *J Infect Dis* 1975;131:543.

Tunkel AR, Wispelway B, Scheld WM. Bacterial meningitis: recent advances in pathophysiology and treatment. *Ann Intern Med* 1990;112:610.

Fever of Unknown Origin

1. What are the definitions of fever and fever of unknown origin?

2. What is the pathogenesis of fever?

3. What are the general categories of disease that can cause fever, and which general categories are the most commonly encountered?

4. Which laboratory tests should routinely be performed in a patient with fever of unknown origin?

5. In most large series, what percentage of patients with fever of unknown origin have been found to evade diagnosis?

Discussion

1. *What are the definitions of fever and fever of unknown origin?*

Fever is defined as an elevation of the body temperature. The normal temperature may vary from person to person, and ranges from 97.0° to 99.2°F

(36.1° to 37.5°C) in healthy people. The temperature can also demonstrate a diurnal variation, in that it tends to be somewhat lower in the early morning. It is important to document a fever over the course of an entire day, and, to do this, patients should be instructed to keep a log of their temperature at home.

An elevated temperature can be the hallmark of infection; however, a patient with a serious infection can be hypothermic or even have a normal temperature, especially if he or she is elderly or immunosuppressed. Not all fevers are caused by infections.

Petersdorf and Beeson originally defined *fever of unknown origin* as fever that exceeds 38.3°C on several occasions, lasts at least 3 weeks, and defies diagnosis after at least 1 week of routine study in the hospital. The 1 week of routine study is thought to eliminate most short-lived fevers (e.g., viral illness, postoperative fever, and factitious fever). It has been suggested that this last criterion (hospital admission) should be modified to "1 week of intelligent and intensive investigation," which for most patients could be done on an outpatient basis. This definition does not apply to immunocompromised patients, however.

2. *What is the pathogenesis of fever?*

The body temperature is closely regulated within a certain normal range, and fever occurs when the core body temperature exceeds this range. There exists a balance between net heat production and heat loss. Heat is produced through body metabolism and muscle activity; heat is lost by means of dissipation through the skin and the lungs.

A central regulator of body temperature is the preoptic nucleus of the anterior hypothalamus. The hypothalamus controls body temperature by stimulating the autonomic nervous system to produce peripheral vasodilation and sweating. The hypothalamus can also cause heat to be conserved by bringing about cutaneous vasoconstriction. Shivering can also increase heat production.

In the setting of infection or other inflammatory states, mononuclear phagocytes produce cytokines such as IL-1 and TNF that are capable of raising the set-point of the hypothalamus. This initiates the operation of complex mechanisms that produce pyrexia. IL-1 appears to stimulate the hypothalamus through a prostaglandin mechanism, which explains why prostaglandin inhibitors such as aspirin are effective antipyretic agents.

3. *What are the general categories of disease that can cause fever, and which general categories are the most commonly encountered?*

Fevers that defy all attempts at diagnosis pose a challenge to the clinician. Because many causes of fever of unknown etiology are obscure on the initial evaluation of a patient, it is helpful to categorize the diagnostic possibilities into groups according to the likelihood of causing the fever.

There are numerous disease states associated with fever, but infections warrant special attention. Most infectious causes are obvious to the evaluating clinician once a careful history and physical examination coupled with routine diagnostic tests are completed. Certain systemic infectious diseases that are particularly associated with fever of unknown origin include tuberculosis (particularly the extrapulmonary form) and bacterial endocarditis. A complete list of infectious causes of fever of unknown origin is beyond the scope of this text; however, pyogenic bacterial, fungal, mycobacterial, viral, rickettsial, parasitic, and spirochetal infections have all been associated with prolonged fever. Localized causes of fever of unknown etiology include intraabdominal, perinephric, prostatic, and tooth abscesses, hepatobiliary infections, and pelvic infections. These sources of infection can be occult and need to be considered in a patient with a perplexing fever.

Other general categories of fever include malignancy and collagen-vascular disorders. Less common miscellaneous disorders include sarcoidosis, inflammatory bowel disorders, pulmonary emboli, thyroiditis, a retroperitoneal hematoma, granulomatous hepatitis, allergic reactions (drug fevers), and inherited diseases (familial Mediterranean fever). Factitious and fabricated fevers have also been described, but these constitute a diagnosis of exclusion. Finally, a significant minority of fevers with an undetermined cause are idiopathic.

4. *What laboratory tests should routinely be performed in a patient with fever of unknown origin?*

Almost nowhere in the practice of medicine are an in-depth history and complete physical examination as essential as in the evaluation of a patient with fever of unknown origin, and, as Petersdorf observed in 1969, it is important to remember that "at the end of the needle, the X-ray tube, and even the scalpel, is a sick patient who deserves the most thoughtful diagnostic approach of which we are capable."

The appropriate evaluation of each patient with fever of unknown origin needs to be individualized. Attention should be paid to the patient's exposure history, travel history, occupation, animal exposure, hobbies, and medications. The examination should be thorough and particular attention should focus on the lymphoid organs, skin, heart, eye grounds, and conjunctivae in a search for evidence of occult disease, such as bacterial endocarditis, malignancy, and vasculitis.

Blood cultures should be done routinely, as well as a complete blood count with a differential. Chest radiographic studies should also be obtained to rule out infection or malignancy. Various other diagnostic studies, including radiologic examinations and blood tests, are also performed as dictated by the nature of the clinical presentation. Certain serologic tests (such as a Lyme antibody test) may be indicated in the appropriate epidemiologic setting. Clearly, a random search for answers is not appropriate.

5. *In most large series, what percentage of patients with fever of unknown origin have been found to evade diagnosis?*

In the few large trials that have examined this question, between 5% and 25% of patients with fever of unknown origin have been found to elude a specific diagnosis. Table 6-1 summarizes the observations from four of the major series of patients with fever of unknown origin.

Table 6-1. Summary of Study Findings in Patients with Fever of Unknown Origin[a]

Cause	Jacoby and Swartz, 1973 (n = 128)	Larson et al., 1982 (n = 105)	Knockaert et al., 1992 (n = 199)
Infection	40	30	23
Neoplasms	20	31	7
Collagen-vascular disease	15	9	19
Miscellaneous[b]	17–20	17	25
Undiagnosed	5–8	12	26
No. of patients	128	105	199

[a]Numbers are percentages.
[b]Includes all diagnoses not fitting into other categories (e.g., sarcoid).

Case

A 61-year-old white man is seen because of a fever. He was well until 2 months before, when he noted the onset of fatigue, fever, chills, and weight loss. Temperatures as high as 40°C have occurred in a cyclic fashion (every 2 to 3 days), but resolve with acetaminophen. He denies headaches, arthralgias, visual disturbances, abdominal pain, and diarrhea. His medical history is remarkable for asthma, environmental allergies for which he is undergoing immunotherapy, and a hiatal hernia. His family history is unremarkable. The patient does not consume alcohol or smoke cigarettes. He is a retired fireman and has not traveled or had exposure to ill contacts. He has no pets or other animal exposures. There are none of the usually recognized risk factors for HIV infection. He is taking no medications.

At physical examination, the patient is found to be a tired-appearing, elderly man. His blood pressure is 146/85 mm Hg; pulse, 106 beats per minute; respirations, 20 per minute; and temperature, 38.3°C. The head, eyes, ears, nose, and throat examination is remarkable for the finding of dry mucous membranes; his oropharynx is clear and the tympanic membranes are normal. There is no lymphadenopathy except for a small, 1.5 × 2–cm, nontender lymph node in the right inguinal area. The heart sounds are unremarkable except for a regular tachycardia. The lungs are clear to auscultation and percussion. Abdominal examination reveals normal bowel sounds, and no hepatosplenomegaly or masses are palpated. Prostate and rectal findings are normal and a test for occult blood is negative. His skin appears jaundiced. The neurologic findings are normal.

A chest radiograph is normal. A CT scan of the abdomen reveals enlarged portacaval lymph nodes. The serum electrolyte values are normal, and the following laboratory data are reported: white blood cell count, 4,000/μL; hemoglobin, 11.4 g/dL; and platelet count, 134,000/mm^3. The differential count reveals 33% segmented neutrophils, 6% band forms, 18% lymphocytes, 4% reactive lymphocytes, 20% mononuclear cells, and 15% eosinophils. The albumin content is 3.1 mg/dL; total bilirubin, 2.8 mg/dL; alanine aminotransferase, 31 IU/L; AST, 35 IU/L; alkaline phosphatase, 242 IU/L; and lactate dehydrogenase, 567 IU/L. All blood cultures are negative. The erythrocyte sedimentation rate is 50 mm per hour. A purified protein derivative of *M. tuberculosis* (PPD) skin test is negative, as is the serum antinuclear antibody test.

A bone marrow biopsy specimen shows mild chronic inflammation and extensive granulomatosis. The granulomatous foci are composed of eosinophils, small lymphocytes with irregular nuclei, and histiocytes. Routine bacterial, acid-fast bacilli, and fungal cultures and stains are negative. A test for urinary *Histoplasma* antigen is negative. A needle biopsy specimen of the liver reveals sinusoidal dilatation, triaditis, bile stasis, and focal periportal fibrosis with granulomas and dilatation of the portal venous channels.

The patient is begun empirically on a regimen of isoniazid, ethambutol, and rifampin for a presumptive diagnosis of extrapulmonary tuberculosis, but there is little attendant improvement in his clinical status.

1. What is the most likely diagnosis in this patient?
2. What diagnostic test should be performed next?
3. What disorders could be causing the granulomas and fever in this patient?

Case Discussion

1. *What is the most likely diagnosis in this patient?*

The most likely cause of this patient's illness is lymphoma. *M. tuberculosis* is one of the most common organisms to be cultured from patients with fever of unknown origin and, therefore, it is important to rule it out, especially considering that the number of cases of *M. tuberculosis* infection have been increasing in the United States since the mid-1980s. However, the diagnosis may be delayed because it can take cultures 4 to 6 weeks to become positive, although smears of sputum or other appropriate clinical specimens may be positive when stained with acid-fast stain. Occasionally, the PPD skin test is negative, especially in patients with disseminated disease. This emphasizes the importance of using control skin tests in addition to the PPD test. This patient reported no exposure to tuberculosis, and his condition did not improve on antituberculous medications, making this disease less likely.

Certain bacterial infections are prone to disseminate and infect the reticuloendothelial system, including *Brucella* and *Listeria* species. Although *Brucella* infections can be associated with lymphadenopathy and fever, this patient had had no contact with large animals or occupational exposures that would place him at risk for brucellosis. In addition, assuming the laboratory is alerted to this possibility, bone marrow cultures can be positive in a large percentage of patients with *Brucella*.

Collagen-vascular disorders and vasculitis are other causes of fever of unknown origin. Among them are diseases such as polymyalgia rheumatica, systemic lupus erythematosus, mixed connective tissue disorders, and juvenile rheumatoid arthritis. The lack of appropriate symptoms in this patient suggesting a collagen-vascular disorder, and a negative antinuclear antibody test, make this category of disease less likely.

Giant cell arteritis deserves special mention because 15% of patients with this disease can present with fever. Often, the sedimentation rate in these patients exceeds 100 mm per hour. The lack of visual disturbances, temporal artery tenderness, or jaw claudication does not completely rule out this diagnosis, and occasionally a temporal artery biopsy is indicated to elucidate the situation. In one large series, giant cell arteritis was found to be the most common cause of fever of unknown origin in patients older than 50 years of age.

Numerous malignancies have been associated with fever. Neoplasms of the reticuloendothelial system are the most common class of tumors causing fever. Fever in a patient of this age who exhibits both weight loss and adenopathy suggests a malignancy. A cyclic pattern of fevers, such as that demonstrated by this patient, suggests but does not clinch a diagnosis of Hodgkin's disease.

Patients with lymphoma can present with recurrent fever that remains obscure. Other malignancies associated with fever include non-Hodgkin's lymphoma, renal cell carcinoma, and atrial myxomas.

2. *What diagnostic test should be performed next?*

The physician should always proceed in a logical and stepwise manner in the evaluation of a patient such as this one. The workup should start with a detailed history and physical examination, followed by directed laboratory evaluations and not a random searching for an answer. This patient underwent a very extensive workup, including routine blood tests, radiologic evaluations, and cultures, that did not yield a diagnosis. The next most logical step would then be to perform an excisional lymph node biopsy. It is important to try to obtain the entire lymph node, for the purposes of both histologic examination and the performance of special stains and cultures. Occasionally, fine-needle aspiration of a lymph node can be a rapid and reliable method for diagnosis, but the amount of material obtained may not be adequate for complete histologic confirmation of lymphoma. If no peripheral lymph nodes are amenable to biopsy, a laparotomy with sampling of intraabdominal nodes may be needed.

A laparotomy is a relatively invasive procedure. CT scans, magnetic resonance imaging, and sonography are noninvasive and the findings yielded can be extremely helpful in the diagnosis of fevers of unknown origin. However, if a CT scan or ultrasound study detects an intraabdominal abnormality that cannot be cultured or sampled for biopsy percutaneously, laparotomy may be essential to obtain adequate material for histologic studies and culture.

In terms of infectious diseases, certain serologic tests can be invaluable in the evaluation of a patient with a fever of undetermined etiology. Rising antibody titers can be diagnostic for certain infectious diseases, but often acute and convalescent titers need to be determined as a pair to confirm the existence of an acute infection. There are specific serologic tests for many infectious diseases, including those caused by *Brucella, Francisella tularensis*, and *Coxiella burnetii*, but results would unlikely be positive in this setting unless there is an exposure history for these organisms.

Infection with HIV must be sought, especially if the accepted epidemiologic risk factors exist (e.g., homosexual exposures, intravenous drug abuse, and blood product transfusion before the widespread screening for HIV).

3. *What disorders could be causing the granulomas and fever in this patient?*

Granulomas in the liver and bone marrow are nonspecific findings. Because these organs are rich in reticuloendothelial cells, they can respond to antigens and form granulomas. Granulomas are known to be associated with a number of febrile diseases such as infections. Among the infectious causes of granuloma are tuberculosis, fungal infections (e.g., histoplasmosis), brucellosis, Q fever, tularemia, schistosomiasis, syphilis, and Whipple's disease.

Among the noninfectious causes of granuloma, sarcoidosis is the most common. Hepatic granulomas can also be found in the setting of connective tissue diseases, hypersensitivity reactions, primary liver diseases, and malignancy. Of the malignancies, hepatic granulomas can be seen with lymphomas. Finally, in nearly a third of the patients with hepatic granulomas, the cause cannot be ascertained, and these cases are deemed idiopathic.

Suggested Readings

Jacoby GA, Swartz MN. Fever of undetermined origin. *N Engl J Med* 1973;289:1407.

Larson EB, Feathersone HJ, Petersdorf RG. Fever of undetermined origin: diagnosis and follow-up of 105 cases, 1970–1980. *Medicine (Baltimore)* 1982;61:269.

Petersdorf RG. Fever of unknown origin. *Ann Intern Med* 1969;70:864.

Petersdorf RG. Fever of unknown origin: an old friend revisited. *Arch Intern Med* 1992;152:21.

Petersdorf RG. Fever of unexplained origin: report on 100 cases. *Medicine (Baltimore)* 1961;40:1

Pneumonia

1. What symptoms and physical, laboratory, and radiographic findings are commonly observed in patients with community-acquired pneumonia?

2. What are the common causes of community-acquired pneumonia?

3. What is the role of the spleen in combating bacterial infections?

Pneumonia

1. *What symptoms and physical, laboratory, and radiographic findings are commonly observed in patients with community-acquired pneumonia?*

The clinical findings in patients with community-acquired pneumonia are diverse, but can often be helpful in formulating a differential diagnosis. In the setting of bacterial pneumonia, the symptoms are often acute in onset. There are frequently shaking rigors, high fever, and cough productive of purulent sputum. On physical examination, the patient may appear ill, and often signs of lobar consolidation are found on chest examination. A complete blood count may reveal a brisk leukocytosis with a left shift, and a chest radiographic study may show segmental or lobar infiltrates.

Atypical pneumonia (e.g., due to viruses or to *Rickettsia*, *Chlamydia*, or *Mycoplasma* organisms) may also be acute in onset, but the cough is usually dry and nonproductive and rigors are absent. Chest examination may reveal fine diffuse rales, or findings may be normal. Skin examination may reveal a rash. A complete blood count may show a mild leukocytosis, or results may be normal. A chest radiographic study typically shows the presence of diffuse infiltrates throughout both lungs.

Pneumonia due to anaerobic organisms (e.g., aspiration pneumonia) is usually insidious in onset and the fever may be low grade. The cough may be productive of foul-smelling sputum. The patient's dentition may be poor and he or she may have foul-smelling breath. Chest examination may reveal consolidation in the lower lung fields. A mild leukocytosis and lower lobe infiltrates (particularly in the right lower lobe) may be seen on chest radiographic films.

Pulmonary tuberculosis is also insidious in onset. The fever may be accompanied by drenching night sweats, and cough is usually productive. Chest auscultation may reveal signs of upper lobe or apical consolidation. The complete blood count is often normal and chest radiographic studies may show upper lobe infiltrates, often with cavitation. Calcified hilar lymph nodes, which are a residual effect from the primary tuberculous infection, are often observed.

2. *What are the common causes of community-acquired pneumonia?*

The differential diagnosis of community-acquired pneumonia is broad, but can be narrowed considerably by the findings obtained from a careful history and physical examination, sputum Gram's staining, and chest radiographic evaluation. Bacterial pneumonia can be caused by *S. pneumoniae, H. influenzae, S. aureus, Branhamella catarrhalis*, and *Legionella pneumophila*. Uncommon causes of bacterial pneumonia include *Yersinia pestis* (plague), *F. tularensis* (tularemia), and *Bacillus anthracis* (anthrax). Atypical pneumonias are commonly due to *Mycoplasma* species or respiratory viruses. Less common causes of atypical pneumonia include *Chlamydia* species (psittacosis), *C. burnetii* (Q fever), *H. capsulatum, C. immitis*, and *M. tuberculosis*. Anaerobic or cavitary pneumonia is most commonly caused by oral anaerobes or by *M. tuberculosis*. Less common causes include *Mycobacterium kansasii, H. capsulatum, C. immitis*, and *Blastomyces dermatitidis*.

The initial assessment of patients with pneumonia should include obtaining a careful occupational and social history to determine whether there has been exposure to water-cooling facilities (*L. pneumophila*), wild animals (tularemia or plague), birds (psittacosis), or farm animals (anthrax or Q fever), and whether there has been a recent loss of consciousness (aspiration pneumonia) or exposure to people with tuberculosis. Likewise, the travel history is also important in narrowing the differential diagnosis. Recent travel to the southwestern deserts of the United States would suggest coccidioidomycosis; exposure to bird droppings or bat guano in the Midwest would suggest histoplasmosis.

3. *What is the role of the spleen in combating bacterial infections?*

The spleen is part of the reticuloendothelial system and is important in clearing certain bacterial pathogens from the bloodstream. Asplenic people are susceptible to sepsis stemming from encapsulated bacteria (pneumococci, *H. influenzae*, and *N. meningitidis*). Asplenic people should therefore be vaccinated against these infections, preferably before splenectomy if done electively, because the spleen is also important in the development of an antibody response to these vaccines.

Case
A 64-year-old woman from Topeka, Kansas, presents with an 8-hour history of fever, rigors, and a cough productive of blood-tinged sputum. She has been in good health all of her life except for abdominal trauma that necessitated a splenectomy 30 years ago. As you are examining her, she experiences shaking rigors and her fever is found to be 39°C; she also complains of a pleuritic pain over the right posterior chest. Physical examination reveals an ill-appearing woman with a persistent cough productive of purulent sputum. There is dullness to percussion, egophony, and moist rales in the right posterior chest. Her white blood cell count is 15,000/mm³ and a chest radiographic study shows a dense consolidation in the right lower lobe with air bronchograms. Gram's staining of a sputum sample reveals numerous neutrophils and abundant intracellular gram-positive diplococci.

1. What is the most likely diagnosis in this patient?
2. What does the differential diagnosis of pneumonia consist of in this patient?
3. Based on the sputum findings, what is the most likely cause of this patient's condition?
4. What would be the most appropriate treatment for this patient?

Case Discussion

1. *What is the most likely diagnosis in this patient?*

   The rapid onset of symptoms and purulent sputum are findings most suggestive of acute bacterial pneumonia. This diagnosis is further indicated by the lobar consolidation depicted on the chest radiographic study. Although a pulmonary embolism can cause the sudden onset of pleuritic chest pain, hemoptysis, and fever, it would be unusual for rigors and purulent sputum to occur in this setting. Tuberculosis would usually assume a more subacute presentation. Bronchogenic carcinoma can present with bronchial obstruction and a postobstructive pneumonia, although a hilar or perihilar mass would likely be found on chest radiographic studies. This patient's presentation would be unusual for atypical pneumonias, such as those caused by viruses or *Mycoplasma* or *Chlamydia* species.

2. *What does the differential diagnosis of pneumonia consist of in this patient?*

   This patient's signs and symptoms are most consistent with those of acute community-acquired bacterial pneumonia. The most common cause of community-acquired bacterial pneumonia is *S. pneumoniae* (pneumococcus). Other potential causes include *H. influenzae*, anaerobes (aspiration pneumonia), and *L. pneumophila* (usually spread by contaminated aerosols generated by air-conditioning systems, humidifiers, and bath showers). The diagnosis of bacterial pneumonia can usually be easily and rapidly made through the examination of a Gram's-stained specimen of expectorated sputum. This simple and inexpensive test would also be a key to determining the most appropriate therapy for this patient. The lack of dominant bacteria on the Gram's-stained sputum sample suggests the possibility of less common causes of acute lobar pneumonia such as *L. pneumophila*, tuberculosis, or fungi (coccidioidomycosis or histoplasmosis). The diagnosis of pneumonia due to *L. pneumophila* is usually made on the basis of sputum culture findings or on those yielded by a direct fluorescent antibody stain of the sputum. Likewise, if pulmonary tuberculosis is suspected, sputum acid-fast staining should be performed. A tuberculin skin test can screen for previous exposure to tuberculosis, but is of little value in the evaluation of active pulmonary infection. Fungal pneumonias should be suspected if the patient has been exposed to bird or bat feces, has been involved in spelunking (histoplasmosis), or has traveled to Sonoran desert areas in the southwestern United States (coccidioidomycosis).

3. *Based on the sputum findings, what is the most likely cause of this patient's condition?*

The presentation and Gram's stain findings are indicative of pneumonia due to *S. pneumoniae* (pneumococcus), the most common cause of bacterial pneumonia in adults. The elderly, debilitated, and immunosuppressed are especially prone to pneumococcal pneumonia. The splenectomy in this patient also predisposes her to sepsis caused by encapsulated bacteria such as *S. pneumoniae*, *H. influenzae*, and *N. meningitidis*.

4. *What would be the most appropriate treatment for this patient?*

Most *S. pneumoniae* strains in the United States are susceptible to penicillin, although in South Africa, Spain, and Eastern Europe, a high level of penicillin resistance in *S. pneumoniae* has been reported. The sensitivity of these highly resistant strains is also reduced to cephalosporins and erythromycin, and they are treated with vancomycin. Given the risk of overwhelming sepsis, it is imperative that appropriate antibiotic therapy be instituted as quickly as possible in splenectomized patients with suspected pneumococcal pneumonia. Corticosteroids have no role in the treatment of uncomplicated pneumococcal pneumonia. A pneumococcal vaccine is administered to prevent pneumococcal infection in high-risk patients (e.g., asplenic people or those with a chronic pulmonary disease or underlying immunodeficiency), but has no role in the management of acute pneumococcal pneumonia. Pneumococcal vaccination is also recommended for all people older than 65 years of age, and some physicians advocate vaccination for all people older than 55 years of age.

Suggested Readings

Bisno AL, Freeman JC. The syndrome of asplenia, pneumococcal sepsis, and disseminated intravascular coagulation. *Ann Intern Med* 1970;72:389.

Broome CV, Breiman RF. Pneumococcal vaccine: past, present and future. *N Engl J Med* 1991;325:1506.

Jacobs MR, Koornhof HJ, Robins-Browne RM, et al. Emergence of multiply resistant pneumococci. *N Engl J Med* 1978;299:735.

Jacoby GA, Archer GL. New mechanisms of bacterial resistance to antimicrobial agents. *N Engl J Med* 1991;324:601.

Marton A, Gulyas A, Munoz R, Tomaz A. Extremely high incidence of antibiotic resistance in clinical isolates of *Streptococcus pneumoniae* in Hungary. *J Infect Dis* 1991;163:542.

Ward J. Antibiotic-resistant *Streptococcus pneumoniae*: clinical and epidemiologic aspects. *Rev Infect Dis* 1981;3:254.

7 Hematology and Oncology

Paul Seligman

Acute Leukemia

1. What is the pathology of acute leukemia?
2. What are the primary classifications of acute leukemia, and why is this differentiation important?
3. What is the French, American, and British (FAB) classification of acute leukemia?
4. Are there any predisposing factors associated with acute leukemia?
5. What workup and other preparation should be done before initiating antileukemic therapy?
6. What are induction, consolidation, maintenance chemotherapy, and meningeal prophylactic therapy, and how do they differ in the treatment of acute lymphocytic leukemia and acute nonlymphocytic leukemia?
7. What are the risks associated with antileukemic therapy, and what results can be expected?

Discussion

1. *What is the pathology of acute leukemia?*

Acute leukemia is the abnormal clonal expansion of blood cell precursors. The abnormality may occur at different stages of maturation of the cell, and this explains the different types of leukemia. Acute leukemia is usually a rapidly progressive disease, although there are occasional patients whose disease remains stable for weeks or even months. In general, however, it is not the leukemic cells per se that cause the morbidity and mortality in this disorder, but a lack of normal blood cells, resulting in anemia, thrombocytopenia, and leukopenia. This is brought about by the leukemic cells "crowding out" the normal cells in the bone marrow. Other data suggest that leukemic cells may have an inhibitory effect on normal marrow cells. This lack of normal cells may thus lead to life-threatening hemorrhage and infection.

2. *What are the primary classifications of acute leukemia, and why is this differentiation important?*

The primary classifications of acute leukemia are acute lymphocytic leukemia (ALL) and acute nonlymphocytic leukemia (ANLL). The distinction is important because the therapy differs for each type (see answer to Question 6). The overall ratio of ALL to ANLL is 1:6. ALL occurs most commonly in children, whereas ANLL more commonly affects adults.

Table 7-1 lists the cytologic features of acute leukemia.

3. *What is the FAB classification of acute leukemia?*

The FAB classification (Table 7-2) is based largely on the morphologic and histochemical characteristics displayed by the leukemic cells, as well as the nature of the cell surface antigens and cytogenetic features. This information may lead to changes in patient management, either by directing the course of therapy or by defining the prognosis better.

4. *Are there any predisposing factors associated with acute leukemia?*

Certain genetic and environmental factors may predispose a person to acute leukemia. Many chromosomal alterations exist in the setting of the leukemias. The incidence of leukemia is increased in patients with congenital disorders associated with aneuploidy, such as Down's syndrome, congenital agranulocytosis, celiac disease, Fanconi's syndrome, and von Recklinghausen's neurofibromatosis.

Environmental factors implicated in the development of acute leukemia, particularly ANLL, include exposure to ionizing radiation and chemicals.

Table 7-1. The Cytologic Features of Acute Leukemia

Cytologic feature	ANLL	ALL
Auer rods	Occasionally positive	Negative
Peroxidase stain	Often positive	Negative
Sudan black stain	Often positive	Negative
Esterase stain	Often positive	Negative
Periodic-acid Schiff	Usually negative	Usually positive
Immunologic features of lymphocytes (cALLa, T- or B-cell features)	Negative	Positive
Terminal deoxynucleotidyl transferase	Rarely positive	Positive

ANLL, acute nonlymphocytic anemia; ALL, acute lymphocytic anemia; cALLa, common acute lymphocytic leukemia antigen.

Table 7-2. The French, American, and British Classification of Acute Leukemia

FAB classification	Description	Comment
ALL		
L1	Small blasts with little cytoplasm, little cell-to-cell variation	Most common morphology in childhood ALL
L2	Larger cells with greater amount of cytoplasm, greater cell-to-cell variation; irregular nuclei with multiple nucleoli	Most common morphology in adult ALL
L3	Large cells, strongly basophilic cytoplasm; often with vacuoles; nucleoli often multiple	Common in leukemia associated with Burkitt's lymphoma
ANLL		
M1	Acute myelocytic leukemia; cells very undifferentiated with only occasional granules	—
M2	Acute myelocytic leukemia; cells more differentiated with granules, and often with Auer rods	—
M3	Acute promyelocytic leukemia; hypergranular promyelocytes	Often associated with disseminated intravascular coagulation, responds to differentiation agents
M4	Acute myelomonocytic leukemia; both monocytes and myelocytes predominate	Often occurs with extramedullary infiltration (gingival hypertrophy, leukemia cutis, and meningeal leukemia)
M5	Acute monocytic leukemia: monoblasts with relatively agranular cytoplasm	Usually affects children or young adults
M6	Erythroleukemia: red blood cell precursors predominate, but myeloid blasts may also be seen	Also called Di Guglielmo syndrome
M7	Megakaryocytic leukemia: extremely variable morphology; may be diagnosed with monoclonal antibodies to platelets	Rare form of leukemia; very poor prognosis

FAB, French, American, and British; ALL, acute lymphocytic leukemia; ANLL, acute nonlymphocytic leukemia.

Occupations and therapy that involve radiation exposure are known to increase the risk for acquiring acute leukemia. Chemicals, particularly the industrial use of benzene, and several therapeutic drugs (chloramphenicol, phenylbutazone, melphalan, chlorambucil, and others) are causal factors in acute leukemia. The findings from animal studies link certain viruses with acute leukemia; however, it is uncertain whether viruses are actually an etiologic factor in human forms of leukemia, except for lymphomas caused by viruses that develop into a form of ALL.

5. *What workup and other preparation should be done before initiating antileukemic therapy?*

The pretreatment evaluation should include the patient's medical and work history, especially the nature of any radiation or chemical exposure. A physical examination should include the patient's temperature, plus examination of the optic fundi, lymph node areas, oropharynx and gingivae, perianal area, and cranial nerves. Laboratory studies should consist of a complete blood count with differential (the physician should examine the smear), as well as a blood chemistry profile that includes the measurement of uric acid, lactate dehydrogenase (LDH), and muramidase (lysozyme). Bone marrow aspirates and biopsy specimens should be obtained, and investigations should include cytogenetic studies. A transfusion workup should include human lymphocyte antigen (HLA) typing. Lumbar puncture should be performed in all patients suspected of having ALL or ANLL-M4, and the cerebrospinal fluid specimen should be subjected to the usual studies, plus cytologic analysis. A dental examination should be performed.

In addition, the patient's condition should be stabilized before antileukemic therapy is initiated. Hemorrhage and infection should be brought under control. The greatly elevated leukocyte counts (e.g., >50,000/mm^3) that occur in the setting of ANLL can lead to pulmonary complications as well as fatal intracerebral leukostasis and hemorrhage. Cranial irradiation, hydroxyurea, and leukapheresis have all been used to decrease rapidly the numbers of circulating leukemic cells, and hence the risk of complications. (Because of the physical properties of the lymphocytic leukemic cell, this is rarely a problem in patients with ALL.)

Renal damage stemming from urate nephropathy may exist at the time of presentation or may occur with therapy, thus urine alkalinization may prevent the need for dialysis. Patients should receive allopurinol (300 to 600 mg) for at least 24 hours before therapy to reduce the uric acid load, and this treatment should be continued until leukopenia and bone marrow hypocellularity has been achieved.

6. *What are induction, consolidation, maintenance chemotherapy, and meningeal prophylactic therapy, and how do they differ in the treatment of ALL and ANLL?*

These are the phases of therapy used for acute leukemia. Induction therapy is usually the initial therapy and is intended to accomplish complete remission (i.e., no signs or symptoms of disease, normal blood counts, and no evidence of leukemia in the bone marrow). This therapy is usually administered on an inpatient basis, and is very toxic. Consolidation therapy is given after complete remission is achieved. It is similarly toxic, and consists of either the same drugs as those used in induction therapy or different ones. Its object is to reduce the now clinically undetectable leukemic cell mass as much as possible. Maintenance therapy is usually given on an outpatient basis and is less toxic, although complications of therapy can and do arise. This phase usually lasts for 2 to 3 years. Meningeal prophylactic therapy is given by means of lumbar puncture or through a reservoir placed under the scalp that cannulates the third ventricle. Its goal is to reduce the recurrence rate of leukemia in the central nervous system (CNS), which is considered a sanctuary site.

All four therapy phases are used in ALL. In the treatment of ANLL, there is controversy over the use of maintenance therapy, although a second consolidation phase may be used. Meningeal prophylaxis is not used in the treatment of adult ANLL. However, CNS leukemia is more common in childhood ANLL, and prophylaxis is sometimes used in this setting. In general, the response to treatment and the prognosis are better in patients with ALL than in those with ANLL.

7. *What are the risks associated with antileukemic therapy, and what results can be expected?*

As already noted, acute leukemia is usually a rapidly progressive disease that is fatal without therapy. Because the therapy itself is toxic, the mortality rate during induction therapy for ANLL may reach as high as 20%. Some toxicities are specific to the drug used, and these are not discussed here. Nearly all therapies provoke nausea and vomiting, which can be controlled with medications. More significantly, antileukemic therapy is intended to deplete the bone marrow, with subsequent repopulation by normal cells. During this period of depletion, the patient becomes severely thrombocytopenic and must be supported by platelet transfusions (given prophylactically at various intervals to keep the platelet count above 10,000) and usually also by red blood cell transfusions.

Patients also become severely leukopenic, and this makes them very susceptible to infection. The typical signs and symptoms of infection (pus and purulent sputum) are often due to the actions of granulocytes, so infection is often subtle. The oral mucosa and perirectal areas are commonly overlooked sites of infection. Fever in a neutropenic patient must be considered infectious in origin until proved otherwise. When this happens, examination and cultures should be carried out and broad-spectrum antibiotic therapy quickly started. Antifungal agents usually are added if no improvement is seen after 4 to 7 days of fever. The patient must be carefully monitored and treated for herpes virus infection because disseminated infection can be rapidly fatal.

If the leukemic cell burden is great, antileukemic therapy may precipitate the tumor lysis syndrome, caused by the rapid release of cell degradation products. It is characterized by hyperuricemia (causing urate nephropathy), hyperkalemia, hyperphosphatemia, and hypocalcemia. Advance recognition of patients at risk and subsequent treatment with vigorous hydration, allopurinol, and urine alkalinization 24 to 48 hours before the start of chemotherapy can usually prevent the syndrome. These patients must have their electrolyte, uric acid, phosphorus, calcium, and creatinine status repeatedly checked. Any metabolic abnormalities should be corrected and, if necessary, renal dialysis instituted early. Once the leukemic cell burden is decreased and degradation products cleared, the syndrome resolves.

Most children with ALL respond to therapy and achieve long-term survival. Although 90% of adults with ALL experience complete remission with initial therapy, the median remission duration ranges from 24 to 48 months, depending on the study. Median survival is 3 to 5 years. However, approximately one third of all patients achieve long-term disease-free survival. Late recurrences are rare.

Patients with ANLL face a worse prognosis. Approximately 75% experience complete remission, but most cases recur within 36 months. Of those who achieve complete remission, 20% to 25% show long-term disease-free survival. Bone marrow or stem cell transplantation with high-dose chemotherapy is often used but still under investigation as a therapy after the initial chemotherapy in both diseases. The timing of transplantation (first remission, first relapse, or second remission), especially in ALL, is controversial.

Case

A 63-year-old white man is seen in the emergency room with complaints of fever, fatigue, and malaise. He reports having intermittent epistaxis during the past week, mouth sores for the past 3 days, and a nonpruritic rash over his lower extremities, which was noted 24 hours before. He has experienced midchest pain for the past day on swallowing only. He denies chemical, drug, or radiation exposure.

Physical examination reveals a temperature of 38.6°C. He has mild tachycardia, at 108 beats per minute. Head, eyes, ears, nose, and throat findings consist of a few petechiae over the soft palate. Multiple white plaques are seen on the oral mucosa, and there is hypertrophy of the gingivae. During examination of the skin, petechiae are found over the distal lower extremities. Other examination findings are normal. Specifically, no lymphadenopathy or hepatosplenomegaly are found. Other sites of possible infection, including the chest and perirectal area, are clear. The chest radiographic study is likewise normal.

Laboratory findings are as follows: white blood cell count, 17,200/mm^3 with 2% polymorphonuclear leukocytes, 1% band forms, 16% lymphocytes, 4% monocytes, 5% metamyelocytes, 4% basophils, and 68% blastocytes; hemoglobin, 11.1 g/dL; hematocrit, 32.6%; and platelets, 14,000/mm^3. His electrolyte, blood urea nitrogen (BUN), creatinine, and aminotransferase levels are normal. His uric acid level is mildly increased at 9.2 mg/dL (normal, 3.5 to 8.0 mg/dL), as are his LDH level at 373 IU/L (normal, 30 to 220 IU/L) and muramidase level at 24.3 mg/L (normal, 3 to 12.8 mg/L). Examination of a peripheral blood smear reveals occasional nucleated red blood cells, few platelets, and many large cells containing finely reticulated nuclei, several nucleoli, cytoplasmic granules, and occasional Auer rods. Large cells with folded nuclei and large, prominent nucleoli are also seen.

1. What is the most likely diagnosis in this patient?
2. How is the absolute neutrophil count (ANC) calculated, and what is it in this patient?
3. Of what importance is the ANC?
4. Do the evaluation findings point to any specific infections?
5. What would you expect this patient's bone marrow to show?
6. Should a lumbar puncture be performed in this patient?

Case Discussion

1. *What is the most likely diagnosis in this patient?*

    Considering the results of this patient's complete blood count and peripheral blood smear, he has ANLL. The granular myelocytes and monocytes in the smear and the clinical evidence of extramedullary leukemic infiltration (gingival hypertrophy) point to a diagnosis of M4, or acute myelomonocytic leukemia. Examination of bone marrow specimens using special stains can help confirm this diagnosis.

2. *How is the ANC calculated, and what is it in this patient?*

    To calculate the ANC, multiply the total white blood cell count by the percentage of polymorphonuclear leukocytes plus the percentage of band forms. In this case, the patient has 17,200 white blood cells, with 2% polymorphonuclear leukocytes and 1% band forms, or: 17,200 (0.02 + 0.01) = 516 absolute neutrophils.

3. *Of what importance is the ANC?*

    The ANC furnishes a rough estimate of the patient's ability to fight infection. A patient with an ANC of less than 500 is considered neutropenic and very susceptible to overwhelming infection. This patient, with an ANC of approximately 500, fever, and a presumed diagnosis of acute leukemia, falls into this category. Careful examination, together with cultures of blood, sputum, oral lesions, and other possible sites of infection, should be done quickly, and the patient started immediately on broad-spectrum antibiotics. Any delay in the workup or institution of antibiotics may result in overwhelming and possibly fatal infection. Cultures are often negative in neutropenic patients, even though clinically they appear to be septic and respond to antibiotics.

4. *Do the evaluation findings point to any specific infections?*

    This patient complains of midchest pain on swallowing and physical examination reveals white oral plaques. A presumptive diagnosis of *Candida* esophagitis can be made on the basis of these findings, and the patient should be started on antifungal agents as well as broad-spectrum antibacterial antibiotics. Neutropenic patients are susceptible to opportunistic infections, and candidiasis is very common in them.

5. *What would you expect this patient's bone marrow to show?*

    The bone marrow in this patient with ANLL would likely exhibit hypercellularity, with cellular elements often constituting 90% or more of the marrow. The numbers of red blood cell precursors and megakaryocytes will be decreased. The morphology may be normal, or there may be dyserythropoiesis (asynchronous maturing of the nuclear and cytoplasmic elements). The marrow will primarily show a monotonous pattern of cells similar to those seen in the peripheral smear. Flow cytometry should show cell surface markers indicative of immature myeloid cells with monocytoid characteristics.

6. *Should a lumbar puncture be performed in this patient?*

    This patient has a presumptive diagnosis of acute myelomonocytic leukemia. Lumbar punctures are routinely done in cases of ALL and ANLL-M4 because these leukemias are associated with meningitis. Nevertheless, any patient with acute leukemia and symptoms of meningitis or cranial nerve palsies should undergo a diagnostic lumbar puncture, regardless of the leukemic type.

However, the platelet count in this patient is only 14,000/mm³, and lumbar punctures should not be performed when the platelet count is less than 50,000/mm³ because of the risk of hemorrhage. Therefore, platelet transfusions must be given before attempting lumbar puncture to bring the count to 50,000/mm³ or more.

Suggested Readings

Baccarani M, Carbelli G, Amadori S, et al. Adolescent and adult acute lymphoblastic leukemia: prognostic features and outcome of therapy—a study of 293 patients. *Blood* 1982;60:677.

Bennett JM, Young ML, Anderson JW, et al. Long-term survival in acute myeloid leukemia. *Cancer* 1997;8:2205.

Burnett A, Goldstone AH, Stevens RMF, Hann IM, Rees JKH, Gray RG. Randomized comparison of addition of autologous bone-marrow transplantation to intensive remission: results of MRC AML 10 trial. *Lancet* 1998;351:700.

Gale RP, Hoelzer D. *Acute lymphoblastic leukemia.* New York: Wiley-Liss, 1990.

Koeffler HP. Syndromes of acute nonlymphocytic leukemia. *Ann Intern Med* 1987;107:748.

Anemia

1. What is the definition of anemia, and what is the differential diagnosis based on the mean corpuscular volume (MCV)?
2. Why is it important to examine the peripheral blood smear, and what are the many diagnostic erythrocyte abnormalities and corresponding clinical conditions?
3. What is a reticulocyte, and how is the reticulocyte count used to characterize an anemia? What is the reticulocyte index, how is it calculated, and how is it used in the differential diagnosis of anemia?
4. What is the difference between α- and β-thalassemia, how are they distinguished clinically, and how is electrophoresis useful?
5. What is sickle cell anemia, and how is it manifested clinically? What is the sickle cell trait, and how is it manifested clinically?

Discussion

1. *What is the definition of anemia, and what is the differential diagnosis based on the MCV?*

Anemia is usually defined as an abnormally low hematocrit or hemoglobin concentration, and occurs when the rate of erythrocyte loss exceeds the rate of erythrocyte production. The differential diagnosis of anemia depends on whether the MCV is low, high, or normal. Table 7-3 lists the various possible diagnoses for each of these categories. Sometimes with mild anemia, a diagnosis may be entertained if the MCV is in the high or low range of normal.

Table 7-3. Differential Diagnosis of Anemia Based on Mean Corpuscular Volume

Low MCV	Normal MCV	High MCV
α-Thalassemia	Acute blood loss	Alcohol abuse
β-Thalassemia	Aplastic anemia	Aplastic anemia
Iron deficiency	Chronic disease	Cobalamin deficiency
Lead poisoning	Combination of macrocytic	Folate deficiency
Sideroblastic anemia	and microcytic causes	Hemolysis
	Hemoglobinopathy	Hypothyroidism
	Hemolysis	Liver disease
	Iron deficiency	Myelodysplastic syndromes

MCV, mean corpuscular volume.

2. *Why is it important to examine the peripheral blood smear, and what are the many diagnostic erythrocyte abnormalities and corresponding clinical conditions?*

Peripheral blood smear examination can reveal erythrocyte abnormalities that point to the correct diagnosis of the anemia. Echinocytes, or burr cells, are seen in uremia and pyruvate kinase deficiency. Elliptocytes are the abnormal erythrocytes seen in patients with hereditary elliptocytosis. Nucleated red cells are found in the setting of stress or hematologic disease with bone marrow involvement. Schistocytes or fragments occur in patients with microangiopathic hemolytic anemia. Sickle cells are found in the setting of sickle cell anemia. Spherocytes occur in immune-mediated hemolytic anemia and hereditary spherocytosis. Target cells form in the presence of liver disease and iron deficiency; they also occur after splenectomy.

3. *What is a reticulocyte, and how is the reticulocyte count used to characterize an anemia? What is the reticulocyte index, how is it calculated, and how is it used in the differential diagnosis of anemia?*

A reticulocyte is a young circulating red blood cell that exhibits basophilia under vital staining. The reticulocyte count is used to characterize the bone marrow's attempt to compensate, if at all, for the anemia present. The reticulocyte index (Table 7-4) is a more useful means of characterizing anemia because it is determined by correcting the reticulocyte count for the hematocrit, assuming a normal hematocrit is 45%. This correction is necessary because reticulocytes are counted per 1,000 red blood cells.

Table 7-4. The Reticulocyte Index

Hematocrit (%)	Correction factor
45	1.0
35	1.5
25	2.0

$$\text{Reticulocyte index} = \frac{\% \text{ Reticulocyte} \times \dfrac{\text{Observed hematocrit}}{45}}{\text{Correction factor}}$$

Correction of the reticulocyte index for shift cells: *shift cells − newly released erythrocytes.*

An index of less than 2 is found in the setting of the **hypoproliferative anemias**. These consist of disorders of heme or globin synthesis, such as iron deficiency, anemia stemming from chronic disease, lead poisoning, sideroblastic anemias, and α, β, and other thalassemias; megaloblastic anemias resulting from cobalamin or folate deficiency; myelodysplastic syndromes; aplastic anemias; and other metabolic causes, such as renal insufficiency and hypothyroidism.

Hyperproliferative anemias are associated with a reticulocyte index greater than 2. These anemias arise as the result of acute blood loss; nutrient replacement, such as cobalamin, folate, or iron replacement, but before the resolution of anemia; both hereditary and acquired hemolysis; and primary or secondary polycythemia.

Newer, automated reticulocyte counts introduced for general clinical practice may be more accurate and automatically calculate the reticulocyte index.

4. *What is the difference between α- and β-thalassemia, how are they distinguished clinically, and how is electrophoresis useful?*

The **α-thalassemias** constitute abnormalities of the gene, or genes, responsible for the synthesis of the α chain of hemoglobin. Humans contain four genes for this purpose and each is responsible for about a fourth of the α chains synthesized. Any combination of from one to four of these α genes may be missing. Thalassemia is unapparent clinically when only one gene is missing, and this is called α_1-*thalassemia*. This defect exists in up to 30% of the American black population. If two of the α genes are missing, the entity is referred to as α_2-*thalassemia*. These patients are usually asymptomatic, although their hematocrit and MCV may be slightly low. This defect affects approximately 2% of African Americans. When three of the α genes are lacking, the patient exhibits the phenotype of α-thalassemia (Hemoglobin H disease) with a low hematocrit and MCV, and β-chain tetramers or hemoglobin H is found in the red blood cells. When all four α genes are missing, the result is usually a stillborn infant with hydrops fetalis.

α-Thalassemia is the most common form of thalassemia in the population of Southeast Asia.

The **β-thalassemias** consist of abnormalities of the gene, or genes, responsible for the β chain of hemoglobin, and they cause insufficient β-chain synthesis. This leads to the formation of α-chain tetramers and inclusions of this hemoglobin attached to the plasma membranes of erythrocytes, resulting in hemolysis. Patients with heterozygous β-thalassemia exhibit a modest decrease in their hematocrit values and a marked decrease in their MCVs. Patients with homozygous β-thalassemia have severe anemia and low MCVs. They require transfusion, and complications may arise stemming from the excess accumulation of iron.

Electrophoresis may be used to suggest the diagnosis of α-thalassemia in patients missing three genes, and thus having sufficient fast-migrating hemoglobin H (α_1- and α_2-thalassemia traits may not be detected). The precise number of missing α genes can be determined in hybridization studies through the use of a complementary DNA probe.

The findings yielded by hemoglobin electrophoresis are usually diagnostic in the setting of β-thalassemia. Because α-chain synthesis is normal in these patients, the other hemoglobins seen in adults, including hemoglobin A_2 and F, are increased in a compensatory fashion. Thus, patients with heterozygous β-thalassemia would have elevated hemoglobin A_2 and F levels with hemoglobin A present. Patients with homozygous β-thalassemia would have no hemoglobin A and markedly elevated hemoglobin F and A_2 levels.

5. *What is sickle cell anemia, and how is it manifested clinically? What is the sickle cell trait, and how is it manifested clinically?*

Sickle cell disease is the most commonly recognized clinically significant hemoglobinopathy. It stems from a substitution of valine for glutamic acid in the β chain of hemoglobin and can be diagnosed by electrophoresis. Sickle cell anemia results when both β chains are abnormal. Sickled cells should be evident on a peripheral blood smear. Hemoglobin S is less soluble than normal hemoglobin at a low oxygen tension, causing the hemoglobin molecules to crystallize, which deforms the red blood cells. These misshapen cells greatly increase the blood viscosity, which leads to small-vessel occlusion and hence pain and organ infarctions, specifically stroke as well as pulmonary, renal, and bone infarction.

Sickle cell disease may be manifested by a variety of crises: **Pain** is the most common symptom, and is thought to be secondary to red blood cell sludging and infarction. **Splenic sequestration and dactylitis** are common in children, but rare in adults. **Aplastic anemia** is uncommon, but is typically associated with infections, which may be mild. **Megaloblastic anemia** is usually secondary to folate deficiency, and arises because abnormal cells have a shortened life span. This increases the turnover of red blood cells and places an increased demand on folate stores. **Hemolytic anemia** occurs rarely in patients with sickle cell anemia.

The sickle cell trait is usually asymptomatic because only one of the two β chains is abnormal. It can also be diagnosed by electrophoresis, and this is most important for the purposes of genetic counseling.

Case 1   A 42-year-old man is seen by his primary care physician because of a rectal urgency. On sigmoidoscopy, a mass is located at 8 cm. He undergoes resection to remove the mass and after surgery he receives 5-fluorouracil and undergoes pelvic radiation therapy. After he completes therapy, he returns to his primary care physician 6 months later with complaints of fatigue and dyspnea on exertion. As part of the evaluation, a complete blood count is obtained and reveals the following findings: white blood cell count, 3.9×10^9/L; hemoglobin, 8.2 g/dL; hematocrit, 24.4%; MCV, 86 femtoliters; reticulocytes, 1%; and platelets, 450,000/mm^3. The patient has a serum iron content of 23 μg/dL, a total iron-binding capacity of 256 μg/dL, and a ferritin level of 10 ng/mL.

1. What is the likely cause of this patient's anemia, and how would you evaluate him further?
2. If the patient is iron deficient, why is his MCV 86 femtoliters?
3. Based on the patient's iron status, what treatment should be prescribed, and how should therapy be monitored?

Case Discussion

1. *What is the likely cause of this patient's anemia, and how would you evaluate him further?*

The cause of this patient's anemia is likely multifactorial. However, the ferritin below 12 ng/mL and the percentage transferrin saturation (total iron-binding capacity/Fe) below 10% are both diagnostic for iron deficiency. He should receive oral iron supplementation, but he should be evaluated for a gastrointestinal source of blood loss (e.g., recurrent tumor, second primary cancer, or some other nonmalignant source).

The patient may also be anemic and leukopenic due to the extensive exposure of the bone marrow to radiation during pelvic radiation therapy. This bone marrow damage may be compounded by the concomitant 5-fluorouracil treatment.

Finally, the possibility of other contributory factors, such as folate and cobalamin deficiency, should also be investigated.

2. *If the patient is iron deficient, why is his MCV 86 femtoliters?*

The MCV may be normal in the settings of early iron deficiency, although the red cell distribution width is high under these circumstances. The MCV may also be normal in iron-deficiency anemia complicated by another nutritional deficiency, such as folate or cobalamin deficiency. In this patient, the MCV is likely higher than expected as a result of his recent 5-fluorouracil treatment.

3. *Based on the patient's iron status, what treatment should be prescribed, and how should therapy be monitored?*

The patient has iron deficiency. Ferrous sulfate (300 mg three times a day) provides 180 mg of elemental iron per day, which should normalize the hematocrit over the course of several months. The hematocrit should increase by 1% to 3% each week and his reticulocyte count should also increase significantly with this treatment.

The status of the absorption of oral iron can be easily demonstrated by determining the fasting serum iron level before and 3 to 4 hours after the ingestion of a single 300-mg tablet of ferrous sulfate. If normal, the level should rise a minimum of two times the baseline (fasting) value.

Case 2   A 67-year-old woman is seen for complaints of mild memory loss and fatigue. On evaluation, she is found to have an anemia, which is characterized by the following laboratory values: white blood cell count, 5,200/mm³; hemoglobin, 9.1 g/dL; hematocrit, 26.9%; MCV, 101 femtoliters; reticulocytes, less than 1%; and platelets, 154/mm³. Her serum cobalamin level is 260 pg/mL and her folate, thyroid-stimulating hormone, and liver function tests are normal. The patient does not abuse alcohol, and her peripheral blood smear is unrevealing.

1. How would you further evaluate this patient's anemia?
2. Based on the laboratory results so far, what test, or tests, might be helpful in diagnosing the cause of this patient's anemia?
3. Why might such a patient be deficient in cobalamin?

Case Discussion

1. *How would you further evaluate this patient's anemia?*

Serum cobalamin and folate levels should be determined. In addition, a search for both ethanol abuse and liver disease should be undertaken and hypothyroidism ruled out. If none of these is found to be a likely cause, other reasons for the anemia (refractory or aplastic anemia) should be explored. A peripheral blood smear should be examined for possible clues such as hypersegmented polymorphonuclear leukocytes (seen in cobalamin deficiency) or target cells (seen in liver disease).

2. *Based on the laboratory results so far, what test, or tests, might be helpful in diagnosing the cause of this patient's anemia?*

This patient likely has cobalamin deficiency, even though her level of 260 pg/mL is within the normal range. Because studies have shown that such deficiency results in methylmalonic aciduria and homocystinemia, these metabolic substrates should be measured in this patient. Other testing that might be considered includes a Schilling test or measurement of anti–intrinsic factor-blocking antibodies.

3. *Why might such a patient be deficient in cobalamin?*

There are various causes of cobalamin deficiency. It can stem from the ingestion of insufficient animal protein, as seen in true vegetarians. Failure to release cobalamin from food binders or failure to secrete intrinsic factor results in pernicious anemia. Failure to absorb the intrinsic factor–cobalamin complex in the distal ileum, as occurs in patients who have undergone an ileal resection or who have regional enteritis, can also lead to cobalamin deficiency. Rare causes are abnormal or absent transcobalamin II, and nitrous oxide abuse.

Suggested Readings

Beutler E, Lichtman MA, Coller BS, Kipps TJ, eds. *Hematology*, 5th ed. New York: McGraw-Hill, 1995.

Wintrobe MM, ed. *Clinical hematology*, 9th ed. Philadelphia: Lea & Febiger, 1993.

Bleeding Disorders

1. What are the major divisions of the coagulation system?
2. What are the general screening tests for evaluating each of the major divisions of the coagulation system?

3. What common disorders are associated with each of the major divisions of the coagulation system?
4. What are the clinical manifestations of various bleeding disorders?
5. What workup is indicated for a bleeding patient?
6. What therapies are available for the management of bleeding disorders?

Discussion

1. *What are the major divisions of the coagulation system?*

   The coagulation system is quite complex, but can be viewed as consisting of at least three major components: the vascular endothelium, the blood coagulation proteins (both those that promote clotting and those that lyse clots by means of the fibrinolytic system), and the platelets. The coagulation cascade represents a series of proteins that, when initiated, forms a fibrin clot. A simple outline of the cascade is shown in Fig. 7-1. Complex issues such as the exact mechanisms by which anticoagulants, such as protein C and protein S, function and how factor VII may activate factor IX are not completely understood.

2. *What are the general screening tests for evaluating each of the major divisions of the coagulation system?*

   Vascular endothelial integrity can be assessed using the bleeding time. In this test, a nick is made in the skin under standardized conditions, and the time to cessation of bleeding is measured.

   The blood coagulation proteins usually are evaluated by *in vitro* studies using the patient's citrate-anticoagulated plasma. This is done by adding back to the patient's plasma various components of the coagulation cascade to induce clot, and the procedure is standardized against plasma from a patient with normal plasma coagulation components. The two most common tests for doing this are the prothrombin time (PT) and the partial tissue thromboplastin time (PTT). The PT measures the extrinsic pathway of the coagulation cascade, and this is done by adding tissue thromboplastin to the patient's plasma. If there is a deficit in any of the common pathway components or factor VII, the clotting time is abnormally prolonged. The PTT measures the intrinsic and common pathways; a deficit in the common or intrinsic pathway proteins results in a prolonged PTT. A third, less commonly used, screening test, is the thrombin time, which measures only the last step in the cascade—the conversion of fibrinogen to fibrin—and is done by adding thrombin to the patient's plasma. Thus, if the patient has too little fibrinogen or a dysfunctional fibrinogen protein, the time is prolonged. Finally, each of the components of the cascade, including factors I to XIII, can be assayed directly to evaluate for deficits.

   Platelets can be evaluated both quantitatively (by the platelet count) and functionally. Platelet function can be assessed by the bleeding time; qualitatively defective platelets do not form an adequate platelet plug and the bleeding time is prolonged. In addition, platelets can be analyzed *in vitro* for their aggregability using platelet stimulants (e.g., ristocetin).

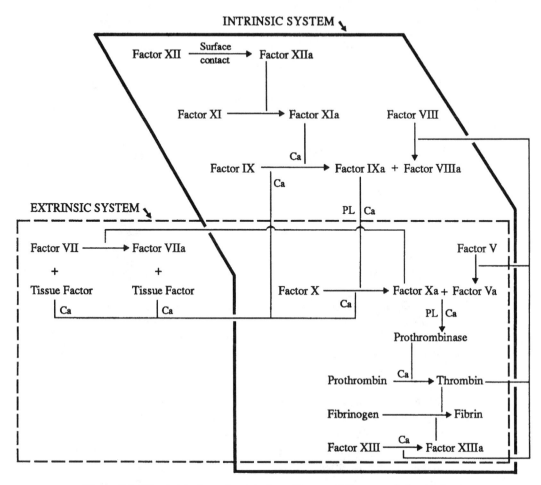

Figure 7-1. The intrinsic and extrinsic pathways of the coagulation system.

3. *What common disorders are associated with each of the major divisions of the coagulation system?*

The vascular endothelium may be fragile in the setting of several acquired conditions, including vasculitis and long-term steroid use. This is important to realize because it may cause the bleeding time to be prolonged despite normal platelet number and function.

Deficits in the blood coagulation proteins may be congenital or acquired. The most common congenital disorders consist of deficiencies in factor VIII (hemophilia A) or factor IX (hemophilia B, or Christmas disease), which are inherited in an X-linked manner. Another common congenital disorder is von Willebrand's disease, in which there is a deficit in von Willebrand's factor. This factor is bound to factor VIII and is necessary for both platelet function and for clotting to take place by the intrinsic pathway.

Deficiencies in various factors can be acquired when their production is antagonized, as occurs with Coumadin (sodium warfarin; Du Pont Pharma, Wilmington, DE) therapy, a substance that inhibits the production of activated vitamin K-dependent factors (II, VII, IX, X, and protein C and S). Another common situation that causes deficiencies in various factors is liver disease; because the liver is the site for the synthesis of nearly all the coagulation factors, severe liver disease results in deficient production of factors. Malnutrition, malabsorption, and liver disease can all lead to a deficit in vitamin K, with a subsequent deficit in the vitamin K-dependent factors. Finally, the overwhelming consumption of all factors can result in a coagulopathy, as occurs in disseminated intravascular coagulation (DIC).

The platelet population can be depressed because of either underproduction or excessive destruction. Underproduction occurs as a consequence of bone marrow suppression (brought about by chemotherapy, infections, drugs, or infiltration with other cells, such as occurs in the setting of leukemia or cancer). Excessive destruction can occur in the setting of an enlarged spleen (sequestration), bleeding (consumption) or consumptive disorders (DIC or thrombotic thrombocytopenic purpura/hemolytic uremic syndrome), and on an autoimmune basis [idiopathic thrombocytopenic purpura (ITP)].

Qualitative defects can be congenital, but more often are acquired and due to drug exposure (aspirin, nonsteroidal antiinflammatory drugs, and some antibiotics) or uremia.

4. *What are the clinical manifestations of various bleeding disorders?*

Although any of the bleeding disorders may result in excessive hemorrhage associated with such events as surgical procedures, trauma, or gastrointestinal bleeding, each displays some characteristic features. Vascular fragility is typically associated with subcutaneous ecchymoses. Plasma coagulation protein deficiencies in patients with hemophilia are associated with spontaneous soft tissue and joint bleeds. Other plasma factor deficiencies, as well as platelet deficits, are associated with diffuse ecchymoses (cutaneous and soft tissue). Platelet deficits are also manifested by petechiae (small capillary hemorrhages in mucosal surfaces and areas of increased hydrostatic pressure, such as the ankles and feet) and purpura (larger areas of hemorrhage). Von Willebrand's disease is unique in that it may present with both soft tissue bleeding (factor VII deficiency) and mucosal bleeding (platelet dysfunction).

5. *What workup is indicated for a bleeding patient?*

Evaluation of the bleeding patient begins with a good history taking. It needs to be determined if the condition is of long standing or is new. Questions about previous bleeding episodes (nosebleeds, bruising, menstrual flow, bleeding with trauma, surgery, and delivery) as well as family history are vital for determining the nature of the disorder. A careful drug history, including over-the-counter drug use, must be taken. The patient's medical history and a review of symptoms may reveal evidence of autoimmune disorders or intercurrent illness.

Physical examination is important in evaluating sites of bleeding (cutaneous, mucosal, soft tissue, or joint bleeding sites, as well as petechiae). An enlarged spleen and evidence of liver disease (e.g., spiders or hemangiomata) or malnutrition should be sought, and the patient's overall medical condition should be assessed.

A screening for bleeding disorders should include a platelet count, PT, and PTT; if any of these results are abnormal or there is evidence of mucosal bleeding, determination of a bleeding time may also be indicated.

If the PT or PTT is prolonged, the next step in the evaluation should be a 1:1 mix in which the patient's plasma is mixed with normal plasma and the PT and PTT are determined again. If the patient is deficient in some factor, the normal patient's plasma partially corrects this deficiency and the PT or PTT are corrected to a normal value. If an inhibitor to a particular factor is present, this inhibitor also blocks the action of the normal plasma, and the PT or PTT are not corrected. The most common inhibitor is the lupus anticoagulant, which is seen in the presence and absence of autoimmune disease; it is usually associated with an elevated PTT that is not corrected with a 1:1 mix. It is associated with an increased risk of clotting, not bleeding.

If the platelet count is very low (20,000/mm^3) and the PT and PTT are normal, a bone marrow biopsy may be indicated to determine whether there are adequate platelet precursors in the bone marrow. If platelet precursors are absent, an underproduction state exists; if precursors are present, this implies the low platelet count stems from peripheral destruction. Using the detection of anti-platelet antibodies as evidence for the autoimmune destruction of platelets is not reliable because some normal people have anti-platelet antibodies without peripheral destruction, whereas the titers in people with ITP may be low.

6. *What therapies are available for the management of bleeding disorders?*

Blood components can be used to correct deficiencies in parts of the coagulation system. Fresh frozen plasma contains various percentages of each of the coagulation proteins and can be used when more than one factor is deficient (e.g., vitamin K-dependent factors). Cryoprecipitate contains von Willebrand's factor, fibrinogen, and factor VIII, but is most commonly used in people with an acquired fibrinogen deficiency (e.g., DIC and liver disease). Because of the risk of viral infection (it is pooled from multiple donors), cryoprecipitate is no longer used as frequently for patients with mild hemophilia and von Willebrand's disease. Instead, DDAVP (desmopressin) is now used in the treatment of these diseases, as well as the platelet dysfunction associated with uremia and other qualitative defects. This drug works by stimulating the release of von Willebrand's factor (factor VIII) from the endothelium. There are also specific heat-treated factor concentrates for factors VIII and IX that can be used for the management of hemophilia.

Quantitative platelet problems caused by underproduction, as well as some consumptive states such as uncontrolled bleeding, can be treated with platelet transfusions. This is often futile in the setting of autoimmune destruction until the autoimmune process is arrested; in fact, platelet transfusion may accelerate destruction by stimulating the immune system. The usual initial treatment for

ITP is high-dose prednisone, followed by splenectomy if the prednisone fails to block the immune destruction. Transfusing platelets into a patient who has uremia or who is taking a drug that renders his or her own platelets dysfunctional is also futile because the transfused platelets quickly become affected as well.

Case 1   A 47-year-old white man comes to the emergency room complaining of hematemesis and a 4-day history of abdominal pain and passing black, tarry stools. He gives a history of peptic ulcer disease that is linked to heavy alcohol use, and this was associated with one previous episode of bleeding. He denies the use of any medications, including over-the-counter medicines, and denies a family history of bleeding. On review of the systems, he describes some increased bruising over the past 2 to 3 months. On physical examination he is found to be jaundiced and in moderate distress; alcohol is smelled on his breath. His skin is remarkable for scattered ecchymoses and spider angiomas. His liver span is 15 cm and there is some tenderness plus a palpable spleen tip. The patient is continuing to pass melena and vomit bright red blood.

The following initial laboratory values are found: white blood cell count, 4,500/mm^3 with a normal differential; hemoglobin, 6.0 g/dL; hematocrit, 18%; platelets, 87,000/mm^3; aspartate aminotransferase (AST), 95 mU/mL (normal, 0 to 35 mU/mL); alanine aminotransferase (ALT), 40 mU/mL (normal, 0 to 38 mU/mL); total bilirubin, 3.5 mg/dL (normal, <1.0 mg/dL); and alkaline phosphatase, 450 mU/mL (normal, 0 to 125).

1. How would you proceed with the evaluation of this patient's bleeding problem?
2. What blood products would you give this patient, if any?
3. What other medicines, if any, would you give to this patient to manage his bleeding?
4. What factors may be contributing to this patient's low platelet count?

Case Discussion

1. *How would you proceed with the evaluation of this patient's bleeding problem?*

While emergency medical management of his bleeding is being provided through the placement of a nasogastric tube, together with the intravenous administration of fluids for blood pressure support as needed and typing and crossmatching in preparation for the administration of packed red blood cells, this patient with apparent chronic liver disease needs to have his coagulation status evaluated. Both the PT and PTT should be determined promptly and measurement of the fibrinogen level should be considered because it can be decreased in the setting of chronic liver failure. In this case, if the PT and PTT prove to be elevated, as expected, there is probably little reason for a 1:1 mix in this acutely ill patient because a deficiency state is very likely.

2. *What blood products would you give this patient, if any?*

If his PT or PTT proves to be elevated, the best blood product for replacing the deficient factors is fresh frozen plasma. In addition, if his fibrinogen level is measured and found to be less than 100 mg/dL, cryoprecipitate may also be indicated. Finally, it may become necessary to administer platelets if his count falls below 20,000/mm³ in the face of active bleeding.

3. *What other medicines, if any, would you give to this patient to manage his bleeding?*

With a history and physical examination findings consistent with alcoholism and liver disease, vitamin K should also be given.

4. *What factors may be contributing to this patient's low platelet count?*

His low platelet count may stem from multiple causes. First, the platelet count can fall in the face of massive bleeding (consumption). Second, he may be chronically underproducing platelets owing to either chronic alcohol suppression of the bone marrow or folic acid deficiency. Finally, he has an enlarged spleen, which may be sequestering his platelets.

Case 2   A 35-year-old Hispanic woman presents to the emergency room complaining of a nosebleed that has persisted for several hours. She denies a history of previous bleeding, though she has noticed some increased bruising over the past week and the appearance of a small, purplish rash on her feet and ankles. She denies any excessive bleeding with the delivery of her three children and has not undergone any surgical procedures. She denies taking aspirin, although she has taken acetaminophen for relief of a mild backache, and is on no other medicines. On review of her symptoms, she denies arthralgias, arthritis, fevers, cold symptoms, or other infectious symptoms; she has been in good health until now. On examination, she is found to be well developed and in no distress. There is some fresh as well as dried blood obscuring the nasal mucosa; she has no conjunctival hemorrhages but does have palatal petechiae. Her spleen is not palpable but there is a petechial rash around both ankles. Her nosebleed requires nasal packing for control.

The following initial laboratory values are found: white blood cell count, 6,700/mm³ with a normal differential; hemoglobin, 14.2 g/dL; hematocrit, 42.2%; MCV, 85 μ^3; platelets, 5,000/mm³; PT, 11.5 seconds (control, 12 seconds); and PTT, 28 seconds (control, 28.5 seconds).

1. What would you do next to evaluate this patient's bleeding?

2. What results would you expect from the further evaluation of this patient's bleeding?

3. What therapy would you institute in this patient?

Case Discussion

1. *What would you do next to evaluate this patient's bleeding?*

With the normal coagulation findings and complete blood count, except for the platelet count, and the absence of other physical findings such as an enlarged spleen, a bone marrow biopsy is not essential to evaluate for mega-karyocytes. Some clinicians may choose to treat for presumptive ITP and evaluate the patient in 24 hours.

2. *What results would you expect on this further evaluation?*

   Her clinical picture is consistent with that of ITP, and, in this setting, an adequate bone marrow specimen would show an increased or normal number of megakaryocytes. If the physician chooses to treat the patient empirically for ITP (see later), the patient should have significant improvement (i.e., platelet count ≥20,000 with less incidence of bleeding) in 24 hours.

3. *What therapy would you institute in this patient?*

   Platelet transfusions would not be helpful in this patient and might even accelerate the destructive process. Prednisone treatment (60 to 100 mg per day) should be initiated once bone marrow findings confirm the diagnosis or if the patient is treated empirically.

Case 3   You are asked to consult on the case of a 65-year-old white man with a history of severe rheumatoid arthritis who has cervical spine instability that now requires orthopedic stabilization. The preoperative laboratory results are as follows: white blood cell count, 10,000/mm^3 with a normal differential; hemoglobin, 12 g/dL; hematocrit, 36%; MCV, 86 femtoliters; platelets, 190,000/mm^3; PT, 12 seconds (control, 11.5 seconds); PTT, 52.2 seconds (control, 32.5 seconds); and bleeding time, 10.5 minutes (normal, 0 to 9.5 minutes).

The patient denies any bleeding history, and underwent a right knee replacement in the past without difficulty. He has taken large doses of aspirin in the past, but is currently on a nonsteroidal agent and takes no other medicines. There is no family history of bleeding disorders. On examination, he exhibits the sequelae of severe chronic rheumatoid arthritis, with deformed joints of the hands. He has no significant skin lesions. His spleen is not palpable and his liver is not enlarged.

1. What further preoperative evaluation would you do to reassure the surgeon that intraoperative hemostasis is adequate?
2. What blood products, if any, would you use in this patient?
3. What changes, if any, would you make in this patient's medications?

Case Discussion

1. *What further preoperative evaluation would you do to reassure the surgeon that intraoperative hemostasis is adequate?*

   The patient's main coagulation abnormalities include a slightly prolonged bleeding time and an elevated PTT. His medications include a nonsteroidal antiinflammatory agent, which can reversibly affect platelet function; this is the most likely source of his mildly increased bleeding time. In the absence of a bleeding history and if no emergency circumstances prevail, a 1:1 mix of his elevated PTT is indicated. His history of a chronic inflammatory condition is a strong indicator to have his lupus anticoagulant level determined.

2. *What blood products, if any, would you use in this patient?*

If a 1:1 mix does not correct in response to normal plasma, this indicates the presence of an inhibitor. His clinical picture is consistent with a lupus anticoagulant, which is actually associated with a risk of clotting, not bleeding, so no blood products are indicated. If his 1:1 mix does correct, implying a deficiency state, then specific assays of factor levels, including factors VIII and IX, may be necessary to identify the specific deficiency. This is highly unlikely in the absence of clinical bleeding.

This patient's slightly prolonged bleeding time does not require any intervention.

3. *What changes, if any, would you make in this patient's medications?*

His nonsteroidal medication should be stopped for at least 5 to 7 days before the spine stabilization procedure to allow normal platelet function to return. Immediately before surgery, his bleeding time should be checked again to confirm this return to normal.

Suggested Readings

Beutler E, Lichtman MA, Coller BS, Kipps TJ, eds. *Hematology*, 5th ed. New York: McGraw-Hill, 1995.

Wintrobe MW, ed. *Clinical hematology*, 9th ed. Philadelphia: Lea & Febiger, 1993.

Breast Cancer

1. What is the incidence of breast cancer?
2. What is the natural history of breast cancer?
3. What are the risk factors for breast cancer?
4. Of what does the screening for breast cancer consist?
5. What is the TNM classification, and what are the stages of breast cancer?
6. What are the prognostic indicators associated with breast cancer?
7. What is the difference between modified radical mastectomy and lumpectomy plus radiation therapy in the treatment of stage I and II breast cancer, and what are the indications for each?
8. What is the role for adjuvant chemotherapy in the treatment of breast cancer?
9. Of what does the treatment of node-negative breast cancer consist?
10. What is the purpose and the underlying principles of endocrine manipulation in the treatment of metastatic breast cancer?
11. What is the role of systemic chemotherapy in the treatment of metastatic breast cancer?

Discussion

1. *What is the incidence of breast cancer?*

Breast cancer is the most common neoplasm in women, with an incidence that continues to rise and currently stands at 1 in 10 women. The incidence rises dramatically with age.

2. *What is the natural history of breast cancer?*

Breast cancer is considered to be a systemic disease from the time of diagnosis, regardless of the stage. The average doubling time varies from 23 to 500 days. Therefore, a 1-cm tumor may have existed for 2 to 17 years before diagnosis.

Despite local control, affected patients continue to die at a rate faster than that seen in age-matched control subjects for the first 20 years after treatment. In addition, patients dying from any cause are found to have evidence of tumor at autopsy. The most common sites of distant metastases are the bone, liver, and lung.

Paraneoplastic conditions that may be associated with breast cancer include hypercalcemia, neuromuscular disorders, dermatomyositis, acanthosis nigricans, and hemostatic abnormalities.

Common secondary malignancies in patients with breast cancer consist of cancer in the opposite breast, ovarian cancer, and colorectal carcinoma.

3. *What are the risk factors for breast cancer?*

High-risk factors (threefold or greater increase) for the development of breast cancer are:

- Age greater than 50 years.
- Previous cancer in one breast, especially that occurring premenopausally.
- Breast cancer in the family, although the risk varies depending on whether the disease was in a first-degree family member, was unilateral or bilateral, and occurred premenopausally or postmenopausally: bilateral and premenopausal disease carries an 8.8 times greater risk; bilateral and postmenopausal disease carries a 5.4 times greater risk; unilateral and premenopausal disease carries a 3 times greater risk; and unilateral and postmenopausal disease carries a 1.5 times greater risk.
- Parity. Women who are nulliparous or who were first pregnant after 31 years of age have a three to four times increased risk.
- Lobular carcinoma *in situ* carries a 30% risk of becoming invasive.
- Certain forms of benign breast disease are associated with an increased risk of cancer. Gross cystic disease with lesions exceeding 3 mm, multiple intraductal papillomas, and atypical hyperplasia are considered premalignant.

Intermediate-risk factors (1.2- to 1.5-fold increase) for the development of breast cancer consist of menstruation (either early menarche or late menopause); oral estrogen therapy; alcohol consumption; diabetes mellitus; history of cancer of the uterus, ovary, or colon; and obesity.

4. *Of what does the screening for breast cancer consist?*

Women older than 20 years of age should perform breast self-examination every month. Premenopausal women should examine their breasts *5 to 7* days after the end of their menstrual cycle, and postmenopausal women should do this on the same day of every month.

Women should have their breasts examined by a physician every *2 to 3* years between the ages of 20 and 40 years and annually thereafter. The

American Cancer Society has recommended that a baseline mammogram should be obtained between the ages of 35 and 39 years, with mammograms obtained every 1 to 2 years in women aged 40 to 49 years and then yearly after the age of 50 years.

5. *What is the TNM classification, and what are the stages of breast cancer?*

The TNM (primary tumor, regional nodes, metastases) classification and the various stages of breast cancer are outlined in Table 7-5.

6. *What are the prognostic indicators associated with breast cancer?*

Table 7-6 summarizes the 5- and 10-year survival statistics associated with the various TNM stages. These statistics do *not* take into account results of adjuvant chemotherapy, but are useful in designing trials using adjuvant chemotherapy.

The patient's hormonal status also has a bearing on her prognosis, in that estrogen- and progesterone receptor-positive tumors possess a 70% to 85%

Table 7-5. The TNM Classification of Breast Cancer

| Stage grouping[a] | Disease Extent | | | |
	Primary tumor (T)	Lymph nodes (N)[d]	Distant metastses (M)	TNM classification
0	Noninvasive carcinoma *in situ*; Paget's disease of the nipple (TIS)	Homolateral axillary nodes negative (N0)	None	TIS N0 M1
I	Greatest dimension ≤2 cm (T1)[b]	Homolateral axillary nodes negative (N0)	None	T1 N0 M0
II	Greatest dimension >2 cm and ≤5 cm (T2)[b]	Homolateral axillary nodes positive but not fixed (N1)	None	T0 or T1, N1, M0 T2 N0 or N1, M0
IIIA	Greatest dimension >5 cm (T3)[b]	Homolateral axillary nodes positive and fixed to one another, skin, or chest wall (N2)	None	T0 or T1 N2 M0 T2 N2 M0 T3 N0–2 M0
IIIB	Any size with (T4)[b] satellite skin nodules, skin ulceration, fixation to skin or chest wall, or edema of breast, including *peau d'orange*[c]	Supraclavicular or infraclavicular nodal involvement; edema of the arm with or without palpable axillary lymph nodes (N3)	None	T4, any N, M0 Any T, N3, M0
IV	Any size	Any status	Present	Any T, any N, M1

[a]The American Joint Committee recognizes two stage groupings: postoperative-pathologic (presented in this table) and clinical-diagnostic.

[b]T0 indicates no tumor demonstrable in breasts; T1, T2, and T3 include tumor fixation to underlying pectoral fascia or muscle, which does not change the classification of lesions. (Inflammatory breast cancer is classified as a separate entity and is not included in T4.)

[c]Skin dimpling and nipple retraction do not affect staging classification.

[d]The clinical-diagnostic stage grouping subdivides movable homolateral axillary lymph nodes into N1a—nodes not considered to contain tumor (approximately 33% are histologically positive); and N1b—nodes considered to contain tumor (approximately 25% are histologically negative).

Adapted from the American Joint Committee for Cancer Staging and End-Results Reporting, 1983.

Table 7-6. Prognostic Indicators for Breast Cancer

Prognostic indicators	Five years (%)	Ten years (%)
Clinical stage		
0	>90	90
I	80	65
II	60	45
IIIA	50	40
IIIB	35	20
IV & inflammatory breast cancer	10	5
Tumor size (cm)		
<1		80
3–4		55
5–7.5		15
Axillary nodes		
None positive	80	65
1–3 positive	65	40
>3 positive	30	15

chance of responding to hormonal therapy; those women with only one-receptor positivity have exhibited a 33% to 50% response rate to hormone manipulation. Even in women with receptor-negative tumors, there is still a 10% to 20% chance of response to hormone manipulation.

7. *What is the difference between modified radical mastectomy and lumpectomy plus radiation therapy in the treatment of stage I and II breast cancer, and what are the indications for each?*

Although mastectomy controls local disease, it has a devastating psychological impact on both the patients and their families; therefore, surgical techniques designed to preserve the breast are warranted. In 1976, the National Surgical Adjuvant Breast Project (NSABP) began a randomized trial comparing total mastectomy, segmental mastectomy, and segmental mastectomy plus radiation. All 1,843 patients underwent axillary node dissection. The 8-year follow-up revealed that lumpectomy in patients with tumors less than 4 cm in diameter and with free surgical margins is an appropriate form of therapy in stage I and II breast cancer. In addition, irradiation plus lumpectomy probably decreases the likelihood of local recurrence.

8. *What is the role for adjuvant chemotherapy in the treatment of breast cancer?*

The lymph node status is the most important prognostic indicator in this disease. Patients with positive nodes are at a high risk for local recurrences as well as metastatic disease.

A prospective, randomized trial showed that the addition of CMF (cyclophosphamide, methotrexate, and 5-fluorouracil) to the treatment protocol improves the 10-year overall survival in both premenopausal and postmenopausal women. If the tumor is receptor positive, adding tamoxifen to the chemotherapy regimen has been shown in multiple trials to increase disease-free survival, and in some studies overall survival benefit has been shown.

9. *Of what does the treatment of node-negative breast cancer consist?*

Some patients thought to be node negative in the past have been found to be node positive by careful analysis using techniques such as sentinel node biopsy. The treatment of node-negative breast cancer is still controversial. Originally, women with negative nodes were thought to have a very good prognosis, but 30% are still found to be dying of the disease. Giving therapy to all such patients is not without hazard; therefore, it would be of great value to have indicators that could predict who would be good candidates for treatment. Tests can predict aggressive tumors such as increased cells in the S phase of the cell cycle and the presence of tumor markers such as Her2. Other factors, such as the size of the primary tumor, the histologic grade, and hormone receptor status may also be influential. Most studies now suggest that patients with tumors larger than 1 cm should be treated with adjuvant chemotherapy, particularly if the tumors are larger than 2 cm or show evidence for aggressive disease. Tamoxifen has been shown to protect selected high-risk patients from development of breast cancer and is effective in preventing recurrence in patients with small tumors that are node negative but positive for estrogen and progesterone receptors.

10. *What is the purpose and the underlying principles of endocrine manipulation in the treatment of metastatic breast cancer?*

It has been known for many years that there is an interrelationship between the ovaries and the breasts. Patients with locally recurrent breast cancer have exhibited a dramatic response to bilateral oophorectomy. More recently, with the ability to identify estrogen receptors in breast tissue, it was natural for antiestrogen therapy to be used for the treatment of breast cancer. The first trials of hormonal agents were conducted in patients with metastatic disease, and they proved that these agents were not only efficacious but well tolerated, with weight gain the only major side effect.

Because of their success in the management of advanced disease, hormonal agents have been instituted as adjuvant therapy and chemoprevention agents. Although the finding of estrogen receptor positivity constitutes the greatest advantage, many women are negative for receptors, or their status is unknown. Thus, many physicians try hormonal manipulation in both the adjuvant or advanced setting, regardless of the receptor status, because the agents are well tolerated and these patients do not have other poor prognostic indicators that would dictate the use of chemotherapy. Trials examining the combination of chemotherapy and hormonal agents are under way.

11. *What is the role of systemic chemotherapy in the treatment of metastatic breast cancer?*

Patients are candidates for chemotherapy if their disseminated disease is highly aggressive, they are hormone receptor negative, or they fail to respond to endocrine manipulation. There are several variations of combination chemotherapy regimens containing cyclophosphamide, methotrexate, 5-fluorouracil, doxorubicin, paclitaxel, carboplatin, and other agents. Also, new monoclonal antibody treatments, including an antibody directed against the Her-2 antigen, are available.

Case 1   A 35-year-old white woman with a family history of breast cancer discovers a lump in her right breast. The lump is confirmed on physical examination and a mammogram is then obtained. A 1.7-cm lesion is identified and sampled for biopsy. Pathologic analysis of the biopsy tissue reveals an infiltrating ductal carcinoma. The patient elects to undergo lumpectomy with axillary node dissection. One of seven lymph nodes is positive, and estrogen and progesterone receptor studies are negative. The histologic grade of the tumor is 3/3, the DNA is diploid, and the percentage S phase is 8.5.

The patient receives local irradiation followed by six cycles of CMF. She has no evidence of disease and is seen every 3 months for follow-up.

1. What is this patient's TNM classification and stage?
2. Was lumpectomy an appropriate treatment?
3. Does this patient have poor prognostic indicators?

Case Discussion

1. *What is this patient's TNM classification and stage?*

   This patient has a T1 lesion because her primary tumor was less than 2 cm. Her nodal status is N1 because one of the nodes showed tumor infiltration, and her metastasis status is graded as M0 because no metastases were found. Therefore, she has stage II disease.

2. *Was lumpectomy an appropriate treatment?*

   Evidence suggests lumpectomy is an alternative to mastectomy in the management of stage II disease. Because of her one positive node, radiation therapy is also recommended to lessen her increased potential for local recurrence. The finding of one positive node also makes her a candidate for systemic chemotherapy to limit distant metastases.

3. *Does this patient have poor prognostic indicators?*

   This patient has several poor prognostic features: her age of 35 years; a high-grade tumor morphology together with a high-percentage S phase, despite a diploid population; negativity for both receptors; and the one positive node. Her chance of surviving 10 years is only approximately 40%.

Case 2   A 62-year-old woman was first seen 7 years ago because of a 4-cm left breast mass. Biopsy results revealed adenocarcinoma, and the patient underwent a modified radical mastectomy and axillary node dissection. Two of 22 nodes were positive, and the tumor was positive for estrogen and progesterone receptors. The patient was placed on tamoxifen therapy.

She did well until 5 years ago, when right hip pain developed. A bone scan revealed the presence of metastatic disease in her spine, ribs, and right hip. She was switched to anastrozole (Arimidex; Zeneca Pharmaceuticals, Wilmington, DE), a second-line hormonal agent. Fourteen months later, pain occurred in her left shoulder and she became increasingly lethargic. A restaging evaluation showed progressive bone scan findings and hypercalcemia. She was started on chemotherapy and fluid diuresis was instituted to treat her hypercalcemia acutely. The patient received six cycles of chemotherapy, with subsequent stabilization of her disease; however, 22 months later, her disease rapidly progressed. She was treated with another chemotherapy regimen, but after initial stabilization of her disease, she died 16 months later.

1. What was this patient's original TNM classification and stage?
2. Is her clinical course typical of breast cancer?
3. Was a second hormonal agent warranted?
4. What was the cause of her hypercalcemia, and how should it be treated?

Case Discussion

1. *What was this patient's original TNM classification and stage?*

    The patient originally had a T2 lesion because her tumor was 4 cm, her nodal status was N1 because axillary dissection revealed seven positive nodes, and her metastasis status was M0 because no obvious metastatic lesions were discovered. Taken together, she originally had stage II disease.

2. *Is her clinical course typical of breast cancer?*

    Breast cancer is considered a chronic disease based on the hypothesis that micrometastases exist at the time of diagnosis. This theory is supported by the observation that women with early-stage breast cancer still exhibit an increased risk of dying from their disease for 20 years, despite curative intent.

3. *Was a second hormonal agent warranted?*

    The best predictor of hormonal response is a response to a previous hormonal agent. In this case, the patient responded to tamoxifen for 2 years; therefore, another hormonal agent was appropriate, and this produced 14 months of further response.

4. *What was the cause of her hypercalcemia, and how should it be treated?*

    Two general mechanisms can bring about hypercalcemia in a patient with cancer: (a) tumor cells in direct contact with bone can induce an osteolytic mechanism; and (b) tumor cells can secrete humoral substances that activate osteoclasts.

    The first mechanism primarily operates in breast cancer. Acute intervention requires fluid diuresis. However, the patient must first be adequately hydrated before diuresis is started, because dehydration only worsens the hypercalcemia. Treatment of the underlying cause should then be instituted, as was done in this patient with chemotherapy. Some agents such as bisphosphonates not only help treat hypercalcemia, but, with continual use, improve symptoms caused by breast metastases to bone *and* may improve survival.

Suggested Readings

Clark GM, Dressler LG, Owens MA, Pounds G, Oldaker T, McGuire WL. Prediction of relapse or survival in patients with node-negative breast cancer by DNA flow cytometry. *N Engl J Med* 1989;320:627.

Fisher B, Costantino JP, Wickerham DL, et al. Tamoxifen for prevention of breast cancer: report of the National Surgical Adjuvant Breast and Bowel Project P-1 Study. *J Natl Cancer Inst* 1998;90:1371.

Fisher B, Redmond C, Poisson R, et al. Eight-year results of randomized clinical trial comparing total mastectomy and lumpectomy with or without irradiation in the treatment of breast cancer. *N Engl J Med* 1989;320:822.

Early Breast Cancer Trialists' Collaborative Group. Polychemotherapy for early breast cancer: an overview of the randomized trials. *Lancet* 1998;352:930.

McGuire WL. Adjuvant therapy for node-negative breast cancer. *N Engl J Med* 1989;320:525.

Chronic Myelogenous Leukemia

1. What is the definition of chronic myelogenous leukemia (CML)?
2. What is the etiology of CML?
3. What is the pathogenic mechanism responsible for CML?
4. What is the epidemiology of CML?
5. What are the clinical characteristics of CML?
6. What are the laboratory findings encountered in the setting of CML?
7. What are the cytogenetic and biochemical abnormalities typically found in patients with CML?
8. What is the treatment for CML?
9. What is the prognosis in patients with CML?

Discussion

1. *What is the definition of CML?*

   Chronic myelogenous leukemia is a hematopoietic stem cell disease characterized by anemia, extreme blood granulocytosis, granulocytic immaturity, basophilia, often thrombocytosis, and splenomegaly.

2. *What is the etiology of CML?*

   The etiology of CML is unknown, but exposure to ionizing radiation has been found to increase the risk of CML above the expected frequency in certain populations. Some of these major populations are (a) the Japanese exposed to radiation from the Nagasaki and Hiroshima atomic bomb explosions; (b) the British with ankylosing spondylitis treated with spinal irradiation; and (c) women with uterine cervical carcinoma who require radiation therapy. The frequency of CML (as well as acute leukemia) in these populations is significantly greater than that expected for comparable unexposed groups. Chemical leukemogens have not been identified as causative agents of CML.

3. *What is the pathogenic mechanism responsible for CML?*

   Chronic myelogenous leukemia results from the acquired (somatic mutation) malignant transformation of a single stem cell whose potency dominates hematopoiesis in the affected person, with the involvement of erythropoiesis, neutrophilopoiesis, eosinophilopoiesis, basophilopoiesis, monocytopoiesis, and thrombopoiesis. Several observations suggest that some lymphocytes may be derived from the primordial malignant cell as well, thus placing the culprit lesion closer if not in the pluripotential stem cell. The exact mechanism that causes the transformation to take place has not been fully elucidated, but the Ph[1] (Philadelphia) chromosome has been implicated. The hematopoietic cells contain a reciprocal translocation between chromosomes 9 and 22 in over 90% of patients. This leads to an overtly foreshortened long arm of one of the chromosome 22 pairs. Chromosome 9 contains the c-*abl* gene at band 34; chromosome 22 has the break point cluster region (bcr) and c-*sis* i genes at band 11. The c-*abl* gene from chromosome 9 is transported to the chromosome 22 bcr, which is the Ph[1] chromosome. As a consequence of these events, a new gene is formed, the bcr-*abl* gene, which codes for a new protein through the formation of a new messenger RNA. This new protein is a phosphoprotein with a molecular weight of 210,000 (P210 bcr-*abl*) and possessing tyrosine kinase activity. Its abnormal activity presumably alters the response of the hematopoietic stem cell so that it continues to proliferate rather than being under the control of hematopoietic growth factors.

4. *What is the epidemiology of CML?*

Chronic myelogenous leukemia accounts for approximately 2% of all cases of leukemia and the mortality rate associated with it is approximately 1.5 per 100,000 population per year. The disease occurs slightly more often in men, but its manifestations and course are similar for both sexes. Approximately 10% of the cases occur in people between 5 and 20 years of age, and CML accounts for approximately 3% of all the childhood leukemias.

5. *What are the clinical characteristics of CML?*

The disease is characterized by three phases: (a) a chronic phase, (b) an accelerated phase, and (c) a blast crisis.

The most frequent complaints seen during the **chronic phase** include easy fatigability, loss of a sense of well-being, decreased tolerance to exertion, anorexia, abdominal discomfort, early satiety, weight loss, and excessive sweating. The symptoms are vague, nonspecific, and gradual in onset. Physical examination may detect pallor and splenomegaly.

Uncommon presenting signs and symptoms of CML include hypermetabolism that simulates thyrotoxicosis, acute gouty arthritis, priapism, tinnitus, stupor, left upper quadrant and left shoulder pain as a consequence of splenic infarction and perisplenitis, diabetes insipidus, and acne urticaria, which is associated with hyperhistaminemia.

In some patients in this phase, the disease is discovered when blood cell counts are determined during a routine medical examination. The symptoms and signs of the disease and the laboratory findings typically remain stable, and the duration of this phase is variable. Usually it lasts approximately 4 years, but it can last from weeks to many years before transforming to the accelerated phase.

In most cases of CML, the patient's disease eventually changes to a more aggressive, symptomatic, and troublesome form (the **accelerated phase**) that responds poorly to therapy that formerly controlled the chronic phase. This metamorphosis is often gradual and manifested by refractory splenomegaly; extramedullary tumor masses; changes in the blood, bone marrow, and differential cell counts; and new cytogenetic abnormalities. The onset of fever without infection, weakness, night sweats, weight loss, arthralgias, and bone or left upper quadrant pain may occur before there is laboratory evidence of the phase. These laboratory abnormalities include a decrease in the hemoglobin content with increasing red blood cell abnormalities, an abrupt increase or fall in the white count without treatment, and an increase in the number of blast or immature cells. Thrombocytosis or thrombocytopenia and an increase in the number of basophils or eosinophils are also seen.

The **blastic phase** can be manifested by an extramedullary blast infiltration or by a bone marrow blast crisis.

An extramedullary blast crisis is the first manifestation of the accelerated phase in approximately 10% of patients, and this principally involves the lymph nodes, serosal surfaces, skin and soft tissue, breasts, and the CNS. Bone involvement may lead to severe pain, tenderness, and radiographic changes. The CNS involvement is usually meningeal and may be preceded by headache, vomiting, stupor, cranial nerve palsies, and papilledema; it is associated with an increase in the number of cells and the protein level, as well as the presence of blast cells in the spinal fluid.

Acute leukemia, the blast phase, develops in most patients with CML, and this can take from days to years to occur after the diagnosis of CML. The signs and symptoms are fever, hemorrhage, bone pain, and lymphadenopathy, as well as the other manifestations already cited. The blastic transformation is usually myeloblastic or myelomonocytic, but can be erythrocytic or lymphoid in nature. Special staining techniques, biochemical assays, or monoclonal antibody determinations are needed to identify the type of transformation once the patient is in the blastic phase. Patients usually die within weeks to months. The median survival in patients in the myeloid blast crisis is approximately 3 to 6 months, and that in patients in the lymphoid blast crisis is 12 months, with survival beyond 2 years unusual. Severe infections, hemorrhage, and organ dysfunction, especially of the liver and kidney, are among the leading causes of death.

6. *What are the laboratory findings encountered in the setting of CML?*

The diagnosis of CML can be made on the basis of the **hematologic findings**, specifically those yielded by the blood count and the blood smear. Common findings are a decrease in the hematocrit; the presence of nucleated red blood cells in the circulation; a leukocyte count that is always elevated, often exceeding $1,000 \times 10^9$/L; the presence of all stages of granulocyte development in the blood with a generally normal appearance; and a blast cell prevalence ranging from 0.5% to 5%. Myelocytes, metamyelocytes, and band forms account for approximately 40%. The number of basophils is increased, as is the total absolute lymphocyte count (mean, approximately 15×10^9/L). In addition, the platelet count is elevated in approximately 50% of patients at the time of diagnosis; platelet counts over $1,000 \times 10^9$/L are not unusual; and neutrophil alkaline phosphatase activity is low or absent in over 90% of patients. The defects in white cell adhesion, emigration, and phagocytosis are mild and compensated for by high neutrophil concentrations, and thus do not predispose patients in the chronic phase to infections. Platelet dysfunction can occur but is not associated with spontaneous or exaggerated bleeding, as with other myeloproliferative disorders.

In terms of the **morphologic findings**, the bone marrow is markedly hypercellular and hematopoietic tissue takes up 75% to 90% of the marrow volume. Granulopoiesis is dominant, with a granulocytic–erythroid ratio of between 10 and 30:1 (normal, 2 to 4:1). Erythropoiesis is usually decreased, the megakaryocytes are normal or increased in number, and the population of eosinophils and basophils may be increased.

7. *What are the cytogenetic and biochemical abnormalities typically found in patients with CML?*

The Ph^1 chromosome, designated t(9;22)(q34;q11), is present in over 90% of patients with CML. During the blast phase, most patients exhibit additional chromosome abnormalities, usually a $+8$, the gain of a second Ph^1 chromosome, or rarely a chromosome loss (-7).

Variant Ph^1 chromosome translocations occur in approximately 5% of patients and usually consist of complex rearrangements. Every chromosome is involved except the Y chromosome. There is a small group of patients with CML who do not have the Ph^1 chromosome, but virtually all patients have an abnormal chromosome 22 with bcr rearrangements. The characteristic biochemical abnormalities consist of an increase in the uric acid level, an increase in the serum level of cobalamin-binding capacity, a raised cobalamin concentration, an increase in the LDH level, pseudohyperkalemia (an *in vitro* hyperkalemia secondary to K^+ release from platelets), pseudohypoglycemia (secondary to leukocyte utilization *in vitro*), hypercalcemia, hypergammaglobulinemia, and low leukocyte alkaline phosphatase activity.

8. *What is the treatment for CML?*

All the biochemical alterations must be corrected. The hyperuricemia must be treated with adequate hydration and allopurinol. However, the specific treatment for the disease depends on the stage and goal of therapy.

For **chemotherapy**, hydroxyurea is used most often because it has fewer side effects than alkylating agents, which can induce aplastic anemia and acute leukemia in patients with CML. Hydroxyurea treatment has a minimal effect on survival, controls the hematologic alterations (without suppressing the Ph^1 chromosome), and improves the patient's quality of life.

Multidrug regimens have been used. They can eradicate the Ph^1 chromosome, but at the expense of high morbidity and without prolonging survival. Thus, they are not generally accepted.

Both **α-** and **γ-interferons** have shown antileukemic activity in the setting of CML; α-interferon produces a normalization of blood counts in approximately 75% of patients and suppresses the Ph[1] chromosome in approximately 15% of treated patients. The Ph[1]-negative cell also lacks the bcr rearrangements.

Drawbacks to interferon treatment are that maintenance therapy is required and it is not free of side effects. Some studies suggest that the prolonged use of interferon (i.e., >1 year) in responders *may* make patients *less* responsive to bone marrow transplantation.

Splenic **irradiation** may be useful to control splenomegaly and to palliate the symptoms resulting from it. **Splenectomy** may be useful in carefully selected patients with symptomatic thrombocytopenia who do not respond to chemotherapy and have a greatly enlarged spleen; however, it is only a palliative measure.

Autologous and allogeneic bone marrow transplantations are useful in the treatment of some patients with CML. This treatment can eradicate the Ph[1]-carrying clone and has led to an apparent cure of some patients with CML. However, the high toxicity resulting from the procedure, particularly in those who lack suitable donors or are of advanced age, limit its use.

Leukapheresis can be useful in two types of patients: pregnant women with a very high white cell count and hyperleukocytic patients who need rapid cytoreduction to alleviate the signs and symptoms of leukostasis.

9. *What is the prognosis in patients with CML?*

In patients with CML who are treated with standard chemotherapy, the median survival ranges from 45 to 60 months. Approximately 25% to 35% of patients survive 5 years, and 8% to 17% survive 8 years. Long-term results with bone marrow transplantation should significantly increase this percentage. Occasional patients have remained in the chronic phase for 10 to 25 years.

Case

A 37-year-old white man is seen because of lack of energy, night sweats, and poor appetite with a sensation of fullness after eating even very small amounts of food.

Physical examination reveals signs of anemia, splenomegaly, and the existence of petechiae. A complete blood count is performed and yields the following findings: hematocrit, 25%; platelets, 300,000/mm³, and white blood cells, 72,000/mm³. A bone marrow biopsy is performed and the specimen is found to exhibit a granulocytic–erythroid ratio of 10:1 with 100% cellularity and 1% blastocytes.

1. What is the differential diagnosis in this patient, based on the physical examination findings?
2. Based on the hematologic findings, what hematopoietic abnormalities would you expect in this patient with suspected CML?
3. What do the bone marrow findings indicate in this patient?

4. What would be the most specific test for establishing the diagnosis of CML in this patient?

5. If the patient is started on single-agent chemotherapy, what would be the likely effect?

Case Discussion

1. *What is the differential diagnosis in this patient, based on the physical examination findings?*

When the diagnosis of CML is considered, other possibilities, such as a solid cancer, lymphomas, and chronic infections must be excluded. These other diseases may cause a leukemoid reaction by increased stimulation of normal myelopoiesis. Usually a leukemoid reaction results in a white blood cell count of less than 100,000/mm^3, and less than 10% of cells are myelocytes or more immature forms.

Because normal hematopoiesis is suppressed, the patient could exhibit the signs and symptoms of anemia, such as headache, palpitations, pallor, and cardiac failure. Very rarely, lymph node enlargement is found in patients with CML. Splenomegaly is almost the rule in patients with CML, and it is the source of poor appetite and upper abdominal pain, such as that seen in this patient. Finally, petechiae, although possible, are not very frequent findings in patients with CML.

2. *Based on the hematologic findings, what hematopoietic abnormalities would you expect in this patient with suspected CML?*

Normal hematopoiesis is suppressed by the leukemic activity in the bone marrow, leading to a decreased number of red blood cells, as well as decreased hemoglobin level and hematocrit. Typically, the anemia of CML is normochromic normocytic. Hypochromic microcytic anemia is typical of iron deficiency.

Although immature, most of the white cells look morphologically normal, and mature neutrophils, band forms, metamyelocytes, and myelocytes constitute most of the white blood cells in this patient. Another characteristic finding is an increased number of basophils. If most of the cells are blasts, this indicates acute leukemia in most cases, although it can also indicate the patient is in the blastic phase of CML.

3. *What do the bone marrow findings indicate in this patient?*

The bone marrow findings are consistent with a diagnosis of CML, and bone marrow biopsy constitutes an important part of the diagnostic evaluation in patients with any kind of leukemia (acute and chronic). Normally, the granulocytic–erythroid ratio ranges from 2 to 4:1, but, in the setting of CML, cells of white lineage predominate and increments of any form of white blood cells, from myeloblasts to mature neutrophils, can be found. An increment in lymphocytes and red blood cell precursors is not characteristic of CML. The normal bone marrow cellularity is 50% fat and 50% or less cells, but, in the leukemias, the accelerated production of abnormal cells causes the fat to be replaced, and the cellularity increases to 100%. Finally, even in normal bone marrow, a very small number of blast cells can be found; in CML, a small percentage of blast cells can be found, but this does not necessarily signify acute leukemia. In blast crisis or acute leukemia, at least 20% of the cells in the bone marrow are blast cells.

4. *What would be the most specific test for establishing the diagnosis of CML in this patient?*

The most specific test for establishing the diagnosis of CML is a cytogenetic investigation for the Ph[1] chromosome, or t(9;22), which is found in 90% of cases of CML.

5. *If the patient is started on single-agent chemotherapy, what would be the likely effect?*

The chemotherapeutic agent most commonly used in the treatment of CML is hydroxyurea. This therapy can improve the patient's quality of life by rapidly decreasing the number of white blood cells and platelets. It does not prolong survival very much, if at all, in patients with CML. Eventually all patients progress to the accelerated phase or blastic crisis and die of the disease. The interferons, particularly α-interferon, have proved useful in the treatment of CML. These agents can induce complete hematologic and cytogenetic remissions, with suppression of the Ph[1] chromosome in patients with CML.

Allogeneic bone marrow transplantation has been the only curative treatment for CML but has a high rate of complications. Advanced age and the lack of suitable donors preclude its use in many patients, but it may be the therapy of choice in this 37-year-old man.

Suggested Readings

Bernstein R. Cytogenetics of chronic myelogenous leukemia. *Semin Hematol* 1988;25:20.

Canellos G. Clinical characteristics of the blast phase of chronic myelogenous leukemia. *Hematol Oncol Clin North Am* 1990;4:359.

Kurzrock R, Gutterman JU, Talpaz M. The molecular genetics of Philadelphia chromosome positive leukemias. *N Engl J Med* 1988;319:990.

Reiter E, Greinix HT, Brugger S, et al. Long term follow up after allogeneic stem cell transplantation for chronic myelogenous leukemia. *Bone Marrow Transplant* 1998;4:S86.

Rodriguez J, Cortes J, Smith T, et al. Determinations of prognosis in late chronic-phase chronic myelogenous leukemia. *J Clin Oncol* 1998;16:3782.

Colon Cancer

1. What is the incidence of colon cancer?
2. What are some of the known risk factors for colon cancer?
3. Should patients be screened for colon cancer?
4. What is the current treatment for primary colon cancer?
5. What staging procedures need to be done to stage adequately a patient with colon cancer?
6. What is the staging system for colon cancer?
7. What is the prognosis for patients with colon cancer, based on their stage?

8. What should the follow-up consist of in patients with colon cancer after they have undergone primary surgical resection for curative intent?
9. Are there any effective adjuvant treatments to decrease the risk of recurrence in patients with colon cancer who have undergone resection?
10. Is there any effective chemotherapy for patients with metastatic disease?

Discussion

1. *What is the incidence of colon cancer?*

   There are more than 140,000 new cases of colon cancer each year in the United States. It affects approximately 1 of every 20 people in Western cultures and accounts for 15% of all cancers. In the United States, the actual incidence rate is approximately 35 cases per 100,000 population per year.

2. *What are some of the known risk factors for colon cancer?*

   There are several inherited colonic polyposis syndromes associated with an increased risk of cancer of the large bowel. The most important one is the familial adenomatosis syndrome, which is inherited as an autosomal dominant trait. In affected people, polyps develop over the entire length of the colon by 30 years of age. If a total colectomy is not performed, the cancer rate escalates to as high as 80% to 90% by 45 years of age. Other, less frequent polyposis syndromes include Gardner's, Oldfield's, and Turcot's syndromes.

   There appears to be a certain genetic tendency toward colon carcinoma that is independent of the inherited polyposis syndromes. First-degree relatives of people with colon cancer have a two- to threefold greater chance of acquiring colon cancer than the general population.

   Patients with inflammatory bowel disease are also at increased risk for colon cancer. Those with ulcerative colitis have approximately a 50% to 60% chance for development of large bowel carcinoma if a colectomy is not performed. Crohn's disease is also associated with an increased risk of colon cancer, but to a much lesser degree than ulcerative colitis.

   The findings from several population studies have suggested that diet plays a large role in the development of colon cancer. Cultures in which the populace consumes a high-fat, low-fiber diet exhibit an increased incidence of colon cancer, compared with cultures in which a low-fat, high-fiber diet is consumed.

3. *Should patients be screened for colon cancer?*

   The prognosis for colon cancer is dramatically improved the earlier it is detected and treated. Screening programs are aimed at detecting colon cancers at an early stage and have led to an improvement in survival and in the risk of relapse. Most screening programs are directed at populations with a high risk for colon cancer, including the groups already mentioned.

   Screening techniques for colon cancer comprise digital rectal examination, the testing of stool for occult blood, sigmoidoscopy with an air-contrast barium enema, and colonoscopy. Recommendations are that people should be checked for occult blood at 50 years of age and yearly thereafter with sigmoidoscopy performed at the same age and every 3 years thereafter. Less well accepted screening procedures, including colonoscopy performed routinely for those at risk based on the diseases described previously or a family history of colon cancer, are performed on a more individual basis.

4. *What is the current treatment for primary colon cancer?*

The primary treatment for colon cancer is surgical. Once the cancer has been diagnosed and preoperative staging performed, the patient should be referred to an oncologic surgeon for definitive treatment. The exact surgical approach used is dictated by the tumor's location in the colon. For true colon cancers (i.e., cancers above the peritoneal reflection), a hemicolectomy is usually performed. For rectal carcinomas (i.e., tumors below the peritoneal reflection), a low anterior resection or an abdominoperineal resection is performed. Regardless of the surgical procedure, a thorough exploration of the entire abdomen, including the liver, should be carried out and any suspect lesions sampled for biopsy.

5. *What staging procedures need to be done to stage adequately a patient with colon cancer?*

The preoperative staging evaluation of patients with colon cancer includes history taking, physical examination, complete blood count, liver function tests, the carcinoembryonic antigen (CEA) level, and a chest radiograph. If liver function tests show elevations, these should be further investigated by computed tomographic (CT) scanning. Surgical and pathologic staging should then be performed to determine the exact stage of the disease. If the preoperative CEA level is elevated, repeat measurement should be performed approximately 1 month after surgery to see if it returns to normal.

6. *What is the staging system for colon cancer?*

There are many staging systems for colon cancer. The most widely used is the Aster-Coller modification of the Dukes staging system (Table 7-7). It is based on the depth of tumor invasion, regional lymph node involvement, and distant metastasis.

7. *What is the prognosis for patients with colon cancer, based on their stage?*

Table 7-8 lists the 5-year survival rates for the various stages of the Aster-Coller modification of the Dukes staging system; this does not take into account improvement in survival with adjuvant chemotherapy regimens.

Table 7-7. The Aster-Coller Modification of the Dukes Staging System

Stage	Depth of invasion	Lymph node status	Distant metastases
A	Invades submucosa	Negative	Absent
B1	Invades muscularis propria	Negative	Absent
B2	Invades serosa	Negative	Absent
B3	Imvades through bowel wall into adjacent organs	Negative	Absent
C1	Invades positive muscularis propria	Positive	Absent
C2	Invades positive serosa	Positive	Absent
C3	Invades through bowel wall into adjacent organs	Positive	Absent
D	Any depth of invasion	Positive or negative	Present

Table 7-8. Five-year Survival Rates for Aster-Coller Stages

Stage[a]	5-year survival (%)
A	95
B1	90
B2	78
B3	63
C1	74
C2	48
C3	38
D	<5

[a]See Table 7-7 for definition of stages.

8. *What should the follow-up consist of in patients with colon cancer after they have undergone primary surgical resection for curative intent?*

Routine scheduled follow-up is very important for the early detection of local and distant recurrences, as well as new primary colon cancer. Patients should be seen every 3 to 4 months for the first 3 years. Follow-up evaluation should include history, physical examination, liver function tests, measurement of the CEA level, and complete blood counts. A chest radiograph should be obtained yearly. CT scanning should be performed for further evaluation of rising liver function tests or CEA levels. After 3 years, the interval between these evaluations can be increased. Patients should undergo colonoscopy at 1-year intervals until they are found to be free of polyps, and then every 3 years after that.

9. *Are there any effective adjuvant treatments to decrease the risk of recurrence in patients with colon cancer who have undergone resection?*

Several studies have shown that 1 year of postoperative treatment with 5-fluorouracil and levamisole can decrease by 41% the likelihood of stage C colon cancer recurrence. The death rate in this setting was reduced by 33%. More recently, selected studies of 5-fluorouracil and leucovorin therapy have shown a decrease in both recurrence and death rates for patients with late stage B colon cancer (i.e., B2 or B3 lesions).

10. *Is there any effective chemotherapy for patients with metastatic disease?*

5-Fluorouracil with the addition of leucovorin, which modulates the activity of 5-fluorouracil, has led to an increase in the response rates in metastatic disease to 40% to 60%. Clinical trials still under way are assessing the most efficacious dose and schedule of combined 5-fluorouracil and leucovorin treatment.

Case   A 72-year-old white man is seen in the emergency room because of severe fatigue and vague abdominal discomfort. He has no significant past medical history other than slight anemia, which was noted during a physical examination 3 years ago. His hematocrit at that time was 37%, and white blood cell and platelet counts were normal. Physical examination was remarkable only for cachexia and a pale appearance. His initial laboratory values at the current time are as follows: white blood cell count, 7,800/mm^3; hemoglobin, 7 g/dL; hematocrit, 21%; platelets, 600,000/mm^3; MCV, 62 femtoliters; AST, 89 mU/mL (normal, 0 to 35 mU/mL); ALT, 129 mU/mL (normal, 0 to 38 mU/mL); alkaline phosphatase, 360 mU/mL (normal, 0 to 125 mU/mL); and total bilirubin, 0.7 mg/dL (normal, <1.0 mg/dL).

The patient is admitted to the hospital for blood transfusion and evaluation of his anemia. The admission chest radiograph shows numerous pulmonary nodules, and a barium enema examination reveals a near-obstructing lesion at the hepatic flexure. A CT scan of the liver depicts numerous low-density lesions in both lobes of the liver. Colonoscopy is performed, and this reveals a mucosal lesion at the hepatic flexure. Biopsy of this lesion reveals adenocarcinoma.

1. What is the cause of this patient's anemia?
2. Would earlier diagnosis of the cause of this patient's anemia have made any difference?
3. What type of treatment would you now advise for the lesion in the hepatic flexure of the colon?
4. Would you recommend any other treatments for the lesions in the lung or liver?
5. What stage is this patient's cancer?
6. What is the prognosis in this patient?

Case Discussion

1. *What is the cause of this patient's anemia?*

    The patient almost certainly has iron-deficiency anemia secondary to the chronic blood loss in the stool stemming from a bleeding colon cancer.
2. *Would earlier diagnosis of the cause of this patient's anemia have made any difference?*

    It is difficult to say whether an earlier diagnosis would have definitely made a difference. It should certainly have been possible to diagnose the colon cancer, and at an earlier stage the prognosis would likely have been better.
3. *What type of treatment would you now advise for the lesion in the hepatic flexure of the colon?*

    The patient needs to undergo a hemicolectomy to prevent obstruction. This is only for palliation and will not affect the overall prognosis.
4. *Would you recommend any other treatments for the lesions in the lung or liver?*

    This patient has metastatic disease and should be offered systemic chemotherapy consisting of 5-fluorouracil and leucovorin, which is the standard approach for metastatic colon cancer. The best doses and schedules of administration are yet to be determined. If at all possible, the patient should be enrolled in a clinical trial.
5. *What stage is this patient's cancer?*

    This patient clearly has metastatic disease, and thus is in stage D according to the Aster-Coller modification of the Dukes staging system.

6. *What is the prognosis in this patient?*

This patient has terminal, incurable cancer. He has approximately a 30% to 45% chance of responding to the combination of 5-fluorouracil and leucovorin. If he responds, he will likely live longer than if he does not respond. He has approximately a 25% to 30% chance of 1-year survival.

Suggested Readings

Midgley R, Kerr D. Colorectal cancer. *Lancet* 1999;353:391.

Steele G Jr. Combined-modality therapy for rectal carcinoma: the time has come. *N Engl J Med* 1991;324:764.

Steele G Jr, Bleday R, Mayer RJ, et al. A prospective evaluation of hepatic resection for colorectal carcinoma metastases to the liver: Gastrointestinal Tumor Study Group Protocol 6584. *J Clin Oncol* 1991;9:1105.

Steele G Jr, Burt R, Winawer SJ, eds. *Basic and clinical perspectives of colorectal polyps and cancer.* New York: Alan R. Liss, 1988.

Erythrocytosis

1. What is erythrocytosis?

2. What are the two major types of erythrocytosis?

3. What are some causes of secondary erythrocytosis due to appropriate erythropoietin secretion?

4. What are some causes of secondary erythrocytosis due to inappropriate erythropoietin secretion?

5. What is polycythemia vera?

6. What are the symptoms of polycythemia vera?

7. How is polycythemia vera diagnosed?

8. What is the likely length of survival in a patient with polycythemia vera?

9. What is the rare hepatic complication that can arise in patients with polycythemia vera?

Discussion

1. *What is erythrocytosis?*

A patient with a hematocrit greater than 55% that is not due to dehydration is considered to have an erythrocytosis. The chromium-151–labeled red blood cell measurement of the total red blood cell mass is, however, the gold standard for establishing the diagnosis.

2. *What are the two major types of erythrocytosis?*

When the elevated hematocrit is due to increased erythropoietin secretion, this constitutes secondary erythrocytosis. Primary erythrocytosis is caused by increased red blood cell production that does not stem from increased erythropoietin secretion.

3. *What are some causes of secondary erythrocytosis due to appropriate erythropoietin secretion?*

Any disorder that causes tissue hypoxia stimulates the renal production of erythropoietin. These disorders include arteriovenous shunts, chronic obstructive lung disease, living at high altitudes, or hemoglobin (Hb Chesapeake and methemoglobin) that does not release oxygen correctly. In relative erythrocytosis, the red blood cell mass is normal, and this occurs in the settings of dehydration or decreased plasma volume.

4. *What are some causes of secondary erythrocytosis due to inappropriate erythropoietin secretion?*

Many disease states can be associated with increased erythropoietin production. Diseased kidneys may secrete erythropoietin inappropriately or tumors may secrete hormones that function like erythropoietin. Renal, adrenal, or hepatic tumors, ovarian carcinoma, or benign uterine myomas all secrete erythropoietin-like substances. Other causes of increased erythropoietin secretion are hydronephrosis, renal cysts, or renal transplantation.

5. *What is polycythemia vera?*

Polycythemia vera is an absolute erythrocytosis secondary to the clonal expansion of red blood cells, making it a myeloproliferative disorder.

6. *What are the symptoms of polycythemia vera?*

Symptoms stem from vascular congestion or obstruction due to increased blood viscosity. Patients complain of headaches, itching and burning feet, or malaise. The retinal veins become engorged and hepatosplenomegaly may be present. The incidence of cardiovascular and cerebrovascular disease is increased in these patients because of the elevated blood viscosity.

7. *How is polycythemia vera diagnosed?*

An increased red blood cell mass, an oxygen saturation of 92% or more, and splenomegaly are the cardinal signs of polycythemia vera. If splenomegaly is not present, to be diagnosed with the disorder, the patient must have a platelet count that exceeds 400,000/mm^3, a white blood cell count greater than 12,000/mm^3, a cobalamin level of 900 pg/mL or greater, or an elevated neutrophil alkaline phosphatase score.

8. *What is the likely length of survival in a patient with polycythemia vera?*

Without treatment, half the patients die within 24 months, usually due to vascular disease. Phlebotomy to maintain a hematocrit of 45% can prolong the life span to over 6 years, and median survival in patients who receive radiation therapy is 12.5 years.

9. *What is the rare hepatic complication that can arise in patients with polycythemia vera?*

Budd-Chiari syndrome is an occlusion of the hepatic veins sometimes seen in patients with polycythemia vera and other diseases that increase blood viscosity. This causes right upper quadrant pain and elevations in the liver enzyme levels. It is very difficult to treat, and is best prevented by aggressively treating the erythrocytosis.

Case   A 55-year-old man who is a smoker and has hypertension sees his internist because of malaise and nasal stuffiness with a full sensation in his frontal sinuses.

On further questioning, the patient also describes having itchy, red feet that worsen in the shower. The patient has no shortness of breath with activity and does not snore or experience daytime drowsiness.

Physical examination reveals a plethoric patient who is in no acute distress. His lungs are clear to auscultation. His liver span is 18 cm and his spleen tip is palpable.

The following laboratory values are reported: hematocrit, 65%; white blood cell count, 8,500/mm³; platelets, 250,000/mm³; and differential: 50% segmented neutrophils, 30% lymphocytes, 5% basophils, and 10% monocytes.

Arterial blood gas determinations performed on room air reveal a partial pressure of oxygen of 65 mm Hg, a partial pressure of carbon dioxide of 38 mm Hg, and an oxygen saturation of 93%.

1. What is the diagnosis in this patient?
2. Why is it important to know whether the patient snores or experiences daytime drowsiness?
3. What is the cause of this patient's nasal stuffiness?
4. What should be the initial treatment in this patient?
5. What is this patient's prognosis?

Case Discussion

1. *What is the diagnosis in this patient?*

    This patient most likely has polycythemia vera. The oxygen saturation greater than 90% and the presence of splenomegaly support the diagnosis. A chromium-151–labeled red blood cell measurement of the red blood cell mass would confirm polycythemia, but is almost always high when the hematocrit is greater than 60%. The presence of mononuclear and basophilic cells also supports the diagnosis of a myeloproliferative disorder, which would be further supported by a bone marrow biopsy that shows trilinear hyperplasia.

2. *Why is it important to know whether the patient snores or experiences daytime drowsiness?*

    Snoring and daytime drowsiness are symptoms of sleep apnea, a cause of secondary erythrocytosis. Although phlebotomy can cure the patient's erythrocytosis, it cannot treat the nighttime hypoxia or sleep apnea, and the patient could go on to have right-sided heart failure.

3. *What is the cause of this patient's nasal stuffiness?*

    Although he may have a sinus infection, the nasal stuffiness is most likely due to increased blood viscosity.

4. *What should be the initial treatment in this patient?*

    Phlebotomy should be performed as soon as possible to decrease the hematocrit to 45% to 50%. The increased blood viscosity puts this patient with two other risk factors for atherosclerotic disease, smoking and hypertension, at risk for a stroke or cardiovascular accident.

5. *What is this patient's prognosis?*

Even with careful treatment of his erythrocytosis by phlebotomy and chemo-therapy, his life expectancy will probably be limited because of his smoking and hypertension.

Suggested Readings

Conley CL. Polycythemia vera, diagnosis and treatment. *Hosp Pract* 1987;22:107.

Ellis JT, Peterson P, Geller SA, et al. Studies of the bone marrow in polycythemia vera and the evolution of myelofibrosis and second hematologic malignancies. *Semin Hematol* 1986;23:144.

Murphy S. Diagnostic criteria and prognosis in polycythemia vera and essential thrombocytopenia. *Semin Hematol* 1999;36:9.

Schwarts RS. Polycythemia vera: chance, death, and mutability [Editorial]. *N Engl J Med* 1998;338:613.

Lymphomas

1. How and when does Hodgkin's disease typically present?
2. What is the relationship between the histologic patterns and the stage in Hodgkin's disease?
3. Of what should the staging evaluation in patients with Hodgkin's disease consist, and how do the findings have an impact on therapy?
4. What are the cure rates and the long-term sequelae of the treatment for Hodgkin's disease?
5. What are the known causes or diseases associated with the development of non-Hodgkin's lymphoma?
6. How does the National Cancer Institute classification of non-Hodgkin's lymphoma differ from the older Rappaport classification?
7. How does the biology of high-grade lymphoma differ from that of low-grade lymphoma, and how does this affect treatment and survival?
8. What type of lymphoma typically involves the skin, and how does this influence staging and treatment?
9. What population of patients is prone to acquiring secondary CNS lymphoma, and can this be prevented?
10. What complication of therapy can occur in the setting of rapidly growing tumors, and how can this be prevented?

Discussion

1. *How and when does Hodgkin's disease typically present?*

Hodgkin's disease typically presents in adolescence or young adulthood. However, a bimodal age distribution has been observed, especially in developed countries. The first peak is in adolescence or young adulthood, whereas the second peak occurs at 55 years of age. Interestingly, the risk of Hodgkin's disease correlates with the level of education.

Hodgkin's disease typically presents as a waxing and waning adenopathy, most commonly in the neck or supraclavicular area. Fifty percent of patients present with a mediastinal mass visible on chest radiography, and 40% present with B symptoms (fever, night sweats, and 10% weight loss in the preceding 6 months).

2. *What is the relationship between the histologic patterns and the stage in Hodgkin's disease?*

There are four distinct histologic patterns seen in Hodgkin's disease, all of which possess the Sternberg-Reed cell. The four histologic patterns and their prevalences are nodular sclerosis (70%), lymphocyte predominance (15%), mixed cellularity (10%), and lymphocyte depletion (5%).

Hodgkin's disease is staged according to the Ann Arbor classification:

Stage I. Involvement of a single lymph node region (I) or a single extralymphatic organ or site (I_E).

Stage II. Involvement of two or more lymph node regions on the same side of the diaphragm (II), or localized involvement of two or more extralymphatic organs or sites (II_E).

Stage III. Involvement of lymph node regions on both sides of the diaphragm (III), or localized involvement of an extralymphatic organ or site (III_E) or spleen (III_S), or both (III_{SE}). III_1 refers to involvement of lymph nodes in the upper abdomen; III_2 refers to involvement of lower abdominal nodes.

Stage IV. Diffuse or disseminated involvement of one or more extralymphatic organs, with or without associated lymph node involvement. The organ, or organs, involved may be identified by a symbol.

Also: A = asymptomatic; B = fever, night sweats, and weight loss exceeding 10% of the total body weight.

Hodgkin's disease spreads through contiguous lymph nodes; however, the spleen is commonly the only site of involvement in the abdomen, and its involvement is thought to be due to hematogenous spread.

Histologic progression in Hodgkin's disease involves the progressive loss of lymphocytes. For example, lymphocyte predominance can progress to mixed cellularity and eventually lymphocyte depletion. Those patients who present with nodular sclerosis may also experience some changes in histologic type, although most do not show obvious histologic progression. The histologic pattern also correlates with the stage of the disease, and thus the prognosis. Nodular sclerosis and lymphocyte predominance are more commonly seen in early disease (stages I and II). Therefore, these histologic patterns are associated with a better outcome. Mixed cellularity and lymphocyte depletion are associated with a poorer prognosis and are often seen in patients with advanced disease.

3. *Of what should the staging evaluation in patients with Hodgkin's disease consist, and how do the findings have an impact on therapy?*

The staging evaluation in patients with Hodgkin's disease includes a complete history and physical examination. Laboratory investigations should include a complete blood count and evaluation of the smear for changes indicating anemia, hemolysis, or abnormal white blood cells as well as a differential, determinations of the sedimentation rate and alkaline phosphatase level, and evaluation of liver and renal function. The radiologic evaluation should always include radiographic studies of the chest, abdomen, and pelvis and a CT scan of the abdomen and pelvis. Head or chest CT scans or bone marrow films should be obtained if symptoms are present. Bilateral lymphograms of the lower extremities are no longer routinely done but may be indicated in some patients even with the new-generation CT scanners.

A diagnosis based on tissue findings is a must. However, a diagnosis based on needle aspiration or cytologic findings is not adequate because the tissue obtained by these methods yields no information about the nodal architecture. It is preferable to obtain a lymph node or wedge of a large mass, but even then it may take more than one lymph node biopsy to document the presence of the disease if only reactive hyperplasia is seen. Bone marrow biopsy is a required part of the staging workup, particularly in symptomatic patients, but should not be substituted for the tissue examination because, again, the nodal architecture cannot be observed. The role of the staging laparotomy is controversial, however. General guidelines suggest performing a staging laparotomy if the results would affect the nature of therapy. This may happen in early stage disease (i.e., stages IB, IIB, and IIIA), when the findings from laparotomy could alter a decision to use radiation therapy alone.

The choice of therapy in patients with Hodgkin's disease is governed by stage. Patients with stage I and II disease can be treated with radiation therapy alone. If there is bulky disease, combined chemotherapy and irradiation should be used. For patients with stage III and IV disease, chemotherapy should be used with radiation delivered to sites of bulky disease. There is still some controversy about what is the best treatment for stage IIB and IIIA disease. Most therapeutic options have high remission rates, and frequently long-term side effects dictate choice.

4. *What are the cure rates and the long-term sequelae of the treatment for Hodgkin's disease?*

Combination chemotherapy and advances in radiation therapy have achieved overall cure rates of approximately 70% in patients with Hodgkin's disease. The cure rates seen for early-stage disease are greater, with a 95% long-term survival rate observed for patients with stage I disease. The great number of survivors has allowed long-term follow-up and a study of the effects of combination chemotherapy and radiation therapy.

Hodgkin's disease is associated with immunologic abnormalities involving changes in both lymphocyte function and humoral immunity. These defects are aggravated by treatment and this increases the risk of such infections as disseminated herpes zoster. This immune dysfunction can last for years after treatment. Treatment with chemotherapy is associated with an increased risk of secondary leukemia, which is further increased in patients older than 40 years of age, heavily treated patients (both chemotherapy and radiation therapy), and patients who undergo prolonged therapy with alkylating agents.

The sequelae of the therapy for Hodgkin's disease are various. It is important to be aware of them, but also important that therapy not be severely modified (i.e., a lower dosage of either chemotherapy or radiation therapy) to minimize risk, because attempting to minimize the risk in this manner may compromise cure.

5. *What are the known causes or diseases associated with the development of non-Hodgkin's lymphoma?*

The risk of lymphoma is increased in patients with certain connective tissue and immunologic disorders. These include Klinefelter's syndrome, acquired hypogammaglobulinemia, Chediak-Higashi syndrome, iatrogenic immunosuppression, ataxia-telangiectasia syndrome, Sjögren's syndrome, Wiskott-Aldrich syndrome, rheumatoid arthritis and systemic lupus erythematosus, Swiss-type agammaglobulinemia, common variable immunodeficiency disease, acquired immunodeficiency syndrome, and the X-linked lymphoproliferative syndrome.

A viral etiology of lymphoma has been proposed, but no clear proof of this exists. Nevertheless, certain types of lymphoma have been associated with a viral etiology (e.g., Burkitt's lymphoma and Epstein-Barr virus). The search to establish a viral cause has implicated oncogenes, leading to the identification of various cytogenetic abnormalities in lymphoma. The common pattern is for a known oncogene to be translocated into an immunoglobulin gene locus. The common translocations are listed in Table 7-9.

6. *How does the National Cancer Institute working formulation of non-Hodgkin's lymphoma differ from the older classifications?*

The non-Hodgkin's lymphomas are classified according to histologic type. In the past, the most commonly used scheme was the Rappaport classification, but, as a greater understanding of the immune system was acquired, newer classifications were developed. The newer Working Formulation is based on the morphologic features of each type of lymphoma. This classification divides the lymphomas into three major subgroups: low grade, intermediate grade, and high grade. Thus, the lymphomas are classified according to both their morphologic features and their behavior. The classification is shown in Table 7-10.

7. *How does the biology of high-grade lymphoma differ from that of low-grade lymphoma, and how does this affect treatment and survival?*

High-grade non-Hodgkin's lymphoma is a group of diseases that behave aggressively, especially compared with the behavior typical of low-grade non-Hodgkin's lymphoma or Hodgkin's disease. The mean survival in patients with high-grade disease who do not respond to therapy is 2 years, whereas patients with low-grade disease can live for up to 10 years.

Table 7-9. Common Translocations in Patients with Lymphoma

Translocation	Histologic type of lymphoma
t(8;14) chromosome	Burkitt's and non-Burkitt's
t(2;8) chromosome	Burkitt's and non-Burkitt's
t(8;22) chromosome	Burkitt's and non-Burkitt's
t(14;18) chromsome	Follicular lymphoma

Table 7-10. Classification of Lymphomas: National Cancer Institute
Working Formulation

Low grade
  Small lymphocytic consistent with chronic lymphocytic leukemia
  Follicular, predominantly small cleaved cell
  Follicular mixed, small cleaved plus large cell
Intermediate grade
  Follicular, predominantly large cell
  Diffuse small cleaved cell
  Diffused mixed, small cleaved and large cell
  Diffused large cell (cleaved and noncleaved cell)
High grade
  Large cell immunoblastic
  Lymphoblastic (convoluted and nonconvoluted cell)
  Small noncleaved cell (Burkitt's and non-Burkitt's)

Patients with high-grade lymphoma can present with localized disease (<20%), but more commonly are in an advanced stage. There can be involvement of either extranodal (35%) or privileged sites (the CNS or testes). Most disease is of B-cell origin (85%), with the remainder of T-cell origin.

Poor prognostic factors include poor performance status, bulky disease (>10 cm), high LDH level (>500 IU/dL), bone marrow involvement, and B symptoms.

High-grade non-Hodgkin's lymphomas are very sensitive to chemotherapy, and aggressive treatment offers the only chance for cure. Up to 60% of patients can be cured with the newer chemotherapy regimens. This is in sharp contrast to the experience with low-grade lymphomas, in which cure rates of less than 20% are seen and survival does not seem to be affected by the type of response to chemotherapy.

8. *What type of lymphoma typically involves the skin, and how does this influence staging and treatment?*

Lymphomatous involvement of the skin is commonly seen in the setting of T-cell lymphoma. It occurs in approximately 10% of all cases of non-Hodgkin's lymphoma, and this group of diseases is called *cutaneous T-cell lymphoma* (CTCL). The low-grade form of CTCL is mycosis fungoides or Sezáry syndrome. Sezáry syndrome is diagnosed in the setting of mycosis fungoides when the malignant cells (Sezáry cells) are found in the peripheral blood.

The staging classification for CTCL differs from that for other forms of non-Hodgkin's lymphoma, and is based on the TNM system, as shown in Table 7-11.

The mainstay of management of early mycosis fungoides and Sezáry syndrome has been topical treatment, but there is little evidence that this prolongs survival. Treatment trials have included systemic chemotherapy as well in the hope of improving survival.

9. *What population of patients is prone to acquiring secondary CNS lymphoma, and can this be prevented?*

Central nervous system involvement is rarely seen in patients with low-grade lymphoma. When seen, a histologic transformation to high-grade lymphoma

Table 7-11. National Cutaneous T-Cell Lymphoma Workshop Staging Classification[a]

T	Skin	N	Lymph nodes	M	Visceral organs
T1	Limited plaques (<10% body surface area)	N0	No adenopathy, histology negative	M0	No involvement
T2	Generalized plaques	N1	Adenopathy; histology negative	M1	
T3	Cutaneous tumors	N2	No adenopathy; histology positive		
T4	Generalized erythroderma	N3	Adenopathy; histology positive		

Stage I. Limited (IA) or generalized (IB) plaques without adenopathy or histologic involvement of lymph nodes or viscera (T1 N0 M0 or T2 N0 M0).

Stage II. Limited or generalized plaques with adenopathy (IIA) or cutaneous tumors with or without adenopathy (IIB); without histologic involvement of lymph nodes or viscera (T1–2 N1 M0 or T2 N0–1 M0).

Stage III. Generalized erythroderma with or without adenopathy; without histologic involvement of lymph nodes or viscera (T4 N0–2 M0).

Stage IV. Histologic involvement of lymph nodes (IVA) or viscera (IVB) with any skin lesion and with or without adenopathy (T1–4 N2–3 M0 for IVA; T1–4 N0–3 M1 for IVB).

[a]Blood involvement should be recorded as absent (B0) or present (B1) but is not currently used to determine final stage.

should be suspected. Within this group, CNS involvement is more common when Waldeyer's tonsillar ring, the bone marrow, or the testes are affected. Among the high-grade lymphomas, there is a group of especially aggressive lymphomas, and these consist of undifferentiated lymphomas (Burkitt's and non-Burkitt's type), lymphoblastic lymphoma, and acute T-cell lymphoma. The incidence of CNS involvement is high in these patients and, therefore the CNS should be treated prophylactically with intrathecal chemotherapy.

10. *What complication of therapy can occur in the setting of rapidly growing tumors, and how can this be prevented?*

The tumor lysis syndrome can occur in the setting of tumors that are exquisitely sensitive to chemotherapy and is seen when there is a large tumor burden. The syndrome is characterized by hyperuricacidemia, hyperphosphatemia, hyperkalemia, and hypocalcemia, and can result in acute renal failure and sudden death if not treated. Fortunately, if the signs are carefully watched for, the patient can be spared its effects. The management of this syndrome includes aggressive hydration, the alkalinization of urine, and allopurinol therapy before and continuing through chemotherapy.

Case

A 42-year-old woman is referred to you by her family physician for the evaluation of bilateral neck adenopathy. She has noticed this swelling intermittently for approximately 6 months. She has occasionally noticed axillary node swelling but denies any other adenopathy. She has noticed that she tires more easily and seems to "pick up every little virus." She admits to experiencing occasional early satiety, but denies any increase in abdominal girth or changes in bowel habits. She denies any fever, chills, night sweats, weight loss, or change in appetite.

Her family history is remarkable for a mother with breast cancer (the patient's last mammogram 1 year ago was normal). She does not smoke or drink.

Physical examination findings are remarkable for bilateral neck and axillary adenopathy. She has no oral or pharyngeal lesions and no breast masses. Her spleen is mildly enlarged but her liver size is normal. She has no other physical abnormalities.

Laboratory findings are remarkable for a mild normochromic, normocytic anemia (hemoglobin, 13.0 g/dL; hematocrit, 39%); the platelet count is 250,000/mm³; and the white blood cell count is 5,200/mm³ with a normal differential. A chemistry panel is remarkable for a slightly elevated LDH level, but the AST, ALT, bilirubin, and alkaline phosphatase values are normal. Her chest radiographic study is normal.

A staging evaluation is done and reveals the following findings. Tissue analysis reveals malignant lymphoma consisting of follicular small cleaved (nodular poorly differentiated) cells that are CD20 positive. Bone marrow biopsy reveals normal cellularity with lymphoid follicles (normal for age), a slight increase in the number of erythroid precursors, normal megakaryocytes, and a decrease in the iron content. Cytogenetic examination identifies a balanced translocation, t(14;18). CT scan of the abdomen depicts moderate splenomegaly and mild retroperitoneal adenopathy. Serum immunoelectrophoresis reveals mild hypogammaglobulinemia with a monoclonal IgM spike.

1. Based on the physical examination and laboratory findings, what is the differential diagnosis in this patient?
2. Based on the findings from the staging evaluation, what stage of non-Hodgkin's lymphoma is this patient in, and what are her treatment options and prognosis?
3. What are the implications of her cytogenetic abnormalities?
4. Is it necessary further to evaluate or treat her hypogammaglobulinemia?
5. What is the significance of the monoclonal IgM spike in this patient?

   The patient is observed to do fine at her 6-month visits, until 4 years later, when painful and enlarging nodes develop.

6. What form of therapy would you offer her when the painful and enlarging nodes are detected, and what outcome can she expect?

   With the onset of therapy consisting of oral alkylating agents, a severe anemia develops in this patient, requiring transfusion.

7. How would you evaluate the anemia that develops with the alkylating agent therapy?

   The results of investigations performed to determine the source of her anemia are as follows: Coombs' direct and indirect test, positive; reticulocyte count, 9%; blood smear, spherocytes and increased reticulocytes; and bone marrow biopsy, increased cellularity with erythroid hyperplasia plus the presence of small lymphocytes, suggesting lymphomatous involvement.

8. Based on the findings yielded by the investigations for her anemia, what are the treatment options at this point?

   This patient does well for 6 months with monthly intravenous chemotherapy and immunoglobulin therapy, as needed. Two years after the start of therapy, increased splenomegaly develops that appears refractory to the previous chemotherapy.

9. With the appearance of increased splenomegaly, what is the differential diagnosis, and how should you confirm it?

10. What are the treatment options in this patient whose disease is now in an advanced stage?

Case Discussion

1. *Based on the physical and laboratory findings, what is the differential diagnosis in this patient?*

    The neck adenopathy in this patient can represent a normal finding; 50% of patients can have nodes that are less than 0.5 cm in diameter. It can also signify acute infection stemming from acute viral infections, mononucleosis, toxoplasmosis, or pulmonary infections, but usually in this setting the nodes are firm and tender and usually recede within 2 to 4 weeks. Solid tumors are also a consideration in the differential diagnosis, and include head and neck cancer, as well as thymic, lung, and breast cancer; lung and breast cancers are more commonly associated with supraclavicular and axillary adenopathy. A fourth possibility is Hodgkin's disease or non-Hodgkin's lymphoma. Patients with lymphoma can have lymph nodes that "come and go."

2. *Based on the findings from the staging evaluation, what stage of non-Hodgkin's lymphoma is this patient in, and what are her treatment options and prognosis?*

    Non-Hodgkin's lymphoma is staged according to the Ann Arbor classification used for Hodgkin's disease. According to this system's criteria, this patient has stage III disease. In the setting of low-grade lymphoma, it is important to identify localized versus disseminated disease as well as any poor prognostic factors. This patient has disease above and below the diaphragm as well as probable splenic involvement. She does not clearly have bone marrow involvement, because lymphoid follicles can be a benign finding.

    In light of these findings, her prognosis is fairly good. The median survival for both treated and untreated follicular small cleaved lymphoma can be up to 8 years. The initial treatment for advanced low-grade lymphoma is very controversial. It responds to both single- and multiple-agent chemotherapy as well as radiation therapy, but there is no overwhelming evidence that early treatment prolongs survival. Attempts to eradicate disease with high-dose chemotherapy (with or without bone marrow rescue) have not been shown to prolong overall survival. It would not be unreasonable to wait until this patient becomes symptomatic before starting treatment.

3. *What are the implications of her cytogenetic abnormalities?*

    The t(14;18) abnormality is a common finding in the setting of follicular small cleaved lymphoma. In this abnormality, the *bc12* oncogene on chromosome 18 has been translocated to the immunoglobulin heavy chain locus on chromosome 14. It is now widely accepted that this abnormality is found in all patients with this histologic pattern. It is also found in approximately 30% of patients with diffuse lymphoma, and, in these cases, it probably represents a histologic transformation from follicular small cleaved lymphoma, and can therefore be considered a poor prognostic indicator. It is not a prognostic factor in the setting of follicular small cleaved lymphoma. The presence of CD20 surface antigen documents that this is a B-cell lymphoma. This finding also predicts that patients will respond to new biologic therapy with anti-CD20 antibodies.

4. *Is it necessary further to evaluate or treat her hypogammaglobulinemia?*

Hypogammaglobulinemia is occasionally found in association with low-grade lymphoma and chronic lymphocytic leukemia. It is not often a problem, as it is in multiple myeloma, but this immunologic defect should be remembered when infections occur in these patients or when neutropenia is precipitated by treatment or bone marrow involvement. Patients with life-threatening infections may benefit from gamma globulin therapy. To date, however, there is no clear role for prophylactic gamma globulin therapy in the prevention of hypogammaglobulinemia associated with lymphoma or leukemia.

5. *What is the significance of the monoclonal IgM spike in this patient?*

Although the size of the spike is not given, it is still important information because of the possibility of hyperviscosity associated with IgM, unlike IgG, for which hyperviscosity is far less likely. Waldenström's macroglobulinemia is associated with lymphoma, and is usually seen in patients with diffuse small lymphocytic lymphoma. A monoclonal gammopathy can affect up to 15% of the patients with low-grade lymphoma and is most commonly seen when the cells have plasmacytoid features.

6. *What form of therapy would you offer her when the painful and enlarging nodes are detected, and what outcome can she expect?*

The decision of when to treat low-grade non-Hodgkin's lymphoma is, as already mentioned, a controversial issue. Most physicians recommend waiting until symptoms appear, consisting of rapidly enlarging nodes, B symptoms, cytopenias due to bone marrow involvement, or an increased adenopathy that threatens organ function.

If the symptomatic disease is localized, radiation therapy that focuses on the site involved is a viable option. For the management of more generalized disease, a single alkylating agent with or without steroids can be very effective. More aggressive combination chemotherapy can also be considered. This form of therapy is clearly more toxic and, although it improves the duration of the disease-free survival, it has not been proved to extend the overall survival period.

In determining the likely outcome of treatment in this patient, complete remissions can be achieved in the setting of low-grade lymphoma, mostly for localized (stage I and II) disease. "Spontaneous remission" can also occur (approximately 5% to 10%). The cure rate for advanced low-grade lymphoma is very low. Even with the institution of aggressive chemotherapy (see earlier), less than 10% of affected patients remain disease free after 5 years.

7. *How would you evaluate the anemia that develops with the alkylating agent therapy?*

During this patient's initial evaluation, she was noted to have a mild anemia with a slight increase in erythroid precursors. Her LDH level was elevated, but her liver enzyme values were normal. In this case, the raised LDH level could represent either a high turnover of tumor cells or the destruction of red blood cells (hemolysis), or both. The slight elevation in the number of red blood cells could also be due to peripheral destruction. This patient should undergo a complete assessment of her anemia, including evaluation for hemolysis; iron, cobalamin, and folate deficiency; and bone marrow involvement by lymphoma, which is an unlikely cause in this setting.

8. *Based on the findings yielded by the investigations for her anemia, what are the treatment options at this point?*

This patient has hemolytic anemia. It is more commonly seen with chronic lymphocytic leukemia (the leukemia phase of follicular small cleaved lymphoma). Often patients have an underlying compensated hemolysis, as this patient did, with anemia, increased erythroids, and an increased LDH level. Beginning the treatment with chemotherapy can unmask the hemolysis because the bone marrow response is retarded by marrow suppressive agents.

The treatment for hemolytic anemia in this setting has two goals: (a) to terminate the hemolytic process, and (b) to treat the underlying disease. Treatment with steroids can address both problems and is considered the standard of care. If the hemolysis is not stopped with high-dose steroids, immunoglobulin therapy should be started. Once the hemolysis is controlled, the same or a more aggressive chemotherapy regimen may be implemented.

9. *With the appearance of increased splenomegaly, what is the differential diagnosis, and how should you confirm it?*

The increased splenomegaly that does not respond to the chemotherapy previously used may represent a transformation to a more aggressive histologic type of lymphoma. This occurs at a rate of approximately 8% per year in patients with follicular small cleaved lymphoma; usually the transformation is to a diffuse large cell lymphoma. Histologic transformation represents a change in the natural history of the disease and signifies a much shortened survival.

Histologic transformation should be documented by tissue examination. Again, a lymph node or mass is the best source of tissue for this purpose.

10. *What are the treatment options in this patient whose disease is now in an advanced stage?*

When histologic transformation occurs, the prognosis is very poor and patients respond poorly to even the most aggressive chemotherapy regimens. In older patients who have concurrent disease, it may be reasonable to use only palliative measures (pain management) and perhaps administer local radiation therapy if needed.

Suggested Readings

Bennett CL, Armitage JL, Armitage GO, et al. Costs of care and outcomes for high-dose therapy and autologous transplantation for lymphoid malignancies: results from the University of Nebraska 1987 through 1991. *J Clin Oncol* 1995;13:969.

Canellos G. Is there an effective salvage therapy for advanced Hodgkin's disease? *Ann Oncol* 1991;2:1.

DeVita VT Jr, Hubbard SM, Longo DL. Treatment of Hodgkin's disease. *J Natl Cancer Inst* 1990;10:19.

Hancock SL, Hoppe RT. Long-term complications of treatment and causes of mortality after Hodgkin's disease. *Seminars in Radiation Oncology* 1996;6:225.

Koh HK, Foss FM, eds. Cutaneous T-cell lymphoma. *Hematol Oncol Clin North Am* 1995;9:943.

National Cancer Institute. Summary and description of a working formulation for clinical usage: the Non-Hodgkin's Lymphoma Pathologic Classification Project. *Cancer* 1982;49:2112.

Waldmann TA, Davis MM, Bongiovanni KF, Korsmeyer SJ. Rearrangements of genes for the antigen receptor on T cells as markers of lineage and clonality in human lymphoid neoplasms. *N Engl J Med* 1985;313:776.

Young RC, Longo DL, Glatstein E, et al. The treatment of indolent lymphomas: watchful waiting v aggressive combined modality treatment. *Semin Hematol* 1988;25:11.

Lung Cancer

1. What are the approximate incidence, death rate, and risk factors for lung cancer?
2. What are the two pathologic categories of lung cancer, and their histologic features?
3. What are some clinical features that may suggest a correlation with a certain pathologic subtype?
4. What is essentially the mainstay of curative therapy in non-small cell lung cancer (NSCLC)?
5. How does the staging and treatment of small cell lung cancer (SCLC) differ from that of NSCLC?
6. What are the two major determinants of prognosis for both NSCLC and SCLC?

Discussion

1. *What are the approximate incidence, death rate, and risk factors for lung cancer?*

   Each year, lung cancer kills more men and women in the United States than any other cancer, and there are approximately 150,000 new cases of lung cancer diagnosed each year. At the time of diagnosis, only 35% of patients have local disease; thus, the disease has spread to regional nodes or distant sites in 65%. However, even in patients with nonmetastatic (local) disease, complete cure is the exception; therefore, the yearly mortality rate approaches the annual incidence, and this was estimated to be 136,000 in 1987.

   Nearly 90% of all patients diagnosed with lung cancer have a smoking history, and the causal relationship between tobacco use and lung cancer makes it a major public health problem and one of the most potentially preventable diseases. Other important risk factors account for less than 10% of cases of lung cancer diagnosed, and these include uranium and radon exposure and passive smoking. The risk of acquiring lung cancer falls significantly in the first 5 years after the cessation of smoking, and, after 20 years, is equal to that in people who have never smoked.

To illustrate the seriousness of the public health problem, the lung cancer incidence has risen by 40% in women between 1940 and 1984, from 7 to 35 per 100,000, and this is mainly due to the increased use of tobacco use in the female population. In addition, a higher-than-expected incidence of lung cancer has been seen in women in the lower pack-year categories, suggesting that women are acquiring lung cancer at a younger age and after smoking fewer years than men.

Furthermore, although overall tobacco use is decreasing in the United States, smoking may be increasing among certain groups of minorities and adolescents, and recent tobacco company advertising campaigns have been directed toward these groups. The years of potential lost life resulting from lung cancer mortality in these groups is probably twice that seen for the remaining population.

2. *What are the two pathologic categories of lung cancer, and their histologic features?*

For both treatment and prognostic purposes, most lung cancers are divided into two clinically useful categories: SCLC, which accounts for 25% of all lung cancers, and NSCLC, which consists of squamous cell carcinomas (40% of the lung cancers), adenocarcinomas (25% of the lung cancers), and large cell carcinomas (10% of the lung cancers).

3. *What are some clinical features that may suggest a correlation with a certain pathologic subtype?*

Patients may present with a variety of symptoms, including cough, hemoptysis, shortness of breath, chest pain, or unexplained weight loss (Table 7-12). Abnormalities revealed by the physical examination may suggest the diagnosis and include signs of lung consolidation resulting from an obstructed bronchus, supraclavicular adenopathy stemming from the local and regional spread of the cancer, or Horner's syndrome, which is due to tumor impingement on the sympathetic nerve fibers that course near the apex of the lung.

Laboratory examination may reveal the presence of hyponatremia due to the syndrome of inappropriate antidiuretic hormone secretion (SIADH); this is a paraneoplastic syndrome caused by inappropriate vasopressin secretion,

Table 7-12. Signs and Symptoms of Lung Cancer

Signs and symptoms	% of patients
Routine chest radiographic study (asymptomatic)	16
Hemoptysis	30
Cough	25
Dyspnea	11
Pneumonitis	8
Pain	6
Wheezing	2
Dysphagia	1
Hoarseness	0.5
Systemic symptoms—weight loss	0.5

and is seen most often in the setting of SCLC. The hyponatremia that presumably results from SIADH can be demonstrated in up to 60% of the patients with SCLC by administering a water load. Cushing's syndrome may develop secondary to the excessive production of adrenocorticotropic hormone by the tumor, and, again, is most commonly seen in SCLC. Both the absolute and ionized serum calcium levels may be high, and this can be due to multiple reasons, including metastases to bone as well as the production of a parathyroid hormone–like substance from the cancer. Hypercalcemia is most often seen in patients with squamous (epidermoid) lung cancer, but may be associated with any histologic subtype. The location of the tumor on chest radiographic studies as well as certain laboratory findings can suggest certain histologic types. Squamous cell carcinomas and SCLCs tend to be found centrally on the chest radiography. Squamous cell lung cancer tends to cavitate, and this can be seen on chest radiographs. Adenocarcinoma tends to occur peripherally in the lung, and this is the most common lung cancer in those who have never smoked.

Although these clinically useful associations cannot establish a diagnosis, they can help the oncologist direct the nature of the evaluation, both before and after the histologic type is known.

4. *What is essentially the mainstay of curative therapy in NSCLC?*

Significant cure rates for NSCLC are achieved only for complete surgical resection of nonmetastatic disease. The staging process defines the extent of disease spread, and the stage correlates with the resectability, and hence with the cure rates and survival. No cures are seen for the current form of chemotherapy, and cure is uncommon with radiation therapy (approximately 5% of stage III cases).

In all cases in which resection is performed with curative intent, the decision to go ahead with this is based on the expectation that no gross residual disease will remain at the conclusion of the procedure. This involves multiple preoperative decisions, including (a) verifying that the patient's lung function can tolerate obligate resection of some normal lung; (b) ensuring there is no pulmonary or extrapulmonary disease that would preclude major surgery and general anesthesia; and (c) accurately staging the extent of disease to select only those patients with a reasonable chance of complete resection. Even with these considerations, however, overall only 10% of all patients with NSCLC survive 5 years, and less than half of patients who undergo successful resection remain free of disease at 5 years.

At present, only stage I and II, and some stage III, patients are considered good candidates for resection with a reasonable chance of cure. This means the tumor cannot be associated with malignant effusion, cannot have spread to contralateral mediastinal lymph nodes, and cannot have metastasized to any distant site. The usual sites of distant metastases in patients with lung cancer include the adrenal glands, bone, brain, lung, lymph nodes, and pleura. Less common sites of metastases are the skin and bone marrow.

The standard treatment for stage IIIb patients (i.e., those without distant metastases but with unresectable and locally advanced disease) is radiation therapy to a total dose of 55 to 60 Gy. Only 4% to 8% of these patients are alive at 5 years, which represents a small fraction of cures (up to 5%). Stage IV patients are those with distant metastases and, by and large, treatment in this setting is for palliation only and consists mostly of chemotherapy using cisplatin-based regimens.

5. *How does the staging and treatment of SCLC differ from that of NSCLC?*

Small cell lung carcinoma differs markedly from the other pathologic types of lung cancer in terms of its natural history, cell biology, and response to therapy, and is distinct from NSCLC. SCLC has a rapid clinical course, and the median survival in untreated patients is only 2 months for metastatic and 4 months for localized disease. Based on autopsy data, 98% of patients with SCLC have distant metastases at the time of diagnosis. This includes the 30% who at diagnosis have no evidence of distant metastases according to the results of the usual staging procedures.

For practical reasons, SCLC is further defined as either limited or extensive. In limited disease, the tumor is confined to the hemothorax of origin and regional lymph nodes, and can be encompassed in a tolerable radiation therapy field. In extensive disease, tumor exists beyond these bounds, usually distant metastases. Surgery (other than for diagnostic biopsy) has no role in the management of SCLC because even most of the patients with limited disease have subclinical distant metastases; complete response rates to chemotherapy in SCLC are as high as 40% to 70%, with complete plus partial response rates as high as 80% to 85%, and survival in the setting of untreated disease is dismal. Instead, most patients should receive combination chemotherapy. With six or more courses of chemotherapy, approximately 10% of patients with limited disease can expect to be alive at 5 years, and these represent probable cures. The current standard of therapy includes irradiation of the involved areas as well as chemotherapy to decrease the chances of relapse locally.

In patients with extensive disease who undergo chemotherapy, the partial plus complete response rates can range from 50% to 85% and the median survival can range from 7 to 11 months; however, there are only anecdotal reports of cure at 5 years.

6. *What are the two major determinants of prognosis for both NSCLC and SCLC?*

For both SCLC and NSCLC, the prognosis depends on (a) the tumor extent (graded as limited or extensive in SCLC and as stage I to IV in NSCLC) and (b) the performance status of the patient. Better responses to therapy and certainly more significant cure rates are seen in patients with lower-stage lung cancers. In addition, the performance status [usually measured by the Karnofsky performance status scale or the Southwest Oncology Group (SWOG) scale] is a major predictor of response to therapy and survival. Patients who are symptomatic or, more significantly, nonambulatory (as indicated by their performance status) are less likely to respond to therapy and have shorter survivals. The performance status scales most often used by clinicians are given in Table 7-13.

Table 7-13. Karnofsky and Zubrod Performance Status Scales

Definition	Karnosfky scale (%)	Zubrod scale
Normal; no complaints; no evidence of disease	100	0
Able to carry on normal activity; minor signs or symptoms of disease	90	1
Normal activity with effort; some signs or symptoms of disease (no special care needed; fully ambulatory)	80	1
Cares for self but unable to carry on normal activity (unable to work; in bed <50%/day)	70	2
Requires occasional assistance but is able to care for most needs (in bed >50%/day but not bedridden)	60	2
Requires considerable assistance and frequent medical care	50	3
Disabled; requires special care and assistance	40	3
Bedridden	30	4
Very sick; hospitalization necessary	20	4
Moribund	10	4
Dead	0	4

Case 1   A 56-year-old real estate broker with a 76 pack-year history of tobacco use (he has smoked two packs of cigarettes per day since 18 years of age) has been followed regularly by his physician. He undergoes yearly chest radiographic studies, and the most recent radiographs obtained 8 months earlier were normal. He is seen by his physician because of 10 days of hemoptysis, consisting of blood-tinged sputum production, in the setting of a chronic cough. He denies weight loss, chest pain, and bone pain, and he experiences no increased dyspnea on exertion. On examination, his lungs are found to be clear; there is neither hepatosplenomegaly nor clubbing and the neurologic findings are grossly nonfocal. Laboratory studies show normal liver function, a calcium level of 11.1 mg/dL, and an albumin level of 3.9 g/dL. His complete blood count is normal. A chest radiographic study demonstrates a new, 2 × 3 cm, right hilar mass.

1. What diagnostic tests should be performed in this patient?
2. Was a yearly chest radiographic study a reasonable screening procedure for this man who smokes, or should this have been done more frequently?
3. What clinical finding suggests (although does not establish) the histologic type of this patient's lung cancer, and what type is it?
4. What stage of lung cancer is this patient in, and what further studies should be performed?
5. If the patient has stage II NSCLC, what is the appropriate treatment?
6. What further measures can be taken to reduce the patient's risk of death from lung cancer?

Case Discussion

1. *What diagnostic tests should be performed in this patient?*
    Most lung cancers are diagnosed on the basis of the findings yielded by

bronchoscopic biopsy of a lung mass. In some situations, however, there is an easier source of tissue. For example, biopsy of an abnormal (palpable) supraclavicular lymph node, if present, will likely yield tissue adequate for histologic study as well as for staging purposes, and the information gained is important to planning treatment.

The clinician must be wary of initial diagnoses of malignancy based on the findings revealed by the fine-needle aspiration (FNA) technique. This method obtains either only single cells or small clumps of cells for cytologic study within the aspirate, and it is almost always difficult or impossible to determine an exact pathologic diagnosis based on the information revealed. FNA biopsy should usually be reserved for confirmation of metastases or recurrences after an initial diagnosis has already been made. In most cases, bronchoscopic biopsy obtains tissue adequate for histologic examination.

Sometimes patients present with symptoms stemming from metastatic disease, and the source of a primary tumor is not as clear as it is in this patient. In such an event, correlation of the pathologic characteristics with the likely sources of the primary cancer can suggest the further radiologic and diagnostic tests to perform to determine the origin of the tumor.

2. *Was a yearly chest radiographic study a reasonable screening procedure for this man who smokes, or should this have been done more frequently?*

Because lung cancer (both NSCLC and SCLC) cure rates are significant only in the setting of earlier-stage disease (stage I and II NSCLC and limited-stage SCLC), it seems reasonable that earlier detection would increase the percentage of cures. In several randomized, controlled trials, mass screening using roentgenographic and sputum cytology has been done in 31,360 high-risk patients (men 45 years of age or older who smoked at least one pack of cigarettes per day). These studies have all shown that intensive screening can detect early lung cancer, but that 45% to 60% of patients so identified actually have stage II or III disease, for whom the 5-year survival rate is 15%. Investigators at all three centers contend that the mortality rates for lung cancer do not differ significantly between the screening group and the control group. Thus, at this time there is no justification for the large-scale application of these screening methods, even in high-risk populations.

The American Cancer Society no longer recommends yearly screening chest radiographic studies in the smoking population, and no study findings support more frequent screening chest roentgenography to decrease the mortality.

3. *What clinical finding suggests (although does not establish) the histologic type of this patient's lung cancer, and what type is it?*

This patient's chest radiograph revealed the lung mass to be central (hilar) in location. The two common tumor types typically found in this location are squamous (epidermoid) cell carcinoma (a type of NSCLC) and SCLC, although biopsy findings are needed to establish the diagnosis. The high calcium value is most often seen with squamous cell carcinoma.

4. *What stage of lung cancer is this patient in, and what further studies should be performed?*

According to the current American Joint Committee on Cancer (TNM) staging system, the stage of this patient's cancer is T2 NX MX (tumor 3 cm in greatest dimension, nodal status unknown, and unknown metastases).

In the setting of NSCLC, normal liver function test results (including aminotransferases, alkaline phosphatase, LDH, and γ-glutamyl transpeptidase) predict reasonably well that no liver metastases will be found on a radionuclide or CT scan. In this patient, a CT scan of the chest should be obtained to evaluate the hilar and mediastinal nodes, and the examination can easily be extended through the liver and adrenals. If the CT findings and the alkaline phosphatase level are normal, and because the patient has no bone pain, these would predict no bone metastases, making a bone scan unnecessary. If findings from a thorough neurologic examination performed by a consulting neurologist are normal, CT scanning of the head can be deferred. In this setting, the patient would clinically be in stage II, graded T2 N0 M0.

5. *If the patient has stage II NSCLC, what is the appropriate treatment?*

For stage II NSCLC, surgical excision (lobectomy or pneumonectomy) with intent of cure is the treatment of choice. If the arterial blood gas values, pulmonary function tests, electrocardiogram, and past medical history indicate the patient has no excess risk for major surgery, a thoracic surgeon is then consulted. Because the patient may still have spread of cancer to the mediastinal or hilar nodes (and not seen on a CT scan as being abnormal), which would make his cancer unresectable, mediastinoscopy should be performed and the mediastinal nodes on the right and left should be sampled for biopsy.

If these findings are negative, a right upper lobectomy through a lateral thoracotomy can be performed with subsequent pathologic study. If, for instance, a 2.8 × 3.2-cm tumor with two peribronchial nodes positive for squamous cell lung cancer is encountered at operation, the patient is in pathologic stage II, designated T2 N1 M0, and his overall chance of 5-year survival ranges from 15% to 30%. If the patient is found to have a pathologic stage I tumor, the 5-year survival would approach 40% to 50%, mostly representing cures.

6. *What further measures can be taken to reduce the patient's risk of death from lung cancer?*

Even patients surgically cured of their lung cancer have a significant chance of acquiring subsequent lung cancers, as well as other tumors. As with those in whom tumors have not yet developed, cessation of smoking can significantly reduce subsequent risk, and this patient should be strongly advised to do so.

Case 2 A 68-year-old woman presents to the emergency room because of a new-onset grand mal seizure. She is lethargic, but neurologic findings are otherwise normal. A head CT scan reveals a 2-cm right parietal and a 0.5-cm left occipital enhancing mass, and a chest radiographic study reveals a 4-cm left hilar mass with distal atelectasis. She has smoked one pack of cigarettes per day for 40 years, but quit 1 month ago. Anticonvulsants are administered, the patient is admitted to the hospital, and bronchoscopy is performed, which shows a mass in the right main-stem bronchus. Biopsy is done and pathologic examination reveals a small cell cancer.

A bone scan shows an abnormality in her left femur, and her alkaline phosphatase level is increased at 214. A CT scan of the abdomen is normal.

1. What stage is this patient's cancer?
2. How should this patient's cancer be treated?
3. If, 6 weeks after diagnosis, physical examination reveals only alopecia, and a chest radiograph and bone scan are normal, what is the likelihood of cure?

Case Discussion

1. *What stage is this patient's cancer?*

    The patient has extensive SCLC with metastases to the brain.

2. *How should this patient's cancer be treated?*

    Most chemotherapy traverses the blood–brain barrier poorly. Therefore, the patient should be started on whole-brain radiation therapy. Because SCLC is a rapidly growing tumor, and radiation therapy lasts 4 to 6 weeks, combination chemotherapy should also be initiated.

3. *If, 6 weeks after diagnosis, physical examination reveals only alopecia, and a chest radiograph and bone scan are normal, what is the likelihood of cure?*

    Small cell lung cancer is responsive to both radiation therapy and chemotherapy. Complete responses are witnessed in 15% to 30% of patients with extensive disease. However, the 5-year survival is only 4% to 8% in this setting, and tumor usually recurs quickly.

Suggested Readings

Bunn PA, Lichter AS, Makuch RW, et al. Chemotherapy alone or chemotherapy with chest radiation therapy in limited stage small cell lung cancer: a prospective randomized trial. *Ann Intern Med* 1987;106:655.

Carney DN, de Leij L. Lung cancer biology. *Semin Oncol* 1988;15:199.

Elderly Lung Cancer Vinorelbine Italian Study Group. Effects of vinorelbine on quality of life and survival of elderly patients with advanced non-small-cell lung cancer. *J Natl Cancer Inst* 1999;91:66.

Lababede O, Meziane MA, Rice TW. TNM staging of lung cancer: a quick reference chart. *Chest* 1999;115:233.

Mountain CF, Luckman JM, Hammer SP, et al. Lung cancer classification: the relationship of disease extent and cell type to survival in a clinical trials population. *J Surg Oncol* 1987;35:147.

Prostate Cancer

1. How common is prostate cancer?
2. How does prostate cancer arise and spread?
3. How is prostate cancer graded and staged, and why is this important?
4. What is the typical clinical presentation of prostate cancer?
5. After a physical examination, how is a suspicion of prostate cancer confirmed?

6. Once prostate cancer is diagnosed, how is a staging evaluation performed?

7. What treatment is recommended for stage A1 prostate cancer?

8. Which category of patients is considered for a radical prostatectomy?

9. Is any alternative therapy available for patients with stage A2 or B prostate cancer?

10. What therapy may be administered to patients with stage C or D disease?

11. In terms of the recommended treatments, what survival can be expected in patients with stage A1, A2, B, or C prostate cancer?

12. What complications attend the use of radical prostatectomy and irradiation that patients should be aware of in advance?

13. What is the treatment for disseminated prostate cancer?

14. Is the prostate-specific antigen level useful in screening asymptomatic men for prostate cancer?

Discussion

1. *How common is prostate cancer?*

Approximately 90,000 new cases of carcinoma of the prostate are identified every year. Of men in their 80s and older than 90 years of age, 50% and 90% of the prostates, respectively, are found to have carcinoma at autopsy. It is the second most common malignancy in American men and the most common cancerous cause of death in men older than 75 years of age. The clinical incidence is higher in blacks than in whites, and it is much lower for Japanese men living in Japan. Thus, racial and environmental factors may be involved in its development.

2. *How does prostate cancer arise and spread?*

Prostate adenocarcinoma arises from the epithelium of the peripheral acinar glands. It is slow growing, and half of all cases of early-stage (A) prostate cancer are found only at autopsy. Prostate cancer extends first locally through its capsule and then invades the lymphatics and blood vessels. Lymph node involvement occurs sequentially, with initial spread to the periprostatic and obturator nodes, and later the iliac and periaortic nodes. Distant hematogenous spread tends to occur late in the disease and frequently involves the axial and proximal skeleton, liver, and lungs. However, more than half of all symptomatic patients with prostate cancer present with metastases.

3. *How is prostate cancer graded and staged, and why is this important?*

Prostate cancer is broadly staged into categories A, B, C, and D. Stage A is carcinoma detected by pathologic examination of glands removed because of clinically benign disease. Stage A1 represents well differentiated tumor involving less than 5% of the surgical specimen, and stage A2 constitutes tumor either involving more than 5% of the surgical specimen or a poorly differentiated tumor. Stage B is clinically detectable disease that is intracapsular and involves one lobe (B1) or more than one lobe (B2). In stage A and B cancer, the serum acid phosphatase and prostate-specific antigen levels are usually not elevated. Stage C is cancer that has invaded through the prostate capsule but is confined to the pelvis. Stage D, or metastatic disease, includes two categories: D1 (local pelvic nodal involvement) and D2 (distant, nodal, bone, or visceral disease), and is frequently associated with elevated serum tumor markers.

4. *What is the typical clinical presentation of prostate cancer?*

Classically, the disease is detected in elderly men with the occurrence of back pain, weight loss, anemia, urinary frequency, and nocturia, and, less often, dysuria, a slow urinary stream, urinary retention, and rarely hematuria.

Prostate cancer can be found during a routine physical examination or screening, or when investigating for a pathologic fracture, bone pain, palpable lymphadenopathy, chronic renal insufficiency, anemia, cachexia, or a number of other seemingly unrelated signs and symptoms. Approximately 50% of the indurated prostatic lesions felt on rectal examination turn out to be adenocarcinoma on biopsy. The most effective screening test remains a careful rectal examination.

5. *After a physical examination, how is a suspicion of prostate cancer confirmed?*

Most often, the diagnosis of prostate cancer is confirmed by needle biopsy findings. The transrectal route has been made accurate and safe through the use of transrectal ultrasound and the biopsy gun. Open biopsy and transurethral biopsy are less frequently used owing to the higher morbidity associated with their use.

6. *Once prostate cancer is diagnosed, how is a staging evaluation performed?*

A thorough physical examination is performed to determine the size of the primary tumor and if any evidence of metastatic tumor is present. Serum prostate-specific antigen level, serum acid phosphatase level, and liver function are assessed. A chest radiographic study and radioisotope bone scan are routinely performed. Depending on the patient, pelvic or other CT scans, ultrasound, bipedal or pelvic lymphadenectomy, and a skeletal radiographic survey may be required. Intravenous pyelography is performed to assess ureteral status.

A complete blood count as well as BUN and serum creatinine measurements are routinely done to detect anemia or obstructive uropathy. The serum acid phosphatase level is elevated in most stage D patients, in approximately 25% of stage C patients, and only rarely in early-stage prostate cancer. False-positive results, however, do occur in a wide variety of malignant and nonmalignant disorders. The prostate-specific antigen level is more sensitive (95%) and equally specific (>95%). A chest radiographic study may reveal metastases to the ribs, lungs, or hilar nodes. The bone scan is more sensitive and has largely supplanted the skeletal radiographic survey, but requires careful interpretation. The abdominal CT scan, together with positive FNA findings in the pelvic nodes, can often eliminate the need for a pelvic lymphadenectomy for staging purposes. The latter is not useful for stage A1 lesions, which almost never metastasize to pelvic nodes, or for poorly differentiated stage C prostate adenocarcinoma with elevated tumor markers, because over 90% of these are metastatic. However, pelvic lymphadenectomy is frequently useful in staging intermediate disease to determine the prognosis and plan treatment.

7. *What treatment is recommended for stage A1 prostate cancer?*

Only observation is recommended by most urologists for patients with stage A1 prostate cancer because of the very slow and infrequent (<10%) progression of the tumor at this stage. The data from follow-up studies have indicated the survival for this group is similar to that of age-matched control subjects.

8. *Which category of patients is considered for a radical prostatectomy?*

A radical prostatectomy is effective in patients with tumor confined to the prostate—stages A2 and B carcinoma. The retropubic approach with a nerve-sparing technique to minimize the risk of impotence is commonly used. This is usually preceded by bilateral pelvic node dissection and frozen-section examination to confirm noninvolvement by the tumor.

9. *Is any alternative therapy available for patients with stage A2 or B prostate cancer?*

If a staging lymphadenectomy reveals no pelvic node metastases or if patients are poor operative risks, prostate cancer may be successfully treated with external-beam irradiation. In some centers, internal radiation combined with some external-beam radiation therapy is the treatment used. In general, the long-term control rate and survival for localized prostate cancer is similar regardless of whether surgery or irradiation is the therapy selected.

10. *What therapy may be administered to patients with stage C or D disease?*

Patients with stage C or D disease often receive external-beam irradiation delivered to the pelvic and periaortic nodes, but this has not been observed consistently and clearly to enhance survival. In some symptomatic patients who have pelvic pain, lower extremity edema, hematuria, or urethral obstruction, palliative external-beam radiation therapy may be used. An alternative is to proceed directly to hormonal ablation therapy.

11. *In terms of the recommended treatments, what survival can be expected in patients with stage A1, A2, B, or C prostate cancer?*

Only 1% of patients with stage A disease die of prostate cancer, and metastases develop in only 5% within 5 to 10 years without treatment. The natural history of this group is determined in the elderly by coexistent disease.

Without treatment, 35% of patients in stage A2 have metastases and 20% die within 5 to 10 years of diagnosis. The results of radical prostatectomy closely approximate the clinical picture seen in untreated patients with stage A1 disease. The same applies to stage B1 and B2 disease, and hence it may be concluded that, with appropriate treatment, survival in patients with early-stage prostate cancer is similar to that of age-matched normal control subjects. Thus, most patients with stage A or B disease, particularly those older than 65 years of age, die of something else.

12. *What complications attend the use of radical prostatectomy and irradiation that patients should be aware of in advance?*

Radical prostatectomy, even using modern nerve-sparing techniques, can cause impotence in 20% to 50% of patients and urinary incontinence in 5%. Radiation therapy is associated with symptoms of radiation proctitis and cystourethritis. None of the immediate postoperative complications occurs, but radiation therapy has a similar incidence of the other side effects, although their onset may take longer.

13. *What is the treatment for disseminated prostate cancer?*

Hormonal manipulation is the standard approach for the treatment of disseminated prostate cancer. Chemotherapy is minimally effective and is considered only if hormonal treatment fails.

The response to treatment in the setting of prostate cancer is typically difficult to assess. It includes physical findings, performance status, bone pain, weight change, and the hemoglobin level. Bone scans and other imaging techniques, serum acid phosphatase, and, most important, prostate-specific antigen levels also predict response.

Orchiectomy leads directly to low testosterone levels. The nonsteroidal estrogen diethylstilbestrol (at an oral dose of 1 to 3 mg per day) achieves the same effect by suppressing gonadotropin release, but diethylstilbestrol is seldom used because it has been associated with increased cardiovascular complications. Luteinizing hormone-releasing hormone agonists (leuprolide and goserelin) bring about suppressed testosterone levels in 2 to 3 weeks and can be conveniently administered at monthly intervals or longer as a subcutaneous depot preparation. Testosterone receptor level antagonism can be achieved by the more recently introduced nonsteroidal agent, flutamide.

Choosing among the commonly used initial hormonal approaches (i.e., leuprolide or flutamide) often depends on individual patient preference with respect to toxicities and cost.

The combination of a luteinizing hormone-releasing hormone agonist and an antiandrogen may bring about an increased response rate in patients with low-volume stage D2 prostate cancer. However, in general, no one hormonal treatment has been conclusively proved to be superior in terms of response. Approximately 40% of patients experience complete or partial responses and, in another 40%, the disease remains stable for at least 3 months. It is not yet clearly proved that treatment of metastatic prostate cancer prolongs survival, although some study findings suggest it may. If initial hormonal manipulation fails, a second hormonal treatment has achieved a response in only 10% to 20% of patients.

Chemotherapy achieves responses (usually partial) in less than 20% of patients; in addition, it can often produce substantial toxicity and does not prolong survival. Thus patients are usually offered palliative or experimental chemotherapy approaches. Some evidence now exists for the efficacy of suramin, which blocks growth factor effects in prostate cancer.

14. *Is the prostate-specific antigen level useful in screening asymptomatic men for prostate cancer?*

An elevated prostate-specific antigen value is useful in the detection of early prostate cancer in asymptomatic men. However, because early prostate cancer is often not associated with clinical disease, studies examining the utility of mass prostate-specific antigen screening are still under way to determine if this screening ultimately improves survival. Most clinicians agree that a proper prostate examination on rectal examination for men older than 50 years of age is a cost-effective and potentially helpful screening method.

Case   A 65-year-old man presents to the emergency room because of a backache that has lasted for several days, which became severe after a fall. Three years before, the patient began to have urinary frequency and dribbling on micturition, and was noted to have a hard, nontender prostate nodule with obliteration of the lateral sulcus and a palpable seminal vesicle on one side, for which he received external-beam irradiation. His prostate-specific antigen level was slightly elevated before therapy but returned to normal thereafter, and was normal 4 months ago.

Physical examination reveals a diffuse tenderness over the lower thoracic and lumbar spines. Rectal examination reveals a hard, irregular prostate. The remainder of the physical examination findings are unremarkable. Laboratory workup shows the following: hemoglobin, 11.5 g/dL; hematocrit, 32%; white blood cell count, 9.8×10^9/L; platelets, 162×10^9/L; white blood cell differential—neutrophils, 68%; lymphocytes, 26%; monocytes, 4%; band forms, 2%; erythrocyte sedimentation rate, 87 mm in the first hour; and alkaline phosphatase, 320 U (normal, up to 150 U). Two nucleated red blood cells are seen per 100 white blood cells.

A chest radiographic study shows increased bone densities in several ribs, and a radiograph of the lumbar spine shows multiple areas of bone sclerosis but no fractures. A bone scan shows multiple areas of increased activity scattered over the axial skeleton.

1. What was the stage of this patient's prostate cancer 3 years ago?
2. Was the treatment given at that time appropriate?
3. How would you go about proving a diagnosis of prostate cancer now?
4. What are the treatment options and prognosis in this patient now?
5. What are the complications of external-beam irradiation for the treatment of prostate cancer?

Case Discussion

1. *What was the stage of this patient's prostate cancer 3 years ago?*

The patient had stage C prostate cancer 3 years ago based on palpable extension of the tumor across the prostatic capsule and a negative bone scan. A palpable seminal vesicle is abnormal.

2. *Was the treatment given at that time appropriate?*

The treatment for stage C prostate cancer is external-beam irradiation or, in selected instances, radical prostatectomy. Adjuvant hormonal treatment, or combined surgery and radiation, are still under investigation.

3. *How would you go about proving a diagnosis of prostate cancer now?*

The presence of immature white and red blood cells in the circulation together with the anemia (a leukoerythroblastic picture) suggests the existence of bone marrow infiltration. A bone marrow biopsy and staining for acid phosphatase and prostate-specific antigen might clinch the diagnosis. An elevated serum prostate-specific antigen level in the presence of sclerotic bone lesions establishes the diagnosis of metastatic prostate cancer.

4. *What are the treatment options and prognosis in this patient now?*

The treatment options for metastatic prostate cancer with predominant bone lesions is to reduce or block testicular androgen production, either by medical or surgical means. Radiation therapy can be used for the management of painful bone lesions not amenable to androgen deprivation. There is no effective chemotherapy. Androgen deprivation can be effected by gonadotropin-releasing hormone analogues like leuprolide. This type of therapy gives a median time to further progression of disease of approximately 15 months and a median survival of 30 months. Bilateral orchiectomy is an option but may not be acceptable to some patients for psychological reasons.

5. *What are the complications of external-beam irradiation for the treatment of prostate cancer?*

The common complications of external-beam irradiation are impotence, suprapubic or perineal edema, proctitis, persistent tumor, and fibrosis of the prostate, making it hard and its substance clinically indistinguishable from that of malignancy.

Suggested Readings

Albertsen PC, Fryback DG, Storer BE, et al. Long-term survival among men with conservatively treated localized prostate cancer. *JAMA* 1995;274:626.

Carvalhal GF, Smith DS, Mager DE, Ramos G, Catalona WJ. Digital rectal examination for detecting prostate cancer at prostate specific antigen levels of 4 ng/mL or less. *J Urol* 1999;161:835.

Crawford ED, Eisenberger MA, McLeod DG, et al. A controlled trial of leuprolide with and without flutamide in prostatic carcinoma. *N Engl J Med* 1989;321:419.

George NJR. Natural history of localized prostatic cancer managed by conservative therapy alone. *Lancet* 1988;1:494.

Gerber GS, Chodak GW. Routine screening for cancer of the prostate. *J Natl Cancer Inst* 1991;83:329.

Gleason DF. Histologic grade, clinical stage, and patient age in prostate cancer. *National Cancer Institute Monographs* 1988;7:15.

8 Pulmonology

Marvin I. Schwarz

Acute Respiratory Distress Syndrome

1. What is the definition of acute respiratory distress syndrome (ARDS)?
2. What are the principles of management in the patient with ARDS?

Discussion

1. *What is the definition of ARDS?*

Although seemingly a simple question, there is no simple answer. Many processes such as congestive heart failure, pneumonia, or the acute interstitial pneumonias can mimic ARDS. A useful definition that has been used in many research settings consists of the following criteria: diffuse pulmonary infiltrates, profound hypoxemia (usually requiring mechanical ventilation), pulmonary compliance less than 20 mL/cm H_2O (stiff lungs), and a pulmonary capillary wedge pressure less than 18 mm Hg (noncardiogenic edema). Etiologies include pneumonia, all forms of shock, aspiration, high-altitude and neurogenic pulmonary edema, transfusion-related acute lung injury, trauma, and burns. The underlying pathologic process is the histologic lesion referred to as diffuse alveolar damage.

2. *What are the principles of management in the patient with ARDS?*

There are no specific therapies for ARDS other than the treatment of the precipitating cause. Trials of biologic modifiers have been disappointing, but new agents are being tested. Management is mainly supportive and treating the underlying initiating cause in the hope that the lung can return to normal. The specific goals of therapy are to maintain tissue oxygenation (maximize oxygen delivery) while preventing complications resulting from mechanical ventilation, such as barotrauma (pneumothorax), and lung injury stemming from high airway pressures or oxygen toxicity.

Case

A 27-year-old white male motorcyclist is transported to the emergency room after he was involved in a high-speed, head-on collision with an oncoming automobile. At the accident scene, he was poorly responsive; his initial blood pressure was 70/40 mm Hg and injuries included a flail chest on the right, several pelvic fractures, an open fracture of the femur, and a closed, displaced fracture of the left tibia. A central and two peripheral catheters are inserted, and normal saline is administered at maximal rates. His blood is typed and crossmatched. He is also intubated in the emergency room, and a chest tube inserted on the right yields a bloody return. Suction is applied and no air leak is noted. Several units of blood are administered, and abdominal lavage fluid proves bloody. He is rushed to the operating room to undergo a laparotomy, and a liver laceration is found and repaired. During surgery he receives 8 units of whole blood, 5 units of platelets, and 8 units of fresh frozen plasma. His orthopedic injuries are appropriately treated and he is transferred to the surgical intensive care unit in critical but stable condition. Chest radiographic study confirms that the endotracheal and chest tubes are in good position and reveals a right lower lobe infiltrate thought to be secondary to a pulmonary contusion. The ventilator is initially set at an inspired oxygen concentration (FIO_2) of 40%, respiratory rate of 12 per minute, and tidal volume of 900 mL in an assist-control mode. Arterial blood gas measurement reveals a pH of 7.46, a partial pressure of carbon dioxide (PCO_2) of 34 mm Hg, and a partial pressure of oxygen (PO_2) of 59 mm Hg, with an oxygen saturation of 92%. On the second hospital day, 12 hours after admission, he becomes agitated while on the ventilator, his respiratory rate rises to 25 per minute, his minute ventilation increases from 8.5 to 18 L/min, and airway pressure rises from 20 to 60 cm H_2O. A repeat chest radiograph now shows diffuse infiltrates that exhibit a "whiteout" pattern. Repeat arterial blood gas analysis reveals a PO_2 of 39 mm Hg.

1. What is the differential diagnosis of this patient's clinical deterioration?
2. What are the risk factors that put this patient at risk for ARDS?
3. How would you manage this patient's hypoxemia?
4. What are the potential problems associated with positive end-expiratory pressure (PEEP)?
5. What is the mortality rate associated with ARDS?

Case Discussion

1. *What is the differential diagnosis of this patient's clinical deterioration?*

   Several possible diagnoses need to be considered in this setting. First, an infection (pneumonia) must always be ruled out. It is possible that the patient aspirated gastric contents at the accident scene while his level of consciousness was impaired, and this could have injured the lung directly due to acid aspiration or set the stage for an overwhelming pneumonia. Alternatively, a nosocomial (hospital-acquired) pneumonia could have been acquired in the surgical intensive care unit, although the early onset of his ARDS makes this unlikely. The massive fluid resuscitation could lead to a fluid-overload congestive heart failure syndrome, even despite a normal-functioning heart before the accident. If a cardiac contusion occurred, this would make him more susceptible to this complication. Pulmonary contusions are worth considering, but are usually more localized and develop within several hours. Airway hemorrhage, perhaps stemming from either bronchial fracture or a traumatic intubation, can occur, but is typically associated with bloody secretions when severe. The ARDS could also have resulted from prolonged hypotension or replacement of blood products or transfusion-related acute lung injury. Regardless, this patient has ARDS and under these circumstances, pathologic study would show diffuse alveolar damage consisting of hyaline membrane formation, alveolar wall edema, and inflammation.

2. *What are the risk factors that put this patient at risk for ARDS?*

   Although the exact etiology of ARDS is unclear, several risk factors have been clearly implicated in the development of the syndrome. This patient's risk factors are:

   Hypotension—usually prolonged and severe (systolic blood pressure <90 mm Hg).

   Hypertransfusion—more than 10 units of blood products in a 24-hour period.

   Aspiration—any patient with depressed mental status is at great risk for gastric aspiration; the resulting chemical burn is a common precursor for ARDS.

   Fat emboli syndrome—this syndrome consists of diffuse pulmonary infiltrates, mental status changes, thrombocytopenia, and conjunctival or axillary petechiae. It occurs most often in the presence of severe and multiple long bone fractures, and is thought to result from fat emboli migrating from the bone marrow to the lungs. However, it usually occurs 24 to 72 hours after admission, making it unlikely in this patient.

   Other risk factors include sepsis, pneumonia, drugs, pancreatitis, lung contusion, toxic fume inhalation, and oxygen toxicity.

3. *How would you manage this patient's hypoxemia?*

   Acutely, the F_{IO_2} should be increased to 100%. However, the prolonged administration of 100% oxygen for 3 or more days is likely to lead to oxygen toxicity and further worsening of ARDS. Accordingly, the F_{IO_2} should be decreased to the lowest level that achieves an oxygen saturation of 90% to

92%. There appears to be a threshold of 50% to 60% below which oxygen toxicity is rare. If an FIO_2 above this range is necessary, then a trial of PEEP is indicated. PEEP appears to improve oxygenation by recruiting collapsed gas-exchange units (atelectasis). Data indicate that putting the patient into the prone position also improves oxygenation.

4. *What are the potential problems associated with PEEP?*

Positive end-expiratory pressure may be lifesaving by improving oxygenation and allowing the FIO_2 to be lowered to "safe" levels; however, it is associated with several potential problems. The first is hypotension. High levels of positive intrathoracic pressure impede venous return to the heart and may be transmitted to the pulmonary arteries, causing pulmonary hypertension. Both these factors serve to decrease cardiac output, which precipitates hypotension.

The risk of barotrauma is greatly increased with PEEP because of the positive airway pressures and may result in pneumothorax or pneumomediastinum. Pneumothorax in a ventilated patient is often a medical emergency because a tension pneumothorax may evolve. PEEP levels above 15 cm H_2O are particularly risky. The prophylactic administration of PEEP, before the onset of ARDS, has been shown to be of no value.

5. *What is the mortality rate of ARDS?*

In 1967, the mortality rate observed for ARDS was 60%. This has decreased to 40% to 50%, mainly due to improved ventilatory management as opposed to the treatment of the ARDS itself. In the survivors, pulmonary function can return to normal, and this usually occurs by 6 months. Persistent abnormalities past this time indicate pulmonary fibrosis and pulmonary impairment.

Suggested Readings

Ashbaugh DG, Bigelow DB, Petty TL, Levine BE. Acute respiratory distress in adults. *Lancet* 1967;2:319.

Fowler AA, Hamman RF, Good JT, et al. Adult respiratory distress syndrome: risk with common predispositions. *Ann Intern Med* 1983;98:593.

Petty TL. Indicators of risk, course, and prognosis in adult respiratory distress syndrome. *American Review of Respiratory Disease* 1985;132:471.

Asthma

1. What is asthma, and how is it classified?
2. How is asthma diagnosed?
3. What conditions are associated with or may complicate asthma?

Discussion

1. *What is asthma, and how is it classified?*

Asthma is not a single disease, but rather a clinical syndrome consisting of (a) an increase in airway responsiveness to a variety of stimuli; (b) variable airflow obstruction, which is usually reversible, either spontaneously or with treatment; and (c) a chronic, multicellular inflammatory response within the airways that produces patchy bronchial epithelial denudation, submucosal edema, hypersecretion of mucus, and sub-basement membrane collagen deposition. The asthmatic response to stimuli may be immediate, occurring within minutes and termed the *early asthmatic response*, or delayed, arising several hours after exposure and termed the *late asthmatic response*. The early asthmatic response primarily results from bronchial smooth muscle constriction; the late asthmatic response is characterized by inflammatory cell infiltration and activation. Both patterns may be triggered by exposure to the same stimuli, and may work in concert to produce sustained narrowing of the airway lumen.

Asthma may be classified based either on the presumptive etiology or on symptom severity and the pattern of airflow obstruction. Historically, attempts have been made to classify asthmatic subjects as having either intrinsic or extrinsic disease. Intrinsic asthmatics have no personal or family history of allergies, their immunoglobulin E (IgE) levels are normal, and they have no easily identifiable environmental precipitants of their symptoms. In contrast, extrinsic asthmatics have allergic or atopic histories, their IgE levels are typically elevated, and they have specific antigenic triggers to their asthma. This traditional etiologic classification is probably now obsolete because individual asthmatic subjects commonly exhibit both IgE- and non–IgE-mediated responses to bronchoprovocative stimuli. Therefore, a classification scheme that is based instead on the severity of symptoms and on lung function is more clinically relevant, and provides a framework on which to base a stepwise treatment approach. One proposed classification scheme is presented in Table 8-1.

Because the severity of an acute asthma attack may be underestimated by both patients and their families, they should make use of home expiratory

Table 8-1. Asthma Classification Scheme

Asthma severity	Clinical features	Pulmonary function
Mild	Intermittent, brief symptoms (<1–2 times per week)	Expiratory flow rates >80% of predicted
	Rare nocturnal symptoms (<2 times per week)	Expiratory flow rate variability <20%
Moderate	Exacerbations >2 times per week	Expiratory flow rates 60%–80% of predicted
	Nocturnal symptoms >2 times per week	Expiratory flow rate variability 20%–30%
Severe	Almost daily bronchodilator use	Expiratory flow rate <60% of predicted
	Frequent, continuous symptoms	Expiratory flow rate variability >30%
	Frequent nocturnal awakenings	
	Physical activities limited by symptoms	
	Hospitalization for asthma within the previous year	

flow rate devices, which can more objectively measure asthma severity. Factors that have been associated with an increased risk of asthma mortality include frequent emergency room visits, hospitalization within the previous year, prior life-threatening episodes, a past need for intubation, a recent reduction in the corticosteroid dosage or cessation of use, noncompliance with medical therapy, the presence of serious depression or psychosocial behavioral problems, and a lower socioeconomic status.

2. *How is asthma diagnosed?*

Because patients with asthma represent a heterogeneous group, the diagnosis requires assessment of a patient's pulmonary function and attention to selected details revealed by the medical history, physical examination, and laboratory tests. Historical clues important in establishing the diagnosis of asthma include the episodic and variable nature of the airflow obstruction and the reversibility of the obstruction. The most common symptoms—cough, wheezing, chest tightness, shortness of breath, and sputum production—are nonspecific and by themselves nondiagnostic. The pattern of symptoms may be suggestive, in that nocturnal (and early morning) symptoms are particularly characteristic of asthma. Commonly reported precipitants of bronchospasm include exercise, cold air, environmental allergens, exposure to occupational or chemical irritants, and upper respiratory tract infections. The differential diagnosis of adult wheezing or cough may include mechanical obstruction of the airway (e.g., foreign body, tumor mass, or granulomatous narrowing), vocal cord dysfunction, congestive heart failure, pulmonary embolus, aspiration injury, pulmonary eosinophilia syndromes, and other forms of chronic obstructive pulmonary disease (e.g., cystic fibrosis, chronic bronchitis, and emphysema).

The physical examination findings may be either unremarkable or suggest the presence of air trapping and hyperinflation, with an increased anteroposterior thoracic diameter and a low diaphragm. Wheezing is the most characteristic breath sound of asthma but is an unreliable indicator of severity. Bronchospasm may produce a prolonged expiratory phase with reduced tidal volumes and minimal air movement. In this setting, faint wheezing paradoxically intensifies as airflow improves. Rhonchi and other adventitious sounds may suggest the presence of secretions in the airways. Signs of severe airflow obstruction may include an increased pulsus paradoxus, supraclavicular retractions with accessory muscle use (sternocleidomastoid and intercostals), and thoracoabdominal paradox (the paradoxical retraction of abdominal musculature with inspiration).

Pulmonary function testing should be pursued in all patients with suspected asthma. Spirometric findings of reduced expiratory flow rates with a normal inspiratory flow–volume curve, lung volumes suggesting increased thoracic gas and residual volumes, and increased airway resistance are all characteristic signs of asthma and may be alleviated by bronchodilator treatment. After an acute exacerbation of asthma, however, pulmonary function may remain abnormal long after the symptoms have returned to their baseline status.

Additional studies and signs that may be useful in the evaluation of asthma include (a) bronchoprovocation testing with methacholine, histamine, or exercise to document increased airway responsiveness to stimuli; (b) eosinophilia; (c) increased IgE levels; (d) Charcot-Leyden crystals (crystallized cationic proteins), eosinophils, or Curschmann's spirals (bronchiolar casts of mucus and cellular debris) in the sputum; and (e) a chest radiograph showing hyperinflation or the presence of barotrauma. No single test or battery of tests is appropriate for every suspected case. Selected studies may provide the objective evidence needed to confirm the diagnosis of asthma when the history and physical examination findings are only suggestive.

3. *What conditions are associated with or may complicate asthma?*

Several conditions may complicate the asthma syndrome, and they require special consideration.

Although a person's clinical course is not predictable, unstable asthma develops during **pregnancy** in approximately one third of asthmatic women, one third experience no change, and symptoms are actually less severe in one third. Poorly controlled asthma during pregnancy may contribute to prenatal mortality, an increased likelihood of prematurity, and low birth weight. Therefore, using medications to obtain optimal control of asthma is appropriate, even if their safety in pregnancy has not been unequivocally proved. Inhaled forms of cromolyn, a corticosteroid preparation, selective β_2 agonists, appropriately monitored theophylline use, and even systemic corticosteroids can be used when necessary to prevent fetal hypoxia. Medications that should be avoided include α-adrenergic compounds, brompheniramine, epinephrine, and some decongestants (oral α agonists), antibiotics (tetracycline and ciprofloxacin), and live virus vaccines.

The likelihood of asthma-related **postoperative complications** depends on the severity of the patient's airway hyperresponsiveness, the degree of airflow obstruction, and the amount of excess airway secretions at the time of operation. In addition, endotracheal intubation and the type of procedure performed (thoracic and upper abdominal) may pose an additional risk. Preoperative corticosteroids may be indicated if expiratory flow rates are reduced (<80% of personal best) or if corticosteroids have been required to control asthma in the previous 6 months.

Maintenance of nasal patency may improve lower airway function and asthma control. Although the mechanisms involved in this relationship are not completely understood, **nasal obstruction**, such as that caused by rhinitis, sinusitis, and nasal polyps, may lead to asthma instability and worsening of symptoms. Nasal β_2 agonists and corticosteroids are sometimes useful in treating nasal obstruction.

Approximately 2% of all cases of asthma are due to **occupational exposure** to specific sensitizing substances. Proteins, organic compounds, and some inorganic chemicals (metal salts) have been implicated. Once the diagnosis is established, complete avoidance of exposure is mandatory because continued exposure to even minute concentrations may provoke severe and potentially fatal bronchospasm. Also, once well established, occupational asthma may not be completely reversible. The pharmacologic therapy used for this type of asthma is similar to that used for other forms of asthma, but is no substitute for diligent avoidance of exposure to the offending agents.

Chemical sensitivities may also provoke asthma attacks. Approximately 5% to 20% of adults with asthma sustain severe and potentially fatal exacerbations of asthma after taking aspirin or other nonsteroidal antiinflammatory drugs. Physical examination in these patients often reveals the existence of nasal polyps, and symptoms of vasomotor rhinitis may precede the development of aspirin-induced bronchospasm. Less commonly, sulfites, which may be used as a food preservative, and tartrazine, a yellow dye that may be used as a food coloring, have been linked to the occurrence of acute bronchospasm.

Although **gastroesophageal reflux** is more common in people with asthma, its relationship to bronchospasm is controversial. Most people with asthma with symptomatic gastroesophageal reflux have hiatal hernias, and the association between the two conditions may be best demonstrated by simultaneously monitoring the esophageal pH and pulmonary function. Medical management consisting of proton pump inhibitor usually is effective in these patients.

Case   A 26-year-old woman presents to the emergency room at 3:00 a.m. complaining of worsening cough with yellow-green sputum, shortness of breath, and wheezing of 5 days' duration. Her symptoms began after an upper respiratory tract infection that was manifested as a low-grade fever, rhinorrhea with postnasal drip, and nasal congestion. She reports poor sleep quality for the prior 2 days because of severe coughing and has used over-the-counter nasal sprays and cough suppressants, but without relief. She is 18 weeks pregnant, but has no significant past medical history. Her physical examination reveals that she is diaphoretic and unable to speak in sentences. Her vital signs reveal a respiratory rate of 30 breaths per minute, a heart rate of 120 beats per minute, a temperature of 37°C, and a pulsus paradoxus of 22 mm Hg. Spirometry is attempted but proves poorly reproducible, with a "best effort" forced expiratory volume in 1 minute (FEV_1) of 30% of predicted. The remainder of her examination findings are noteworthy for the presence of supraclavicular retractions with inspiration, diffusely diminished breath sounds with scattered, high-pitched inspiratory and expiratory wheezes, and a palpable subcutaneous crepitation over her anterior thorax. She is quite anxious, but alert and cooperative.

1. What additional studies may be important for the proper management of this patient?
2. What are the initial management considerations in this patient?
3. What are the treatment considerations for ongoing management in this patient?

Case Discussion

1. *What additional studies may be important for the proper management of this patient?*

The patient's clinical presentation suggests acute, severe bronchospasm, and the immediate focus of the emergency room effort should be therapeutic rather than diagnostic. Although this is the initial episode of asthma for this patient, numerous factors suggest it is a dangerously severe attack. Dyspnea at rest, an inability to speak, and the use of accessory muscles are important observations. Objective measures of attack severity are an increased pulsus paradoxus and expiratory flow rates less than 40% of predicted. The intensity of wheezing is an unreliable indicator. The presence of subcutaneous emphysema suggests an associated pneumothorax or pneumomediastinum. Based on this presentation, chest radiography and arterial blood gas measurement are indicated, although treatment should not be delayed to do these. The chest radiographic findings may exclude the diagnosis of pneumonia and delineate the source of the subcutaneous emphysema. A pneumomediastinum can typically be watched without specific therapy, whereas a pneumothorax would likely require insertion of a chest tube with water-seal suction to bring about reexpansion. The arterial blood gas studies would likely show hypoxemia with hypocapnia. Hypoxemia with an elevated alveolar-arterial oxygen gradient is the result of mismatched ventilation and perfusion. Acute bronchospasm results in hyperventilation, and the arterial blood chemistry data should reflect a respiratory alkalosis with a reduced $Paco_2$. If the attack is severe and prolonged, the $Paco_2$ may rise as a result of increased dead space ventilation (high ventilation–perfusion ratio) and respiratory muscle fatigue. A normal or elevated $Paco_2$ in the setting of severe airway obstruction suggests impending respiratory failure and warrants intensive care unit observation, with consideration given to mechanical ventilation.

2. *What are the initial management considerations in this patient?*

The immediate goals of therapy are to ensure adequate oxygenation and gas exchange while reducing the bronchospasm and the work of breathing. In this case, the patient is "breathing for two" and fetal hypoxia is an important concern. At a minimum, adequate supplemental oxygen should be given immediately to ensure a Pao_2 exceeding 65 mm Hg and an oxygen saturation greater than 90%. The decision to use ventilatory support consisting of intubation and mechanical ventilation is a difficult one, but may be lifesaving in patients with mental status deterioration, worsening respiratory distress from exhaustion, or progressively increasing $Paco_2$ levels with respiratory acidosis.

Frequent dosing with an inhaled β_2-adrenergic agonist delivered by nebulizer or metered-dose inhaler is the most effective bronchodilator therapy for acute, severe asthma (status asthmaticus). Asthmatic patients who are initially unresponsive to intensive inhaled therapy may respond to the subcutaneous delivery of β_2 agonists, but oral administration is not indicated for acute management. Epinephrine should be avoided in this patient because it is a teratogen.

In addition to inhaled β_2 agonists and supplemental oxygen, systemic corticosteroids should be instituted early in the emergency room management. Corticosteroids reduce airway obstruction by interrupting the inflammatory cascade at one or more critical steps in its genesis, and may also have a synergistic effect on β-adrenergic receptor activity. In general, systemic corticosteroids should be considered if significant improvement is not seen within the first 30 to 60 minutes of intensive bronchodilator treatment. Early corticosteroid use has been shown to lead to a reduction in both the rate of hospitalization and the rate of return to the emergency room after discharge. Inhaled corticosteroids are not indicated for the management of acute, severe asthma. Theophylline preparations offer little additional benefit when added to inhaled β_2 agonist treatment in the emergency room, but they may augment respiratory muscle function during hospitalization. The use of inhaled β_2 agonists, systemic corticosteroids, and even theophylline preparations (with serum levels kept at <12 μg/mL) may be considered appropriate in the setting of pregnancy and unstable asthma. Cautious hydration is also appropriate because insensible water losses increase with hyperventilation. The use of antibiotics is commonly reserved for objectively documented infections. The sputum production, even though it is yellow-green, does not mandate antibiotic treatment unless there is Gram's stain evidence of a dominant organism.

3. *What are the treatment considerations for ongoing management in this patient?*

   The optimal management of chronic asthma relies on four interrelated principles: objective assessment of lung function, pharmacologic therapy, environmental control, and patient education. The goals of effective management are to maintain near-normal pulmonary function and physical activity levels, minimize symptoms and prevent exacerbations, and avoid the adverse effects of asthma medications. Spirometry, based on the peak expiratory flow rates or FEV_1, provides an objective measure of asthma control and can be useful in adjusting medications (particularly tapering systemic corticosteroids) and assessing the need for intervention. Pharmacologic therapy is typically prescribed in a stepwise manner. In recognition that asthma is a chronic inflammatory disease, trends in therapy have placed a greater emphasis on the use of inhaled corticosteroids or cromolyn as first-line medications, with inhaled β_2 agonists used to bring about acute relief of bronchospasm, as needed. Theophylline preparations and oral β-adrenergic agonists are often used as second-line agents, and are particularly useful for controlling the nocturnal worsening of asthma. Short "bursts" of oral corticosteroids are best used in the early treatment of acute, severe exacerbations, and every effort should be made to avoid chronic dependence on oral corticosteroids once the acute attack is controlled.

   In selected cases, the identification and avoidance of specific triggers of bronchospasm may have significant impact on asthma control. Avoidance of aeroallergens (dust mites, cat dander, pollens, and molds), chemicals (sulfites and tartrazine), certain medications (aspirin, beta blockers, and acetylcholinesterase inhibitors), and strong aeroirritants (tobacco smoke, household sprays, and wood smoke) may be helpful for certain patients. Although exercise is a common precipitating factor, the use of inhaled β_2 agonists or cromolyn before exercise may minimize the associated bronchospasm. Last, patient education should begin at the time of diagnosis and be encouraged throughout the continued care of the patient with asthma. Learning to identify important signs and symptoms of asthma, the correct use of the peak expiratory flow rate meter and metered-dose inhaler, and addressing issues related to medication effects and environmental control may minimize patient misunderstandings regarding the ongoing management of asthma. In this patient, a warning regarding the avoidance of α-adrenergic agonists until the completion of the pregnancy is also warranted.

Suggested Readings

International report: international consensus report on diagnosis and treatment of asthma. Publication no. 923091. Washington, DC: U.S. Department of Health and Human Services, Public Health Service, National Institutes of Health, June 1992.

National Asthma Education Program. *Executive summary: guidelines for the diagnosis and management of asthma.* Publication no. 913042 A. Bethesda, MD: Office of Prevention, Education, and Control, National Heart, Lung and Blood Institute, National Institutes of Health, July 1991.

National Asthma Education Program. *Executive summary: management of asthma during pregnancy.* Publication no. 933279 A. Bethesda, MD: Office of Prevention, Education, and Control, National Heart, Lung and Blood Institute, National Institutes of Health, October 1992.

Chronic Obstructive Pulmonary Disease

1. What is chronic obstructive pulmonary disease (COPD)?
2. What are the epidemiologic trends in COPD?
3. What is the most commonly held theory explaining the development of emphysema?
4. What are the common signs and symptoms of COPD?
5. What are the common laboratory and radiographic findings in the setting of COPD?

Discussion

1. *What is COPD?*

    The term *COPD* is commonly applied to two disorders: emphysema and chronic bronchitis. Most patients with COPD have a combination of these two diseases. Some authors also include chronic obstructive asthma and other disorders associated with chronic airflow limitations (e.g., bronchiolitis obliterans) under the heading of COPD.

2. *What are the epidemiologic trends in COPD?*

    There has been an approximate 60% increase in the prevalence of COPD since the late 1970s. Although emphysema is a common postmortem finding in adults, its prevalence is strongly correlated with smoking. COPD is more commonly diagnosed in men than women, but, as more adolescent girls than boys are beginning to smoke, this trend may change. A heavy smoker exhibits an average decline in FEV_1 of 40 to 45 mL per year; this decline is only 20 mL per year in a nonsmoking adult.

3. *What is the most commonly held theory explaining the development of emphysema?*

In part based on observations gleaned in people with α_1-antitrypsin deficiency, most authorities believe that the destruction of the alveolar wall and airspace enlargement seen in the setting of emphysema is due to an imbalance between the proteases and antiproteases in the lower respiratory tree (α_1-antitrypsin being the major protein in this category). Cigarette smoke inactivates the normal antiproteases in people who do not have α_1-antitrypsin deficiency.

4. *What are the common signs and symptoms of COPD?*

Although the initial complaint is usually dyspnea, some patients seek medical care because of chronic cough or sputum production, wheezing, recurrent pulmonary infections, or, in rare circumstances, weight loss or lower extremity swelling. Early in the disease, physical examination findings may be normal. Later, auscultation of the chest may reveal wheezing, rhonchi, or, in patients with predominant emphysema, decreased breath sounds. Percussion of the chest typically reveals hyperinflation and low diaphragms. In advanced cases, the point of maximal impulse may be felt in the subxiphoid area. Cyanosis, a right-sided third heart sound (S_3), jugulovenous distention, and lower extremity edema are late findings.

5. *What are the common laboratory and radiographic findings in the setting of COPD?*

There are no specific laboratory values seen in the setting of COPD. The routine blood count is normal, although patients with chronic hypoxia may show elevated hematocrits. The finding of eosinophilia should raise the possibility of concomitant asthmatic bronchitis. Typically in COPD the flow rates are reduced, the lung volumes are increased due to hyperinflation as measured by increased thoracic gas volume and functional residual capacity, and the diffusing capacity is decreased in emphysema. Reductions in both the FEV_1 and forced vital capacity (FVC) are routinely seen, although the FEV_1 is reduced out of proportion to the FVC. Early on, the chest radiograph is usually normal. As emphysema develops, the lungs show hyperinflation, flattening of the diaphragms, and an increased retrosternal airspace. Occasionally, frank bullae can be seen. The electrocardiogram tends to be normal, except in advanced disease, when it may show low voltage in the limb leads, early R waves in V_1 and V_2, and peaked P waves (P pulmonale).

Case   A 65-year-old man is seen because of a 5-day history of progressive shortness of breath and dyspnea on exertion. He also complains of a cough productive of green sputum, as well as vague right-sided chest pain. He has felt feverish at home, but denies any shaking chills, sore throat, nausea, vomiting, diarrhea, edema, or exposure to anyone with a similar illness.

The patient has been smoking two packs of cigarettes per day for the past 30 years. However, he recently decreased his habit to one pack per day. He was seen by a physician approximately half a year ago and told that he had emphysema. He has not been hospitalized previously. He is a retired bus driver and lives at home with his wife. They have no pets. Although he has noted some dyspnea on exertion over the past 3 to 4 years, he continues to maintain an active lifestyle and can still mow the lawn without much difficulty. He can walk 1 to 2 miles on a flat surface at a modest pace. The patient rarely drinks alcohol. He denies any other significant past medical history, including a history of childhood asthma or allergic diseases, significant cough, sputum production, or exposure to asbestos. His medications include sustained-release theophylline and over-the-counter vitamins.

At physical examination, the patient is found to be a somewhat thin but well developed man in moderate respiratory distress. His blood pressure is 150/98 mm Hg with a pulsus paradoxus of 20 mm Hg, his pulse is 110 beats per minute, his temperature is 37.9°C orally, and his respiratory rate is 24 breaths per minute and labored. Head, eye, ears, nose, and throat findings are unremarkable. No adenopathy is found in his neck, and the neck veins are flat. His chest is hyperexpanded, and there is use of the accessory muscles of respiration. Hyperresonance to percussion is noted. His breath sounds are distant with an occasional scattered wheeze. During the cardiac evaluation, the point of maximal impulse is located in the epigastric area. There is a regular tachycardia with a systolic fourth sound (S_4) heard best at the right lower sternal border. No murmurs or rubs are noted. His abdomen is scaphoid, bowel sounds are normal, and no tenderness or organomegaly is noted. His extremities are free of clubbing, cyanosis, and edema. Pulse oximetry shows a 91% saturation on room air.

1. What tests and studies would you order in this patient?

    A chest radiographic study reveals the presence of hyperexpanded lung fields, a small cardiac silhouette, evidence of bullous disease in both lungs, and an alveolar infiltrate in the right middle lobe with some degree of volume loss. No effusions are seen.

    Arterial blood gas measurement performed on room air reveals a pH of 7.50, a $Paco_2$ of 23 mm Hg, a Pao_2 of 51 mm Hg, and an oxygen saturation of 92%. Results of a complete blood count are as follows: white blood cells, 14,300/mm^3 with 8% band forms and 8.4% polymorphonuclear leukocytes; the hematocrit reading is 44%. A chemistry panel reveals the following findings: sodium, 139 mEq/L; potassium, 4.1 mEq/L; chloride, 108 mEq/L; bicarbonate, 20 mEq/L; blood urea nitrogen, 21 mg/dL; and creatinine, 0.9 mg/dL. His theophylline level is 3.7 μg/mL. The electrocardiogram reveals sinus tachycardia with low voltage in the limb leads, and no acute changes.

2. What is your diagnosis based on the information you have, and how would you manage this patient?

3. What therapy should you institute while the patient is in the hospital?

    The patient is started on inhaled agents and intravenous ampicillin. After 2 days of treatment, his condition fails to improve and respiratory fatigue requiring emergent endotracheal intubation and ventilation develops. His wife states that she does not want to prolong the patient's life "by artificial means" and is worried that the patient will require indefinite mechanical ventilation. Another option would be the use of noninvasive ventilation with bi-pap (i.e., nasal positive airway pressure during inspiration and expiration).

4. How would you respond to the patient's wife's concern about the need for indefinite mechanical ventilation?

   The patient's sputum culture grows *Hemophilus influenzae* that is resistant to ampicillin. His antibiotics are changed, and 4 days later he is successfully extubated. After 14 days in the hospital, he is ready to be discharged.

5. After the patient is discharged, how would you follow him, and what are your treatment options now?

Case Discussion

1. *What tests and studies would you order in this patient?*

   A **chest radiographic study** should be obtained. Although the value of a routine chest radiographic study in patients with an exacerbation of COPD has been debated, this patient has a productive cough, low-grade temperature, and localizing chest pain, all of which indicate the existence of an intrathoracic abnormality, and making a chest radiograph important.

   Despite a pulse oximetry reading of 91%, **arterial blood gas measurements** are called for in this patient. There are several factors that can cause a poor correlation between the pulse oximetry value and the Pao_2, as measured by arterial blood gas determinations. It is poor in patients with jaundice or dark skin pigmentation, as well as in those with poor peripheral circulation. Furthermore, under various physiologic and pathologic conditions (e.g., changes in the pH or 2,3-diphosphoglyceric acid level), the oxyhemoglobin dissociation curve can be shifted to the right or left. Therefore, the oximeter can either underpredict or overpredict the actual Pao_2. Finally, in a patient with a moderately severe pulmonary process, knowledge of the $Paco_2$ and pH is imperative.

   A **complete blood count** and **chemistry panel** should be obtained. The complete blood count can provide useful information regarding the severity of the infectious process (e.g., leukocytosis). Furthermore, significant polycythemia may indicate the existence of long-standing hypoxia, which signifies the chronicity and severity of the disease. The chemistry profile can provide valuable information concerning electrolyte imbalance (e.g., hyponatremia in the syndrome of inappropriate antidiuretic hormone secretion) or volume depletion. Knowledge of the serum bicarbonate level is useful in conjunction with the arterial blood gas findings to assess the chronicity of any respiratory acid–base disorders.

   In a patient of advanced age with risk factors for coronary artery disease (tobacco abuse and hypertension) and chest pain, an **electrocardiogram** is called for. Furthermore, many types of arrhythmias (e.g., multifocal atrial tachycardia) are seen predominantly in the setting of decompensated pulmonary disease.

The **theophylline level** must be determined. Because this drug has a narrow therapeutic index, close monitoring of the serum levels is essential in acutely ill patients.

2. *What is your diagnosis based on the information you have, and how would you manage this patient?*

The patient has a right middle lobe pneumonia and, as a result, an exacerbation of his COPD. Given the lack of cough and sputum production in his past history, as well as the bullae noted in the chest radiographic study, his clinical picture is consistent with emphysema, as opposed to chronic bronchitis. Most patients have a combination of both disorders. He should be admitted to the hospital.

3. *What therapy should you institute while the patient is in the hospital?*

Blood and sputum cultures should be obtained. A Gram's-stained sputum specimen should be examined both by the primary physicians and by the laboratory technician.

Inhaled β-adrenergic agonists (e.g., 0.5 mL of albuterol in 1.5 mL of saline) are the mainstay of treatment for a COPD exacerbation. The initial dosing frequency of this medication depends on the severity of the disease; it can be administered every 1 to 3 hours. As the patient's condition improves, the dosing frequency can be reduced to every 4 to 6 hours. Although metered-dose inhalers can be used with a similar degree of success, their efficacy depends on the ability of the patient to coordinate the timing of the inhalation and the activation of the inhaler, making them a less-than-optimal tool in an acutely ill patient.

The role of **theophylline** in the management of an acute exacerbation of COPD remains controversial. Most authorities agree that theophylline is a weak bronchodilator with a low therapeutic index. In a randomized, controlled study, the addition of aminophylline to a well formulated therapeutic regimen in hospitalized patients with COPD failed to show any benefit in terms of improvement in lung function or the dyspnea scale. If used, theophylline levels should be monitored closely and the patient observed for any signs or symptoms of toxicity.

Inhaled anticholinergics may also be useful. Ipratropium bromide (Atrovent; Boehringer Ingelheim, Ridgefield, CT) is the agent of choice. Atrovent is available in a metered-dose inhaler formulation, and can be given in-line into ventilator tubing. Occasional blurred vision or urinary retention has been noted in patients using it. For the treatment of a patient with *stable* COPD, Atrovent is superior to β agonists. The combination of the two can modestly improve the bronchodilation achieved, as well as prolong the effective duration of action of each agent. The starting dose of Atrovent is two inhalations four times a day.

The use of **systemic corticosteroids**, like that of theophylline, is controversial. A stronger case for their use can be made if the patient has exhibited a previously documented steroid response, has eosinophilia, or has shown a significant bronchodilator response to the inhaled agents. A reasonable starting dose is 40 to 60 mg of intravenous methylprednisolone every 6 hours. This regimen is changed to an oral form (e.g., prednisone, 40 to 60 mg per day) with rapid tapering. Monitoring of the side effects (e.g., hyperglycemia, mental status changes, and gastritis) is crucial. Inhaled corticosteroids have no role in the acute management of this patient.

Antibiotics are indicated even when an infiltrate is not found on the chest radiograph. In a well designed, controlled clinical trial, patients with COPD treated with broad-spectrum oral antibiotics (the newer cephalosporins, macrolides, and fluoroquinolones) did better than the control patients. In this situation, the choice of antibiotic depends on the sputum Gram's stain findings. Bacteria commonly responsible for lower respiratory tract infections in this patient population include *Streptococcus pneumoniae, H. influenzae*, and *Branhamella catarrhalis*. The latter two usually produce β-lactamase.

4. *How would you respond to the patient's wife's concern about the need for indefinite mechanical ventilation?*

The condition of patients with COPD frequently deteriorates to the point where they require ventilatory support. The prognosis for being able to wean the patient from the ventilator, as well as his or her future quality of life, depends on the patient's premorbid lung function and functional state. Although the status of this patient's pulmonary function is unknown, given his high quality of life and functional status before this episode, the odds are overwhelmingly in his favor that he can be successfully extubated. Therefore, very aggressive treatment is indicated.

5. *After the patient is discharged, how would you follow him, and what are your treatment options now?*

Every attempt should be made to encourage him to stop smoking. The rate of pulmonary function loss in smokers who quit smoking gradually reverts toward the rate seen in the normal population. The risk of lung cancer and heart disease also declines significantly.

Among the therapeutic interventions now available are well designed smoking cessation therapy groups, such as the one offered by the American Lung Association, as well as the supervised use of nicotine gum. It is also important that a follow-up chest radiographic study be obtained within 4 to 6 weeks to demonstrate disappearance of the infiltrate. An unresolved infiltrate could be due to lung cancer (especially with the volume loss seen earlier on his chest radiograph). The incidence of lung cancer is much higher in smokers with COPD than in those without. This risk also diminishes significantly with the cessation of smoking. The patient should also receive annual influenza vaccines and, although a controversial measure, a one-time polyvalent pneumococcal vaccine. His medications should include an inhaled β agonist or Atrovent, or both. The judicious use of sustained-dose oral theophyllines and steroids (inhaled if possible) may be indicated. Finally, a repeat arterial blood gas measurement on room air should be performed when the patient's condition is clinically stable. Supplemental oxygen for patients with a Pao$_2$ of 55 mm Hg or less can improve a patient's cognitive ability, exercise tolerance, and right heart function, as well as prevent the development of pulmonary hypertension. Ultimately, it can lengthen the patient's life span.

Suggested Readings

Anthonisen NR. Hypoxemia and O_2 therapy. *American Review of Respiratory Diseases* 1982;126:729.

Petty TL, ed. *Chronic obstructive pulmonary disease*, 2nd ed. New York: Marcel Dekker, 1985.

Snider GL. Emphysema: the first two centuries and beyond. *American Review of Respiratory Diseases* 1992;146:1615.

Idiopathic Pulmonary Fibrosis

1. What are the basic pathologic events that lead to interstitial lung disease (ILD)?

2. What are the classic pulmonary function test abnormalities observed in the setting of idiopathic pulmonary fibrosis (IPF)?

3. What is the outcome if IPF is left untreated, and is the diagnosis one of exclusion?

4. What are the presenting symptoms of IPF?

Discussion

1. *What are the basic pathologic events that lead to ILD?*

Regardless of the underlying cause of ILD, the morphologic pattern of progression is similar. In a common sequence of events, a known or unknown stimulus or insult precipitates an alveolitis, defined as the influx of inflammatory cells into the alveolar structure. Unlike acute insults, as seen in bacterial pneumonia (which results in a transient inflammatory infiltrate), the alveolitis of ILD is chronic. The persistence of this alveolitis injures the parenchymal cells and the alveolar capillary membrane. Inflammation and abnormal repair then lead to mesenchymal cell proliferation, with the attendant production of excess collagen and connective tissue elements in the extracellular matrix. Ultimately, the normal architecture of the lung is replaced by cystic spaces separated by thick bands of fibrous tissue, indicative of end-stage honeycomb lung. IPF is the prototypic ILD whose underlying pathologic process is usually interstitial pneumonia.

2. *What are the classic pulmonary function test abnormalities observed in the setting of IPF?*

The characteristic pulmonary function test abnormalities include a reduction in lung volumes and airflow (FEV_1 and FVC), with preservation of the FEV_1/FVC ratio. This normal or increased ratio is due to the increased elastic recoil of the stiff lung parenchyma. Patients with certain interstitial lung diseases (e.g., chronic hypersensitivity pneumonitis, pulmonary eosinophilic granuloma, and cystic fibrosis) may initially exhibit normal or increased lung volumes secondary to small airway involvement with airflow obstruction (a reduced FEV_1/FVC ratio) and air trapping. In addition, the development of emphysema in conjunction with *any* type of ILD may initially be associated with relatively mild abnormalities on routine pulmonary function tests. It is thus important to remember that the absence of classic PFT abnormalities *does not* rule out IPF or any other ILD. The gas exchange at rest is initially normal in many patients with IPF; however, exercise-induced desaturation is one of the earliest signs and the most sensitive means to detect the disease. The diffusion capacity is typically reduced but may be normal, especially in the early stages of the disease.

3. *What is the outcome if IPF is left untreated, and is the diagnosis one of exclusion?*

Idiopathic pulmonary fibrosis is an inflammatory disorder that steadily progresses if untreated. With time, the chronic inflammatory response (alveolitis) produces fibrosis, along with the classic physiologic abnormalities already described. Although the etiology is unknown, the clinicopathologic manifestations are specific, and, therefore, it is *not* a diagnosis of exclusion.

4. *What are the presenting symptoms of IPF?*

The insidious onset of breathlessness and nonproductive cough is common to most cases. Fatigue, low-grade feverishness, arthralgias, and myalgias are also relatively common, but nonspecific, symptoms. The occurrence of frank arthritis, myositis (muscle tenderness and weakness), photosensitivity, Raynaud's phenomenon, visual problems, and so on, suggests the existence of other systemic processes, such as collagen-vascular disease, vasculitis, or sarcoidosis. Dry inspiratory crackles may be the only physical finding, although digital clubbing is seen in 40% to 70% of cases. A chest radiograph usually reveals reticular (linear) or reticulonodular opacities in the lower lung zones. The high-resolution CT scan indicates peripheral and basilar interstitial infiltrates and honeycombing.

Case   A 58-year-old woman is referred for the evaluation of breathlessness and cough. She first began noticing dyspnea on exertion approximately 3 to 4 years ago when using her floor sweeper. However, she noted no limitation when performing any of her other usual activities. Her dyspnea worsened slightly over the ensuing years without any other symptoms until 9 months ago, when a nonproductive cough developed. This was treated with antibiotics and inhaled bronchodilators, without improvement. Over the past 9 months, her breathlessness has worsened and she now has trouble climbing one flight of stairs. She tires easily and occasionally feels feverish, but has not experienced arthralgias, myalgias, night sweats, or other constitutional symptoms. She has experienced no chest pain or hemoptysis and has no history of cardiopulmonary disease. Her past medical history is unremarkable. Medications include Atrovent and theophylline (Theo-Dur; Schering-Plough, Kenilworth, NJ). She is married and has never smoked. She has worked as a retail sales clerk for 17 years without exposures. She has had no pet birds, leaky pipes, or moldy conditions in her home.

Physical examination reveals a respiratory rate of 20 unlabored breaths per minute with dry inspiratory rales heard over the lower third of the posterior lung fields. She shows no clubbing or edema. Laboratory evaluation reveals a normal hemogram and biochemical profile. Anti-nuclear antibodies show weak positivity at 1:80. Testing for the rheumatoid factor is negative.

A chest radiograph shows dense reticular opacities that are most prominent in the lower lung zones as well as small lung volumes. Pulmonary function tests reveal a total lung capacity of 70% of predicted and a functional residual capacity that is 66% of predicted. The FEV_1 is 50% of predicted with an FVC that is 58% of predicted. The FEV_1/FVC ratio is 88%. Her diffusion capacity is 85% of predicted. The Pao_2 on room air while resting is 60 mm Hg, which drops to 38 mm Hg with exercise.

1. How would the diagnosis of IPF best be confirmed in this patient?
2. If the thoracoscopic lung biopsy specimen reveals the presence of the usual interstitial pneumonitis, what are the treatment options for this patient?

Case Discussion

1. *How would the diagnosis of IPF best be confirmed in this patient?*

Although the clinical, radiologic, and physiologic picture in this patient is most suggestive of IPF, other interstitial lung diseases, such as chronic hypersensitivity pneumonitis, bronchiolitis obliterans organizing pneumonia, respiratory bronchiolitis, and stage III sarcoidosis, may present in an identical fashion. Therefore, lung tissue is needed to make a definitive diagnosis. Unfortunately, transbronchial biopsies yield only small fragments of tissue that are inadequate to establish the diagnosis of IPF. Open lung biopsy or the less invasive video-assisted thoracoscopic lung biopsy are required to obtain sufficient tissue to demonstrate the characteristic pathologic process of the usual interstitial pneumonitis. Biopsy specimens in this setting show variable degrees of cellular infiltration and fibrosis. A predominance of cellular lesions is associated with better responsiveness to therapy.

2. *If the thoracoscopic lung biopsy specimen reveals the presence of the usual interstitial pneumonitis, what are the treatment options for this patient?*

Corticosteroids have long been the initial drug of choice in patients with IPF in an attempt to suppress active, ongoing alveolar and interstitial inflammation and injury. High doses of 1 mg/kg (60 to 100 mg per day) for 6 to 8 weeks followed by a *slow* taper to 0.5 mg/kg (30 to 50 mg per day) over the next 3 months are recommended. Response to treatment is often not seen for 3 to 6 months, and responders usually require at least a year of therapy and often much longer. Unfortunately, the response rates are low, with only 20% to 25% of patients showing improvement with therapy. In patients who fail a trial of steroids, approximately 20% either may show improvement or the disease process may stabilize with cytotoxic therapy. Supplemental oxygen therapy is important in the treatment of hypoxic patients with IPF because it improves exercise tolerance and prevents or delays the onset of cor pulmonale.

Suggested Readings

Crystal RG, Gadek JE, Ferrans VJ. Interstitial lung disease: current concepts of pathogenesis, staging and therapy. *Am J Med* 1981;70:542.

King TE. Idiopathic pulmonary fibrosis. In: Schwarz MI, King TE, eds. *Interstitial lung disease*, 2nd ed. Toronto: BC Decker, 1993 p. 367.

Turner-Warwick M, Burrows B, Johnson A. Cryptogenic fibrosing alveolitis: response to corticosteroid treatment and its effect on survival. *Thorax* 1980;35:593.

Pleural Disease

1. What is a pleural effusion?
2. What are the physical findings associated with a pleural effusion?
3. What is the significance of differentiating between transudative and exudative pleural effusions?
4. What diagnostic laboratory tests can be performed on pleural fluid to distinguish transudates from exudates?
5. What is empyema?
6. How do you develop a treatment plan in the patient with a pleural effusion?

Discussion

1. *What is a pleural effusion?*

   A pleural effusion is an abnormal collection of fluid in the potential space between the visceral and parietal pleura. Normally, this space contains only a few milliliters of fluid, which helps to lubricate these surfaces.

2. *What are the physical findings associated with a pleural effusion?*

   Pleural effusions can be appreciated on physical examination when they are large enough to produce a fluid level in the chest and compress underlying lung tissue. Dullness to percussion with decreased or absent breath sounds in a dependent anatomic location is typical of effusions. Egophony is an important finding that distinguishes an effusion stemming from atelectasis secondary to bronchial obstruction. Lobar consolidation with a patent bronchus, such as in some pneumonias, may be difficult to distinguish from an effusion on examination, particularly because these two abnormalities often coexist. A whisper pectoriloquy may be heard in the setting of consolidation but is absent in the setting of effusions. In addition, physical findings that suggest a systemic illness, such as congestive heart failure, cirrhosis, and lupus erythematosus, provide important clues to the potential cause and nature of a pleural effusion discovered on physical examination or radiographic study.

3. *What is the significance of differentiating between transudative and exudative pleural effusions?*

   This division is an important first step in the diagnostic evaluation of a pleural effusion. In the context of a transudative pleural effusion, the pleura itself is not diseased but fluid is accumulating because of the effect of abnormal Starling forces stemming from a systemic illness, such as congestive heart failure, cirrhosis, and nephrosis. In these conditions, pleural fluid accumulates for the same reasons that peripheral edema and ascites develop. In the setting of an exudative effusion, the pleura is primarily involved by the disease. Examples include malignancies in the pleura (usually metastatic), infections, collagen-vascular diseases, and pulmonary infarctions. In these processes, the pleural surface is damaged and fluid accumulates independent of Starling forces.

4. *What diagnostic laboratory tests can be performed on pleural fluid to distinguish transudates from exudates?*

There are a number of simple laboratory tests that can help in distinguishing transudative from exudative pleural effusions. Exudates have a higher protein content and lactate dehydrogenase (LDH) level than transudates because the lining cells of the pleura are affected by the disease process. A fluid protein level greater than 50% of the patient's corresponding plasma protein level, an LDH level greater than 180 IU, or an LDH level greater than 60% of the patient's corresponding plasma level has been shown to distinguish exudates from transudates. If any of these three values are present, it is more than 90% likely that the effusion is an exudate. The finding of a high cell count in the pleural fluid suggests the presence of an exudate but is a less reliable indicator than the protein and LDH values. Once an exudate has been identified, other studies can be performed to help elucidate its cause. These include cytologic analysis, microbiologic stains and cultures, pH determination, and serology tests such as an anti-nuclear antibody profile.

5. *What is empyema?*

Empyema is an infection in the pleural space. This infection may be bacterial, mycobacterial, or fungal in origin. Occasionally, intermediate organisms such as *Actinomyces* and *Nocardia* can also cause empyema. Empyemas often must be distinguished from parapneumonic effusions, in which pneumonia in tissue adjacent to the pleura can cause an inflammatory response in the pleura with the development of an inflammatory exudate. The diagnostic hallmark of empyema is identification of the causative organism either by special staining of the fluid or by culture. Often such information is not obtained despite careful evaluation, and a clinical diagnosis of empyema is made based on the overall clinical presentation. A low glucose level (<50 mg/dL) or a low pH (<7.30), or both, suggest the presence of empyema, but are also seen in the settings of malignancy, esophageal rupture, and rheumatoid arthritis (low glucose level only). Empyemas are difficult infections to cure with antimicrobial therapy alone, particularly when bacterial in origin. These empyemas are essentially intrapleural abscesses and, like most abscesses, require drainage to achieve resolution.

6. *How do you develop a treatment plan in the patient with a pleural effusion?*

The most important aspect in planning treatment is to understand the etiology of the effusion. If it is a transudate, you need to determine which of the systemic edematous conditions is present. Effective treatment of the congestive heart failure, nephrosis, or cirrhosis, if possible, resolves the effusion. If the effusion is associated with an infection, such as a parapneumonic effusion or an empyema, definitive treatment of the infection is indicated. Malignant effusions must be addressed in the context of the underlying malignancy. Thus, the treatment of a pleural effusion depends on the information gleaned during an appropriate clinical evaluation of the patient as a whole.

Case

A 43-year-old man with long-standing rheumatoid arthritis presents to the emergency room complaining of right pleuritic chest pain. He has severe seropositive disease requiring ongoing aspirin and intramuscular gold therapy. He was started on prednisone by his physician 1 week earlier for an acute flareup of synovitis in his wrists and hands. For several days before the onset of the pleuritic pain, the patient has noted malaise, anorexia, and fevers. The night before presentation, he noted the onset of sharp, nonradiating pain in the right chest, which worsens with coughing or deep breathing. His cough is nonproductive. He denies cigarette or alcohol use.

On physical examination, he is found to be in moderate distress because of his chest pain. His blood pressure is 120/70 mm Hg, pulse is 120 beats per minute and regular, the respiratory rate is 20 breaths per minute, and temperature is 38°C orally. His examination findings are remarkable for good dentition; a normal jugular venous pressure; a regular tachycardia without murmurs, gallops, or rubs; and no peripheral edema. Lung examination reveals dullness to percussion at the right base with absent breath sounds in that area. Egophony is present at the right base but whisper pectoriloquy is not noted. The left lung is clear except for a small area of decreased breath sounds at the base, without egophony.

A complete blood count reveals a mild normocytic anemia with a hemoglobin level of 12.5 g/dL. The white blood cell count is 13,000/mm^3 with an increase in the number of band forms. A chest radiograph shows a moderate right pleural effusion, a small left pleural effusion, and a normal cardiac silhouette.

Thoracentesis of the right pleural effusion yields 250 mL of yellow, slightly cloudy fluid. The white blood cell count in the fluid is 3,500/mm^3 with 90% neutrophils. The red blood cell count is 1,000/mm^3. The protein level is 4.0 g/dL, the LDH level is 400 IU, the glucose content is 10 mg/dL, and the pH is 7.12.

1. What is the most likely cause of the right pleuritic chest pain?
2. What further tests would you do to verify your diagnosis?
3. How would you manage this patient's acute problem?
4. What are the intrathoracic manifestations of rheumatoid arthritis?

Case Discussion

1. *What is the most likely cause of the right pleuritic chest pain?*

The presentation consisting of fever, the acute onset of pleuritic pain, and an exudative pleural effusion with a predominance of neutrophils is most consistent with a bacterial infection of the pleural space, or empyema. Empyema is usually the result of a pneumonia that extends to and involves the adjacent pleura. The pleural fluid may have a low glucose level and usually has a low pH (<7.30). The most common causes include anaerobic bacteria (often resulting from an aspiration pneumonia), *Staphylococcus aureus*, pneumococcus, and tuberculosis. In immunocompromised hosts, the differential diagnosis includes fungi and other opportunistic pathogens.

In this patient, the diagnosis of pulmonary embolism with subsequent pulmonary infarction certainly cannot be absolutely excluded. This can present with fever and pleuritic pain as well. However, the pleural fluid is usually frankly bloody as a result of local tissue infarction. In addition, hemoptysis may be an associated finding. This patient's effusion had a low red blood cell count and he has no risk factors for pulmonary emboli, such as prolonged bed rest or recent trauma.

Rheumatoid involvement of the pleura is actually quite common. Most patients with rheumatoid arthritis have a pleural effusion at some time in their life. The classic characteristics of the fluid are an exudate with a low glucose level and a high rheumatoid factor level. The presentation is typically subacute when the effusion becomes large enough to cause symptoms or, in most cases, is noted on examination or a radiographic study in an asymptomatic patient.

Constrictive pericarditis may be a rare consequence of rheumatoid involvement of the pericardium. However, it is usually manifested by a right-sided congestion with an elevated jugular venous pressure (usually with a Kussmaul's sign), hepatomegaly, and peripheral edema.

2. *What further tests would you do to verify your diagnosis?*

Gram's staining and culture of the pleural fluid in a patient with empyema is important to identify a causative organism and direct the choice of antibiotic therapy. The Gram's stain findings are often positive and can narrow the differential diagnosis and the antibiotic choices. When tuberculous empyema is suspected, acid-fast staining of a sample of pleural fluid is indicated. Subsequent cultures and sensitivities are useful in adjusting drug therapy. In the event of empyema caused by anaerobic bacteria, the Gram's stain findings are more often than not negative, and cultures may yield negative results unless the fluid is carefully handled and processed anaerobically. When anaerobic empyema is suspected, empiric therapy is often necessary if an organism cannot be identified.

A ventilation–perfusion scan is used to screen for pulmonary emboli. The classic feature of a pulmonary embolus is absence of perfusion to a substantial area of lung with preserved ventilation (i.e., a mismatch). If a pulmonary embolus is suspected on the basis of the scan findings and there is a significant clinical suspicion for this diagnosis as well, empiric anticoagulation is indicated.

Determination of the rheumatoid factor level in the pleural space can be performed to ascertain whether a pleural effusion in a patient with rheumatoid arthritis is related to the underlying rheumatoid process. However, the presence of a high rheumatoid factor does not exclude a secondary complication of a rheumatoid effusion such as infection.

An echocardiogram is a useful way to assess the pericardium when pericardial disease, such as constrictive pericarditis, is suspected.

3. *How would you manage this patient's acute problem?*

The therapy for emphysema always involves antimicrobial drugs directed toward the known or presumed causative organism, or organisms. For instance, if the Gram's stain findings and culture show pneumococcus, this calls for intravenous penicillin treatment. In patients with bacterial empyemas, traditional therapy also involves chest tube, smaller catheter, or surgical drainage of the pleural space because this essentially represents an abscess cavity and antibiotic therapy alone is usually ineffective. Drainage is not done in the event of tuberculous empyema, however. The therapy for this is prolonged (6 to 12 months) treatment with antituberculous drugs. Some clinicians have recommended that, in the event of pneumococcal empyema, antibiotic therapy alone is often effective when the fluid is not loculated and the patient is doing well. In this patient, the low pH of the fluid and significant pleuritic pain would prompt placement of a small percutaneous catheter into the right pleural space to drain the empyema completely. Intravenous heparin for 2 weeks followed by long-term oral sodium warfarin is the traditional therapy for pulmonary emboli. Pericardiocentesis is the treatment for pericardial tamponade, but is not indicated for constrictive pericarditis. Prednisone can be administered to suppress a flareup of rheumatoid disease involving the joints, although it does not appear to have any effect on pleural or pericardial involvement.

4. *What are the intrathoracic manifestations of rheumatoid arthritis?*

Rheumatoid arthritis is truly a systemic illness. As already noted, most patients with this disease have pleural involvement at some time. Pericardial involvement is less common and, fortunately, is rarely clinically significant. Pulmonary nodules can also form, particularly in patients with rheumatoid nodules on their extremities. These nodules are similar histologically to the peripheral nodules, they wax and wane with the intensity of the systemic disease, and are rarely significant clinically. In addition to these manifestations, rheumatoid disease can cause pulmonary fibrosis that, if progressive, can be fatal. Rarely, bronchiolitis obliterans may occur in rheumatoid arthritis. This is characterized by a progressive, irreversible illness similar to emphysema in its radiographic appearance and physiologic abnormalities, and is usually fatal within 5 years of presentation.

Suggested Readings

Hunninghake GW, Fauci AS. State of the art: pulmonary involvement in the collagen vascular diseases. *American Review of Respiratory Diseases* 1979;119:471.

Light RW. *Pleural diseases*. Philadelphia: Lea & Febiger, 1983:101–118.

Light RW. Disorders of the pleura. In: Murray J, Nadel J, eds. *Textbook of respiratory medicine*. Philadelphia: WB Saunders, 1988, p. 671.

Pulmonary Complications of Human Immunodeficiency Virus Infection

> **1.** What are the pulmonary complications in a patient with human immunodeficiency virus (HIV) infection?
>
> **2.** What tests would help you establish a specific diagnosis?

Discussion

> **1.** *What are the pulmonary complications in a patient with HIV infection?*
>
> Human immunodeficiency virus is a lymphotropic retrovirus that infects T4 (helper) lymphocytes, B cells, and monocytes, leading to a defect in cell-mediated immunity, which then predisposes to the development of a variety of neoplasms and opportunistic infections. The lung is one of the primary target organs in HIV disease, and pulmonary complications are the leading cause of hospitalization and death in HIV-infected patients. The spectrum of pulmonary disorders associated with HIV infection includes both infectious and noninfectious diseases. The infectious causes of pulmonary disease include both opportunistic and nonopportunistic agents. The most common opportunistic organisms are *Pneumocystis carinii*, cytomegalovirus, and *Mycobacterium avium-intracellulare* (MAI). Although opportunistic infections are common in HIV-infected patients, these patients are also more susceptible to nonopportunistic infections, including pyogenic organisms (*S. pneumoniae* and *H. influenzae*), *Mycobacterium tuberculosis*, and fungal infections. The specific infection the patient acquires depends on the degree of immune deficiency and his or her exposure to specific organisms. The noninfectious pulmonary disorders include Kaposi's sarcoma, non-Hodgkin's lymphoma, lymphocytic interstitial pneumonitis, nonspecific interstitial pneumonia, alveolar proteinosis, bronchiolitis obliterans organizing pneumonia, primary pulmonary hypertension, and emphysema.
>
> **2.** *What tests would help you establish a specific diagnosis?*
>
> A chest radiographic study, arterial blood gas determinations, a complete blood count, LDH measurement, and sputum studies should all be carried out in an HIV-infected patient presenting with fever and increasing shortness of breath. Although the chest radiograph can be helpful, the radiographic manifestations of pulmonary disease significantly overlap in this group of patients. Most patients with *P. carinii* pneumonia (PCP) are hypoxic and hypocapnic, and exhibit a widened alveolar-arterial gradient, often before any abnormality is detected on a chest radiograph. The complete blood count in HIV-infected patients typically demonstrates an absolute lymphopenia, which primarily stems from a decrease in the number of T4 cells. The LDH level is elevated in 95% of the patients with PCP and has been shown to increase with worsening symptoms and decline in response to therapy. Sputum in patients with pyogenic bacterial infections is often purulent, and the Gram's

stain and culture findings should dictate the antibiotic choice. Patients with PCP often have a nonproductive cough, making it necessary to obtain a sputum specimen that is induced by the inhalation of hypertonic saline. Sputum and blood cultures for MAI infection and tuberculosis are also indicated. This has a yield of between 25% to 85%, depending on the experience of the person performing the test. Methenamine silver staining is the traditional method to identify the organism's cyst.

Case   A 37-year-old homosexual man, known to be HIV positive, is seen for evaluation of progressive dyspnea and fever. He was well until 7 to 8 months ago, when he noted the onset of weight loss, diffuse adenopathy, and night sweats. Over the past month, he has noted progressive dyspnea, a dry, nonproductive cough, and daily fever spikes. He has smoked 20 cigarettes a day from the age of 18 years, denies alcohol or drug abuse, and has lived in the Ohio River valley as well as the Southwest. Physical examination reveals a blood pressure of 110/65 mm Hg, pulse of 100 beats per minute, respiratory rate of 32 breaths per minute, and temperature of 39°C. Throat examination findings are remarkable for a white exudate on the posterior pharyngeal wall. The lymph nodes are diffusely enlarged and nontender. During chest examination, bilateral crackles are noted. The remainder of the examination findings are unremarkable. A chest radiograph reveals the presence of diffuse bilateral interstitial infiltrates.

1. What is the differential diagnosis in this patient, and do the chest radiograph findings influence this?
2. If the initial test results do not confirm your diagnosis, what test would you do next?
3. What therapy would you initiate, and is there a role for prophylactic therapy?

Case Discussion

1. *What is the differential diagnosis in this patient, and do the chest radiograph findings influence this?*

   Although malignancy and a chronic infectious process such as tuberculosis could account for these chronic and subacute symptoms, this patient's clinical picture is most consistent with a complication of HIV infection. Besides the spectrum of pulmonary disorders associated with HIV infections, primary cardiac disorders should also be considered when dyspnea and bilateral rales are encountered. The fever and chills in this patient indicate an infectious cause. The differential diagnosis in this patient would include PCP, tuberculosis, and infection with nonopportunistic pulmonary pathogens, such as *S. pneumoniae, H. influenzae,* and *S. aureus.*

   As already mentioned, the chest radiograph can be helpful in making the diagnosis, even though there is significant overlap in the radiographic manifestations of the various pulmonary diseases. In PCP, the most common finding is a diffuse increase in the interstitial and alveolar markings, although nodular infiltrates, cavities, pneumatoceles, and, more recently, pneumothoraces and pleural effusions have all been observed in this setting. In addition, 20% of patients with PCP can have a normal radiograph. Kaposi's sarcoma often presents with nodular infiltrates, with or without a pleural effusion. The effusion is either serosanguineous or hemorrhagic and is due to pleural involvement by the sarcoma. The presence of intrathoracic adenopathy suggests tuberculosis, non-Hodgkin's lymphoma, Kaposi's sarcoma, or MAI infection.

2. *If the initial test results do not confirm your diagnosis, what test would you do next?*

If the sputum specimen findings are nondiagnostic, the next diagnostic procedure would be fiberoptic bronchoscopy with bronchoalveolar lavage and, in some cases, a transbronchial biopsy. This allows the alveolar tissue to be directly sampled. Bronchoalveolar lavage is performed by placing the bronchoscope in the distal airway and instilling 100 to 200 mL of saline into the airway, then immediately removing the solution. The lavage technique has a yield of 75% to 95% in the setting of PCP, and transbronchial biopsy has a yield of 85% to 95%. Kaposi's sarcoma, however, is difficult to diagnose using bronchoscopy. If bronchoscopic findings are nondiagnostic, an open lung biopsy should be done. This involves an open thoracotomy and is rarely needed.

3. *What therapy would you initiate, and is there a role for prophylactic therapy?*

Treatment with trimethoprim-sulfamethoxazole should be started in conjunction with intravenous corticosteroids. The role of prophylactic therapy is under investigation. It also appears that prophylactic oral therapy with trimethoprim-sulfamethoxazole is highly efficacious in preventing recurrence of PCP. However, many patients are unable to endure prolonged therapy because of adverse side effects. Aerosolized pentamidine is also used for PCP prophylactic treatment, and has been shown to be effective.

Suggested Readings

Hopewell PC, Luce JM. Pulmonary manifestations of the acquired immunodeficiency syndrome. *Clin Immunol Allergy* 1986;6:489.

Murray JF, Mills J. Pulmonary infectious complications of human immunodeficiency virus infection: part I. *American Review of Respiratory Diseases* 1990;141:1356.

Murray JF, Mills J. Pulmonary infectious complications of human immunodeficiency virus infection: part II. *American Review of Respiratory Diseases* 1990;141:1582.

Solitary Pulmonary Nodule

1. What is a solitary pulmonary nodule (SPN)?

2. What percentage of SPNs are benign?

3. What clinical and radiologic findings are associated with a higher incidence of malignancy in an SPN?

4. What is the most common cause of an SPN?

Discussion

1. *What is an SPN?*

   Solitary pulmonary nodules are single opacities located entirely within the lung parenchyma and usually less than 4.0 cm in diameter. They are not associated with atelectasis or hilar adenopathy on plain chest roentgenograms.

2. *What percentage of SPNs are benign?*

   Seventy-five to 85% of SPNs are benign, and 15% to 25% are malignant (either primary or metastatic disease). The physician's role is to expedite the workup and resection of potentially curable malignant SPNs, while avoiding costly evaluations and painful thoracotomies for SPNs that are benign or already unresectable (i.e., metastatic).

3. *What clinical and radiologic findings are associated with a higher incidence of malignancy in an SPN?*

   There are several features that suggest malignancy:

   Age. Virtually all SPNs in adults younger than 35 years of age are benign. The risk of malignant disease increases with increasing age.

   Nodule size. More than 80% of the SPNs larger than 3.0 cm in diameter are malignant; 20% or fewer of the SPNs less than 2.0 cm in diameter are malignant.

   Presence and pattern of calcification. Calcification, particularly that with a central, laminated, or diffuse pattern, is suggestive of benign disease. Malignant disease only rarely shows evidence of calcification, and more frequently exhibits an eccentric pattern.

   History of prior malignancy. As many as 30% of malignant SPNs are metastases from extrathoracic malignancies.

   Smoking history. Although the effect of smoking on malignancy in the setting of SPNs has not been specifically determined, there is a well known association between smoking and the development of primary bronchogenic carcinoma. This risk returns to that of the general nonsmoking population between 10 and 15 years after smoking cessation.

4. *What is the most common cause of an SPN?*

   Over half of all SPNs are found to be granulomas on pathologic examination. Hamartomas represent the next most common benign cause, but constitute less than 10% of the total causes of SPNs.

Case   A 40-year-old woman is seen for a preoperative evaluation before undergoing laparoscopic cholecystectomy. Her medical history is remarkable for mild untreated hypertension. She has undergone no previous surgical procedures. She had a 5-pack-year history of smoking, but quit 8 years ago. She was born and raised in Cincinnati before moving to Denver 3 years ago with her husband and four children. She works as a paralegal in a downtown law firm. She takes no medications other than an occasional aspirin for headache.

A thorough review reveals symptoms referable to her cholelithiasis. Specifically, she denies any systemic or chest complaints, including fever, malaise, weight change, myalgias or arthralgias, chest pain, shortness of breath or dyspnea on exertion, cough, and hemoptysis.

Physical examination reveals a mildly obese woman in no distress. Vital signs are normal except for a blood pressure of 170/90 mm Hg. Head and neck findings are normal, and her lungs are clear. Heart findings are also normal. Abdominal examination reveals right upper quadrant tenderness in response to deep palpation without rebound or guarding. There are no masses or hepatosplenomegaly. Stool is guaiac negative. Her extremities are normal, as are the findings from a thorough neurologic examination. There is no adenopathy.

Laboratory examination, including a complete blood count, chemistry panel 22, arterial blood gas measurement, and urinalysis, all yield findings that are within normal limits. An electrocardiogram is normal. A chest radiographic study reveals a 1.8-cm, round opacity in the left lower lobe, but is otherwise normal.

1. What is the most important next diagnostic step at this time?
2. What are the major possible diagnoses of this patient's nodule?
3. What noninvasive diagnostic test may help to distinguish between the possible diagnoses in this patient?
4. If the test results up to this point have been nondiagnostic or indeterminate, what options should be presented to the patient at this time?

Case Discussion

1. *What is the most important next diagnostic step at this time?*

An old chest radiographic study should be obtained, if possible. If the nodule was present and is unchanged in size on a study from at least 2 years before, it is very likely that this represents a benign lesion, and no further workup is necessary. Malignant lesions usually have a doubling time of weeks to months. In other words, a lesion that grows either very rapidly (days) or very slowly (years) is likely to be benign. In the event of very rapid growth, the patient usually has other pulmonary symptoms consistent with a benign diagnosis, such as infection or pulmonary infarction.

2. *What are the major possible diagnoses of this patient's nodule?*

The differential diagnosis for this patient includes granulomatous disease, bronchogenic carcinoma, hamartoma, pulmonary metastasis from an unknown primary tumor, and "round" pneumonia.

Infectious granulomatous diseases resulting in SPNs include histoplasmosis, coccidioidomycosis, and tuberculosis. Granulomas can also appear as SPNs in the settings of sarcoidosis, rheumatoid arthritis, and vasculitides such as Wegener's granulomatosis. Primary bronchogenic carcinoma is the most frequent source of resected malignant SPNs. Metastatic disease, often originating from extrapulmonary adenocarcinomas of the breast, prostate, or colon, frequently present as SPNs. "Round" pneumonia is an uncommon presentation of acute pulmonary infections in which the alveolar space-filling disease assumes a more rounded, nodular appearance. In the absence of other signs or symptoms, this might be confused with an SPN. Other, rarer causes of SPNs include arteriovenous malformations, bronchogenic cysts, pulmonary infarction, and parasitic disease.

3. *What noninvasive diagnostic test may help to distinguish between the possible diagnoses in this patient?*

Computed tomography, with thin sections through the nodule, should be performed in this patient. SPNs are often found to be multiple on closer examination by CT, suggesting the presence of either granulomatous disease or pulmonary metastases. Less than 1% of primary lung cancers present as multiple and synchronous lesions. CT is also very sensitive in defining the density and configuration of an SPN. The finding of a fat density in the nodule strongly suggests the diagnosis of hamartoma. Central, laminated, or diffuse patterns of calcification also suggest a benign diagnosis (particularly granulomatous disease or hamartoma), whereas eccentric calcification can be found in either benign or malignant disease. Less helpful is the configuration of the SPN. Poorly marginated or spiculated nodules are often malignant, but well marginated spherical nodules can be either benign or malignant. Ipsilateral mediastinal or hilar adenopathy (defined by most radiologists as lymph nodes >1 cm in transverse diameter) can be associated with either benign or malignant lesions. However, adenopathy involving the hemithorax contralateral to the SPN is highly suggestive of nonresectable malignant disease.

4. *If the test results up to this point have been nondiagnostic or indeterminate, what options should be presented to the patient at this time?*

There are three options at this point.

Observation is appropriate in many patients, particularly those with a very low likelihood of malignancy or those for whom an invasive diagnostic procedure would carry an unacceptably high risk of morbidity and mortality. The course of the SPN can be monitored with serial chest radiographic studies obtained every 3 months for the first year, every 6 months for the second year, and yearly thereafter.

Biopsy can be performed using either CT or fluoroscopy-guided transthoracic FNA or fiberoptic bronchoscopy with transbronchial biopsy. The latter procedure is associated with a lower diagnostic yield, particularly for small (<2 cm) peripheral SPNs. In any event, if no diagnosis is reached, more aggressive attempts to obtain definitive tissue must be pursued. Nondiagnostic tissue findings should not be construed as evidence of a benign lesion.

Open lung biopsy is a third option. Thoracotomy has the advantage of being both a diagnostic and often a therapeutic procedure. Unfortunately, however, it is also associated with higher morbidity. Many surgeons perform mediastinoscopic lymph node biopsy before open thoracotomy, especially in cases of CT-proven mediastinal adenopathy, to avoid the more extensive procedure if possible. Finally, the SPN, if very peripheral, may produce a dimpling of the visceral pleura, allowing a limited thoracoscopic approach for removal.

Suggested Readings

Lillington GA, Caskey CI. Evaluation and management of solitary and multiple pulmonary nodules. *Clin Chest Med* 1993;14:111.

Midthun DE, Swensen SJ, Jett JR. Approach to the solitary pulmonary nodule. *Mayo Clin Proc* 1993;68:378.

Midthun DE, Swensen SJ, Jett JR. Clinical strategies for solitary pulmonary nodule. *Annu Rev Med* 1992;43:195.

Webb WR. Radiologic evaluation of the solitary pulmonary nodule. *AJR Am J Roentgenol* 1990;154:701.

Acute Pulmonary Embolism

1. What is a pulmonary embolism?
2. What are the common sources of pulmonary emboli?
3. What are the risk factors for pulmonary emboli?
4. Are all acute pulmonary emboli similar?

Discussion

1. *What is a pulmonary embolism?*

A pulmonary embolism is the migration of venous blood clots from the systemic veins to the lungs, resulting in either complete or partial obstruction of the pulmonary arterial blood flow. The incidence of pulmonary emboli exceeds 500,000 per year, with a mortality rate of approximately 10%. If this goes undiagnosed or is improperly diagnosed, the mortality rate can reach 30%.

2. *What are the common sources of pulmonary emboli?*

Close to 90% of pulmonary emboli originate in the deep venous systems of the legs. The upper extremities can also be a source of venous thrombi. Usually related to trauma, congenital fibromuscular bands, or the use of central venous catheters, 12% of all upper extremity thrombi result in pulmonary emboli. In addition, blood clot formation in the pelvic veins may cause either septic or bland pulmonary emboli, especially in the setting of complicated obstetric procedures or gynecologic surgery.

Certain materials can be a source of pulmonary emboli, including air introduced during intravenous injections, hemodialysis, or the placement of central venous catheters; amniotic fluid secondary to vigorous uterine contractions; fat as a result of multiple long bone fractures; parasites; tumor cells; or foreign materials in intravenous drug abusers. These forms of pulmonary emboli are often treated differently than those due to thrombus, and are not discussed further here.

3. *What are the risk factors for pulmonary emboli?*

Three basic risk factors, known collectively as *Virchow's triad*, are associated with thrombus formation and subsequent pulmonary emboli: stasis, hypercoagulability, and endothelial injury. Most clinical risk factors can stem from one of these three pathogenic mechanisms, and these are listed in Table 8-2.

Table 8-2. Risk Factors for Venous Thrombosis

Stasis	Hypercoagulability	Endothelial injury
Congestive heart failure	Deficiency of antithrombin III	Extensive pelvic surgery
Obesity	Deficiency of proteins C and S	Prior injury
Prolonged bed rest	Malignancies	Trauma
Prolonged travel	Oral contraceptives	
	Presence of a lupus anticoagulant	
	Factor V Leiden deficiency	

4. *Are all acute pulmonary emboli similar?*

Kelley and Fishman have divided acute pulmonary emboli into three categories. The rarest, **acute massive occlusion**, is defined as an embolism that occludes enough of the pulmonary circulation to produce circulatory collapse. At autopsy in these patients, large emboli are often found in the vicinity of the bifurcation of the main pulmonary artery, called *saddle emboli*. **Pulmonary infarction** occurs when the embolism obstructs enough blood flow to a specific section of the lung to cause death of lung tissue. This occurs in only 10% of cases of acute pulmonary embolism. The third and most common category is **pulmonary embolism without infarction**. These emboli are the most difficult to diagnose because they manifest no specific symptoms. Because most emboli are multiple, both infarcted and noninfarcted areas in the lung can coexist.

Case

A 27-year-old woman presents to the emergency room after 24 hours of right-sided chest pain, which is worse with inspiration. She is also experiencing shortness of breath and exhibits anxiety. The patient denies sputum production, hemoptysis, coughing, or wheezing, but states that she felt warm at home but did not take her temperature. She denies any recent injury or swelling of her legs, and is a very active person. The patient has also never had or been treated for respiratory problems.

Her past medical history is negative. Her only medication is oral contraceptives, and she has no known drug allergies. She has undergone no surgical procedures.

She smokes one pack of cigarettes per day, and does not consume alcohol. She does not use intravenous drugs and has no other risk factors for HIV disease. She works as an accountant. Her family history is negative for asthma and heart disease.

Physical examination reveals a mildly obese woman in moderate respiratory distress. Her temperature is 38.0°C, her pulse is 115 beats per minute, her blood pressure is 140/80 mm Hg, and her respiratory rate is 26 breaths per minute. No jugular venous distention is observed. Her chest is clear.

Cardiac examination reveals regular rate and rhythm, with normal systolic first and second sounds, and no systolic third or fourth sounds, murmurs, or rubs. Abdominal examination reveals positive bowel sounds and no hepatosplenomegaly. Her extremities show no cyanosis, clubbing, or edema.

Her laboratory values are as follows: hemoglobin, 14.5 g/dL; hematocrit, 42%; white blood cells, 6,000/mm^3 with 74% segmented neutrophils and 26% lymphocytes. Peak expiratory flow is 450 L per minute, which is normal.

1. What is the differential diagnosis in this patient?

    A chest radiographic study reveals a normal cardiac silhouette and clear lung fields, except for a small peripheral infiltrate in the lower left lobe. An electrocardiogram shows sinus tachycardia but no ischemic changes. Arterial blood gas measurement performed on room air (in Denver) reveals a pH of 7.49, a P_{CO_2} of 32 mm Hg, a P_{O_2} of 60 mm Hg, and an alveolar-arterial oxygen gradient of 40. A Gram's-stained sputum specimen exhibits normal flora.

2. What additional tests should be done to help narrow the differential diagnosis?
3. How do you interpret the additional test results?
4. What is the next step in diagnosing an acute pulmonary embolism?
5. Of what should the acute management of this patient's pulmonary embolism consist?
6. How long should anticoagulation therapy be continued?
7. What role would thrombolytic therapy have in this patient?
8. When should a vena caval filter be placed?

Case Discussion

1. *What is the differential diagnosis in this patient?*

    The differential diagnosis in this young woman with acute onset of shortness of breath and chest pain is lengthy. Not all breathing disorders are due primarily to pulmonary disease because ischemic cardiac disease can present with dyspnea when associated with cardiogenic pulmonary edema. However, the nature and location of the pain, the lack of substantial cardiac risk factors, and the patient's age make cardiac ischemia unlikely.

    Several pulmonary disorders can present in this manner. Patients with acute bacterial pneumonia complain of shortness of breath, low-grade fever, and chest pain. However, pneumonia usually also causes sputum production and an elevated white blood cell count, which are not seen in this patient. With the increasing prevalence of the acquired immunodeficiency syndrome (AIDS), dyspnea in a 27-year-old patient should suggest the diagnosis of PCP. Although this patient has no risk factors for HIV disease, this atypical pneumonia must be considered because it may not produce all of the characteristic signs and symptoms of an acute pulmonary infection. Asthma can also present insidiously with acute shortness of breath. However, the lack of a history of asthma, exposure to known triggers of asthmatic symptoms, and a normal peak expiratory flow make this diagnosis unlikely. A spontaneous pneumothorax can cause similar symptomatology, yet it would be unusual for this to be accompanied by a low-grade fever.

    The most common symptoms of pulmonary emboli include shortness of breath, pleuritic pain, cough, and hemoptysis. Pulmonary emboli should always be considered in a patient with acute shortness of breath and a known risk factor for thrombosis (oral contraceptives). Pleuritic chest pain, as seen in this patient, and hemoptysis occur only when the embolism causes a pulmonary infarction. Fevers as high as 39°C have also been reported in the setting of infarction or a concurrent infection. On physical examination, the most common sign is isolated sinus tachycardia; however, in those patients with massive embolism, evidence of acute right ventricular failure may be found. When diagnosing pulmonary embolism, remember that no clinical findings are universal and the absence of specific findings does not rule out the diagnosis.

2. *What additional tests should be done to help narrow the differential diagnosis?*

To help differentiate between the various diagnoses, a chest radiographic study, electrocardiogram, arterial blood gas analysis, and Gram's staining of a sputum sample should be done.

3. *How do you interpret the additional test results?*

In the setting of an acute pulmonary embolism, the arterial blood gas measurement classically reveals a low P_{CO_2}, low P_{O_2}, and a widened alveolar-arterial oxygen gradient. However, many other disorders cause similar abnormal arterial blood gas results, and 10% to 15% of patients with proven pulmonary emboli maintain a normal alveolar-arterial oxygen gradient.

The chest radiograph findings in patients with documented pulmonary emboli are nonspecific. Typically, infiltrates, atelectasis, effusions, or any combination of these are encountered. However, the film can also be completely normal. A peripheral wedge-shaped infiltrate, called a *Hampton's hump*, can be seen when the embolism is associated with infarction, and occasionally decreased pulmonary vascular markings are noted (Westermark's sign), indicative of decreased blood flow to a section of the lung. Both of these classic signs are rare, however.

The electrocardiogram is helpful to rule out ischemic heart disease. In patients with pulmonary emboli, the electrocardiogram usually demonstrates sinus tachycardia or is normal. Only in the presence of massive embolization is a right axis deviation and an S_1, Q_3, T_3 pattern seen.

These test results help to narrow the differential diagnosis. The chest radiograph findings rule out a pneumothorax, and a true bacterial pneumonia is less likely in light of the normal sputum findings. In addition, a small peripheral infiltrate would be unusual in a patient with PCP. The lack of ischemic findings on the electrocardiogram make a primary cardiac abnormality unlikely. With the presentation of shortness of breath, a widened alveolar-arterial oxygen gradient, and chest radiograph findings consistent with an infarction, a pulmonary embolism is now the most likely diagnosis.

4. *What is the next step in diagnosing an acute pulmonary embolism?*

A radionuclide or ventilation–perfusion scan should be obtained in patients with suspected pulmonary emboli. In some centers, a helical CT scan of the thorax has replaced ventilation–perfusion scanning. Measurement of the serum D-dimer, a fibrin degradation product, that demonstrates a level below 500 μg/L excludes the diagnosis of pulmonary embolism. The results of the ventilation–perfusion scan are usually separated into four categories: high probability, indeterminate probability, low probability, and normal. As reported in the Prospective Investigation of Pulmonary Embolism Diagnosis study, high-probability scans correctly diagnose pulmonary emboli in 97% of cases and normal scans are truly negative in 96% of cases. Therefore, if the scan indicates high probability, the patient should be treated for a pulmonary embolism, whereas a normal scan rules out the diagnosis. If the results of the scan are indeterminate or indicate low probability but there is a coexistent high clinical suspicion, other studies are indicated.

One approach when a ventilation–perfusion scan is inconclusive is to perform venous imaging of the lower extremities. Although the absence of thrombus in the legs does not rule out a pulmonary embolism as the cause of the shortness of breath, the presence of deep venous thrombosis is an indication for therapy and obviates the need for further testing.

The gold standard test for the diagnosis of pulmonary embolism is still pulmonary arteriography, and it should be performed in the setting of low-probability or indeterminate ventilation–perfusion scan findings and a high clinical suspicion. This method provides radiopaque images of the pulmonary arteries and is relatively safe in the absence of pulmonary hypertension or severe cardiac disease. Although best performed soon after the onset of symptoms, it is worth considering doing pulmonary arteriography within the first 7 days of presentation. Positive angiographic findings include an intraluminal filling defect or the abrupt cutoff of a vessel.

5. *Of what should the acute management of this patient's pulmonary embolism consist?*

The goal of therapy is to prevent further embolic episodes, and heparin is the initial drug of choice for accomplishing this. First, a large intravenous loading bolus should be given, followed by continuous-drip infusion, maintained for at least 5 and often 7 to 10 days. Anticoagulation should not be withheld pending the results of further studies unless the patient's risk of bleeding complications is greater than the clinical suspicion of pulmonary emboli. The partial thromboplastin time should be monitored and the heparin dosage adjusted to keep the time between 1.5 to 2.0 times the control.

The conventional approach has been to initiate oral anticoagulation on the fifth day of heparin therapy, and then to continue both drugs for another 4 to 5 days, thereby ensuring an adequate transition period. Driven by the desire to shorten the hospital stay, more recent studies have revealed that warfarin can be started 24 to 48 hours after heparin therapy has been initiated. During the first 3 days of warfarin therapy, the prothrombin time is increased before the onset of true anticoagulation. Therefore, before discontinuing the heparin, the prothrombin time should be therapeutic (1.5 times normal) for approximately 2 to 3 days. Low–molecular-weight heparins are excellent for prophylaxis in postoperative patients and probably have a role in the management of acute pulmonary embolism and deep venous thrombosis because they do not require monitoring of the anticoagulation effects.

6. *How long should anticoagulation therapy be continued?*

Long-term anticoagulation is usually achieved with warfarin, although low–molecular-weight heparins can also be used. Patients with reversible risk factors that are subsequently eliminated should undergo anticoagulation for a total of 3 months. If this is an initial episode of embolism and the patient has no clear risk factors, treatment should probably be maintained for 3 to 6 months. Finally, those patients with recurrent emboli and nonreversible risk factors (e.g., incurable adenocarcinoma) should be treated for life. When it is uncertain how long to maintain therapy, impedance plethysmography can help in identifying recurrent deep vein thrombosis.

7. *What role would thrombolytic therapy have in this patient?*

The role of thrombolytic agents (streptokinase, urokinase, and tissue plasminogen activator) is yet to be elucidated in the management of acute pulmonary embolism. There appear to be no significant differences between the three agents in the treatment of pulmonary emboli, except for their respective costs. Thrombolytic agents do accelerate the resolution of the pulmonary artery clot, but they have not been clearly shown to improve survival versus the results observed for conventional heparin therapy. The only adopted use of these agents is for patients with massive embolism and systemic hypotension. When used, thrombolytic therapy must be followed by a standard course of heparin.

8. *When should a vena caval filter be placed?*

The purpose of vena caval filters is both to trap emboli and maintain the patency of the inferior vena cava. These filters are largely viewed as an alternative therapy for thromboembolism when anticoagulation is unacceptable. The three most common indications for filter placement are (a) a contraindication to anticoagulation, (b) failure of proper anticoagulation to prevent the formation of further emboli, and (c) a complication of anticoagulation therapy.

Suggested Readings

Fishman AP, Kelley MA. Pulmonary thromboembolism (including prophylaxis, treatment, sickle cell disease, and multiple pulmonary thrombi). In: Fishman AP, ed. *Pulmonary diseases and disorders*, 2nd ed. New York: McGraw-Hill, 1987.

Hurewitz AN, Bergofsky EH. Pulmonary embolism. In: Cherniack RM, ed. *Current therapy of respiratory disease*. Toronto: BC Decker, 1989, p. 259.

Perrier A, Desmaris S, Goehring C, et al. D-dimer testing for suspected pulmonary embolism in outpatients. *Am J Respir Crit Care Med* 1997;136:492.

PIOPED Investigators. Value of the ventilation/perfusion scan in acute pulmonary embolism: results of the Prospective Investigation of Pulmonary Embolism Diagnosis (PIOPED). *JAMA* 1990;263:2753.

Sarcoidosis

1. What are the symptoms and signs of sarcoidosis?
2. What tests are used to establish the diagnosis?
3. What are the therapeutic options?

Discussion

1. *What are the symptoms and signs of sarcoidosis?*

   Sarcoidosis is a systemic disorder characterized histologically by the presence of noncaseating granulomas. The granulomas can be found in any tissue, such as the lung, skin, myocardium, central nervous system, and kidneys. The symptoms and signs most commonly seen stem from the involvement of the reticuloendothelial system and the lung. Typically, patients present with fatigue, a pigmented papulonodular skin rash, splenomegaly, and chest radiographic findings indicating bilateral hilar adenopathy or patchy nodular pulmonary infiltrates, or both. Laboratory abnormalities include anemia, leukopenia, hypercalcemia, elevation of the liver enzyme levels in a cholestatic pattern, and a polyclonal gammopathy.

2. *What tests are used to establish the diagnosis?*

   The most definitive test to establish the diagnosis of sarcoidosis is tissue biopsy. Sites for biopsy include the skin (if a rash exists) or lung. The sensitivity of bronchoscopy with transbronchial biopsy exceeds 90% in obtaining noncaseating granulomas in patients with sarcoidosis who present with hilar adenopathy and pulmonary infiltrates. However, noncaseating granulomas are only suggestive, but not pathognomonic, evidence for the disease. Other diseases that produce granulomas, such as mycobacterial and fungal diseases, must also be considered. These entities can be ruled out by bronchoscopy with biopsy and bronchoalveolar lavage.

   The serum level of the angiotensin-converting enzyme (ACE) is elevated in some patients with sarcoidosis, but this is neither a sensitive nor specific enough finding for it to serve as a diagnostic test. The level is elevated in approximately 66% of patients with sarcoidosis, but this also occurs in a variety of disorders such as tuberculosis, coccidioidomycosis, hyperthyroidism, and diabetes mellitus. However, the ACE level has been shown to decrease with therapy, and this may thus be a useful objective measure for monitoring the effectiveness of treatment.

3. *What are the therapeutic options?*

   Sarcoidosis is a very heterogeneous disease, with approximately one third of patients improving without treatment, one third progressing clinically, and one third remaining in relatively stable condition. Unfortunately, there is no reliable way to predict in which group patients will fall. Factors that suggest an unfavorable prognosis include extensive pulmonary parenchymal involvement, restrictive physiology on pulmonary function testing, an elevated ACE level, involvement of at least three organ systems, and black race. Organ involvement that mandates the institution of therapy includes eye, central nervous system, or cardiac involvement, as well as hypercalcemia.

Treatment consists of corticosteroids, usually prednisone or its equivalent initiated at a dosage of 30 to 40 mg per day. There is no evidence that any one steroid preparation is superior to another. Inhaled corticosteroids have not been found to be beneficial in the treatment of sarcoidosis. Between 80% and 90% of patients respond to steroid therapy. When effective, a clinical and radiographic response is usually witnessed within 2 to 4 weeks. This high dosage is usually continued for 1 to 2 months, then gradually tapered over the course of the next 1 to 6 months. Many patients can then discontinue taking steroids, but others require ongoing steroid therapy at a dosage of 10 to 15 mg daily or every other day. The response to therapy is confirmed by symptomatic and radiographic improvement, supported by a decreasing ACE level and stable or improving pulmonary function. Although there is symptomatic and radiographic improvement with corticosteroids, there is little evidence that they influence the natural course of the disease.

Case

A 34-year-old black woman is referred to the pulmonary clinic for evaluation of a 2-month history of dry cough, a rash on her forehead and arms, a 5-pound (2.25-kg) weight loss, and an abnormal chest radiographic study. She has an 8-pack-year smoking history and a history of prior intravenous cocaine use, and 6 months ago traveled to Bakersfield, California, for a vacation.

Physical examination reveals a thin woman in no distress. Her temperature is 99°F (37.2°C), pulse is 80 beats per minute, blood pressure is 110/70 mm Hg, and respiratory rate is 20 breaths per minute. A pigmented, papulonodular rash is present on her forehead and upper arms. Funduscopic findings are normal. Bibasilar crackles are heard on chest examination. Abdominal examination reveals an 8-cm liver and palpable spleen tip. There is no cyanosis, clubbing, or edema on examination of her extremities.

The chest radiographic study reveals bilateral hilar adenopathy and diffuse alveolar and nodular infiltrates. Laboratory findings are as follows: white blood cell count, 4,000/mm³ with 70% polymorphonuclear leukocytes, 10% monocytes, 2% eosinophils, and 17% lymphocytes; hemoglobin, 11 g/dL; hematocrit, 33%; platelet count, 300,000/μL; normal serum electrolyte levels; calcium, 10 mg/dL; albumin, 3.8 g/dL; and total protein, 8.0 g/dL.

1. What is the differential diagnosis in this patient?
2. What tests should be done to establish the diagnosis in this patient?

Pulmonary function testing reveals the following lung volumes: total lung capacity, 3.32 L (72% of predicted); thoracic gas volume, 1.63 L (64% of predicted); and residual volume, 0.72 L (59% of predicted). Spirometry shows an FVC of 2.72 L (70% of predicted) and FEV_1 of 2.12 L (75% of predicted). The diffusing capacity for carbon monoxide (DLCO) is 15.6 (46% of predicted) and the DLCO/Alveolar Ventilation (VA) is 4.97 (85% of predicted). Arterial blood gas measurements on room air reveal a pH of 7.41, $Paco_2$ of 32 mm Hg, Pao_2 of 68 mm Hg, and oxygen saturation of 94%.

3. How would you interpret the results of the pulmonary function tests?

Case Discussion

1. *What is the differential diagnosis in this patient?*

As is true for many pulmonary disorders, the radiographic pattern combined with the patient's clinical history and physical examination findings narrows the differential diagnosis. In a patient who presents with this clinical scenario and normal cellular immunity, the differential diagnosis is broad and includes various indolent infectious processes such as tuberculosis; fungal infections such as histoplasmosis, coccidioidomycosis, and *Cryptococcus neoformans* infection; idiopathic immunologic disorders such as sarcoidosis; and, less commonly, metastatic neoplastic disease, Hodgkin's disease, non-Hodgkin's lymphoma, and occupational lung diseases such as berylliosis and silicosis. However, in a patient infected with HIV, the differential diagnosis is skewed differently and includes a higher probability of mycobacterial infection, fungal infection, and Kaposi's sarcoma.

2. *What tests should be done to establish the diagnosis in this patient?*

A serum HIV test should be done in this patient because of her history of intravenous drug abuse. For most people with possible sarcoidosis, however, this test is not necessary.

A sputum sample should be obtained for acid-fast staining and mycobacterial culture. In patients with extensive pulmonary infiltrates due to *M. tuberculosis* infection, three separate morning sputum samples are highly sensitive for detecting the pathogen. In most normal hosts with active pulmonary tuberculosis, the PPD (purified protein derivative) skin test is positive. Patients with sarcoidosis are frequently anergic in response to a variety of skin tests, including the PPD test.

Sputum specimens for fungal staining and culture should also be obtained. The fungi that mimic sarcoidosis are restricted to certain endemic areas. For instance, histoplasmosis is found in the midwestern and southeastern United States. Coccidioidomycosis is endemic to the desert Southwest and arid regions of California, such as the Mojave Desert and the San Joaquin Valley. Given the patient's recent trip to Bakersfield, California, it is necessary to exclude possible infection with coccidioidomycosis. A thorough travel and occupational history always should be taken to exclude any atypical fungal exposure.

Tissue also should be obtained for the purpose of excluding infection and neoplasm, and to support the diagnosis of sarcoidosis. As already discussed, skin biopsy or bronchoscopy with transbronchial biopsy would be helpful if the results revealed noncaseating granulomas. Acid-fast and silver staining can be performed on the biopsy specimens to exclude mycobacterial and fungal infections. In this patient, most clinicians would recommend fiberoptic bronchoscopy with bronchoalveolar lavage and transbronchial biopsy. In the setting of sarcoidosis, the bronchoalveolar lavage fluid characteristically shows an increased percentage of lymphocytes with a predominant CD4 phenotype. In addition, stains and cultures for mycobacterial and fungal diseases can be performed on the bronchoalveolar lavage fluid.

3. *How would you interpret the results of the pulmonary function tests?*

The pulmonary function tests show restricted lung volumes. Spirometry shows a mild degree of obstruction, particularly given the underlying restrictive physiology. The DLCO is reduced.

Pulmonary function tests, including lung volumes, DLCO, spirometry, and arterial blood gas measurement, should be performed for every patient with sarcoidosis and pulmonary parenchymal involvement. The most frequent abnormalities encountered are a reduction in lung volumes (restrictive physiology), often accompanied by a reduction in DLCO. It is not uncommon also to find reduced expiratory flow rates, indicating airway involvement with sarcoidosis. The arterial oxygen saturation usually remains relatively normal at rest, unless advanced disease is present. With exercise, the Pao_2 frequently falls.

Suggested Readings

Gilman MJ, Wang KP. Transbronchial lung biopsy in sarcoidosis. *American Review of Respiratory Diseases* 1980;122:721.

Hillerdal G, Nou E, Osterman K, Schmekel B. Sarcoidosis: epidemiology and prognosis: a 15-year European study. *American Review of Respiratory Diseases* 1984;130:29.

Rust M, Bergmann L, Kuhn T. Prognostic value of chest radiograph, serum angiotensin-converting enzyme and T helper cell count in blood and in bronchoalveolar lavage of patients with pulmonary sarcoidosis. *Respiration* 1985;48:231.

Tuberculosis

1. What is the contemporary epidemiology of tuberculosis?

2. What symptoms and radiographic features are associated with tuberculosis?

3. Who should receive treatment (prophylaxis) for tuberculosis infection?

Discussion

1. *What is the contemporary epidemiology of tuberculosis?*

Despite numerous medical advances in the past century, tuberculosis is still the cause of at least 1 million deaths worldwide each year, and its incidence, although increasing in the 1980s and early 1990s primarily because of AIDS, is again decreasing. Elderly patients now constitute nearly half of the newly diagnosed cases of tuberculosis in the United States because these people were exposed to the tuberculosis epidemic in the first quarter of the 20th century and have been harboring latent infection for many decades. The case fatality rate in the elderly is also disproportionately high, and they face a higher risk of complications with treatment. Others at risk for tuberculosis include medically underserved, low-income, ethnic minority populations, especially African Americans, Native Americans, and Hispanics; institutionalized people; patients with chronic renal failure, silicosis, diabetes mellitus, or lymphoreticular malignancies; alcoholics or those with other substance abuse habits; those with malnutrition; those who have undergone gastrectomy; and those undergoing immunosuppressive or long-term corticosteroid therapy.

2. *What symptoms and radiographic features are associated with tuberculosis?*

Diversity characterizes the clinical manifestations of tuberculosis. Although many patients have constitutional symptoms consisting of weight loss, fatigue, fever, and night sweats, as well as pulmonary symptoms such as cough, intermittent hemoptysis, chest pain, and dyspnea, none of these is uniformly present. In addition, the elderly and patients with AIDS often have extrapulmonary disease and the symptoms and signs are atypical.

The classic chest radiograph in an adult with pulmonary tuberculosis demonstrates fibronodular infiltration of the posterior or apical segments of the upper lobe. There may also be cavitation. Tuberculosis can, however, produce almost any form of pulmonary radiographic abnormality. Moreover, normal radiographic findings do not exclude a diagnosis of disseminated tuberculosis in an elderly or immunocompromised patient. Hilar adenopathy on a chest radiograph in a patient seropositive for HIV is deemed tuberculosis until proven otherwise.

3. *Who should receive treatment (prophylaxis) for tuberculosis infection?*

The tuberculin skin test is the traditional method of demonstrating infection with *M. tuberculosis*, and is based on the principle that infection elicits delayed-type hypersensitivity to certain antigens in culture extracts called *tuberculins*. The tuberculin most commonly used is PPD; it is injected intracutaneously on the volar aspect of the forearm in a dose of 5 tuberculin units. Induration of the site at 48 to 72 hours indicates delayed hypersensitivity to infection with *M. tuberculosis*, but does not necessarily signify the presence of active disease, only infection.

Preventive therapy with isoniazid (INH) given for 6 to 12 months clearly decreases the risk of future tuberculosis—in other words, the progression from an infected state to an actively diseased state manifesting the clinical, radiographic, and microbiologic profile. The goal of INH monotherapy is therefore to treat subclinical infection brought to light by the positive tuberculin skin test. By strict definition, it is not true prophylaxis, but it is often referred to as such. The dosage of INH in adults is 5 mg per kg, up to a total of 300 mg orally per day. People who have contact with a patient with newly diagnosed pulmonary tuberculosis, and whose tuberculin skin test is positive, should undergo INH preventive therapy. If a chest radiograph shows inactive parenchymal tuberculosis (upper lobe scarring), the skin test is positive, and active disease has been excluded by negative sputum findings, such patients should receive INH therapy. People younger than 35 years of age with a positive skin test and a normal chest radiograph should also be treated. Patients whose skin test is positive and in whom the following clinical situations apply should receive 6 to 12 months of preventive therapy: HIV positivity; silicosis;

diabetes mellitus, especially poorly controlled insulin-dependent diabetes; steroid therapy, especially more than 15 mg of prednisone per day; chronic renal failure; lymphoreticular malignancies: leukemia, lymphoma, and Hodgkin's disease; immunosuppressive therapy; gastrectomy; jejunoileal bypass; and weight loss of 10% or more of the ideal body weight.

Case

A 68-year-old black man with a long history of tobacco and ethanol abuse is brought in by his family for evaluation of weight loss, low-grade fevers, and failure to thrive. The patient reports a 2- to 3-month history of progressive 20-pound (9-kg) weight loss, as well as fevers, nonproductive cough, and generalized weakness. His cough became productive of white sputum 2 days earlier. The patient denies chest pain, hemoptysis, ill contacts, recent travel, or HIV risk factors. He has smoked one pack of cigarettes per day for 40 years. He drinks approximately one pint (half a liter) of alcohol a day and has done so for many years. Careful review of his old records reveals a PPD test was positive approximately 12 years ago.

Physical examination discloses a cachectic, ill-appearing, elderly black man in moderate respiratory distress. His oral temperature is 38.5°C, with a respiratory rate of 30 breaths per minute, heart rate of 126 beats per minute, and blood pressure of 100/60 mm Hg. Examination findings are remarkable for poor dentition, and rales and rhonchi throughout the right chest, but otherwise findings are unremarkable. Initial laboratory evaluation reveals a white blood cell count of 16,000/mm³ with a leftward shift and a hematocrit of 35%. His oxygen saturation is 80% on room air. A chest radiograph shows a large interstitial and alveolar infiltrate with air bronchograms in the right upper lobe; no cavitation, pleural effusion, or volume loss is noted. Arterial blood gas measurements on the night of admission show worsening hypoxemia and hypercapnea.

The patient is placed in respiratory isolation and is electively intubated on the night of admission. Stains of his sputum done the next morning reveal a pathogen.

1. What is the differential diagnosis of this patient's respiratory failure?
2. What is the diagnostic strategy at this point in his illness?
3. What is the correct therapeutic plan?

Case Discussion

1. *What is the differential diagnosis of this patient's respiratory failure?*

This patient's history is consistent with an infectious process, perhaps superimposed on an underlying malignancy. Bacterial pathogens such as *S. pneumoniae*, *Legionella pneumophila*, and *H. influenzae* are possible causes. Because of his history of ethanol abuse and poor dentition, aspiration pneumonia (with anaerobic pathogens) is also a possibility, but the location of the infiltrates in the upper lobe makes this less likely because aspiration pneumonia tends to favor dependent portions of the lung, such as the superior segments of both lower lobes. Bacterial pneumonia distal to an obstructing lesion such as a cancer is clearly a possibility given his long-standing tobacco use and age; however, the absence of volume loss and presence of air bronchograms on his radiograph somewhat militate against this diagnosis. Viral infection is less likely given his history and the lobar infiltrate. Fungal infection, particularly with *Histoplasma capsulatum*, is a possibility, but less likely given his negative geographic history and the absence of adenopathy on the radiograph. He has no HIV risk factors.

An important clue to the diagnosis is the positive PPD skin test. Because most active cases of pulmonary tuberculosis in adults constitute either postprimary disease or the reactivation of a protracted, even lifelong, infection with the tubercle bacillus, this plus his positive PPD test point to the diagnosis. The important point here is that the clinician should suspect reactivation of tuberculosis even without a history of a positive PPD test. This patient has several currently recognized epidemiologic risk factors for tuberculosis: he is elderly, African American, and a substance abuser (ethanol), and he has poor nutritional status. He has an upper lobe infiltrate, but this does not rule out tuberculosis because the classic fibronodular infiltration of the posterior or apical segments of the upper lobe (right greater than left) may not be present in the elderly or, especially, in HIV-infected patients. Tuberculosis probably needs to be considered in the differential diagnosis of pneumonia in every patient older than 60 years of age. This patient's respiratory failure with hypoxemia and respiratory muscle fatigue (hypercapnea) could be due to any one of the processes discussed, but tuberculosis is the most likely diagnosis.

2. *What is the diagnostic strategy at this point in his illness?*

A careful search for the culprit pathogen, or pathogens, should be undertaken. Blood cultures, Gram's staining and culture of sputum samples, plus sputum stains for acid-fast organisms (mycobacteria) and *Legionella* indicate a fluorescent antibody test should be performed. The value of sputum examination cannot be overemphasized. Gram's staining, especially of a tracheal aspirate or sputum produced by a strong, deep cough, can help in the diagnosis of virtually any bacterial infectious agent in the differential diagnosis. (*Legionella* is difficult to see, but a large number of neutrophils without organisms suggest this diagnosis.) In addition to the stains for acid-fast bacilli (AFB), tuberculosis can be diagnosed with a fluorochrome technique called Auramine O. This patient's sputum was positive for AFB. Approximately 10^4 organisms per mL of sputum are required for an AFB smear to be positive, and only 50% to 80% of patients with pulmonary tuberculosis have positive sputum smear findings. A rapid radiometric technique known as BACTEC allows the recovery and identification of tuberculosis in 10 days, which is an advantage over conventional culture methods that can take 3 to 6 weeks to grow mycobacteria.

A PPD test with two controls should be placed and an induration of 10 mm or more is considered a positive result. However, in the setting of HIV infection, HIV risk factors, recent close contact with infectious people, or chest radiographic findings consistent with old healed tuberculosis (upper lobe scarring), an induration of 5 mm or more is considered a positive reaction. However, as already mentioned, a negative result does not exclude tuberculosis because up to 25% to 30% of newly diagnosed patients with tuberculosis have a negative ($\leq$9 mm) skin test. A booster effect is more powerful ($\geq$6 mm increase) in the cutaneous reaction, and is achieved by performing a second PPD test 7 to 10 days after the first. A second PPD should therefore be considered in this patient, but especially in an elderly patient with a negative PPD, in whom the clinical suspicion for tuberculosis is high. However, the *sine qua non* test for tuberculosis remains the sputum smear and culture.

Additional diagnostic tests that should be part of the evaluation of this patient include an HIV test and comparison of previous and current chest radiographs, if possible. The latter would constitute an important part of the evaluation in this patient. Fiberoptic bronchoscopy could also help in determining if there is an endobronchial lesion, or extrinsic compression from a mass, as well as enable sampling of secretions and biopsies for microbiologic evaluation.

3. *What is the correct therapeutic plan?*

After appropriate culture results are obtained, treatment needs to be directed toward the most likely pathogens in this man's illness. Based on the differential diagnosis, you would need to provide antibiotic coverage for *S. pneumoniae, H. influenzae*, possibly anaerobes, and possibly *Legionella* species. The severity of this patient's illness mandates aggressive, but well considered, therapy. His initial regimen should include coverage for community-acquired pneumonia and *Legionella*. Antituberculous therapy should be initiated only after his AFB smears prove positive. It was also very important that on admission the patient was placed in respiratory isolation to prevent the spread of tuberculosis, which is transmitted almost exclusively by means of aerosolized respiratory secretions, not only to other patients but to health care workers as well. His sputum smear positivity for *M. tuberculosis* constitutes a state of infectiousness. People receiving therapy promptly become noninfectious as their cough subsides and the concentration of organisms in their sputum decreases. Most authorities believe that treatment reverses infectiousness within approximately 2 weeks of the start of therapy; until then, isolation measures should be maintained.

His antituberculous chemotherapy should consist of a four-drug regimen, comprising INH, rifampin, pyrazinamide, and streptomycin, and maintained for 6 months. Many studies have convincingly demonstrated the curative efficacy of multidrug regimens given for 6 to 9 months. A standard treatment is effective when given for 6 months in a supervised setting. Compliance with antituberculous therapy is absolutely critical for cure. Noncompliance is also one of the major reasons for the emergence of drug resistance. Multidrug therapy is always used in the treatment of tuberculosis because of the potential for primary or spontaneous resistance, which occurs in 1×10^6 organisms. Extrapulmonary tuberculosis is treated like pulmonary tuberculosis, and tuberculosis contracted in the setting of AIDS is also treated with standard regimens, and is still curable.

Suggested Readings

Bass JB, Farer LS, Hopewell PC, et al, for the American Thoracic Society, Medical Section of the American Lung Association. Diagnostic standards and classification of tuberculosis. *American Review of Respiratory Diseases* 1990;142:725.

Bass JB, Farer LS, Hopewell PC, Jacobs RF, for the American Thoracic Society, Medical Section of the American Lung Association. Treatment of tuberculosis and tuberculous infection in adults and children. *American Review of Respiratory Diseases* 1986;134:355.

Cohn DL, Catlin BJ, Peterson KL, et al. A 62-dose, 6-month therapy for pulmonary and extrapulmonary tuberculosis: a twice-weekly, directly observed, and cost-effective regimen. *Ann Intern Med* 1990;112:407.

Heffner JE, Strange C, Sahn SA. The impact of respiratory failure on the diagnosis of tuberculosis. *Arch Intern Med* 1988;148:1103.

Iseman M. Tuberculosis. In: *Synopsis of clinical pulmonary disease*, 4th ed. St. Louis: Mosby-Year Book, 1989.

9 Nephrology

Tomas Berl and Isaac Teitelbaum

Acute Renal Failure

1. Under what circumstances is the serum creatinine a reliable marker for glomerular filtration rate (GFR)? How is the creatinine clearance estimated from the serum creatinine?
2. What clinical findings most commonly suggest the presence of acute renal failure?
3. What processes need to be considered when attempting to ascertain the cause of acute renal failure?
4. What are the most common causes of acute renal failure in hospitalized patients and in outpatients?
5. What are the urinary findings that assist in differentiating prerenal azotemia from intrarenal acute renal failure?
6. What are the complications of acute renal failure?

Discussion

1. *Under what circumstances is the serum creatinine a reliable marker for GFR? How is the creatinine clearance estimated from the serum creatinine?*

   The serum creatinine is a reliable marker for creatinine clearance and GFR only in the steady state, that is, when the serum creatinine is neither increasing nor decreasing. In a steady state, the creatinine clearance (C_{cr}) may be estimated from the serum creatinine (S_{cr}) by the Cockroft-Gault equation:

$$C_{cr} = \frac{(140 - \text{age}) \times \text{weight (kg)}}{72 \times S_{cr}} (\times 0.85 \text{ for female subjects})$$

Table 9-1. Causes of Prerenal Azotemia

Reduced extracellular and intravascular volume
   Gastrointestinal losses (vomiting, diarrhea, nasogastric suction)
   Dehydration
   Burns
   Hemorrhage
Reduced intravascular volume but increased extracellular volume
   Cirrhosis
   Nephrotic syndrome
   Congestive heart failure
   Third-space fluid accumulation (postoperative from abdominal surgery, severe pancreatitis)
Hemodynamically mediated acute renal failure
   Nonsteroidal antiinflammatory agents (due to renal prostaglandin inhibition)
   Angiotensin-converting enzyme inhibition (due to a decrease in efferent arteriolar tone)
   Hepatorenal syndrome

From *MKSAP IX*. Philadelphia: American College of Physicians, 1992. Reprinted with permission.

2. *What clinical findings most commonly suggest the presence of acute renal failure?*

A rise in the blood urea nitrogen (BUN) and serum creatinine levels and the development of oliguria (<400 mL per day) or anuria (<100 mL per day) are the common clinical findings that suggest the presence of acute renal failure. However, the absence of oliguria does not exclude acute renal failure because the process may also be nonoliguric. In fact, 20% to 30% of patients with acute renal failure are nonoliguric.

3. *What processes need to be considered when attempting to ascertain the cause of acute renal failure?*

In patients with acute renal failure, a prerenal, postrenal, and intrarenal process needs to be considered. The respective causes of prerenal and postrenal azotemia as well as intrinsic renal disease are listed in Tables 9-1 to 9-3.

Table 9-2. Causes of Postrenal Azotemia

Intratubular obstruction
   Uric acid nephropathy
   Methotrexate crystal deposition
Ureteric obstruction
   Retroperitoneal carcinoma (cervix, prostate, uterus) or sarcoma
   Retroperitoneal fibrosis
Intrinsic causes
   Nephrolithiasis
   Necrotic papillae (papillary necrosis)
   Blood clots
Urethral obstruction
   Prostatic hypertrophy
   Blood clots
   Bladder dysfunction (e.g., flaccid bladder in diabetics)

From *MKSAP IX*. Philadelphia: American College of Physicians, 1992. Reprinted with permission.

Table 9-3. Most Common Causes of Intrarenal Acute Renal Failure

---

Glomerular diseases
   Rapidly progressive glomerulonephritis
   Postinfectious glomerulonephritis
   Focal glomerulosclerosis associated with acquired immunodeficiency syndrome
Tubulointerstitial nephritis
   Hypersensitivity reactions: penicillins, sulfonamides, fluoroquinolones
   Associated with systemic infections (*Legionella,* systemic exposure to organic solvents,
     Toxoplasma)
Acute tubular necrosis
   Ischemia, hypotension, septicemia, postoperative patients
   Direct drug toxicity: aminoglycosides, cisplatin, amphotericin, contrast agents, cyclosporine
   Myoglobin or hemoglobin
   Renal cortical necrosis
   Acute tubular necrosis in pregnancy
   Hypercalcemia
Vascular diseases
   Renal artery occlusion
   Acute vasculitis
   Malignant hypertension
   Atheroembolic disease, multiple cholesterol emboli syndrome

---

From *MKSAP IX.* Philadelphia: American College of Physicians, 1992. Reprinted with permission.

4. *What are the most common causes of acute renal failure in hospitalized patients and in outpatients?*

In hospitalized patients, the most common cause of acute renal failure (45%) is acute tubular necrosis, followed by prerenal azotemia and obstruction; glomerulonephritis, vasculitis, interstitial nephritis, and atheroembolic disease comprise most of the remaining causes. In contrast, acute renal failure in outpatients is most commonly due to prerenal azotemia (70%), followed by obstruction. Drug nephrotoxicity [e.g., angiotensin-converting enzyme (ACE) inhibitors and nonsteroidal antiinflammatory drugs (NSAIDs)] accounts for most of the remaining cases.

5. *What are the urinary findings that assist in differentiating prerenal azotemia from intrarenal acute renal failure?*

The urinary findings that can be used to help differentiate between prerenal azotemia and intrarenal acute renal failure are listed in Table 9-4.

6. *What are the complications of acute renal failure?*

The various complications of acute renal failure are listed by category in Table 9-5.

Case　　A 65-year-old diabetic woman presents to the emergency room with right upper quadrant pain that radiates around to the back, together with nausea, vomiting, anorexia, lightheadedness, and a diminished urine output over the past 24 hours. She has no previous history of renal dysfunction. Her temperature is 37.5°C, her supine blood pressure is 110/70 mm Hg, and her pulse is 80 beats per minute; upright, her blood pressure is 85/60 mm Hg and her pulse is 110 beats per minute.

Table 9-4. Urine Findings in Prerenal Azotemia and Acute Renal Failure

Laboratory test	Prerenal azotemia	Intrarenal acute renal failure
Urinary osmolality (mOsm/kg)	>500	<400
Urinary sodium (mEq/L)	<20	>40
Urine–plasma creatinine ratio	>40	<20
Renal failure index: $U_{Na}/U_{Cr}/P_{Cr}$	<1	>2
Fractional excretion of sodium:		
$U_{Na}/P_{Na}/U_{Cr}/P_{Cr} \times 100$	<1	>2
Urinary sediment	Normal or occasional granular casts	Brown granular casts, cellular debris

U_{Na}, urinary sodium level; U_{Cr}, urinary creatinine level; P_{Cr}, serum creatinine level; P_{Na}, serum sodium level.

From Yaqoob MM, Alkhurnaizi AM, Edelstein CL, et al. Acute renal failure: pathogenesis, diagnosis, and management. In: Schrier RW, ed. *Renal and electrolyte disorders,* 5th ed. Boston: Little, Brown, 1997. Reprinted with permission.

The physical examination findings are otherwise remarkable for the presence of decreased skin turgor, dry mucosal membranes, flat neck veins, and absence of axillary sweat. Her lungs are clear and the cardiac findings are normal. There is exquisite right upper quadrant abdominal tenderness that worsens with inspiration, her stool is guaiac negative, and no edema is noted. Neurologic examination reveals nonfocal findings.

The following laboratory data are obtained: hematocrit, 50.2%; white blood cell count, 19,500/mm³ with 82% polymorphonuclear leukocytes, 16% band forms, and 2% lymphocytes; platelets, 312,000/mm³; sodium, 146 mEq/L; potassium, 4.1 mEq/L; chloride, 111 mEq/L; carbon dioxide, 22 mEq/L; glucose, 195 mg/dL; BUN, 35 mg/dL; creatinine, 1.6 mg/dL; total bilirubin, 1.8 mg/dL; alkaline phosphatase, 289 IU; and aspartate aminotransferase (AST), 35 U/L.

Urinalysis reveals a pH of 5, a specific gravity of 1.028; 1+ glucose, trace

Table 9-5. Complications of Acute Renal Failure

Metabolic
  Hyponatremia, hyperkalemia, hypocalcemia, hyperphosphatemia, hypermagnesemia, and
    hyperuricemia
Cardiovascular
  Pulmonary edema, arrhythmias, hypertension, pericarditis
Neurologic
  Asterixis, neuromuscular irritability, somnolence, coma, seizures
Hematologic
  Anemia, coagulopathies, hemorrhagic diathesis
Gastrointestinal
  Nausea, vomiting
Infectious
  Pneumonia, urinary tract infection, wound infection, septicemia

From Yaqoob MM, Alkhurnaizi AM, Edelstein CL, et al. Acute renal failure: pathogenesis, diagnosis, and management. In: Schrier RW, ed. *Renal and electrolyte disorders,* 5th ed. Boston: Little, Brown, 1997. Reprinted with permission.

ketones, occasional nonpigmented granular casts, and no cellular casts or bacteria. The urine sodium level is 10 mEq/L and the urine creatinine level is 80 mg/dL.

Abdominal ultrasound reveals the existence of gallstones and dilatation of the biliary tree. The kidneys measure 11 cm but exhibit no hydronephrosis or increased echogenicity.

While in the emergency room, the patient's fever spikes to 39°C, which is accompanied by 3 minutes of rigors and a decrease in blood pressure to 80/50 mm Hg. She is admitted to the hospital with a diagnosis of acute cholecystitis for the purpose of observation and eventual cholecystectomy. She is given gentamicin [2 mg per kg intravenously (IV)] and ampicillin (2 g IV every 6 hours). Her urine output over 12 hours is 100 mL. The next morning, the following laboratory values are reported: sodium, 140 mEq/L; potassium, 5 mEq/L; chloride, 100 mEq/L; carbon dioxide, 15 mEq/L; glucose, 130 mg/dL; BUN, 40 mg/dL; and creatinine, 2.5 mg/dL. Urinalysis now reveals a pH of 5 and a specific gravity of 1.010 with occasional renal tubular epithelial cells and a rare, muddy-brown granular cast. The urine sodium level is 80 mEq/L and the urine creatinine level is 40 mg/dL. Blood cultures are positive for a gram-negative bacillus.

Over the next 3 days, the patient remains oliguric and mild congestive heart failure develops. The BUN and creatinine levels rise steadily to 100 and 5.5 mg/dL, respectively.

1. At the time of arrival in the emergency room, what is the most likely explanation for this patient's acute renal dysfunction, and why?
2. At the time of the patient's arrival in the emergency room, what treatment would you prescribe, and why?
3. What is the cause of the continuing rise in the serum creatinine level after the patient is admitted to the hospital, and why?
4. What is the role for diuretics in this patient, and what is the proper dosage?
5. What is the appropriate approach to fluid management when the patient becomes oliguric?
6. What are the indications for acute dialysis in acute renal failure, and what alternative extracorporeal procedures could be considered?

Case Discussion

1. *At the time of arrival in the emergency room, what is the most likely explanation for this patient's acute renal dysfunction, and why?*

There is no evidence for a postrenal cause of the acute renal failure in this patient, given the renal ultrasound study showing no obstruction. This leaves prerenal and intrarenal causes as the source of the acute renal failure. The history and physical examination findings suggest prerenal azotemia stemming from volume depletion. The laboratory data that corroborate this diagnosis include a BUN–creatinine ratio that exceeds 20 and a fractional extraction of sodium (FENa) of 0.13%. The FENa is calculated as follows: $U_{Na}/P_{Na}/U_{Cr}/P_{Cr} \times 100\% = 10/146/80/1.6 \times 100\% = 0.13\%$, where U_{Na} and P_{Na} are the urine and serum sodium levels, respectively, and U_{Cr} and P_{Cr} are the urine and serum levels of creatinine, respectively. In the setting of oliguria (<400 mL of urine per day), an FENa of less than 1% implies prerenal azotemia, whereas an FENa of greater than 2% implies an intrarenal process.

2. *At the time of the patient's arrival in the emergency room, what treatment would you prescribe, and why?*

    In this clinical setting, repletion of the extracellular fluid volume is the most critical element of therapy. This can be accomplished by the administration of either normal saline or lactated Ringer's solution; 250 to 500 mL can be given rapidly over 1 to 2 hours. These solutions, which are devoid of colloid, distribute in both intravascular and extravascular spaces. Fluid infusion should be continued until the blood pressure changes are no longer evident and a euvolemic state has been restored. This will also be accompanied by the reappearance of sodium in the urine. In the setting of prerenal azotemia, this maneuver should promptly return renal function to baseline.

3. *What is the cause of the continuing rise in the serum creatinine level after the patient is admitted to the hospital, and why?*

    After she is admitted to the hospital, the patient's clinical picture becomes more consistent with an intrarenal cause of acute renal failure, such as acute tubular necrosis. This is supported by the presence of tubular epithelial cells and brown granular casts in the urine. In addition, both the decrement in the U_{Cr}/P_{Cr} to 16 and the increase in the FENa to 3.57% strongly support this diagnosis. As to the cause of the intrarenal injury itself, gram-negative sepsis appears to be the most likely culprit. Aminoglycosides can also cause acute renal failure; however, this patient received only one dose of the antibiotic and, more commonly, the associated renal failure is nonoliguric. Ampicillin can cause acute interstitial nephritis, which has been reported for a number of antibiotics, especially penicillin. The urinalysis would be expected to show white blood cells, red blood cells, white blood cell casts, and eosinophils.

4. *What is the role for diuretics in this patient, and what is the proper dosage?*

    Diuretics have been used in an attempt to convert oliguric patients with acute renal failure to a nonoliguric state, which is associated with a better outcome and simpler fluid management. Whether this "conversion" truly alters the prognosis has not been settled. Diuretics can play a major role in the treatment of fluid overload that accompanies the patient's diminished urine output. Because loop diuretics need to reach the luminal membrane in this setting, very high doses are required (240 to 300 mg IV of furosemide or 8–12 mg IV of bumetanide). Doses higher than these have been used, but are not associated with an improved outcome and can cause permanent ototoxicity.

5. *What is the appropriate approach to fluid management when the patient becomes oliguric?*

    When a patient is oliguric (urine volume ≤500 mL), fluid restriction is needed and intake should not exceed 1 L because daily insensible losses are estimated to be between 500 and 700 mL. Likewise, sodium and potassium restriction is necessary. Thus, the administration of 1 L of 0.5 N NaCl (i.e., approximately 75 mEq of sodium) without potassium supplementation is likely to prevent expansion of the extracellular fluid volume, hyponatremia, and hyperkalemia. If the episode of acute renal failure is more prolonged, nutritional support is also important.

6. *What are the indications for acute dialysis in acute renal failure, and what alternative extracorporeal procedures could be considered?*

Dialysis is undertaken whenever any of the complications of acute renal failure ensue. These are listed in Table 9-5. Most commonly, dialysis is instituted for the management of fluid overload that is refractory to diuretic therapy, hyperkalemia that is resistant to therapy, or metabolic acidosis that cannot be adequately treated with bicarbonate. In oliguric, catabolic patients, dialysis has also been used to prevent rather than treat uremic symptoms, so-called "prophylactic dialysis." Continuous arteriovenous hemofiltration and continuous arteriovenous hemodialysis are alternatives to hemodialysis, and are being increasingly used.

Suggested Readings

Cadnapaphornchai P, Alavalapati RK, McDonald F. Differential diagnosis of acute renal failure. In: Jacobson HR, Striker GE, Klahr S, eds. *The principles and practice of nephrology*, 2nd ed. St. Louis: Mosby, 1995.

Yaqoob MM, Alkhunaizi AM, Edelstein CL, Conger JD, Schrier RW. Acute renal failure: pathogenesis, diagnosis, and management. In: Schrier RW, ed. *Renal and electrolyte disorders*, 5th ed. Philadelphia: Lippincott–Raven, 1997, p. 449.

Metabolic Acidosis

1. What is the definition of metabolic acidosis?
2. What compensatory mechanism is triggered by metabolic acidosis?
3. How is the anion gap calculated, and how is it helpful in evaluating metabolic acidosis?
4. What are the causes of a metabolic acidosis with an increased anion gap, and what is the anion responsible for the increased anion gap?
5. How is the osmolar gap calculated, and how is this value useful in evaluating patients with a metabolic acidosis?
6. What are the causes of a metabolic acidosis with a normal anion gap?
7. What is the difference between proximal and distal renal tubular acidosis (RTA), and how are these two forms of RTA differentiated?

Discussion

1. *What is the definition of metabolic acidosis?*

Metabolic acidosis is a disorder that results from either the addition of hydrogen ion or the loss of bicarbonate, which, if unopposed, results in acidemia. However, metabolic acidosis is not defined either as a decrement in the serum bicarbonate level or any given systemic arterial pH because, in the

Table 9-6. Causes of Metabolic Acidosis with an Increased Anion Gap

Cause	Anion
Increased acid production	
Diabetic ketoacidosis	BHB, AcAc
Lactic acidosis	Lactate, pyruvate
Starvation	—
Alcoholic ketoacidosis	BHB > AcAc
Nonketotic hyperosmolar coma	—
Inborn errors of metabolism	—
Ingestion of acid-generating toxic substances	
Salicylate overdose (>30 mg/dL)	Variety
Methanol ingestion	Formate, lactate
Ethylene glycol ingestion	Lactate, glycolate, oxalate
Solvent inhalation	—
Failure of acid excretion	
Acute renal failure	Variety, SO_4, PO_4
Chronic renal failure	—

BHB, betahydroxybutyrate; AcAc, acetoacetate.

setting of mixed acid–base disorders, the serum bicarbonate level or pH, or both, can be normal and even elevated despite the presence of metabolic acidosis.

2. *What compensatory mechanism is triggered by metabolic acidosis?*

When metabolic acidosis develops, any decrease in pH activates carotid chemoreceptors and central nervous system receptors to stimulate ventilation. The increase in the minute ventilation lowers the partial pressure of carbon dioxide (P_{CO_2}), thereby returning the pH toward normal.

3. *How is the anion gap calculated, and how is it helpful in evaluating metabolic acidosis?*

Metabolic acidosis is broadly classified on the basis of the presence or absence of an anion gap. The anion gap (in millimoles per liter) is calculated using the following formula: plasma sodium − (plasma chloride + plasma bicarbonate). In most laboratories, a normal anion gap is considered to be 12 ± 2 mmol/L. A normal anion gap results from either the addition of hydrochloric acid or the loss of bicarbonate with the concomitant retention of chloride. Because chloride is retained and is included in the calculation, the anion gap is maintained in the normal range. An increased anion gap results from the addition of an exogenous or endogenous acid. The anions produced by these acids are not measured and chloride is not retained. The anion gap increases because bicarbonate is consumed to buffer the organic acid. For example, organic anion + H^+ + $NaHCO_3^- \rightarrow H_2O + CO_2 +$ Na organic anion + organic acid. Because the organic anion is not measured or included in the calculation, the anion gap increases.

4. *What are the causes of a metabolic acidosis with an increased anion gap, and what is the anion responsible for the increased anion gap?*

The various causes of metabolic acidosis with an increased anion gap are listed in Table 9-6.

Table 9-7. The Causes of a Metabolic Acidosis with a Normal Anion Gap

---

Gastrointestinal loss of HCO_3^-
  Diarrhea
  Small bowel or pancreatic drainage or fistula
  Ureterosigmoidostomy, long or obstructed ileal loop conduit
  Anion exchange resins
  Ingestion of $CaCl_2$ or $MgCl_2$
Renal loss of HCO_3^-
  Carbonic anhydrase inhibitors
  Renal tubular acidosis
  Hyperparathyroidism
  Hypoaldosteronism
Miscellaneous
  Recovery from ketoacidosis
  Dilutional acidosis
  Infusion of HCl or its congeners
  Parenteral alimentation acidosis[a]

---

[a]Some formulas contain excess organic cations (balanced by Cl^-), which yield H^+ on metabolism.

5. *How is the osmolar gap calculated, and how is this value useful in evaluating patients with a metabolic acidosis?*

The plasma osmolality is calculated using the following formula: Calculated osmolality $= 2[Na] + [glucose]/18 + [BUN]/2.8 + [ethanol]/4.6$. The osmolar gap is equal to the measured osmolality minus the calculated osmolality. A normal osmolar gap is less than 10 mOsm/kg. When the osmolar gap is elevated in an acidemic patient, ethylene glycol or methanol intoxication must be strongly suspected.

6. *What are the causes of a metabolic acidosis with a normal anion gap?*

The causes of metabolic acidosis with a normal anion gap are listed in Table 9-7.

7. *What is the difference between proximal and distal RTA, and how are these two forms of RTA differentiated?*

Renal tubular acidosis is one of the common causes of metabolic acidosis with a normal anion gap. Proximal RTA results from a failure to resorb the normal amount of bicarbonate in the proximal tubule, whereas distal RTA results from a defect in hydrogen ion secretion in the distal tubule. These two forms of RTA can be differentiated by determining the urine pH during systemic acidosis. In proximal RTA, when the serum bicarbonate, and there-fore the filtered bicarbonate level, is lowered to one that allows for proximal resorption of the filtered load, thereby preventing excessive distal delivery, the urine can be maximally acidified (pH <5.4). In contrast, in distal RTA, the urine cannot be maximally acidified independent of the serum bicarbonate concentration.

Case A 29-year-old man has been hospitalized in the psychiatry service for 2 months because of depression. The patient leaves the hospital on a pass and, on returning, complains of abdominal pain and vomiting. Over the next several hours, he becomes more agitated and is then found in an unarousable state and posturing.

Physical examination reveals a temperature of 102°F (38.8°C), pulse of 102 beats per minute, respiratory rate of 35 breaths per minute, and blood pressure of 160/100 mm Hg. The patient is unresponsive to pain. Funduscopic findings are within normal limits. No odors are noted on his breath.

Laboratory findings reveal the following: sodium, 142 mEq/L; potassium, 4.7 mEq/L; chloride, 111 mEq/L; bicarbonate, 10 mmol/L; serum calcium, 9.4 mg/dL; BUN, 12 mg/dL; and creatinine, 1.3 mg/dL. Arterial blood gas measurements performed on room air show a pH of 7.2, P_{CO_2} of 17 mm Hg, and partial pressure of oxygen (P_{O_2}) of 100 mm Hg.

1. What is this patient's acid–base disturbance, and what are the possible causes?
2. Why is the patient tachypneic, and is the compensation appropriate?
3. What other tests or laboratory findings would be useful in making the specific diagnosis?

    In this patient, the serum glucose level proves to be normal and no serum ketones are detected. The plasma osmolality is 347 mOsm/kg and the osmolar gap is calculated to be 51 mOsm/kg.
4. With the new information yielded by these additional tests, what possible diagnoses still remain?
5. How would you proceed to determine which substance is responsible for this patient's presentation?
6. How would you treat this patient?

Case Discussion

1. *What is this patient's acid–base disturbance, and what are the possible causes?*

    The patient has an acidemia because the pH is 7.2. This could result from either a metabolic or a respiratory acidosis. The combination of a low P_{CO_2} and a low serum bicarbonate concentration confirms the presence of a metabolic acidosis. In addition, the anion gap is elevated. The most likely causes of a metabolic acidosis with an increased anion gap, as outlined in Table 9-7, include diabetic ketoacidosis, lactic acidosis, starvation, alcoholic ketoacidosis, salicylate overdose, methanol or ethylene glycol ingestion, and renal failure.

2. *Why is the patient tachypneic, and is the compensation appropriate?*

    The patient is tachypneic as a compensatory response to the metabolic acidosis. If the patient were not tachypneic, the pH would be even lower and this would suggest an additional respiratory disorder. This patient is exhibiting an appropriate respiratory compensatory response. The serum bicarbonate level is decreased by 14 mmol/L from normal. Therefore, the P_{CO_2} should be decreased by 14 to 21 mm Hg (Table 9-8). The patient has a P_{CO_2} that is decreased by 21 mm Hg from normal, and this compensation is appropriate for the degree of metabolic acidosis involved. Table 9-8 summarizes the general expected compensatory responses to acid–base disorders.

Table 9-8. Rules of Thumb for Beside Interpretation of Acid–Base Disorders

Metabolic acidosis
  $Paco_2$ should fall by 1.0 to 1.5 × the fall in plasma $[HCO_3^-]$
Metabolic alkalosis
  $Paco_2$ should rise by 0.25 to 1.0 × the rise in plasma $[HCO_3^-]$
Acute respiratory acidosis
  Plasma $[HCO_3^-]$ should rise by approximately 1 mmol/L for each 10–mm Hg increment in
    $Paco_2$ (±3 mmol/L)
Chronic respiratory acidosis
  Plasma $[HCO_3^-]$ should rise by approximately 4 mmol/L for each 10–mm Hg increment in
    $Paco_2$ (±4 mmol/L)
Acute respiratory alkalosis
  Plasma $[HCO_3^-]$ should fall by approximately 1–3 mmol/L for each 10–mm Hg decrement
    in $Paco_2$, usually not to less than 18 mmol/L
Chronic respiratory alkalosis
  Plasma $[HCO_3^-]$ should fall by approximately 2–5 mmol/L per 10–mm Hg decrement in
    $Paco_2$, but usually not to less than 14 mmol/L

$Paco_2$, arterial carbon dioxide tension; $[HCO_3^-]$, bicarbonate ion concentration.
From Shapiro JI, Kaehny WD. Pathogenesis and management of metabolic acidosis and alkalosis. In: Schrier RW, ed. *Renal and electrolyte disorders,* 5th ed. Boston: Little, Brown, 1997. Reprinted with permission.

3. *What other tests or laboratory findings would be useful in making the specific diagnosis?*

   The patient clearly has a metabolic acidosis with an increased anion gap, but it is necessary to identify the specific cause with further testing. Initial tests that might elucidate the cause of the process include (a) the serum glucose level to determine whether hyperglycemia is present; (b) serum ketone levels to ascertain if acetoacetate is present; (c) serum salicylate and lactate levels to determine whether salicylate intoxication or lactic acidosis is present; and (d) serum osmolality to determine if the osmolar gap is elevated.

4. *With the new information yielded by these additional tests, what possible diagnoses still remain?*

   With this additional information, you know that the patient has metabolic acidosis with an increased anion and osmolar gap. This limits the possible diagnoses to either methanol or ethylene glycol ingestion.

5. *How would you proceed to determine which substance is responsible for this patient's presentation?*

   To determine which substance is responsible for this patient's presentation, both methanol and ethylene glycol levels should be assayed in the blood. In addition, the urine could be examined for the presence of calcium oxalate crystals, which are frequently present in the setting of ethylene glycol ingestion because of the metabolic conversion of the ethylene glycol to oxalate. In the setting of methanol intoxication, visual disturbances could ensue.

6. *How would you treat this patient?*

   The treatment of metabolic acidosis involves treating the underlying disorder. In acute metabolic acidosis, the rapid correction of pH through the administration of bicarbonate appears to produce derangements in cardiovascular function, probably caused by a paradoxical intracellular acidosis. The use of bicarbonate in this setting is therefore controversial. More specifically, two goals become important in a patient who has ingested ethylene glycol. The first is to inhibit the metabolism of ethylene glycol. Although ethylene glycol itself is not a toxic substance, the metabolites produced by the liver are quite toxic and can precipitate acute renal failure and even cause death. Alcohol dehydrogenase is the enzyme responsible for the metabolism of ethylene glycol, and it can be competitively inhibited by ethanol. Therefore, the first step in treating ethylene glycol ingestion is the infusion of ethanol. The second goal is to remove the ethylene glycol from the body. Ethylene glycol is excreted very slowly by the kidneys and, if the blood level is very high, hemodialysis may become necessary to improve removal of this substance from the blood. A similar approach is used for methanol ingestion.

Suggested Readings

Bushinsky, D. A. Metabolic acidosis. In: Jacobson HR, Striker GE, Klahr S, eds. *The principles and practice of nephrology*, 2nd ed. St. Louis: Mosby, 1995, p. 924.
Shapiro JI, Kaehny WD. Pathogenesis and management of metabolic acidosis and alkalosis. In: Schrier RW, ed. *Renal and electrolyte disorders*, 5th ed. Philadelphia: Lippincott–Raven, 1997, p. 130.

Metabolic Alkalosis

1. What is the definition of metabolic alkalosis?
2. What are the processes involved in the generation of metabolic alkalosis?
3. What are the processes involved in the maintenance of metabolic alkalosis?
4. What are the two major categories of metabolic alkalosis, and what laboratory test is used to differentiate between the two?
5. What are the causes of NaCl-responsive metabolic alkalosis?
6. What are the causes of NaCl-resistant metabolic alkalosis?
7. What are the causes of metabolic alkalosis that are unclassified?
8. What is the compensatory mechanism that is stimulated by metabolic alkalosis?

Discussion

1. *What is the definition of metabolic alkalosis?*
   Metabolic alkalosis is a disorder that results from either the loss of hydrogen ions or the addition of bicarbonate, which, if unopposed, results in alkalemia. Metabolic alkalosis is not defined by either an increment in the serum bicarbonate concentration or a given systemic arterial pH because, in the setting of mixed acid–base disorders, the serum bicarbonate level or the pH, or both, could be either normal or even decreased in the presence of metabolic alkalosis.

2. *What are the processes involved in the generation of metabolic alkalosis?*

Pathophysiologically, the development of metabolic alkalosis involves two phases. The first involves the generation of metabolic alkalosis. As follows from the definition just given, metabolic alkalosis can be generated as a result of either a net loss of hydrogen ions from the extracellular fluid, most commonly from either the upper gastrointestinal tract or more rarely through the kidneys, or from the net addition of bicarbonate or substances that generate bicarbonate (e.g., lactate, citrate, and acetate). In addition, the loss of fluid containing concentrations high in chloride and low in bicarbonate, as occurs with diuretic use and certain gastrointestinal tract diseases such as villous adenoma, generates a metabolic alkalosis.

3. *What are the processes involved in the maintenance of metabolic alkalosis?*

The kidney provides the corrective response to metabolic alkalosis by excreting excess bicarbonate. When the serum bicarbonate level exceeds 28 mEq/L, the anion appears in the urine, thus preventing a further increase in its concentration. The maintenance of alkalosis therefore requires an alteration in renal bicarbonate resorption. Several factors constrain the kidney's ability to excrete bicarbonate and are important in the maintenance phase of metabolic alkalosis. Probably the most important factor in this regard is extracellular fluid volume depletion, which serves to stimulate increased sodium resorption and bicarbonate reclamation in the proximal tubule. Another important factor in the maintenance of metabolic alkalosis is the chloride concentration. When the plasma bicarbonate concentration rises, the chloride concentration must fall. Because chloride is the only anion other than bicarbonate that can accompany sodium resorption, bicarbonate resorption is enhanced in its absence. Therefore, chloride must exist in sufficient quantity to allow for bicarbonate excretion. The hormone aldosterone stimulates the exchange of sodium ions for hydrogen ions or potassium ions in the distal tubule. With the exchange of hydrogen ions, bicarbonate generation occurs in the plasma. Potassium ion depletion directly enhances bicarbonate resorption. An elevation in the P_{CO_2} also stimulates bicarbonate resorption, and is important in the compensatory mechanism that keeps respiratory acidosis in check.

4. *What are the two major categories of metabolic alkalosis, and what laboratory test is used to differentiate between the two?*

Metabolic alkalosis can be divided into two groups: NaCl responsive and NaCl resistant. The former is found in alkalemic patients who are volume depleted, and the latter in those with volume expansion. The most useful laboratory test for discriminating between the two groups is a spot urine chloride determination done before the initiation of therapy. In NaCl-responsive states, the urine chloride concentration is usually less than 20 mEq/L, and frequently even less than 10 mEq/L; in NaCl-resistant states, the urine chloride level exceeds 20 mEq/L. However, although metabolic alkalosis is routinely divided into these two categories, there are several disorders that are unclassified.

Table 9-9. Causes of NaCl-Responsive Metabolic Alkalosis

Gastrointestinal disorders
  Vomiting
  Gastric drainage
  Villous adenoma of the colon
  Chloride diarrhea
Diuretic therapy
Correction of chronic hypercapnia
Cystic fibrosis

5. *What are the causes of NaCl-responsive metabolic alkalosis?*
    The causes of NaCl-responsive metabolic alkalosis are listed in Table 9-9.
6. *What are the causes of NaCl-resistant metabolic alkalosis?*
    The causes of NaCl-resistant metabolic alkalosis are listed in Table 9-10.
7. *What are the causes of metabolic alkalosis that are unclassified?*
    The unclassified causes of metabolic alkalosis are listed in Table 9-11.
8. *What is the compensatory mechanism that is stimulated by metabolic alkalosis?*
    When metabolic alkalosis develops, the alkalemia is sensed by chemoreceptors in the respiratory system. This leads to hypoventilation and an increase in P_{CO_2}. As a general rule, the ΔP_{CO_2} mm Hg $= 0.25 - 1.0$ M$\times$ [HCO_3^-] mEq/L, where ΔP_{CO_2} is the change in the P_{CO_2}. This hypoventilatory response is not as efficient as the hyperventilatory responses that accompany a metabolic acidosis, however.

Case

A 25-year-old man with no previous medical history presents to the emergency room because of abdominal pain and severe vomiting of 2 days' duration, during which time he has been unable to eat or drink. He is taking no medications.

Physical examination reveals the following: temperature, 37.6°C; pulse, 120 beats per minute; respiratory rate, 18 breaths per minute; and blood pressure, 120/80 mm Hg. Orthostatic changes in the pulse and blood pressure are found, and there is mild, diffuse abdominal tenderness.

The following laboratory findings are reported: sodium, 140 mEq/L; potassium, 3.4 mEq/L; chloride, 90 mEq/L; bicarbonate, 35 mmol/L; and creatinine, 1.5 mg/dL. Arterial blood gas measurements on room air reveal a pH of 7.55, P_{CO_2} of 42 mm Hg, and P_{O_2} of 77 mm Hg.

Table 9-10. Causes of NaCl-Resistant Metabolic Alkalosis

Excess mineralocorticoid
  Hyperaldosteronism
  Cushing's syndrome
  Bartter's syndrome
  Excessive licorice intake
Profound potassium depletion (800–1,000 mEq deficit)

Table 9-11. Unclassified Causes of Metabolic Alkalosis

Alkali administration
Recovery from organic acidosis
Antacids and exchange resins administered in renal failure
Milk-alkali syndrome
Massive blood or plasmanate (human plasma protein faction) transfusions
Nonparathyroid hypercalcemia
Glucose ingestion after starvation
Large doses of carbenicillin or penicillin

1. What acid–base disturbances are present in this patient?
2. What are the possible causes of this patient's metabolic alkalosis, and what laboratory test might be useful to elucidate the nature of the cause?
3. What factors are responsible for the generation and maintenance of the metabolic alkalosis in this patient?
4. If the patient's vomiting were to stop spontaneously, would the acid–base disturbance also resolve?
5. How would you treat this patient?

Case Discussion

1. *What acid–base disturbances are present in this patient?*

    The patient is alkalemic (pH, 7.55). Therefore, either a metabolic alkalosis, a respiratory alkalosis, or both, exists. The serum bicarbonate level is elevated to 35 mEq/L, and this indicates a metabolic alkalosis. In the setting of a respiratory alkalosis, the P_{CO_2} would be decreased, which is not the case in this patient. In the setting of metabolic alkalosis, the expected respiratory compensation (hypoventilation) would increase the P_{CO_2}. Because the P_{CO_2} of 44 mm Hg is an increased value, this further supports the presence of a simple metabolic alkalosis with appropriate respiratory compensation.

2. *What are the possible causes of this patient's metabolic alkalosis, and what laboratory test might be useful to elucidate the nature of the cause?*

    As already discussed, metabolic alkalosis can be divided into two broad categories: NaCl-responsive and NaCl-resistant states. The hallmark of NaCl-responsive metabolic alkalosis is intravascular volume depletion. In this patient, the history of severe vomiting plus the vital signs that exhibit orthostatic changes are very suggestive of an NaCl-responsive metabolic alkalosis with intravascular volume depletion. The other causes of an NaCl-responsive metabolic alkalosis are nasogastric drainage, villous adenoma of the colon, chloride diarrhea, and diuretic therapy. Measurement of a spot urine chloride concentration would help to confirm the diagnosis. In this patient, it would likely be low (<20 mEq/L).

3. *What factors are responsible for the generation and maintenance of the metabolic alkalosis in this patient?*

    In the metabolic alkalosis associated with vomiting, the loss of hydrogen ions in the vomitus is responsible for generating the alkalosis. Maintenance

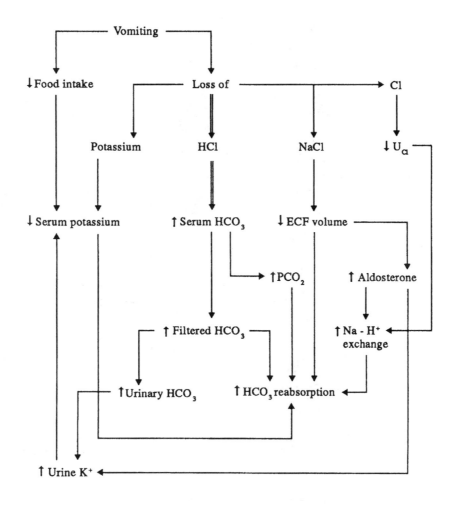

Figure 9-1. The factors responsible for the generation and maintenance of metabolic acidosis. (From Gabow PA. Metabolic alkalosis. In: Gabow PA, ed. *Fluids and electrolytes: clinical problems and their solutions.* Boston: Little, Brown, 1983. Reprinted with permission.)

of the metabolic alkalosis is perpetuated by several factors. The NaCl lost with vomiting leads to a state of intravascular volume depletion, which, in turn, stimulates proximal tubule resorption of both NaCl and NaHCO$_3$. It also stimulates the renin–angiotensin–aldosterone system. The resultant increased aldosterone secretion stimulates Na$^+$/H$^+$ and Na$^+$/K$^+$ exchange in the kidney. The former increases bicarbonate resorption, whereas the latter leads to potassium ion depletion, which also accelerates proximal bicarbonate resorption. The increased PCO$_2$ associated with the compensation for metabolic alkalosis also increases bicarbonate resorption. These events are depicted in Fig. 9-1.

4. *If the patient's vomiting were to stop spontaneously, would the acid–base disturbance also resolve?*

Cessation of vomiting would not necessarily restore the acid–base balance. The patient's vomiting is only the precipitating cause of his metabolic alkalosis. At this point, if his vomiting were to stop, several factors would still prevail (as discussed earlier) and maintain the metabolic alkalosis. Only when both the generating and maintaining factors are eliminated can the acid–base disturbance resolve.

5. *How would you treat this patient?*

In all cases, the treatment of metabolic alkalosis involves management of the underlying process. However, the process that has been the source of the metabolic alkalosis may have resolved, and other factors may be maintaining the metabolic alkalosis. Therefore, treating those factors that are maintaining the metabolic alkalosis may be most important. This patient should receive dual therapy. First, the vomiting (which is the source of the metabolic alkalosis) should be treated using an antiemetic agent. Second, the intravascular volume and potassium depletion must be corrected. This is accomplished by the administration of normal saline plus supplemental potassium. The normal saline is administered until the orthostatic changes in the pulse and blood pressure resolve.

Suggested Readings

Gennari FJ. Metabolic alkalosis. In: Jacobson HR, Striker GE, Klahr S, eds. *The principles and practice of nephrology*, 2nd ed. St. Louis: Mosby, 1995, p. 932.

Seldin D, Rector F. The generation and maintenance of metabolic alkalosis. *Kidney Int* 1972;1:306.

Shapiro JI, Kaehny WD. Pathogenesis and management of metabolic acidosis and alkalosis. In: Schrier RW, ed. *Renal and electrolyte disorders*, 5th ed. Philadelphia: Lippincott–Raven, 1997, p. 130.

Secondary Hypertension

1. What are the major causes of hypertension, and what is the nature of the pathophysiologic mechanism, or mechanisms, responsible for causing the elevation in blood pressure?

2. What should the initial evaluation of a patient who presents with an elevation in blood pressure consist of, and, based on the evaluation findings, what specific clinical features would point toward a particular secondary cause of hypertension?

3. If a secondary cause of hypertension is suspected, what would the further diagnostic evaluation comprise, and what would be the likely findings for each cause?

4. What are the respective treatment options for renal artery stenosis, pheochromocytoma, Cushing's syndrome, and primary hyperaldosteronism?

Discussion

1. *What are the major causes of hypertension, and what is the nature of the pathophysiologic mechanism, or mechanisms, responsible for causing the elevation in blood pressure?*

Essential hypertension is the most common cause of hypertension and accounts for approximately 90% of all cases. It is usually asymptomatic. The usual age of onset is between 30 and 50 years and patients usually have a genetic predisposition for acquiring it. Other forms of hypertension must be ruled out by an initial screening evaluation before this diagnosis is confidently assigned, however. The regulation of arterial pressure involves a complex, and as yet not fully understood, interaction among neurohumoral mechanisms, sodium excretion, and baroreceptor reflexes. There is evidence to suggest that the mechanism responsible for the elevation in blood pressure in essential hypertension may involve inherited abnormalities in sodium excretion. This limitation in the ability to excrete sodium may amplify the mechanisms that cause a rise in arterial pressure, thereby producing an abnormal response. These mechanisms include (a) an increment in the extracellular fluid volume and cardiac output, with secondary autoregulation causing an increment in peripheral vascular resistance; (b) an increase in the circulatory Na^+/K^+-adenosine triphosphatase inhibitor, which elevates the intracellular sodium and calcium levels, thereby also augmenting peripheral vascular resistance; and (c) an increase in the vascular response to vasoconstriction.

The following are the major secondary causes of hypertension.

The exact prevalence of **renal artery stenosis** is not known, but it probably accounts for approximately 5% of the general hypertensive population. It is an important diagnosis to make because it is the most common treatable form of secondary hypertension at any age, and it is one of the few potentially reversible causes of chronic renal failure. The diagnosis must be considered in any patient with severe hypertension refractory to therapy or in any patient who experiences the onset of hypertension either when very young or very old. Atherosclerotic plaques on the renal arteries cause most cases, particularly in patients older than 50 years of age. Fibromuscular dysplasia, an entity seen in younger patients, particularly women, is the second most common cause of renovascular hypertension. There is evidence to suggest that both renin- and volume-dependent mechanisms play a role in the pathophysiology of renovascular hypertension in humans. The following evidence supports the interplay of both mechanisms: (a) the plasma renin activity is usually normal or high in patients with renal artery stenosis, but never low; (b) there is unilateral hypersecretion of renin from the affected kidney with contralateral suppression; (c) in patients with unilateral renal artery stenosis, removal of the constriction or treatment with an ACE inhibitor usually restores the blood pressure to normal or near-normal values; and (d) the effect of angiotensin blockade and salt restriction on blood pressure in patients with bilateral renal artery stenosis is frequently additive.

Primary hyperaldosteronism is an uncommon cause of secondary hypertension, with a prevalence of approximately 1% in the hypertensive population. This disease can occur at any age. The classic form (Conn's syndrome) results from a unilateral adrenocortical adenoma, and accounts for approximately half of the cases of hyperaldosteronism. The other half of the patients have bilateral adrenal hyperplasia. A small percentage have overproduction that can be suppressed with glucocorticoids. As in other forms of hypertension, the exact pathogenesis is unclear. The findings from early studies suggested that the expected salt and water retention secondary to the aldosterone excess raises the intravascular volume and subsequently cardiac output, thereby raising the blood pressure. However, hypervolemia is not a universal finding in patients with primary hyperaldosteronism. The results of studies in animals have suggested that the more important mechanism is an increase in sodium stores and total peripheral vascular resistance. The mechanism responsible for this is uncertain, but some study findings suggest that excess mineralocorticoids induce membrane changes in vascular smooth muscle, leading to abnormal cation turnover (possibly sodium and calcium), which, in turn, augments vasoconstriction and increases peripheral vascular resistance.

Pheochromocytoma is also a rare cause of hypertension. It is estimated to affect 0.1% of patients with diastolic hypertension. Pheochromocytoma can occur at any age, but it arises most frequently in the fourth and fifth decades. In adults, most pheochromocytomas affect women. Pheochromocytomas are tumors of neuroectodermal origin. If they go undiagnosed, they carry a high risk of causing morbidity and mortality secondary to hypertensive crisis, shock, arrhythmias, cardiac arrest, and stroke. The hypertension of pheochromocytoma is a function of the norepinephrine released into the synaptic cleft. Circulating levels of norepinephrine have little direct involvement in the cause or maintenance of the hypertension.

Hypertension complicates both **acute and chronic renal parenchymal diseases**, and affects approximately 80% to 90% of patients on dialysis. There are several mechanisms that may be involved in producing the hypertension in this setting, and these include (a) a markedly impaired ability of the diseased kidney to excrete salt and water; (b) the production of an unidentified vasopressor substance by the kidney; (c) absent production of a necessary humoral vasodilator substance by the kidney; (d) failure of the kidneys to inactivate circulating vasopressor substances; and (e) activation of the renin–angiotensin system.

The blood pressure in the upper extremities is elevated in 80% of children and adults with **coarctation of the aorta**. The mechanism responsible for this hypertension is an inappropriate activation of the renin–angiotensin system in the presence of an expanded body fluid volume.

Hypertension affects 80% of patients with idiopathic **Cushing's syndrome**. Other clinical features of the disorder include glucose intolerance, menstrual disorders, sterility, loss of libido, acne, striae, osteoporosis, muscle weakness and wasting, edema, polyuria, and renal stones. However, the mechanism whereby adrenocorticotropic hormone and cortisol raise blood pressure in humans has not been elucidated, although there is evidence to suggest that glucocorticoids possess a "hypertensinogenic" action that is separate from their glucocorticoid activity.

In the setting of **renin-producing tumors**, hypertension results from the excess secretion of renin by either a juxtaglomerular cell tumor or nephroblastoma. This causes the peripheral renin levels to be elevated, which mediates the hypertension.

2. *What should the initial evaluation of a patient who presents with an elevation in blood pressure consist of, and, based on the evaluation findings, what specific clinical features would point toward a particular secondary cause of hypertension?*

The initial evaluation of patients with hypertension should include history taking, physical examination, and laboratory tests directed toward uncovering a correctable form of secondary hypertension.

In terms of the **history**, a strong family history, as well as past observations of intermittent blood pressure elevations, suggest essential hypertension. Secondary hypertension often develops either before 30 or after 55 years of age. Other pertinent general questions should elicit information about steroid use, including oral contraceptives, and whether there have been recurrent urinary tract infections or a history of proteinuria, nocturia, trauma, or weight gain or loss.

Physical examination should divulge further diagnostic clues as to the possible cause of the hypertension. The examination should focus on the patient's general appearance, muscular development, blood pressure and pulses in both upper extremities and a lower extremity, the supine and standing blood pressure, funduscopy, palpation and auscultation of the carotid arteries, cardiac and pulmonary examination, auscultation of the abdomen for bruits and palpation for an abdominal aneurysm and enlarged kidneys, and examination of the lower extremities for edema.

Laboratory evaluation at the initial workup should include urinalysis for the presence of protein, blood, and glucose, together with a microscopic examination; the serum creatinine and BUN levels; hematocrit; the serum potassium level; the white blood cell count; the serum glucose, cholesterol, triglyceride, calcium, phosphate, and uric acid levels; electrocardiography; and a chest radiographic study.

The clinical features that suggest renal vascular hypertension are listed in Table 9-12. The clinical features suggesting other secondary causes of hypertension are listed in Table 9-13.

3. *If a secondary cause of hypertension is suspected, what would the further diagnostic evaluation comprise, and what would be the likely findings for each cause?*

A number of tests have evolved to assess the likelihood of **renal vascular hypertension**. Anatomically, this is best confirmed by arteriography. However,

Table 9-12. Clinical Features Suggestive of Renal Vascular Hypertension

Epidemiologic features
  Hypertension in the absence of family history
  Age <25 years or >45 years
  Cigarette smoking
  White race
Features of the hypertension
  Abrupt onset of moderate to severe hypertension
  Sudden onset of hypertension after abdominal trauma
  Recent acceleration of severity of hypertension
  Headaches
  Resistance or escape of blood pressure control with usual therapy
  Development of severe or malignant hypertension
  Retinopathy out of proportion to severity of blood pressure
  Excellent antihypertensive response to angiotensin-covering enzyme inhibitor
  Deterioration in renal function in response to angiotensin-converting enzyme inhibitor
  Blood pressure unaffected or increased with diuretic therapy
Associated features
  Unprovoked hypokalemia
  Hypokalemia in response to a thiazide diuretic
  Abdominal or flank systolic-diastolic bruits
  Carotid bruits or other evidence of large-vessel disease
  Elevated peripheral plasma renin activity in absence of alternative explanation

From Ploth DW. Renovascular hypertension. In: Jacobson HR, Striker GE, Klahr S, eds. *The principles and practice of nephrology.* Philadelphia: Decker, 1991, p. 379. Reprinted with permission.

the finding of renal artery stenosis provides no information concerning the pathophysiology of the vascular lesion. A postcaptopril (25 mg) elevation in plasma renin activity or a decrease in renal perfusion postcaptopril as assessed by scintillation techniques or renal vein renins can provide pathophysiologic information.

If there are clinical features highly suggestive of a **pheochromocytoma**, the evaluation should begin with an assay of the total plasma catecholamine level, as measured through an indwelling 21-gauge butterfly needle in a patient who has been resting supine for 30 minutes. Values over 2,000 pg/mL warrant performance of abdominal computed tomography (CT). Values between 1,000 and 2,000 pg/mL require performance of the clonidine suppression test to determine whether a pheochromocytoma is present. Clonidine does not suppress the release of catecholamines in patients with a pheochromocytoma, as it does in patients with essential hypertension. If the plasma catecholamine values are below 1,000 pg/mL, and the patient is hypertensive, the clonidine suppression test should be performed, but, if the patient is normotensive, the glucagon stimulation test may be helpful. For the glucagon test to be positive, the plasma catecholamine level must increase by threefold, or to greater than 2,000 pg/mL, 1 to 3 minutes after administration of the drug. If any of these test results are positive, abdominal CT should be performed. In patients whose clinical presentation suggests a pheochromocytoma but who have only a slight or moderate rise in the catecholamine level (<1,000 pg/mL), repeat testing,

Table 9-13. Clinical Features of Other Secondary Causes of Hypertension

Primary hyperaldosteronism
  History
    Proximal muscle weakness, polyuria, nocturia, polydipsia, paresthesis, tetany, muscle
    paralysis, frontal headaches.
  Laboratory features
    The diagnostic hallmark of this disease is hypokalemic metabolic alkalosis.
    Hyperglycemia may also be present.
Pheochromocytoma
  Symptoms
    Patients may present in a wide variety of clinical settings, including transient ischemic
    attacks, stroke, headache (usually pounding and severe), palpitations with or without
    tachycardia, and excessive sweating. Less common symptoms include tremor, pallor,
    nausea, weakness, fatigue, weight loss, and chest or abdominal pain.
  Physical examination
    Postural hypotension occurs in 50%–75% of patients. Paroxysmal episodes of
    hypertension occur in about one third of patients. Sweating and muscular weakness
    may be evident.
  Laboratory features
    Hyperglycemia or hypercalcemia may be present.
Coarctation of the aorta
  Symptoms
    Epistaxis, throbbing headache, leg fatigue, cold extremities, and occasional claudication.
  Physical examination
    Disparity in the pulsations and blood pressure between the arms and legs. The pulsations
    in the upper extremities are pounding; those in the lower extremities are weak,
    delayed, or absent. The blood pressure in the arms exceeds that in the legs. There is
    collateral arterial circulation. Murmurs are usually present but vary in location.
  Laboratory features
    Chest radiograph may show prominence of the left ventricle, notching of the inferior
    border of the ribs from collateral vessels, and poststenotic dilatation of the aorta.
Cushing's symdrome
  Symptoms
    Menstrual disorders, loss of libido, hirsutism, acne, striae, muscle weakness, easy bruising,
    edema, polyuria.
  Physical examination
    Hirsutism, acne, striae, muscle weakness and wasting, purpura, bruising, edema, and poor
    wound healing.
  Laboratory features
    Hyperglycemia, impaired glucose tolerance, neutrophilia, lymphopenia, and hypokalemia.
Renal parenchymal disease
  Symptoms
    Uremia and anemia; associated with renal failure.
  Physical examination
    If any findings, those associated with renal failure.
  Laboratory features
    Several laboratory abnormalities may be present. These include elevation of the BUN
    and creatinine levels, anemia, hypocalcemia, hyperphosphatemia, hyperkalemia,
    metabolic acidosis, proteinuria, and hematuria.

BUN, blood urea nitrogen.

including measurement of the urinary catecholamine levels, should be performed.

Echocardiography can visualize the area of **aortic coarctation**, but this is best confirmed by cardiac catheterization.

Historically, **Cushing's syndrome** has been diagnosed based on the following findings: elevated levels of urinary 17-hydroxycorticosteroids and urinary free cortisol, loss of diurnal rhythm in the plasma cortisol concentrations, and failure of plasma cortisol levels to suppress overnight after a single 1-mg dose of dexamethasone. Because the overnight dexamethasone suppression test may not elicit suppression in obese and acromegalic patients, the low-dose dexamethasone suppression test (1.5 mg every 6 hours for 2 days) should be done to distinguish patients with Cushing's syndrome from normal subjects. The high-dose dexamethasone suppression test (2 mg every 6 hours for 2 days) can distinguish Cushing's disease from an adrenal tumor, which does not suppress.

If the cause of **renal parenchymal disease** cannot be identified with certainty based on the history, physical examination, and laboratory findings, renal biopsy may be indicated. The biopsy results may shed light on whether the process is reversible, and thereby point toward treatment options, if any.

In the setting of **renin-producing tumors**, determination of the plasma renin activity by renal vein sampling usually shows a unilateral increase in the absence of a renal artery lesion.

4. *What are the respective treatment options for renal artery stenosis, pheochromocytoma, Cushing's syndrome, and primary hyperaldosteronism?*

The treatment options for **renal artery stenosis** are either surgical or medical, and the choice depends on the patient involved. The surgical options include revascularization of the affected kidney using saphenous vein, autogenous artery, or synthetic (Dacron or polytetrafluoroethylene) grafts. A renal artery endarterectomy may be performed in patients with ostial atheromatous lesions. The most popular method of treatment, at least initially, is percutaneous transluminal balloon angioplasty. If these procedures are either unsuccessful or cannot be undertaken, medical management must be instituted. Beta blockers, ACE inhibitors, and clonidine are the most effective agents for controlling blood pressure in this setting.

Cure of a **pheochromocytoma** consists of surgical removal of the tumor, and proper preoperative preparation helps reduce the attendant morbidity and mortality. In the presence of hypertension, administration of an adrenergic-blocking agent such as phenoxybenzamine (10 to 20 mg twice per day, increasing to 100 mg per day if tolerated). Prazosin is not as effective. However, if the location of the tumor is in doubt or if multiple tumors are suspected, it is best not to administer α-adrenergic blocking agents before surgery. The intravascular volume should be expanded both before and after operation. In patients with inoperable malignant pheochromocytomas, drug therapy is needed. Alpha and beta blockers may be used to control arrhythmias, or methyltyrosine may be prescribed to inhibit catecholamine synthesis.

The best surgical approach in a patient with Cushing's disease is selected excision of the **pituitary adenoma** through a transsphenoidal approach. Surgical removal is sometimes followed by pituitary irradiation to prevent recurrence. A variety of drugs have also been used to treat patients with Cushing's disease. Adrenal tumors are best treated surgically.

Hyperaldosteronism can be treated by either medical or surgical means. Mild aldosterone excess due to an adenoma, and all cases of bilateral hyperplasia, should be managed with aldosterone antagonists such as spironolactone because this disorder is not amenable to surgical treatment. Aldosterone-producing adenomas can be removed to effect cure once they have been appropriately localized by radiologic (CT) techniques.

Case   A 38-year-old adopted white man is seen by his family physician for the management of hypertension of 2 years' duration. Current medications include amiloride (5 mg) and hydrochlorothiazide (50 mg), with good blood pressure control until now. Review of his systems reveals increasing fatigue, headaches, and muscle cramps. Physical examination reveals a blood pressure of 140/100 mm Hg in the left arm and 136/100 mm Hg in the right arm. No disparity in the blood pressure between the arms and the legs is found. The remainder of the examination findings are otherwise unremarkable.

The following laboratory data are reported: sodium, 145 mEq/L; potassium, 2.7 mEq/L; chloride, 109 mEq/L; bicarbonate, 29 mEq/L; BUN, 10 mEq/L; creatinine, 1.2 mg/dL; calcium, 9.1 mg/dL; cholesterol, 213 mg/dL; triglycerides, 163 mg/dL; uric acid, 6.1 mg/dL; phosphate, 2.1 mg/dL; and glucose, 99 mg/dL. Results of urinalysis, including microscopic examination, are normal.

The diuretics are stopped and the patient is placed on potassium supplements. Repeat laboratory work reveals his sodium level is 147 mEq/L, his potassium level is 3 mEq/L, and his blood pressure is 146/104 mm Hg.

1. What is the differential diagnosis of this patient's hypertension?
2. What symptoms are related to the patient's hypokalemia?
3. What diagnostic steps would help confirm the diagnosis in this patient?
4. What are the treatment options in this patient?

Case Discussion

   1. *What is the differential diagnosis of this patient's hypertension?*
      The differential diagnosis includes essential hypertension, primary hyperaldosteronism, pheochromocytoma, Cushing's syndrome, a renin-producing tumor, and renal artery stenosis. Renal parenchymal disease and coarctation of the aorta can be largely excluded as a cause of this patient's hypertension

because the serum creatinine level and urinalysis findings are normal, as are the physical examination findings. The striking feature of this patient's hypertension is the hypokalemia despite treatment with a potassium-sparing diuretic plus potassium supplementation. Hypokalemia may be a feature of primary hyperaldosteronism, Cushing's syndrome, renal artery stenosis, and renin-producing tumors. Pheochromocytoma is considered a possibility because of the patient's complaints of headache and fatigue, although the clinical suspicion for this is low. Although hypokalemia occurs in Cushing's syndrome, the other clinical features of the disorder appear to be lacking. Renal artery stenosis is also unlikely unless the patient has fibromuscular dysplasia. Because the patient's family history is unknown, his genetic propensity for atherosclerosis is not known, but he does not appear to have other evidence of arteriosclerotic disease (e.g., bruits, angina, and claudication). Therefore, the most likely causes include primary aldosteronism and a renin-producing tumor. Essential hypertension can be diagnosed only after the most likely secondary causes have been excluded.

2. *What symptoms are related to the patient's hypokalemia?*

Hypokalemia could explain this patient's headaches, muscle cramps, and fatigue. Additional symptoms may include muscle weakness, polyuria, and paresthesias.

3. *What diagnostic steps would help confirm the diagnosis in this patient?*

Patients with a history of spontaneous hypokalemia, marked sensitivity to potassium-wasting diuretics, and refractory hypertension should be evaluated for primary hyperaldosteronism. The initial screening test is to determine the status of aldosterone excretion during prolonged salt loading. To perform this, 10 to 12 g of NaCl is added to the patient's daily intake. After 5 to 7 days of increased salt intake, the serum potassium concentrations and a 24-hour urine excretion of sodium, potassium, and aldosterone are measured. The serum and urine potassium values indicate whether there is inappropriate kaliuresis (a serum potassium level of <3 mEq/L with a urine potassium level >30 mEq/24 hours). The 24-hour urine sodium level verifies compliance with the prescribed salt intake (≥250 mEq per day). If, under these conditions, the patient's rate of aldosterone excretion fails to show suppression below 14 μg per 24 hours, this makes him a prime candidate for additional studies. The presence of hypokalemia and suppressed plasma renin activity further supports the diagnosis of primary hyperaldosteronism. If a renin-producing tumor were the cause of this patient's hypertension, the plasma renin activity would be elevated. If primary hyperaldosteronism is suspected, adrenal CT scanning should be performed. The finding of an adrenal mass would establish the diagnosis. Adrenal scintigraphy should be done if the CT findings are inconclusive. If the results of scintigraphy are also ambiguous, then adrenal vein sampling should be performed to measure the aldosterone levels. Adrenal vein sampling is still the most accurate test to localize aldosterone-producing tumors.

4. *What are the treatment options in this patient?*

The hypertension associated with primary hyperaldosteronism can be managed adequately in most cases by means of salt and water depletion. The combination of spironolactone with hydrochlorothiazide or furosemide has been used successfully. However, if the adrenal adenoma is confined to one gland and there are no contraindications, the tumor should be removed. Only approximately half of patients are normotensive 5 years after surgery, but normal potassium homeostasis is restored permanently. If primary hyperaldosteronism stems from bilateral hyperplasia of the adrenal gland, this is best managed medically because surgical removal of too much of the adrenal gland can result in adrenal insufficiency.

Suggested Readings

Ploth DW. Renovascular hypertension. In: Jacobson HR, Striker GE, Klahr S, eds. *The principles and practice of nephrology*, 2nd ed. St. Louis: Mosby, 1995, p. 379.

Smith MC, Dunn MJ. The patient with hypertension. In: Schrier RW, ed. *Manual of nephrology*, 4th ed. Boston: Little, Brown, 1995, p. 215.

Nephrolithiasis

1. What are the four major types of kidney stones, and which are radiopaque?

2. What is the shared pathogenesis for the formation of all types of kidney stones?

3. What are the fundamental causes of oversaturation of the urine?

4. What are the acute and chronic sequelae of kidney stones?

5. In the setting of uric acid kidney stones, is the oversaturation of urine with uric acid conditioned primarily by the urine pH or by the amount of uric acid excreted?

6. What are the three types of kidney stones that may present in the form of staghorn calculi, and what are the respective mechanisms responsible for their formation?

7. What are the principal causes of calcium stones?

8. What are the routine outpatient studies that should be performed in patients with recurrent stones?

9. What is the indication for measuring the excretion of uric acid in the setting of hyperuricosuria?

10. What are the potential sources of hypercalciuria?

Discussion

1. *What are the four major types of kidney stones, and which are radiopaque?*

The principal types of kidney stones are composed of calcium salts, uric acid, cystine, and struvite. All except uric acid stones are radiopaque. Calcium-containing stones account for 80% of all stones, 15% are composed of struvite, 5% are made up of uric acid, and cystine stones are very rare.

2. *What is the shared pathogenesis for the formation of all types of kidney stones?*

All kidney stones result from an excessive supersaturation of the urine. The ion concentration product at which salts in solution are in equilibrium with their solid phase is called the *equilibrium solubility product*. In the absence of a solid phase, salts may exist in a supersaturated state, above the equilibrium solubility product. In this setting, crystals composed of other compounds may act as heterogeneous seed nuclei that foster the formation of stones. If the ion product is sufficiently high, then new crystals form. Because an increase in urine volume leads to a decrease in the concentration of all solutes in the urine, an increased fluid intake to 2.5 to 3 L per day is part of the treatment for all kidney stones.

3. *What are the fundamental causes of oversaturation of the urine?*

There are three major reasons for the oversaturation of urine: (a) hyperexcretion of a substance that is relatively insoluble in urine, (b) low urine volume, and (c) an abnormal urine pH. Low citrate excretion has also been implicated as an independent cause of calcium stone formation.

4. *What are the acute and chronic sequelae of kidney stones?*

The acute consequences of kidney stones are urinary tract obstruction, infection, hematuria, pain, and, uncommonly, acute renal failure. Chronic consequences of nephrolithiasis are infection, renal tubular acidosis, and chronic renal insufficiency.

5. *In the setting of uric acid kidney stones, is the oversaturation of urine with uric acid conditioned primarily by the urine pH or by the amount of uric acid excreted?*

Because monosodium urate is more soluble than uric acid, urate stones are rare. There is a significant risk for such stones only when the urinary form is mainly uric acid. Uric acid is a weak acid that has one proton that is dissociable under physiologic conditions with a pK (the negative logarithm of the ionization constant of an acid) of 5.3. Therefore, urate may exist in urine as either monosodium urate or uric acid. The concentration ratios of these two forms is a function of the ambient pH. A change in the urinary pH from 5 to 6.5 alters the undissociated acid concentration eightfold, whereas the urinary excretion of uric acid can increase only up to threefold. Thus, changes in the urine pH play a greater role in uric acid stone formation than do changes in the amount of uric acid excreted.

6. *What are the three types of kidney stones that may present in the form of staghorn calculi, and what are the respective mechanisms responsible for their formation?*

Uric acid, cystine, and struvite kidney stones may form in the renal collecting system and assume a staghorn configuration.

Struvite kidney stones, which are the most common staghorn calculi, are a consequence of infection of the urinary tract by bacteria, usually *Proteus* species, that contain urease. This causes urea to be broken down to $2NH_3 + H_2O + CO_2$. Ammonia reacts with a proton, forming ammonium. This reaction raises the urine pH, resulting in an increased concentration of phosphate ions.

These conditions spawn the formation of struvite ($MgNH_4PO_4 \cdot 6H_2O$), and may also lead to the formation of carbonate apatite ($Ca_{10}[PO_4]_6 \cdot CO_3$) crystals; thus, struvite stones may contain variable proportions of carbonate apatite and struvite.

Cystine stones are a manifestation of cystinuria, a rare hereditary disorder that is characterized by defects in dibasic amino acid transport. Normally, amino acids are almost completely resorbed by the proximal tubule. The urinary excretion of cystine is abnormally high in people with cystine stones, however, and this predisposes them to the formation of cystine stones. The urine pH has little effect on the solubility of cystine. The mechanism responsible for the formation of uric acid stones is discussed in the preceding question.

7. *What are the principal causes of calcium stones?*

There are numerous specific causes of calcium kidney stones, but the major causes can be grouped into the following categories: low urinary volume, hypercalciuria, hyperoxaluria, hyperuricosuria, and alkaline urine. Hypocitruria may also be an independent cause of calcium stone formation, although a low urinary excretion of citrate may actually be a consequence of an alkaline urine.

8. *What are the routine outpatient studies that should be performed in patients with recurrent stones?*

The urine pH and volume should be assessed, and the 24-hour urinary excretion of calcium, uric acid, citrate, oxalate, phosphate, and creatinine should be determined.

9. *What is the indication for measuring the excretion of uric acid in the setting of hyperuricosuria?*

In the setting of hyperuricosuria, uric acid crystals may act as seed crystals that initiate the precipitation of calcium oxalate from the urine. If patients are found to be hyperuricosuric, allopurinol treatment might be warranted.

10. *What are the potential sources of hypercalciuria?*

Most commonly, hypercalciuria is idiopathic in origin. Before making such a diagnosis, however, other causes of hypercalciuria (i.e., sarcoidosis, immobilization, vitamin D excess, hyperthyroidism, Paget's disease, and malignant tumors with metastasis) need to be excluded (Table 9-14).

Case   A 48-year-old man presents to a local emergency room because of right flank pain radiating to his right testicle that has lasted for 2 hours. The pain was initially mild, then became progressively more severe over an hour's time. He has no nausea or vomiting, fever or chills, dysuria, hesitancy, or decreased stream. He has no history of previous kidney stones or urinary tract infections. His past medical history is remarkable only for a history of Crohn's disease, which required resection of a portion of his ileum. He takes no medications.

On examination, he is found to be in obvious discomfort. His abdomen is soft and nontender with no masses. There is mild costovertebral angle tenderness.

Table 9-14. Causes of Hypercalciurea

Cause	Serum calcium level	Other serum values	Usual stone type
Idiopathic hypercalciuria[a]	Normal	Normal	Calcium oxalate or calcium phosphate
Primary hyperparathyroidism	High	Hypophosphatemia, occasionally hyper-chloremic acidosis	Calcium oxalate or calcium phosphate
Renal tubular acidosis	Normal	Hyperchloremic acidosis	Calcium phosphate

[a]Sarcoidosis, Cushing's syndrome, alkali abuse, immobilization, vitamin D excess, hyperthyroidism, Paget's disease, rapidly progressive bone disease, and malignant tumors (which cause hypercalciuria, although not stones) must be excluded on clinical grounds.
From Coe FL. The patient with renal stones. In: Schrier RW, ed. *Manual of nephrology,* 4th ed. Boston: Little, Brown, 1995, p. 90. Reprinted with permission.

His testicles are normal. The remainder of his examination findings are unremarkable. The urine pH is 6, and urinalysis shows 1+ protein and 2+ heme. The sediment contains 10 to 15 red blood cells, 0 to 5 white blood cells per high-power field, and a moderate amount of amorphous crystals. There are no casts. His complete blood count and electrolyte levels are normal. A chest radiographic study and kidney, ureter, and bladder (KUB) film are interpreted as normal.

The following laboratory data are reported: calcium, 10 mg/dL; phosphorus, 3.7 mg/dL; albumin, 4.1 g/dL; creatinine, 1 mg/dL; and BUN, 12 mg/dL. His blood pressure is 140/85 mm Hg, his pulse is 95 beats per minute, his respiratory rate is 20 breaths per minute, and his temperature is 37.2°C.

1. What are some of the possible renal causes of this patient's symptoms?
2. What is the significance of the crystalluria?
3. Does the absence of a colic-like pain suggest that this patient's pain is not due to a kidney stone?
4. What would be the appropriate test for confirming the diagnosis of a kidney stone in this patient?
5. Once the diagnosis of a kidney stone is established, what is the appropriate management that should be implemented in the emergency room?
   Excretory urography reveals a radiopaque stone at the left ureteropelvic junction. Subsequently, the patient passes the stone in his urine while in the emergency room. Laboratory analysis reveals that the stone is composed primarily of calcium oxalate.
6. What are the possible causes and the treatments of hyperoxaluria as seen in this patient?

Case Discussion

1. *What are some of the possible renal causes of this patient's symptoms?*
   Kidney stones, renal infarction, and papillary necrosis may all present with the acute onset of flank pain together with hematuria. However, renal infarc-

tion usually occurs in a patient who has either a local or systemic cause for thrombosis (e.g., trauma, aneurysm, or vasculitis involving the renal artery) or thromboembolism (e.g., endocarditis, mural thrombi, or fat emboli). Papillary necrosis typically occurs in patients with either advanced diabetic nephropathy or sickle cell disease. Kidney stones often arise in people who have no known contributory medical illness.

2. *What is the significance of the crystalluria?*

Except for the finding of cystine crystals, which indicates cystinuria, crystalluria is of no diagnostic value when evaluating a patient for nephrolithiasis.

3. *Does the absence of a colic-like pain suggest that this patient's pain is not due to a kidney stone?*

No. Typically, the pain associated with kidney stones is a steady pain that gradually worsens; it does not fluctuate, as the term *renal colic* suggests.

4. *What would be the appropriate test for confirming the diagnosis of a kidney stone in this patient?*

Although in some cases nephrolithiasis can be diagnosed on the basis of the KUB radiographic findings, it is usually necessary to perform *excretory urography*, as in this patient, to establish the diagnosis. It allows the location, size, shape, and radiolucency of kidney stones to be determined. Although retrograde pyelography can yield the same information, it is a more expensive and invasive procedure. Ultrasonography is not as sensitive as excretory urography for detecting kidney stones. More recently, *noncontrast helical CT* has become the procedure of choice in many centers.

5. *Once the diagnosis of a kidney stone is established, what is the appropriate management that should be implemented in the emergency room?*

The patient should be kept well hydrated, usually with intravenous fluids, to maintain a brisk urine flow, which may promote passage of the stone, and to diminish the risk of nephrotoxicity from the radiocontrast agent. All of the patient's urine should be strained to determine if the patient has passed any stones. If any stones are obtained, they should be sent for analysis. Patients almost always require narcotic analgesics for management of the pain. Patients should be admitted to the hospital if inadequate pain relief is obtained with oral analgesics, or in the event of urinary tract infection or acute renal failure.

6. *What are the possible causes and the treatments of hyperoxaluria as seen in this patient?*

Hyperoxaluria can result in sufficient suprasaturation of the urine with calcium oxalate to cause the precipitation of kidney stones. Over 80% of urinary oxalate is derived from endogenous production, primarily as a breakdown product of glyoxylate. The remainder of urinary oxalate is obtained from dietary sources. Thus, hyperoxaluria can be caused by primary overproduction, intestinal disease, and diet. Overproduction of oxalate (primary hyperoxaluria) is hereditary and severe, but rare. Injury of the bowel wall inflicted by fatty acids or bile salts can result in an increased permeability to oxalate. The most usual clinical setting, as in this patient, is Crohn's disease, ileal resection, or jejunoileal bypass. A high dietary intake of oxalate may be due to the ingestion of foods such as chocolate, nuts, rhubarb, tea, and some fruit juices, as well as the intake of vitamin C in excess of 1,000 mg per day. Treatment usually involves the combination of a low-oxalate and low-fat diet together with oral calcium and cholestyramine administration to "bind" oxalate in the intestine.

Suggested Readings

Coe FL. The patient with renal stones. In: Schrier RW, ed. *Manual of nephrology*, 4th ed. Boston: Little, Brown, 1995, p. 90.

Preminger GM, Pak CYC. Nephrolithiasis. In: Jacobson HR, Striker GE, Klahr S, eds. *The principles and practice of nephrology*, 2nd ed. St. Louis: Mosby, 1995, p. 1015.

Nephrotic Syndrome

1. What is the definition of the nephrotic syndrome?

2. What are the causes of the nephrotic syndrome?

3. What are the clinical and histologic features of the primary (idiopathic) nephrotic syndrome?

4. What are the possible complications of the nephrotic syndrome?

5. What are the treatment options for the nephrotic syndrome?

Discussion

1. *What is the definition of the nephrotic syndrome?*

The nephrotic syndrome is a clinical entity characterized by (a) proteinuria in excess of 3.5 g/1.73 m^2 of body surface area (or 50 mg/kg of body weight) at a time when neither the serum albumin level nor glomerular filtration is decreased; (b) hypoalbuminemia (<3 g/dL), which is a consequence of the renal losses coupled with inadequate hepatic compensatory synthesis; (c) edema, which is a consequence of both the hypoalbuminemia and the sodium retention; and (d) hyperlipidemia, which is probably due to the increased hepatic synthesis of very–low-density lipoproteins, which are converted to cholesterol-carrying low-density lipoproteins. Impaired removal plays an important but probably secondary role in this setting.

2. *What are the causes of the nephrotic syndrome?*

The causes of the nephrotic syndrome can be easily divided into two broad categories. The primary, or idiopathic, forms of nephrotic syndrome are those for which a specific cause cannot be identified despite a reasonably thorough evaluation. The five major histologic subtypes of primary nephrotic syndrome include minimal-change disease (also called *lipoid nephrosis* or *nil disease*), membranous glomerulonephritis, membranoproliferative glomerulonephritis (also called *mesangiocapillary glomerulonephritis*), focal glomerular sclerosis, and proliferative glomerulonephritis. The secondary forms of the nephrotic syndrome are those associated with specific etiologic events or in which glomerular disease arises as a complication of another disease or systemic process. These may be broadly categorized into those stemming from infections, neoplasia, medications, allergens, multisystem diseases, and heredofamilial diseases, and also include various miscellaneous causes (Table 9-15). *Secondary nephrotic syndrome may be associated with any of the major histologic subtypes found in the idiopathic nephrotic syndrome.* The idiopathic nephrotic syndrome is more common than the secondary form.

3. *What are the clinical and histologic features of the primary (idiopathic) nephrotic syndrome?*

   The clinical and histologic features of the primary nephrotic syndrome are listed in Table 9-16.

4. *What are the possible complications of the nephrotic syndrome?*

   The complications of the nephrotic syndrome include accelerated atherosclerosis, increased susceptibility to infections, osteomalacia, and an increased incidence of deep vein and renal vein thrombosis.

5. *What are the treatment options for the nephrotic syndrome?*

   The treatment of the nephrotic syndrome depends on its cause. Certainly, in the case of the secondary nephrotic syndrome, if the primary disorder is treated effectively, the nephrotic syndrome tends to resolve as well. In the case of the primary nephrotic syndrome, certain histologic subtypes (i.e., minimal-change disease and possibly membranous nephropathy) respond to treatment with steroids, with or without cytotoxic agents. Other lesions may be refractory to any type of therapy. Drugs such as the ACE inhibitors or NSAIDs may be useful in reducing the proteinuria by affecting intrarenal hemodynamics, but they cannot in any way alter the primary glomerular abnormality involved.

Case

A 40-year-old woman is referred for evaluation of proteinuria. Aside from occasional arthralgias, she has felt well but is concerned about progressive weight gain and marked swelling of her lower extremities. She has no personal or family history of renal disease, no known chronic systemic illness, nor is she taking any medications. Physical examination findings, including blood pressure, are normal, except for the presence of edema, which is most notable in dependent areas. Laboratory evaluation reveals a normal hematocrit, as well as serum glucose, BUN, and creatinine levels, but she has profound hypoalbuminemia (1.9 g/dL) and hypercholesterolemia (490 mg/dL). Urinalysis shows 4+ proteinuria, oval fat bodies, and free fat droplets but no cellular elements or casts. Her 24-hour urinary excretion of protein is found to be 8.6 g.

1. What is the most common cause of the secondary nephrotic syndrome in adults in the United States? In patients with this disorder, what early finding serves as a harbinger for the subsequent development of nephrotic syndrome and renal insufficiency?

2. What features of the history and physical examination are important in determining if this patient has a primary (idiopathic) or secondary form of the nephrotic syndrome?

Table 9-15. Disorders Associated with Secondary Nephrotic Syndrome

Infectious diseases
  Bacterial: poststreptococcal glomerulonephritis, infective endocarditis, "shunt" nephritis, syphilis, leprosy
  Viral: hepatitis B and C, cytomegalovirus, Epstein-Barr virus, herpes zoster, human immunodeficiency virus
  Protozoal: malaria, toxoplasmosis
  Helminthic: schistosomiasis, trypanosomiasis, filariasis
Neoplastic diseases
  Solid tumors (carcinoma and sarcoma): colon, lung, breast, stomach, kidney
  Hematologic malignancies (leukemias and lymphomas)
Medications
  Nonsteroidal antiinflammatory agents
  Organic, inorganic, elemental mercury
  Organic gold
  Penicillamine
  "Street" heroin
  Probenecid
  Bismuth
  Captopril
Multisystem diseases
  Systemic lupus erythematosus
  Mixed connective tissue disease
  Dermatomyositis
  Dermatitis herpetiformis
  Sarcoidosis
  Henoch-Schönlein purpura
  Goodpasture's syndrome
  Rheumatoid arthritis
  Amyloidosis
  Polyarteritis
Allergic reactions
  Bee sting
  Pollens
  Poison ivy and poison oak
  Serum sickness (antitoxins)
Metabolic diseases
  Diabetes mellitus
  Myxedema
  Graves' disease
Heredofamilial diseases
  Alport's syndrome
  Fabry's disease
  Nail-patella syndrome
  Sickle cell disease
  α_1-antitrypsin deficiency
  Congenital nephrotic syndrome (Finnish type)
  Hereditary amyloidosis (familial Mediterranean fever)
Miscellaneous
  Chronic renal allograft rejection
  Pregnancy-associated (preeclampsia, recurrent or transient)
  Vesicoureteric reflex

Table 9-16. The Clinical and Histologic Features of the Primary (Idiopathic) Nephrotic Syndrome

Glomerular disease	Distinguishing clinical and laboratory findings	Characteristic morphologic features
Minimal-change disease	Most common cause in children (75%); 20% of adults; steroid- or cyclophosphamide-sensitive (80%); nonprogressive; normal renal function; scant hematuria	LM: normal IF: negative EM: podocyte effacement; no immune deposits
Focal and segmental glomerulosclerosis	Early-onset hypertension; microscopic hematuria; progressive renal failure (75%)	LM: early—segmental sclerosis in some glomeruli with tubular atrophy; late—sclerosis of most glomeruli
Membranous nephropathy	Most common cause in adults (40%–50%); peak incidence, fourth and sixth decades; male–female 2–3 : 1; early hypertension (30%); spontaneous remission (20%); progressive renal failure (30%–40%)	LM: early—normal; late—GBM thickening IF: granular IgG and C3 EM: subepithelial deposits and GBM expansion
Membranoproliferative glomerulonephritis	Peak incidence, second and third decades; mixed nephrotic–nephritic features; slowly progressive in most, rapid in some; hypocomplementemia	LM: hypercellular glomeruli with duplicated GBM EM: type I—subendothelial immune deposits; type II—dense GBM
Proliferative	See Table 9-18	

LM, light microscopy; IF, immunofluorescence; EM, electron microscopy; GBM, glomerular basement membrane. From *MKSAP IX.* Philadelphia: American College of Physicians, 1992. Reprinted with permission.

3. What additional laboratory tests would you order either to establish or refute a secondary cause of the nephrotic syndrome?

In this patient, the anti-nuclear antibody (ANA) test is positive and the complement levels are low, indicating that she may have systemic lupus erythematosus (SLE) as the cause of her nephrotic syndrome.

4. How should this patient's evaluation proceed?

Case Discussion

1. *What is the most common cause of the secondary nephrotic syndrome in adults in the United States? In patients with this disorder, what early finding serves as a harbinger for the subsequent development of nephrotic syndrome and renal insufficiency?*

Diabetes mellitus is the most common cause of secondary nephrotic syndrome in adults in the United States. In patients with type I diabetes, the onset of microalbuminuria (albumin excretion of 20 to 200 μg per minute or 30 to 300 mg per day) predicts the subsequent development of nephrotic syndrome and renal insufficiency. These patients should begin treatment with an ACE inhibitor. The clinical significance of microalbuminuria in type II diabetes remains to be determined.

2. *What features of the history and physical examination are important in determining if this patient has a primary (idiopathic) or secondary form of the nephrotic syndrome?*

Differentiating between the primary and secondary forms of the nephrotic syndrome depends on a careful review of the patient's history and physical examination findings and the performance of selected laboratory tests that can identify underlying disease states. It is imperative to determine if there is a family or personal history of diabetes mellitus or connective tissue disease, hereditary conditions such as sickle cell disease or Alport's syndrome, allergen exposure, and so forth. A complete medication list must be obtained, including the use of nonprescription medicines such as NSAIDs. A history of illicit drug use is equally important because heroin nephropathy is not rare in drug abusers. In addition, a travel history is a crucial part of the history taking because, for example, malaria is a well known cause of the nephrotic syndrome and should be considered in those patients who have traveled to endemic areas. Risk factors for hepatitis and human immunodeficiency virus (HIV) infection must also be sought because high-risk populations should be screened for these disorders. In this particular patient (a young woman), the history of occasional arthralgias brings up the possibility of a multisystem disease as the source of the nephrotic syndrome.

3. *What additional laboratory tests would you order either to establish or refute a secondary cause of the nephrotic syndrome?*

Laboratory tests that are useful in establishing a secondary cause of the nephrotic syndrome include the serum glucose level, an ANA determination, complement levels, hepatitis screen, Venereal Disease Research Laboratory test, HIV test, sickle cell preparation, an antistreptolysin titer, throat culture, and serum and urinary protein electrophoresis. The findings yielded by the history and physical examination dictate which of these tests should be performed in a particular patient.

4. *How should this patient's evaluation proceed?*

In the setting of SLE, a kidney biopsy should be performed in an effort to establish the nature of the underlying disorder responsible for the nephrotic syndrome. This patient most likely has either diffuse proliferative glomerulonephritis or membranous nephropathy with SLE. The therapy for the former calls for treatment with steroids and cytotoxic agents, although the latter does not.

Suggested Readings

Bernard DB. Extrarenal complications of the nephrotic syndrome. *Kidney Int* 1988;33:1184.

Bernard DB, Salant DF. Clinical approach to the patient with proteinuria and the nephrotic syndrome. In: Jacobson HR, Striker GE, Klahr S, eds. *The principles and practice of nephrology*, 2nd ed. St. Louis: Mosby, 1995, p. 110.

Kaysen GA. Proteinuria and the nephrotic syndrome. In: Schrier RW, ed. *Renal and electrolyte disorders*, 5th ed. Philadelphia: Lippincott–Raven, 1997, p. 640.

Glomerulonephritiss

1. What is the definition of hematuria?
2. What is the definition of the nephritic syndrome?
3. What are the major causes of hematuria?
4. What can help point toward a glomerular origin as the source of the hematuria?
5. What are the primary diseases of the kidney associated with glomerular hematuria (nephritic syndrome)?
6. What systemic diseases are associated with glomerular hematuria?
7. How is rapidly progressive glomerulonephritis (RPGN) defined?
8. What clinical disorders cause RPGN?

Discussion

1. *What is the definition of hematuria?*

    Hematuria refers to the presence of an abnormally high number of red blood cells in the urine. This is most commonly detected by a dipstick (Hemastix) method, which identifies the presence of hemoglobin. The hematuria is considered macroscopic when the urine is obviously red due to the presence of blood, and it is deemed microscopic when the urine grossly appears normal. A number of foods (such as beets) and some drugs (such as phenazopyridine hydrochloride) as well as porphyria can turn the urine red. In these circumstances, the dipstick result is negative.

2. *What is the definition of the nephritic syndrome?*

    The nephritic syndrome is defined by a constellation of urinary findings that include the presence of hematuria, proteinuria, and red blood cell casts. These findings indicate the presence of a glomerular lesion and are frequently accompanied by azotemia, hypertension, and edema.

3. *What are the major causes of hematuria?*

    The causes of hematuria are best approached in terms of their being either extrarenal or renal in origin. Extrarenal bleeding can occur in the ureters due to calculi or carcinoma; in the bladder due to hemorrhagic cystitis stemming from infection (including *Schistosoma haematobium* in endemic areas), as well as from cyclophosphamide use, carcinoma, catheterization, or calculi; in the prostate due to hypertrophy, carcinoma, or prostatitis; and in the urethra due to urethritis or trauma. Renal causes of hematuria can be classified as either glomerular or nonglomerular and are listed in Table 9-17.

4. *What can help point toward a glomerular origin as the source of the hematuria?*

    The following findings point toward a glomerular cause as the source of hematuria: (a) the presence of dysmorphic red blood cells on phase-contrast microscopy; (b) the presence of red blood cell casts, which is a virtually diagnostic finding; and (c) proteinuria exceeding 500 mg per day.

5. *What are the primary diseases of the kidney associated with glomerular hematuria (nephritic syndrome)?*

    The primary diseases associated with glomerular hematuria are immuno-

Table 9-17. Glomerular and Nonglomerular Renal Parenchymal Causes of Hematuria

Glomerular
  Proliferative glomerulonephritis
    Primary
    Secondary
  Familial diseases of the glomerulus
    Alport's syndrome
    Recurrent benign hematuria (thin basement membrane disease)
  Malignant hypertension
Nonglomerular
  Neoplasms
    Renal cell carcinoma
    Wilms' tumor
    Benign cysts
  Vascular
    Renal infarct
    Renal vein thrombosis
    Malignant hypertension
    Arteriovenous malformation
    Capillary necrosis
    Loin-pain hematuria syndrome
  Metabolic
    Hypercalciuria
    Hyperuricosuria
  Familial
    Polycystic kidney disease
    Medullary sponge kidney
  Papillary necrosis
    Analgesic abuse
    Sickle cell disease and trait
    Renal tuberculosis
    Diabetes
    Obstructive uropathy
  Drugs
    Anticoagulants (heparin, coumarin)
    Drug-induced acute interstitial nephritis
  Trauma

Adapted from Lieberthal W. Hematuria and the acute nephritic syndrome. In: Jacobson HR, Striker GE, Klahr S, eds. *The principles and practice of nephrology.* Philadelphia: Decker, 1991.

globulin A (IgA) nephropathy, poststreptococcal glomerulonephritis, membranoproliferative glomerulonephritis, and idiopathic RPGN.

6. *What systemic diseases are associated with glomerular hematuria?*

Systemic lupus erythematosus, Henoch-Schönlein purpura, Goodpasture's syndrome, vasculitis (including polyarteritis nodosa and Wegener's granulomatosis), and essential mixed cryoglobulinemia are all associated with glomerular hematuria.

7. *How is RPGN defined?*

Rapidly progressive glomerulonephritis is primarily defined in clinical terms as a glomerular disease characterized by progression to end-stage renal disease within weeks to months. The pathologic correlate is extensive crescent formation in the glomeruli, as seen in kidney biopsy specimens.

Table 9-18. Immunopathogenetic Classification of Rapidly Progressive Glomerulonephritis

Anti-GBM antibody (linear immune deposits)
   With lung hemorrhage (Goodpasture's syndrome)
   Without lung hemorrhage
   Complicating membranous nephropathy
Immune complex (granular immune deposits)
   Postinfectious
      Poststreptococcal
      Visceral abscess
      Other
   Collagen-vascular disease
      Lupus nephritis
      Henoch-Schönlein purpura
      Mixed cryoglobulinemia
   Primary renal disease
      IgA nephropathy
      Membranoproliferative glomerulonephritis
      Idiopathic
No immune deposit
   Vasculitis
      Polyarteritis
      Wegener's granulomatosis
      Hypersensitivity vasculitides
   Idiopathic

GBM, glomerular basement membrane.
From Couser WG. Rapidly progressive glomerulonephritis. In: Jacobson HR, Striker GE, and Klahr S, eds. *The principles and practice of nephrology.* Philadelphia: Decker, 1991. Reprinted with permission.

8. *What clinical disorders cause RPGN?*

A number of disorders cause RPGN. These are best defined in immunopathologic terms, depending on the absence or presence (and pattern) of immune deposits (Table 9-18).

Case A 21-year-old college student is referred to the renal clinic for further evaluation of microscopic hematuria, which was discovered during a preemployment physical examination. There is no history of recent infections, trauma, or intravenous drug abuse. She denies any history of rashes, arthralgia, myalgias, fevers, or episodes of gross hematuria.

Physical examination reveals a well developed, well nourished woman who is in no acute distress. Her blood pressure is 125/85 mm Hg; pulse, 72 beats per minute; and respiratory rate, 16 breaths per minute. No rashes, lymphadenopathy, or joint tenderness is noted. The remainder of the physical examination findings are within normal limits.

The following laboratory data are reported: serum sodium, 135 mEq/L; potassium, 4.5 mEq/L; chloride, 105 mEq/L; carbon dioxide, 25 mEq/L; glucose, 98 mg/dL; BUN, 12 mEq/L; and creatinine, 0.8 mg/dL. Urinalysis shows a specific gravity of 1.015, pH of 5.0, 1+ heme, and 1+ protein on dipstick examination.

Microscopic examination of the urine reveals 5 to 10 red blood cells per high-power field, and possibly one red blood cell cast is noted on close scrutiny of the entire slide. The 24-hour urine excretion consists of 1.5 L total volume, with 1,200 mg of creatinine and 1,200 mg of protein.

On further laboratory examination, no secondary systemic cause for the nephritic syndrome is identified. Specifically, ANA and anti-neutrophil cytoplasmic antibody tests are negative, as are tests for hepatitis B and C. Likewise, both the C3 and C4 complement levels are normal. Consequently, a renal percutaneous renal biopsy is performed. The histologic, immunofluorescence, and electron microscopy findings are all consistent with IgA nephropathy.

1. What are the clinical entities that have been associated with prominent mesangial IgA deposits?
2. What clinical findings indicate a poor prognosis in IgA nephropathy?
3. What is the clinical course of IgA nephropathy?
4. What would you advise this patient if she were to contemplate pregnancy?
5. What treatment options are available for this patient?

Case Discussion

1. *What are the clinical entities that have been associated with prominent mesangial IgA deposits?*

   Henoch-Schönlein purpura, chronic liver disease, dermatitis herpetiformis, and Berger's disease have all been found in the setting of mesangial IgA deposits.

2. *What clinical findings indicate a poor prognosis in IgA nephropathy?*

   The clinical findings that portend a poor prognosis in IgA nephropathy are a persistent proteinuria of greater than 1 g per day, elevated blood pressure, male sex, an elevated serum creatinine level, and the absence of macroscopic hematuria.

3. *What is the clinical course of IgA nephropathy?*

   Patients with IgA nephropathy may experience intermittent episodes of gross hematuria, and 5% to 10% of the patients may have early nephrotic syndrome. End-stage renal disease develops in approximately 10% of affected patients by 10 years, and by 20 years in 20% of affected patients. In addition, another 20% to 30% may experience some decline in renal function within 20 years.

4. *What would you advise this patient if she were to contemplate pregnancy?*

   Despite early reports to the contrary, no evidence has been revealed by rather large retrospective surveys indicating that pregnancy unfavorably alters the course of IgA nephropathy. In addition, the chances for a successful pregnancy are excellent if the patient remains free of hypertension or renal insufficiency.

5. *What treatment options are available for this patient?*

   There is no proven treatment for IgA nephropathy. The results of two trials of steroids conducted in East Asia (where the disease is very prevalent) have suggested that they are somewhat effective in patients with persistent proteinuria. However, controlled, prospective trials are needed to ascertain their actual efficacy.

Suggested Readings

D'Amico G. Immunoglobulin A nephropathy. In: Jacobson HR, Striker GE, Klahr S, eds. *The principles and practice of nephrology*, 2nd ed. St. Louis: Mosby, 1995, p. 133.

Glassock RJ. The glomerulopathies. In: Schrier RW, ed. *Renal and electrolyte disorders*, 5th ed. Philadelphia: Lippincott–Raven, 1997, p. 685.

Lieberthal W, Mesler DE. Hematuria and the acute nephritic syndrome. In: Jacobson HR, Striker GE, Klahr S, eds. *The principles and practice of nephrology*, 2nd ed. St. Louis: Mosby, 1995, p. 102.

Hyperkalemia

1. What are the causes of factitious hyperkalemia?
2. What are the primary mechanisms that underlie hyperkalemia, and what are the causes of each?
3. At what level of renal insufficiency does hyperkalemia occur?
4. What are the clinical consequences of hyperkalemia?
5. What therapeutic options are available for hyperkalemic patients, and how rapidly do they reverse the process?

Discussion

1. *What are the causes of factitious hyperkalemia?*

   The causes of factitious hyperkalemia (pseudohyperkalemia) comprise hemolysis of the blood sample, a marked leukocytosis (white blood cell count >50,000/mm^3), thrombocytosis (platelet count >800,000/mm^3), and an excessively tight tourniquet. Hematomas and rhabdomyolysis can precipitate true hyperkalemia by generating an increased release of potassium from cellular stores. Renal insufficiency is associated with a decreased potassium excretory ability.

2. *What are the primary mechanisms that underlie hyperkalemia, and what are the causes of each?*

   The primary mechanisms that bring about hyperkalemia are an increased potassium input from either endogenous or exogenous sources, a transcellular redistribution of potassium, and a decreased excretion of potassium. The respective causes of these potassium-related abnormalities are listed in Table 9-19.

3. *At what level of renal insufficiency does hyperkalemia occur?*

   In the absence of other factors, hyperkalemia supervenes in patients with renal disease when the GFR is less than 10 mL per minute. The adaptive response to decreased renal mass involves the increased excretion of potassium per nephron; this maintains normokalemia despite an unchanged potassium

Table 9-19. The Causes of Hyperkalemia

Causes of increased potassium input
  Exogenous potassium loads
    Rapid intravenous potassium administration
    High potassium intake with severe sodium restriction
  Endogenous potassium loads
    Rhabdomyolysis
    Hemolysis
    Tumor lysis syndrome
    Hematomas
    Increased catabolism
    Burns
Causes of transcellular shift
  Insulin deficiency
  Metabolic acidosis due to mineral acid retention
  Hypertonicity (glucose or mannitol)
  Exercise
  Hyperkalemic periodic paralysis
  Digitalis intoxication
  β-Adrenergic antagonists
Causes of impaired renal excretion
  Diffuse adrenal insufficiency (Addison's disease)
  Selective mineralocorticoid (aldosterone) deficiency
  Primary renal tubular secretory defect
    Obstructive uropathy
    Sickle cell disease
    Systemic lupus erythematosus
    Renal transplant
    Tubulointerstitial nephropathy
  Drug induced
    Spironolactone
    Triamterene
    Amiloride
    Cyclosporine
    Angiotensin-converting enzyme inhibitors
    Pentamidine
    Nonsteroidal antiinflammatory drugs

intake (usually 60 to 80 mEq per day). However, in the presence of the processes listed in the previous question, hyperkalemia arises when the GFR is higher (as high as 40 mL per minute).

4. *What are the clinical consequences of hyperkalemia?*

The most immediate and important impact of hyperkalemia is on the cells possessing excitable membranes (nerve and muscle) because it depolarizes such cells. The most important effect of hyperkalemia is on the heart. The typical sequence of electrocardiographic changes seen with increasing degrees of hyperkalemia include tall, peaked T waves; P-wave abnormalities (including loss of the P wave); prolongation of the QRS complex, sinus arrest, atrioventricular dissociation, ventricular fibrillation, and cardiac arrest.

5. *What therapeutic options are available for hyperkalemic patients, and how rapidly do they reverse the process?*

Table 9-20. Therapeutic Approach to Severe Hyperkalemia

Medication	Dosage	Peak effect
Calcium gluconate[a]	10–30 mL of 10% solution	<5 min
Insulin and glucose[a]	Insulin (5 U IV bolus) followed by 0.5 mU/kg of body weight per minute in 50 mL of 20% glucose	30–60 min
Sodium bicarbonate	100 mL of 1.4% solution	Variable
Kayexalate	Enema (50–100 g)	2–4 h
	Oral (30 g)	12–24 h
Hemodialysis[b]		30–60 min

[a]Recommended initial therapy

[b]Hemodialysis is not listed as immediate therapy because it is not usually available within the first hour or so of arrival to the hospital. If available, it could replace insulin therapy.

From Rombola G, Batlle DC. Hyperkalemia. In: Jacobson HR, Striker GE, Klahr S, eds. *The principles and practice of nephrology.* Philadelphia: Decker, 1991. Reprinted with permission.

The various therapeutic options for hyperkalemia are listed in Table 9-20. As shown, calcium gluconate has the most rapid onset and should therefore be the first-line treatment to protect against the neuromuscular effects of hyperkalemia. Note also that the use of calcium gluconate, insulin with glucose, or sodium bicarbonate does not decrease total body potassium content; unless a decrease in total body potassium is achieved (e.g., with kaliuresis, kayexelate, or dialysis), hyperkalemia will recur when the therapeutic effect of these agents dissipates.

Case   A 30-year-old white man has both diabetes mellitus and hypertension. The diabetes was diagnosed at 8 years of age when ketoacidosis developed. He has since had proliferative retinopathy, nephropathy, and peripheral and autonomic neuropathy. The nephropathy was recognized when the nephrotic syndrome developed 3 years ago, and there has also been a gradual increase in his serum creatinine level over the past 18 months. Hypertension was first detected a year ago. Although his serum glucose levels have in general been well controlled with the twice-daily administration of insulin, blood pressure control has been suboptimal despite treatment with captopril and hydrochlorothiazide.

The following physical examination findings are noted: supine heart rate of 76 beats per minute and blood pressure of 160/110 mm Hg; standing heart rate of 80 beats per minute and blood pressure of 130/90 mm Hg. Funduscopy reveals the presence of hemorrhages, exudates, and neovascularization. His lung fields are clear, no cardiac murmur is present, and there is trace lower extremity edema, decreased sensation to pinprick and vibration in the distal lower extremities, and absent deep tendon reflexes in the lower extremities.

The following laboratory values are reported: sodium, 138 mEq/L; potassium, 7.2 mEq/L; chloride, 110 mEq/L; carbon dioxide, 20 mEq/L; glucose, 129 mg/dL; creatinine, 2.4 mg/dL; BUN, 30 mEq/L; hemoglobin A_{1c}, 8.8%. Electrocardiography demonstrates regular sinus rhythm at 76 beats per minute with a normal axis. The P waves are flattened, the QRS complex is 0.12 seconds in duration, and there are peaked T waves in the precordial leads. Urinalysis reveals a specific gravity of 1.015, pH of 5.0, 3+ protein, and hyaline casts. A 24-hour urine sample shows a creatinine clearance of 35 mL per minute and 4.6 g of protein.

1. What do the electrocardiographic findings signify? How should the patient be treated?
2. What are the most likely factors contributing to this patient's hyperkalemia?
3. What are the drugs that can cause hypoaldosteronism?
4. What is appropriate subsequent therapy for this patient?

Case Discussion

1. *What do the electrocardiographic findings signify? How should the patient be treated?*

   The electrocardiographic findings are characteristic of hyperkalemia. The patient should be treated immediately with calcium gluconate followed by measures to lower the serum potassium, as outlined in Table 9-20.

2. *What are the most likely factors contributing to this patient's hyperkalemia?*

   The major contributory factors responsible for the hyperkalemia in this patient include a decrement in the GFR, the use of captopril, and hyporeninemic hypoaldosteronism. Dietary potassium excess may be operant as well.

   The patient also has a metabolic acidosis that is probably contributing to the hyperkalemia. The development of hyperkalemia when the renal insufficiency is only moderate makes it likely that other factors are involved in the process. The syndrome of hyporeninemic hypoaldosteronism is common in patients with diabetes, and the presence of hyperchloremic acidosis further supports this possibility.

3. *What are the drugs that can cause hypoaldosteronism?*

   Angiotensin-converting enzyme inhibitors, heparin, NSAIDs, and spironolactone can all precipitate hypoaldosteronism. β-Adrenergic blockers may contribute to hypoaldosteronism by impairing renin secretion. Spironolactone is a competitive inhibitor of aldosterone's cytosolic receptor, whereas miloride inhibits potassium secretion through the operation of an aldosterone-independent mechanism. Calcium channel blockers have not been reported to inhibit aldosterone synthesis, but spironolactone is known to inhibit aldosterone action. Trimethoprim has been reported to have an amiloride-like effect in patients with the acquired immunodeficiency syndrome.

4. *What is appropriate subsequent therapy for this patient?*

   This patient should restrict his dietary potassium intake and take loop diuretics to manage the hyporeninemic hypoaldosteronism.

   The dose of his ACE inhibitor needs to be decreased. Mineralocorticoid replacement can worsen the hypertension and sodium retention, and should therefore be avoided. Sodium restriction should also be avoided because it attenuates the kaliuretic effect of the diuretic; sodium delivery is important to potassium excretion.

Suggested Readings

Rosa M, Peterson LN, Levi M. Disorders of potassium metabolism. In: Schrier RW, ed. *Renal and electrolyte disorders*, 5th ed. Philadelphia: Lippincott–Raven, 1997, p. 192.

Rosa M, Batlle DC. Hyperkalemia. In: Jacobson HR, Striker GE, Klahr S, eds. *The principles and practice of nephrology*, 2nd ed. St. Louis: Mosby, 1995, p. 911.

Tannen RL. Potassium disorders. In Kokko JP, Tannen RL. *Fluids and Electrolytes.* Philadelphia: Saunders, 1986, p. 150.

Hyponatremia

1. What does the serum sodium concentration reflect, and what factors can alter the way in which it is interpreted? In what setting is pseudohyponatremia observed?
2. What is the underlying pathogenesis of hyponatremia?
3. What is the diagnostic approach to hyponatremia, and what are its major causes?
4. What are some of the drugs that produce hyponatremia?
5. What are the most common disorders associated with the syndrome of inappropriate antidiuretic hormone secretion (SIADH)?

Discussion

1. *What does the serum sodium concentration reflect, and what factors can alter the way in which it is interpreted? In what setting is pseudohyponatremia observed?*

Hyponatremia represents a decrease in the concentration of sodium relative to that of water in the serum. Total body sodium content may be decreased, unchanged, or even increased. The serum sodium concentration is a measure of the tonicity of body fluids, and it is the major contributor to the serum osmolality, as shown by the equation: $P_{osm} = 2 \times P_{Na} + (glucose/18) + (urea/3)$, where P_{osm} is the serum osmolality and P_{Na} is the serum sodium concentration.

Hyperglycemia can cause a decrement in the serum sodium level by shifting intracellular water out of cells. Because glucose is not freely movable across cell membranes, when the extracellular glucose concentration is elevated in insulin-deficient or -resistant patients, water moves out of cells to equalize osmolality on both sides of the membrane. The movement of water dilutes the serum sodium concentration, but the serum osmolality is maintained. Clinically, hyperglycemia-induced hyponatremia is frequently encountered in the settings of diabetic ketoacidosis and nonketotic hyperosmolar coma. To determine whether a patient has a sodium or water deficit, the serum sodium level should be estimated as if the patient were normoglycemic. The correction factor is as follows: for each 100 mg/dL increase in the serum glucose level, the serum sodium concentration decreases by 1.6 mEq/L. For example, if the sodium concentration is 109 mEq/L and the serum glucose content is 1,600 mg/dL, the corrected sodium concentration (Na_c) would be calculated as follows:

Increase of glucose = 1600 mg/dL − 100 mg/dL = 1,500 mg/dL

Decrease of sodium secondary to hyperglycemia = 1.6 × 1,500/100 = 24 mEq/L

Na_c = 109 + 24 = 133 mEq/L

Therefore, the serum sodium concentration always needs to be interpreted in light of the glucose concentration. Events identical to these occur with exogenous mannitol administration.

In pseudohyponatremia, the serum sodium concentration is low but the serum osmolality is normal. It occurs in settings of severe hyperlipidemia and hyperproteinemia, and is rare. The mechanism responsible for the low serum sodium concentration caused by hyperlipidemia and hyperproteinemia differs from that of hyperglycemia. At extremely elevated concentrations, both lipid and protein cause the sodium distribution space (i.e., plasma water space) to be decreased. Although the sodium concentration in plasma water is normal, it is decreased in the total plasma because of excess lipid or protein.

2. *What is the underlying pathogenesis of hyponatremia?*

Hyponatremia arises when urinary dilution is abnormal. The ability to excrete a lost volume of free water depends on three factors: (a) normal fluid delivery to the distal nephron (i.e., normal GFR and normal proximal tubule resorption); (b) normal functioning of the thick ascending limb of Henle and the cortical diluting segments, which are sites of urinary dilution; and (c) the absence of vasopressin in the circulation, thus allowing the collecting duct to remain water impermeable. In the presence of vasopressin, the tubular fluid equilibrates osmotically with the isotonic or hypertonic urine, thus preventing the excretion of dilute urine.

3. *What is the diagnostic approach to hyponatremia, and what are its major causes?*

Once hyponatremia is confirmed, the next step is to determine whether it is associated with a low, normal, or high total body sodium concentration. Usually a physical examination can distinguish among these possibilities. Orthostatic hypotension and flat neck veins are seen in patients with a low total-body sodium content. Edema and ascites are common findings in patients with a high total-body sodium content. Patients with normal total-body sodium exhibit neither orthostatic changes nor edema. The major causes of each category of sodium concentration are summarized in Table 9-21.

4. *What are some of the drugs that produce hyponatremia?*

Drugs can impair water excretion either by enhancing the renal action of vasopressin or by causing release of the hormone. Some of the more common agents are listed in Table 9-22.

5. *What are the most common disorders associated with SIADH?*

In hospitalized patients, SIADH is the most common cause of hyponatremia. This is broadly due to a malignancy, pulmonary disorder, or central nervous system disorder, as shown in Table 9-23.

Table 9-21. Causes of Hyponatremia

Hypovolemia (decreased total body sodium)	Euvolemia (near-normal total body sodium)	Hypervolemia (increased total body sodium)
Extrarenal sodium losses	Diuretics	Extrarenal disorders
Vomiting (steady state)	Hypothyroidism	Congestive heart failure
Diarrhea	Glucocorticoid deficiency	Hepatic cirrhosis
Fluid sequestration in "third space"	Drugs	Renal disorders
	Pain or emotional stress	Nephrotic syndrome
Peritonitis	Respiratory failure	Acute renal failure
Pancreatitis	Positive-pressure breathing	Chronic renal failure
Rhabdomyolysis	Syndrome of inappropriate antidiuretic hormone secretion	
Burns		
Renal sodium losses		
Diuretics		
Osmotic diuresis (glucose, urea, mannitol)		
Mineralocorticoid deficiency		
Salt-losing nephritis		

From Veis JH, Berl T. Hyponatremia. In: Jacobson HR, Striker GE, Klahr S, eds. *The principles and practice of nephrology.* Philadelphia: Decker, 1995. Reprinted with permission.

Case   A 68-year-old man is hospitalized because of a persistent cough and 25-pound (9-kg) weight loss during the past 3 months. He has a 40-pack-year smoking history. On physical examination, he is found to be slightly confused and slow to respond. There are no orthostatic changes in his blood pressure or pulse. Chest examination reveals findings compatible with a left pleural effusion. Abdominal examination reveals no masses or organomegaly. There is no edema. He weighs 60 kg.

Table 9-22. Drugs Associated with Hyponatremia

Antidiuretic hormone analogues
   Deamino-D-arginine vasopressin
   Oxytocin
Drugs that enhance antidiuretic hormone release
   Chlorpropamide
   Clofibrate
   Carbamazepine
   Vincristine
   Nicotine
   Narcotics
   Antipsychotics or antidepressants[a]
Drugs that potentiate renal action of antidiuretic hormone
   Chlorpropamide
   Cyclophosphamide
   Nonsteroidal antiinflammatory drugs

[a]Antidiuretic hormone release may be secondary to underlying psychosis.
From Veis JH, Berl T. Hyponatremia. In: Jacobson HR, Striker GE, Klahr S, eds. *The principles and practice of nephrology.* Philadelphia: Decker, 1995. Reprinted with permission.

Table 9-23. The Most Common Disorders Associated with the Syndrome of Inappropriate Secretion of Antidiuretic Hormone

Malignancy
  Lung
  Duodenum
  Pancreas
  Lymphoma
Pulmonary disorders
  Pneumonia
  Abscess
  Aspergillosis
  Respiratory failure
  Positive-pressure breathing
Central nervous system disorders
  Neoplasm
  Encephalitis
  Meningitis
  Brain abscess
  Head trauma
  Guillain-Barré syndrome
  Subdural or subarachnoid hemorrhage
  Acute intermittent porphyria
  Acute psychosis
  Stroke

From Veis JH, Berl T. Hyponatremia. In: Jacobson HR, Striker GE, Klahr S, eds. *The principles and practice of nephrology.* Philadelphia: Decker, 1991. Reprinted with permission.

The following laboratory values are reported: sodium, 109 mEq/L; potassium, 3.4 mEq/L; chloride, 78 mEq/L; bicarbonate, 24 mEq/L; BUN, 4 mg/dL; glucose, 85 mg/dL; uric acid, 3.5 mg/dL; serum osmolality, 230 mOsm; and urine osmolality, 300 mOsm. A chest radiographic study shows a left pleural effusion. Purified protein derivative testing is positive.

The patient's serum sodium concentration increases to 133 mEq/L within 24 hours. At that time, the patient is noted to be alert and his behavior appropriate. However, by the next day, he has become uncommunicative and agitated.

1. What are the most likely causes of hyponatremia in this patient, and why?
2. How do the serum potassium, BUN, and uric acid levels help in the assessment of this patient?
3. What are the primary considerations in treating patients with hyponatremia, and how should this patient's condition be managed?
4. What could account for this patient's neurologic deterioration after his initial improvement?

Case Discussion

1. *What are the most likely causes of hyponatremia in this patient and why?*

   This patient appears to have hyponatremia associated with a normal total-body sodium concentration because there are neither orthostatic changes nor edema. He therefore has euvolemic hyponatremia. Adrenal insufficiency appears unlikely clinically, making SIADH the most likely cause of the hypo-natremia. The two leading diagnoses are lung cancer or pulmonary tuberculo-sis. In SIADH, a patient is slightly volume expanded. Thus, as in this patient, the BUN and uric acid levels tend to be low. From the clinical point of view, SIADH is the most likely diagnosis in this patient, but hypothyroidism should also be considered.

2. *How do the serum potassium, BUN, and uric acid levels help in the assessment of this patient?*

The serum potassium concentration of 3.4 mEq/L and the BUN value of 5 mg/dL virtually rule out adrenal insufficiency because this is characterized by a hyperkalemic acidosis and an elevation in the BUN and serum creatinine levels as a consequence of volume contraction. Although the low serum potas-sium concentration brings into question the use of diuretics, the low uric acid level makes this unlikely. A low uric acid level is commonly observed in the setting of SIADH.

3. *What are the primary considerations in treating patients with hyponatremia, and how should this patient's condition be managed?*

The optimal treatment for severe hyponatremia is still controversial because although profound hyponatremia is associated with high mortality and morbid-ity, its rapid correction may cause the formation of neurologic lesions, which are usually irreversible. The primary considerations in the therapy are the acuteness or chronicity of the process and the presence or absence of neuro-logic symptoms attributable to hyponatremia. The following are general treat-ment guidelines.

In the setting of **acute symptomatic hyponatremia** with a change in mental status or seizures, the risk for complications stemming from cerebral edema exceeds the risk of complications from rapid treatment. The patient should receive furosemide and hypertonic saline until convulsions subside.

Asymptomatic hyponatremia is almost always chronic, and rapid correction is likely to do more harm than good. The treatment in these patients should consist of water restriction regardless of their serum sodium status.

In the setting of **symptomatic hyponatremia** of chronic or unknown duration, the serum sodium level should be raised promptly by approximately 10 mEq/L through the administration of saline, then water restriction. A correc-tion rate of 2 mEq/L per hour at any given time or an increase in the serum sodium level by more than 15 mEq per day should not be exceeded.

In the present case, because the patient is symptomatic, it is prudent to correct the serum sodium level to approximately 120 mEq/L in 8 to 12 hours. The solute-free water loss needed to accomplish this may be estimated by multiplying total-body water $\times$ (1 $-$ actual serum sodium/desired serum so-dium). Thus, to correct the serum sodium in this 60-kg man from 109 to 120 mEq/L, he must have a negative water balance of $60 \times 0.6 \times (1 - 109/120) =$ 3.3 L. This may be accomplished by infusing normal saline at a rate of 250 mL per hour while replacing urinary sodium losses with 3% saline so as to achieve a net solute-free water loss. A single injection of furosemide (20 mg

IV) may be administered to promote diuresis; urinary potassium losses should be repleted. The serum sodium concentration may be raised by 1.0 to 1.5 mEq/L per hour. Once the serum sodium level has increased by approximately 10 mEq/L, this regimen should be discontinued.

As for the long-term management of this patient, water restriction to 1,000 mL per day is the treatment of choice. However, because compliance may be difficult to achieve, demeclocycline can be given. This drug interferes with the antidiuretic hormone effect on the kidney and results in a more dilute urine. If the patient's primary disease, lung cancer, or tuberculosis responds to treatment, this would likely promote resolution of the SIADH.

4. *What could account for this patient's neurologic deterioration after his initial improvement?*

This patient's serum sodium level increased by 24 mEq/L in the first 24 hours. This therefore puts him at risk for development of central pontine myelinolysis (CPM), which is characterized by a flaccid quadriparesis, impaired speech and swallowing, facial weakness, and poor response to painful stimuli. Pathologically, loss of myelin around nerve sheaths can be seen in pontine as well as extrapontine areas. The pathogenesis of this lesion remains unknown. There are several risk factors for development of CPM, including alcoholism, malnutrition, and burns, and it is also seen in women taking thiazide diuretics. The results of human and animal studies suggest that rapid correction of severe chronic hyponatremia is associated with CPM, whereas the hyponatremia itself is unrelated.

The findings from studies on idiogenic osmoles may have implications for the pathogenesis of CPM. Idiogenic osmoles in the brain are intracellular organic compounds such as amino acids, myoinositol, and methylamines. The intracellular levels of osmoles decrease slowly during the adaptation to changes in extracellular osmolality so that the cell volume is maintained. Therefore, in the setting of chronic hyponatremia, the rapid increase in extracellular osmolality may shrink brain cells, which have diminished osmotically active osmoles as a consequence of adaptation to the chronic hyponatremia.

Suggested Readings

Berl T, Schrier RW. Disorders of water metabolism. In: Schrier RW, ed. *Renal and electrolyte disorders*, 5th ed. Philadelphia: Lippincott–Raven, 1997, p. 1.

Veis JH, Berl T. Hyponatremia. In: Jacobson HR, Striker GE, Klahr S, eds. *The principles and practice of nephrology*, 2nd ed. St. Louis: Mosby, 1995, p. 888.

10 Rheumatology

Robert W. Janson

Ankylosing Spondylitis

1. What are three possible causes of low back pain in young men?
2. What are four characteristics of muscular low back pain?
3. What are four characteristics of inflammatory low back pain?
4. What four diseases are classified as seronegative spondyloarthropathies?
5. What is the definition of sciatica, and what are three possible causes of it?

Discussion

1. *What are three possible causes of low back pain in young men?*

   Three possible causes of back pain in young men include lumbosacral muscle spasm, a ruptured intervertebral disc, and ankylosing spondylitis or another seronegative spondyloarthropathy. All three conditions may be manifested by low back pain, and they commonly affect young men. Forms of common autoimmune and chronic inflammatory diseases, such as rheumatoid arthritis or systemic lupus erythematosus (SLE), rarely involve the joints of the low back, and thus low back pain is not one of the initial symptoms of these disorders.

2. *What are four characteristics of muscular low back pain?*

Typically, muscular low back pain is sudden in onset, it favors no particular age group, it is worse with use or exercise, and there is local tenderness. Muscular low back pain is often worsened by a change in position and relieved by rest. It usually resolves spontaneously within a few days.

3. *What are four characteristics of inflammatory low back pain?*

Inflammatory low back pain is typically insidious in onset, associated with morning stiffness, it abates with exercise, and it persists for between 3 to many months. In addition, inflammatory low back pain usually starts in late adolescence or early adulthood, with onset after 40 years of age uncommon. Patients with inflammatory low back pain often initially notice a small amount of pain and stiffness in the back in the morning that eases during the day with use. These early symptoms may be intermittent for a few months until they become persistent. Inflammatory low back pain may be relieved to a significant degree by nonsteroidal antiinflammatory drugs (NSAIDs).

4. *What four diseases are classified as seronegative spondyloarthropathies?*

The spondyloarthropathies consist of ankylosing spondylitis, Reiter's syndrome, arthritis secondary to inflammatory bowel disease, and psoriatic arthritis.

5. *What is the definition of sciatica, and what are the three possible causes of it?*

Sciatica is defined as back pain that radiates down one leg below the knee. Sciatica usually occurs as a consequence of lumbar spondylosis (degenerative disc or facet joint disease) and can be associated with a ruptured intervertebral disc or idiopathic sciatic nerve irritation. Infectious, neoplastic, and infiltrative disorders should always be considered.

Case

A 34-year-old white man is seen because of neck pain. Medical history taking reveals that 12 years ago, at the age of 22 years, the patient first noted low back, buttock, and spine pain. He had been involved in a motor vehicle accident and attributed some of his back pain to that. At that time, he saw a number of physicians, who diagnosed mechanical back pain and recommended bed rest, which the patient observed for the next year. However, he found this only seemed to make his back and buttock pain worse. Typically, he was very stiff in the morning for over 2 hours, but in the afternoon he felt better with movement and exercise. He also noted increasing fatigue and some weight loss. Ten years ago, his right hip started hurting. Eight years ago, pain suddenly developed in his right eye and he saw an ophthalmologist, who diagnosed acute iritis and placed him on steroid eye drops. Two years ago, his knees started to swell intermittently. His lumbar and thoracic spine regions became fused, and, to stand up and look straight ahead, he had to bend his knees. He finally had to quit his job as a truck driver because it required prolonged sitting, which made his back pain and stiffness worse. One year later, he was on disability.

Musculoskeletal examination reveals no obvious swelling in any joint, and no movement in the lumbar or thoracic spine is noted while the patient is bending over. His right hip is found to be painful on flexion with internal rotation.

Radiographic studies of the lumbosacral spine are obtained and interpreted to show almost complete obliteration of both sacroiliac joint spaces. The posterior elements in the distal lumbar area are also found to be obliterated, together with bridging or "bambooing" of the spine. A chest radiographic study shows squaring off of the mid-portion of the thoracic vertebrae but no significant syndesmophyte formation.

1. Where is the primary site of disease in ankylosing spondylitis?
2. What five organs can be involved in ankylosing spondylitis, and what are the clinical manifestations?
3. What are three characteristic clinical findings in patients with ankylosing spondylitis that help to distinguish it from rheumatoid arthritis?
4. What is the characteristic family history, gender incidence, and human lymphocyte antigen (HLA) pattern found in the context of ankylosing spondylitis?
5. What are three types of treatment that might be helpful in ankylosing spondylitis?

Case Discussion

1. *Where is the primary site of disease in ankylosing spondylitis?*

   In ankylosing spondylitis, inflammation occurs at the attachment of ligaments to bones, a structure known as the *enthesis*. The cause of this localized inflammation remains unknown. Inflammation may also be seen in the synovium, the tissue lining the joints.

2. *What five organs can be involved in ankylosing spondylitis, and what are the clinical manifestations?*

   Peripheral joint involvement (particularly hips and shoulders) can occur in approximately 30% of patients. Neurologic involvement includes atlantoaxial subluxations and cauda equina syndrome. Pulmonary involvement includes upper lobe fibrosis and restrictive changes. Cardiac involvement includes aortic insufficiency, aortitis, conduction abnormalities, and pericarditis. Ocular involvement presents as anterior uveitis (25% to 30% of patients).

3. *What are three characteristic clinical findings in patients with ankylosing spondylitis that help to distinguish it from rheumatoid arthritis?*

   The three clinical manifestations characteristic of ankylosing spondylitis consist of inflammatory arthritis of the spine, Achilles tendinitis, and plantar fasciitis. These three findings are extremely rare in patients with rheumatoid arthritis.

4. *What is the characteristic family history, gender incidence, and HLA pattern found in the context of ankylosing spondylitis?*

   Typically there is a family history of ankylosing spondylitis, particularly in male family members. In fact, it occurs more commonly in men than women (3:1). This disease is very highly associated with the presence of HLA-B27.

5. *What are three types of treatment that might be helpful in ankylosing spondylitis?*

The treatment of ankylosing spondylitis includes NSAIDs, extension exercises for the back, and heat and physical therapy. It is recommended that all three forms of therapy be used in affected patients. It is thought that extension exercises for the back may help patients maintain a more normal upright posture as the back fuses over time. Sulfasalazine or low-dose weekly methotrexate therapy may be beneficial in patients with progressive disease with peripheral arthritis. Oral corticosteroids are of no value. Local corticosteroid injections may be useful in the treatment of enthesopathies and recalcitrant peripheral synovitis.

Suggested Readings

Inman RD. Seronegative spondyloarthropathies: treatment. In: Klippel JH, ed. *Primer on the rheumatic diseases*, 11th ed. Atlanta: Arthritis Foundation, 1997, p. 193.

Kahn MA. Seronegative spondyloarthropathies: ankylosing spondylitis. In: Klippel JH, ed. *Primer on the rheumatic diseases*, 11th ed. Atlanta: Arthritis Foundation, 1997, p. 189.

Van der Linden S. Ankylosing spondylitis. In: Kelley WN, Harris ED Jr, Ruddy S, Sledge CB, eds. *Textbook of rheumatology*, 5th ed. Philadelphia: WB Saunders, 1997, p. 969,

Crystal-Induced Arthritis

1. What are three different forms of crystal-induced arthritis, and what are the crystals involved?
2. What are three different diseases that characteristically present with arthritis of a single joint?
3. What three joints are most commonly involved in acute attacks of gout?
4. What are some historical features often found in patients with gout?
5. What are three laboratory test findings that may be abnormal in the setting of gout?

Discussion

1. *What are three different forms of crystal-induced arthritis, and what are the crystals involved?*

Gout is a crystal-induced arthritis due to the deposition of monosodium urate crystals. Pseudogout results from the formation and release of calcium pyrophosphate dihydrate crystals. The deposition of hydroxyapatite crystals can induce acute inflammatory arthritides such as calcific tendinitis and the Milwaukee shoulder syndrome.

2. *What are three different diseases that characteristically present with arthritis of a single joint?*

Arthritis of a single joint (monoarticular arthritis) may be the initial symptom of gout, pseudogout, and septic arthritis. Other historical and clinical features may be used to distinguish among these three diagnoses. A definitive diagnosis is made on the basis of the findings yielded by synovial fluid examination, including culture, cell count with differential, and polarized light microscopy for crystal analysis.

3. *What three joints are most commonly involved in acute attacks of gout?*

    Acute gout most commonly arises in the first metatarsophalangeal (MTP) joint; this is known as *podagra*. The next most commonly involved sites are the instep and ankle. Gout has a predilection for cool, peripheral joints.

4. *What are some historical features often found in patients with gout?*

    Patients with gout may have a positive family history for the disease, particularly in male members. Gout is also more common in people who have a history of obesity or alcoholism. Acute attacks of gout may occur during or after an episode of excessive alcohol ingestion, and the attacks commonly begin abruptly during the night or early morning hours.

5. *What laboratory test findings may be abnormal in the setting of gout?*

    Patients with acute attacks of gout often have a mild leukocytosis and an elevated erythrocyte sedimentation rate (ESR). In addition, these patients are hyperuricemic, defined as a serum uric acid level greater than 7.0 mg/dL in men and 6.0 mg/dL in women.

Case   A 52-year-old white man comes to the emergency room complaining of pain in his big toe. He was well until 5:00 this morning, when he was awakened by an aching pain in his right great toe. Within a few hours, the joint was dusky red and hot, and was exquisitely tender to the point that even the weight of the bedding hurt his toe. By 8:00 a.m., the patient could bear only partial weight on the foot. The patient reports a few self-limited, trivial episodes of twinges of pain in this toe over the past year. The patient describes feeling feverish without rigors or chills. There is no history of trauma to the foot, nor is there a family history of arthritis or similar attacks. He is taking hydrochlorothiazide for control of hypertension.

On physical examination, the patient is found to be a stocky, overweight, and red-faced man. His blood pressure is 170/100 mm Hg, his pulse is 90 beats per minute and regular, and his temperature is 38°C. Skin examination discloses no lesions or nodules. On examination of his joints, all show a normal range of motion without synovitis or deformity, except for the right first MTP joint, which shows synovitis, 2+/4; warmth, 4+/4; tenderness, 4+/4; and erythema at the base of the toe and extending onto the dorsal aspect of the forefoot with slight edema.

The following laboratory values are reported: white blood cell count, 12,500 cells/mm^3 with 92% polymorphonuclear leukocytes and 2% band forms; uric acid, 9.0 mg/dL; creatinine, 1.0 mg/dL. Urinalysis reveals no red blood cells or protein. A radiographic study of the right foot discloses soft tissue swelling around the right first MTP joint, but no erosions.

1. What are four different diagnostic procedures that should be performed in every patient with a suspected first attack of acute gout?

2. What are four different factors that may contribute to chronic secondary hyperuricemia?

3. What are the four clinical stages of gout?
4. What three predisposing conditions may each foster acute attacks of gout?
5. What are the appropriate therapies for an acute attack of gout and chronic symptomatic hyperuricemia?

Case Discussion

1. *What are four different diagnostic procedures that should be performed in every patient with a suspected first attack of acute gout?*

   In the setting of a suspected first attack of gout, a complete blood count with differential, a serum uric acid measurement, and serum creatinine determination with urinalysis to exclude underlying renal disease should be performed. Acute gout is diagnosed by joint fluid aspiration, with tests of the sample to include a complete cell count with differential, Gram's staining, cultures, and polarized microscopic examination for crystals.

2. *What are four different factors that may contribute to chronic secondary hyperuricemia?*

   Factors that may predispose to chronic secondary hyperuricemia include the use of several medications, including diuretics and cyclosporine, obesity, lead intoxication, polycystic kidney disease, and myeloproliferative diseases. Each of these factors may cause the blood uric acid level to be elevated through different mechanisms. Consequently, gout may be seen more commonly in people affected by these predisposing factors. The hyperuricemia frequently seen in chronic renal failure is not typically linked to an increased incidence of gout.

3. *What are the four clinical stages of gout?*

   The four stages of gout are asymptomatic hyperuricemia, acute gouty arthritis, intercritical gout (the asymptomatic interval between attacks), and chronic tophaceous gout. Many patients with asymptomatic hyperuricemia do not acquire gouty arthritis. There may not be sharp demarcations between the last three stages of gout because some patients have both chronic tophaceous gout as well as intermittent acute attacks.

4. *What three predisposing conditions may each foster acute attacks of gout?*

   People with particular inborn errors of purine metabolism may be more susceptible to gout. These metabolic abnormalities should be suspected in young men (<30 years of age) presenting with gout who may have a family history of the disorder. The chemotherapy for acute leukemia or lymphoma may also lead to a large uric acid load unless the patient is pretreated with allopurinol, which blocks uric acid formation. Finally, patients with extensive postoperative tissue breakdown with dehydration may also experience transient elevations in their uric acid levels with attendant acute attacks of gout.

5. *What are the appropriate therapies for an acute attack of gout and chronic symptomatic hyperuricemia?*

   The preferred treatment for an acute attack of gout is an oral NSAID. This should be given in high doses for a few days, followed by a taper with discontinuation by 7 to 10 days. Oral colchicine can be used in nonelderly patients with normal renal and hepatic function. Its use is limited by the high incidence of acute gastrointestinal side effects. Both orally and intraarticularly administered corticosteroids are effective in the management of acute attacks of gout in patients who are intolerant of or have contraindications to the aforementioned medications. Patients with chronic symptomatic hyperuricemia require lifelong therapy with probenecid if they are a renal underexcretor of uric acid, or allopurinol if they are overexcretors (overproducers), have uric acid or calcium stones, or tophi.

Suggested Readings

Edwards NL. Gout: clinical and laboratory features. In: Klippel JH, ed. *Primer on the rheumatic diseases*, 11th ed. Atlanta: Arthritis Foundation, 1997, p. 234.

Kelley WN, Wortmann RL. Gout and hyperuricemia. In: Kelley WN, Harris ED Jr, Ruddy S, Sledge CB, eds. *Textbook of rheumatology*, 5th ed. Philadelphia: WB Saunders, 1997, p. 1313.

Pratt PW, Ball GV. Gout: treatment. In: Klippel JH, ed. *Primer on the rheumatic diseases*, 11th ed. Atlanta: Arthritis Foundation, 1997, p. 240.

Fibromyalgia

1. What is the definition of nonarticular rheumatism, and what are four forms of the disorder?
2. What are four clinical types of tendinitis and bursitis, and what is the major structure involved in each type?
3. What are the four main clinical characteristics of fibromyalgia?
4. What are five medical illnesses that may exhibit symptoms similar to those of fibromyalgia?
5. On what basis can fibromyalgia be distinguished from diseases exhibiting similar symptoms?

Discussion

1. *What is the definition of nonarticular rheumatism, and what are four forms of the disorder?*

   Nonarticular rheumatism refers to aches and pains that arise from structures outside of joints, so it is not actually a true form of arthritis. Four forms of nonarticular rheumatism comprise tendinitis, bursitis, fibromyalgia, and the myofascial pain syndrome. Tendinitis involves inflammation and pain in specific tendons, and is usually due to stress or overuse. Bursae are synovium-lined sacs that either overlie or are adjacent to joints and may also become inflamed secondary to overuse. Fibromyalgia is a specific disorder that is discussed in a later question. The myofascial pain syndrome consists of localized tender and painful muscles in the absence of any evidence of an inflammatory muscle disease or fibromyalgia.

2. *What are four clinical types of tendinitis and bursitis, and what is the major structure involved in each type?*

"Tennis elbow" is pain over the lateral epicondyle due to inflammation of the tendons of the wrist extensor muscles that insert at this location. "Golfer's elbow" is pain over the medial epicondyle, again due to inflammation of the tendons that insert at this location. The "shoulder impingement syndrome" results from impingement of the tendons of the rotator cuff with shoulder abduction or flexion and can be associated with supraspinatus tendinitis, subacromial bursitis, or rotator cuff tears. "Housemaid's knee" is prepatellar bursitis brought about by repetitive trauma or overuse such as kneeling.

3. *What are the four main clinical characteristics of fibromyalgia?*

Characteristics of fibromyalgia include diffuse musculoskeletal pain, morning stiffness, nonrestorative sleep, and severe fatigue. These four characteristics are fairly nondescript, often making the diagnosis of fibromyalgia one of exclusion.

4. *What are five medical illnesses that may exhibit symptoms similar to those of fibromyalgia?*

Illnesses that may exhibit symptoms similar to those of fibromyalgia include hypothyroidism, hyperparathyroidism, early rheumatoid arthritis, polymyositis, and polymyalgia rheumatica. However, each of these illnesses is associated with characteristic historical, clinical, and laboratory abnormalities that distinguishes it from fibromyalgia. In addition, it is often difficult to differentiate the symptoms of fibromyalgia from chronic fatigue syndrome. Fibromyalgia has been associated with obstructive sleep apnea.

5. *On what basis can fibromyalgia be distinguished from diseases exhibiting similar symptoms?*

Fibromyalgia can be distinguished from other diseases exhibiting similar symptoms based on a characteristic onset of symptoms in the absence of historical features typical of other diseases. In addition, a physical examination in patients with fibromyalgia reveals completely normal findings except for characteristic tender points over specific muscle groups, as outlined in the following case and discussion.

Case   A 38-year-old white woman is referred for evaluation because of a positive lupus test result. She complains of 6 months of fatigue, difficulty sleeping, morning stiffness, and intermittent swelling of her fingers. She notes that "the swelling feels like it is there now." The stiffness is worse in the morning, but she can put no definite time limit on it. Symptoms are much worse premenstrually.

She was first seen by her family physician complaining of "pain all over." She has been treated with indomethacin without relief. She was subsequently treated by another physician, first with diclofenac and later with piroxicam, but again without relief.

She is a divorced mother of three children who works full time as a licensed practical nurse. She has no history of a rash, oral ulcers, seizures, blood disorder, or a known kidney disease.

Physical examination reveals normal vital signs, as well as normal head, ear, eyes, nose, throat, neck, skin, chest, and abdominal findings. Her fingers and joints are normal, and her muscle strength is normal. Sensation is normal. Several tender or trigger points are identified.

1. What are two characteristics of the sleep disorder that commonly accompanies fibromyalgia?
2. What are the characteristic physical findings in fibromyalgia?
3. Are there any laboratory test abnormalities characteristic of fibromyalgia?
4. What is the therapy for fibromyalgia?
5. Which psychological disorders are often associated with fibromyalgia?

Case Discussion

1. *What are two characteristics of the sleep disorder that commonly accompanies fibromyalgia?*

The sleep disorder seen in the context of fibromyalgia is characterized by early morning awakening and not feeling rested (nonrestorative sleep). Disruption of delta-wave sleep (non-REM stage IV sleep) occurs due to alpha-wave intrusion, and is termed the *alpha-delta sleep pattern of fibromyalgia.*

2. *What are the characteristic physical findings in fibromyalgia?*

Patients with fibromyalgia have a normal physical examination except for tender points in precise locations. These tender points are typically located at the occiput, at the mid-portion of the trapezius, over the supraspinatus, low anterior cervical region, second costochondral junction, lateral epicondyle, outer upper quadrant of the buttocks, greater trochanter region, and medial knee area. These areas are usually tender bilaterally in patients with fibromyalgia. Control points such as the mid-forearm and anterior mid-thigh are not normally painful in patients with fibromyalgia.

3. *Are there any laboratory test abnormalities characteristic of fibromyalgia?*

All laboratory test results in the setting of fibromyalgia are usually completely normal. To exclude disorders that may mimic fibromyalgia, a complete blood count, ESR, creatinine, liver function tests, thyroid-stimulating hormone, creatine phosphokinase (CPK), and urinalysis should be performed.

4. *What is the therapy for fibromyalgia?*

The appropriate therapy for fibromyalgia includes NSAIDs, low-dose tricyclic antidepressants at bedtime to improve the sleep cycle, and nonimpact aerobic exercises. This is a very frustrating disease for both the patient and physician. Many patients may be helped by this multipronged approach to therapy, the most important element of which is an exercise program.

5. *Which psychological disorders are often associated with fibromyalgia?*

Functional psychiatric disorders such as the somatoform disorders and organic psychiatric disorders such as major depression have been associated with fibromyalgia. The anxiety and mild depression often present in fibromyalgia may be secondary to chronic pain and concerns regarding personal independence and debility.

Suggested Readings

Bennett RM. The fibromyalgia syndrome. In: Kelley WN, Harris ED Jr, Ruddy S, Sledge CB, eds. *Textbook of rheumatology*, 5th ed. Philadelphia: WB Saunders, 1997, p. 511.

Freundlich B, Leventhal L. Signs and symptoms of musculoskeletal disorders: diffuse pain syndromes. In: Klippel JH, ed. *Primer on the rheumatic diseases*, 11th ed. Atlanta: Arthritis Foundation, 1997, p. 123.

Nonsteroidal Antiinflammatory Drugs

1. What is considered one primary mechanism of action of aspirin [acetylsalicylic acid (ASA)] and other NSAIDs?
2. The NSAIDs are considered a primary form of therapy for what three general types of arthritis?
3. The beneficial effects of ASA and other NSAIDs include what three primary actions?

Discussion

1. *What is considered one primary mechanism of action of ASA and other NSAIDs?*

    One general effect of ASA and NSAIDs is to reduce the production of prostaglandins from the precursor arachidonic acid by inhibiting the enzyme cyclooxygenase (COX). Each NSAID to a varying degree inhibits both isoenzyme forms of COX: COX-1 is constitutively present in many tissues and is responsible for the production of regulatory prostanoids in the gastric mucosa, platelets, endothelium, and kidneys; COX-2 is produced by stimulated cells and catalyzes the synthesis of proinflammatory prostaglandins. NSAIDs reversibly block COX activity and ASA irreversibly inactivates this enzyme by acetylation. However, these medications have many other actions on inflammatory cells. Their clinical antiinflammatory effects may be due to a multiplicity of actions, rather than to one specific mechanism.

2. *The NSAIDs are considered a primary form of therapy for what three general types of arthritis?*

    The general indications for NSAIDs include forms of inflammatory arthritis, the spondyloarthropathies, and osteoarthritis. However, additional medications are usually prescribed for most patients with inflammatory arthritis, as well as those with some forms of spondyloarthropathy. In addition, patients with osteoarthritis may realize an equivalent benefit from analgesic medications such as acetaminophen.

3. *The beneficial effects of ASA and other NSAIDs include what three primary actions?*

    These medications confer pain relief through their analgesic effect and fever reduction through their antipyretic actions; they also have general antiin-flammatory effects.

Case

A 45-year-old Hispanic woman is admitted for a renal biopsy. She has had rheumatoid arthritis for 5 years and has been treated with various NSAIDs. During the first year, she took up to 3.6 g of ASA per day, but stopped taking it because of gastrointestinal symptoms and inefficacy. She was next prescribed indomethacin (25 mg orally three times daily), but this precipitated severe head-aches and an elevation in her liver function tests. The patient was switched to meclofenamate (50 mg orally three times daily) but had to stop taking this medication after 2 months because of diarrhea. She stopped taking all NSAIDs for 2 years because she was tired of the side effects, but because of continued joint pain and swelling, she has been taking fenoprofen (600 mg orally four times per day) for the past year. In the 2 months before admission, her creatinine level has increased to 3.5 mg/dL and urinalysis has revealed a white blood cell count of 30 cells per high-power field.

On physical examination, mild synovitis without deformity is noted in all proximal interphalangeal (PIP) and metacarpophalangeal (MCP) joints of both hands. Her wrists and ankles are also involved. She has 2+ pretibial pitting edema bilaterally. Her lungs are clear and cardiac findings are normal.

1. What medications used to treat rheumatoid arthritis may be responsible for causing an abnormal urinalysis?
2. What are five possible side effects of non-ASA NSAIDs?
3. What are four drug–drug interactions that may be seen with the use of ASA?
4. What is one agent in each category of NSAID (short, medium, or long duration of action), and what is its usual dosage schedule?
5. Which specific NSAIDs are thought to be most effective in the treatment of rheumatic fever or acute gout?

Case Discussion

1. *What medications used to treat rheumatoid arthritis may be responsible for causing an abnormal urinalysis?*

   Aspirin, other NSAIDs, gold injections or pills, and penicillamine are all medications used in the treatment of rheumatoid arthritis that can cause abnormal urinalysis findings.

2. *What are five possible side effects of non-ASA NSAIDs?*

   Some side effects of non-ASA NSAIDs include headaches, gastrointestinal bleeding resulting from erosive gastritis, decreased platelet function, an in-creased serum creatinine level, and interstitial nephritis. Hepatocellular toxic-ity can occur. These side effects are typically reversible if the medications are withdrawn soon enough. NSAID-associated upper gastrointestinal complica-tions can be decreased with the concomitant use of misoprostol, a synthetic gastroprotective prostaglandin analogue. New, highly selective COX-2 inhibi-tors may prove to be less ulcerogenic than current NSAIDs.

3. *What are four drug–drug interactions that may be seen with the use of ASA?*

Use of ASA may cause the prothrombin time to be prolonged in patients taking sodium warfarin. In addition, ASA may block the effects of uricosuric drugs such as probenecid, and has the potential of worsening gastrointestinal bleeding when taken with alcohol. ASA may also enhance bone marrow suppression in patients taking large doses of methotrexate.

4. *What is one agent in each category of NSAID (short, medium, or long duration of action), and what is its usual dosage schedule?*

Indomethacin is an NSAID with a short duration of action that is taken three times a day. Naproxen has a medium duration of action and is taken twice a day. Piroxicam has a long duration of action and is taken once a day.

5. *Which specific NSAIDs are thought to be most effective in the treatment of rheumatic fever or acute gout?*

Patients with rheumatic fever usually respond dramatically to ASA, and patients with acute gout are treated preferentially with indomethacin.

Suggested Readings

Clements PJ, Paulus HE. Nonsteroidal antirheumatic drugs. In: Kelley WN, Harris ED Jr, Ruddy S, Sledge CB, eds. *Textbook of rheumatology*, 5th ed. Philadelphia: WB Saunders, 1997, p. 707.

Paulus HE, Bulpitt KJ. Nonsteroidal anti-inflammatory drugs. In: Klippel JH, ed. *Primer on the rheumatic diseases*, 11th ed. Atlanta: Arthritis Foundation, 1997, p. 422.

Osteoarthritis

1. Why is pain at the base of the thumb and the gradual onset of pain in a knee with minimal swelling more characteristic of osteoarthritis than of rheumatoid arthritis?

2. What are four situations in which previous or ongoing mechanical joint damage may predispose to the development of osteoarthritis of the knee?

3. What are some of the characteristic findings encountered during physical examination in patients with osteoarthritis?

4. What are three different types of joint disease that may predispose to osteoarthritis, and what is one example of each?

5. What is the joint structure that is primarily involved in osteoarthritis?

Discussion

1. *Why is pain at the base of the thumb and the gradual onset of pain in a knee with minimal swelling more characteristic of osteoarthritis than of rheumatoid arthritis?*

Pain at the base of the thumb represents arthritis of the first carpometacarpal joint. This joint is commonly involved in the setting of osteoarthritis because of frequent mechanical damage incurred during normal use of the hand. It would be very unusual for there to be isolated involvement of this joint with minimal swelling in rheumatoid arthritis. Early osteoarthritis may be characterized by joint pain on use without signs of inflammation. Osteoarthritis is noninflammatory and can involve the distal interphalangeals, PIPs, and first carpometacarpals of the hand; the spine; hips; and knees. Rheumatoid arthritis is inflammatory and involves bilateral MCPs and PIPs in a symmetric fashion and can also involve the MTPs and other synovium-lined joints.

2. *What are four situations in which previous or ongoing mechanical joint damage may predispose to the development of osteoarthritis of the knee?*

A previous ski injury with surgical removal of damaged cartilage and surgical repair of a ruptured medial meniscus resulting from a football injury, with a subsequent unstable knee, are both examples of situations that can predispose to the development of osteoarthritis of the knee. A 20-year occupation as a carpet layer or long-standing obesity may also predispose to osteoarthritis.

3. *What are some of the characteristic findings encountered during physical examination in patients with osteoarthritis?*

Typical findings encountered during physical examination in patients with osteoarthritis include bony overgrowth (osteophytes), joint line tenderness, crepitus on passive motion, and limitation of motion with pain on extremes of motion.

4. *What are three different types of joint disease that may predispose to osteoarthritis, and what is one example of each?*

Metabolic joint diseases, such as hemochromatosis, may involve the articular cartilage and predispose to the development of osteoarthritis. Osteoarthritis also develops later in life in patients who have mechanically unstable joints, such as those with a congenital dislocation of the hip or other bony dysplasias. Forms of inflammatory arthritis, such as long-standing rheumatoid arthritis, may also predispose to the later development of osteoarthritis.

5. *What is the joint structure that is primarily involved in osteoarthritis?*

Osteoarthritis begins in the articular cartilage and later involves other joint structures, particularly the subchondral bone.

Case   A 56-year-old white male construction worker complains of chronic pain in his knees and intermittent pain at the base of his thumb. When gripping something forcefully, the pain at the base of the thumb (first carpometacarpal joint) is sometimes so sharp that he is forced momentarily to stop what he is doing. His knees ache diffusely when he has been on them a lot. These complaints keep him from working as often as he would like. His family history is unremarkable. Medical history reveals the patient has mild essential hypertension for which he has been taking hydrochlorothiazide for 8 years.

Physical examination reveals slight quadriceps atrophy on the right with slight genu varum and a pes anserinus bursitis, flattened arches, and moderate obesity. There is mild crepitus heard in both knees, but without ligamentous instability or abnormalities. No effusion or erythema is present. There is moderate tenderness of the first carpometacarpal joint bilaterally. There are no Heberden's or Bouchard's nodes.

1. What are four characteristic radiographic findings encountered in patients with osteoarthritis?
2. What are some characteristic changes that affect the articular cartilage in patients with osteoarthritis?
3. Osteoarthritis occurring after joint trauma may be due to what three different mechanisms?
4. What two classes of medications are used to treat osteoarthritis?
5. What therapies beside oral medications are used to manage osteoarthritis?

Case Discussion

1. *What are four characteristic radiographic findings encountered in patients with osteoarthritis?*

   Radiographic findings typically encountered in patients with osteoarthritis include loss of joint space, cysts in subchondral bone, subchondral sclerosis or eburnation, and osteophytes (bony spurs) at the joint margins.

2. *What are some characteristic changes that affect the articular cartilage in patients with osteoarthritis?*

   The characteristic changes in articular cartilage that occur in osteoarthritis include pits, clefts, and ulcerations in the surface; changes in the proteoglycan structure and concentration; an increased water content; increased amounts of proteolytic enzymes; and decreased amounts of enzyme inhibitors.

3. *Osteoarthritis occurring after joint trauma may be due to what three different mechanisms?*

   Joint trauma may damage the articular cartilage or the underlying bone, or it may cause instability with altered biomechanics. Each of these three abnormalities may predispose to the later development of osteoarthritis.

4. *What two classes of medications are used to treat osteoarthritis?*

   Acetaminophen, an analgesic, should be the first-line therapy for osteoarthritis. If this is unsuccessful, NSAIDs can be used. Under investigation are oral glucosamine and chondroitin sulfate, cartilage derivatives, and doxycycline.

5. *What therapies beside oral medications are used to manage osteoarthritis?*

   Other therapeutic modalities helpful in the management of osteoarthritis consist of heat or cold application, weight loss, physical therapy that focuses on muscle-strengthening exercises, intraarticular injections of corticosteroids, and orthopedic surgical repair in selected patients. Topical application of capsaicin cream or intraarticular injection of hyaluronate may be beneficial in some patients.

Suggested Readings

Brandt KD. Management of osteoarthritis. In: Kelley WN, Harris ED Jr, Ruddy S, Sledge CB, eds. *Textbook of rheumatology*, 5th ed. Philadelphia: WB Saunders, 1997, p. 1394.

Hochberg MC. Osteoarthritis: clinical features and treatment. In: Klippel JH, ed. *Primer on the rheumatic diseases*, 11th ed. Atlanta: Arthritis Foundation, 1997, p. 218.

Solomon L. Clinical features of osteoarthritis. In: Kelley WN, Harris ED Jr, Ruddy S, Sledge CB, eds. *Textbook of rheumatology*, 5th ed. Philadelphia: WB Saunders, 1997, p. 1383.

Polymyositis and Dermatomyositis

1. What three general categories of joint or muscle disease need to be considered in a patient presenting with diffuse aches and muscle weakness?
2. What are five subgroups of inflammatory muscle disease?
3. What historical information would suggest the presence of inflammatory muscle disease?
4. What two laboratory test results might be abnormal in patients with inflammatory muscle disease?
5. What four diagnostic tests or procedures should be performed in any patient with suspected inflammatory muscle disease?

Discussion

1. *What three general categories of joint or muscle disease need to be considered in a patient presenting with diffuse aches and muscle weakness?*

   A patient with diffuse aches and muscle weakness may have a form of inflammatory arthritis, particularly rheumatoid arthritis; a form of thyroid disease, either hyperthyroidism or hypothyroidism; or a form of inflammatory muscle disease.

2. *What are five subgroups of inflammatory muscle disease?*

   Inflammatory muscle disease can be divided into the following disorders: primary idiopathic polymyositis, primary idiopathic dermatomyositis, polymyositis and dermatomyositis associated with neoplasia, childhood dermatomyositis associated with vasculitis, and polymyositis and dermatomyositis associated with collagen vascular disease such as SLE or scleroderma.

3. *What historical information would suggest the presence of inflammatory muscle disease?*

   The muscle disease in patients with suspected inflammatory muscle disease may be preceded by a flu-like illness. The patients may then experience the insidious onset of proximal muscle weakness, characterized by difficulty climbing stairs or getting out of chairs. Inflammatory myopathies typically involve proximal muscle groups (e.g., shoulder/pelvic girdles and neck flexors).

4. *What two laboratory test results might be abnormal in patients with inflammatory muscle disease?*

   Two abnormal test findings in patients with polymyositis or dermatomyositis are an elevation in the ESR and in the serum CPK level. Approximately 50% of patients have a positive anti-nuclear antibody (ANA). Myositis-specific antibodies can occur in a subset of patients and can predict clinical manifestations and prognosis.

5. *What four diagnostic tests or procedures should be performed in any patient with suspected inflammatory muscle disease?*

   The diagnostic evaluation of patients with suspected inflammatory muscle disease should include serologic testing for ANA subtypes, electrocardiography, electromyography, and muscle biopsy to confirm the suspected diagnosis.

Case   A 47-year-old white woman is seen by her physician with a chief complaint of muscle weakness, along with vague complaints of decreased energy and diffuse aches and pains. She describes a flu-like illness that occurred 3 months earlier, from which she has never quite recovered. Routine physical examination findings are unremarkable, and the results of a baseline biochemical screen (including thyroid function studies) are within normal limits. Electrocardiography, a chest radiographic study, and pulmonary function test results are also unrevealing. She is given an empiric trial of naproxen (375 mg orally twice a day).

Three months later, she begins to experience actual muscle tenderness and difficulty climbing the two flights of stairs to her apartment. On questioning, she also complains of pain and difficulty chewing meats and an 8-pound (3.6-kg) weight loss. She denies fevers, chest pain, shortness of breath, a change in bowel habits, or skin rashes. She has noted mild puffiness of both her hands and feet.

Physical examination reveals grade 4/5 strength in the proximal muscle groups of both the upper and lower extremities without atrophy. There is also grade 4/5 weakness of the neck flexors. Her distal strength is normal. Her reflexes are symmetric. Her skin is clear, and breast and pelvic examination findings are unremarkable.

The following laboratory results are reported: hematocrit 34%; ESR 63 mm per hour; ANA 1:256 fine speckled pattern; rheumatoid factor negative; CPK 987 U/L (normal, <150 U/L).

She is scheduled to undergo electromyography and muscle biopsy of the left triceps.

1. What four different skin lesions are seen in patients with dermatomyositis?
2. What are some of the clinical characteristics of involved muscles in the setting of polymyositis or dermatomyositis?
3. What other organs beside muscle may be involved in patients with polymyositis or dermatomyositis?
4. What diagnostic evaluation is indicated to search for a possible malignancy in patients with polymyositis or dermatomyositis, and what may happen to the muscle disease when the malignancy is treated?
5. What two forms of medications are most effective in treating inflammatory muscle disease?

Case Discussion

1. *What four different skin lesions are seen in patients with dermatomyositis?*
   The skin lesions seen in patients with dermatomyositis include an erythematous rash over the anterior chest and neck (V-sign rash), an erythematous rash over the shoulders and proximal arms (shawl-sign rash), erythematous raised lesions over the knuckles (Gottron's papules), and a periorbital lilac-colored rash (heliotrope rash).

2. *What are some of the clinical characteristics of involved muscles in the setting of polymyositis or dermatomyositis?*

The muscle weakness seen in the setting of polymyositis or dermatomyositis is usually proximal and symmetric, and the affected muscles may be tender to palpation. Neck flexors may be involved.

3. *What other organs beside muscle may be involved in patients with polymyositis or dermatomyositis?*

The lungs, heart, and joints may also be involved in patients with polymyositis or dermatomyositis. Pulmonary involvement includes interstitial lung disease, aspiration pneumonia, respiratory muscle weakness, and pulmonary hypertension. Cardiac manifestations are dysrhythmias, conduction blocks, and myocarditis. Patients may experience arthralgias or an inflammatory arthritis.

4. *What diagnostic evaluation is indicated to search for a possible malignancy in patients with polymyositis or dermatomyositis, and what may happen to the muscle disease when the malignancy is treated?*

Malignancies may develop in patients with polymyositis or dermatomyositis, either before or after the onset of inflammatory muscle disease. The diagnostic evaluation for a possible malignancy in this setting usually includes only a good history and physical examination (including breast, pelvis, and prostate), a chest radiographic study, a stool guaiac test, and routine laboratory tests. The malignancies found in these patients include carcinomas of the lung, gastrointestinal tract, breast, and ovaries. If the malignancy is treated, the muscle disease may improve.

5. *What two forms of medications are most effective in treating inflammatory muscle disease?*

The treatment of polymyositis and dermatomyositis should first consist of systemic corticosteroids given in high doses. If patients show a poor response to steroids or if the dosage cannot be decreased, immunosuppressive drug treatment with such agents as azathioprine or methotrexate may be instituted.

Suggested Readings

Olsen NJ, Wortmann RL. Inflammatory and metabolic diseases of muscle. In: Klippel JH, ed. *Primer on the rheumatic diseases*, 11th ed. Atlanta: Arthritis Foundation, 1997, p. 276.

Wortmann RL. Inflammatory disease of muscle and other myopathies. In: Kelley WN, Harris ED Jr, Ruddy S, Sledge CB, eds. *Textbook of rheumatology*, 5th ed. Philadelphia: WB Saunders, 1997, p. 1177.

Reiter's Syndrome

1. In what two diseases is arthritis associated with diarrhea?
2. What two possible diagnoses are suggested when acute arthritis occurs in a patient with urethral discharge?
3. What are four types of a seronegative spondyloarthropathy?
4. What are the four clinical manifestations of Reiter's syndrome?

5. What are the history and physical examination findings typically observed in patients with Reiter's syndrome?

Discussion

1. *In what two diseases is arthritis associated with diarrhea?*

Arthritis associated with diarrhea may be seen in the setting of either Reiter's syndrome or inflammatory bowel disease. In Reiter's syndrome, the diarrhea may precede the arthritis by a few weeks. In inflammatory bowel disease, the peripheral arthritis and diarrhea arise at the same time and the clinical activity of the arthritis may correlate with the activity of the inflammatory bowel disease.

2. *What two possible diagnoses are suggested when acute arthritis occurs in a patient with urethral discharge?*

Acute arthritis occurring in a patient with a urethral discharge suggests a diagnosis of either disseminated gonococcal infection or Reiter's syndrome. These diagnoses can be differentiated on the basis of characteristic clinical features as well as by a positive urethral or cervical culture for *Neisseria gonorrhoeae*.

3. *What are four types of a seronegative spondyloarthropathy?*

Four types of seronegative spondyloarthropathy include ankylosing spondylitis, Reiter's syndrome, arthritis associated with inflammatory bowel disease, and psoriatic arthritis. The back involvement in these three disorders may be clinically indistinguishable, but they can be differentiated on the basis of skin findings and other associated clinical manifestations.

4. *What are the four clinical manifestations of Reiter's syndrome?*

Besides the asymmetric arthropathy typically of joints of the lower extremities, patients with Reiter's syndrome can exhibit four secondary clinical manifestations. These comprise urethritis or cervicitis, dysentery, eye disease (conjunctivitis or uveitis), and mucocutaneous disease.

5. *What are the history and physical examination findings typically observed in patients with Reiter's syndrome?*

Reiter's syndrome is diagnosed on the basis of history and physical examination findings, and not on the basis of any laboratory result. These clinical findings include the development of an acute arthritis in one or a few joints after an episode either of diarrhea or of painless urethritis or cervicitis. The diagnosis may be further strengthened by the presence of conjunctivitis or urethritis, as well as characteristic skin findings of circinate balanitis or keratoderma blennorrhagicum (see later).

Case A 32-year-old man is seen because of increasing right knee pain and swelling over the past 3 days. On further questioning, it is discovered that the patient had an episode of fever and diarrhea 14 days ago that was associated with mucus and blood in the stool. This illness resolved spontaneously after 4 days and the patient was again well until 1 week ago, when dysuria developed acutely at the same time as a clear penile discharge. He has not been exposed to untreated water and has one sexual partner, his wife of 5 years. Six days ago, painless, shallow ulcerations of the glans penis developed. During this period, he also noted the onset of bilateral redness and pruritus of the eyes, along with a clear discharge. Three days ago, acute swelling of the right knee associated with pain arose spontaneously and, since then, has steadily worsened. At the same time, the bilateral eye inflammation and dysuria with discharge have abated.

Physical examination reveals mild injection of the conjunctival vessels bilaterally. His visual acuity and retina are normal. Slit-lamp examination demonstrates no evidence of anterior uveitis. Examination of the skin reveals discrete hyperkeratotic nodules over the soles of his feet bilaterally and there are three shallow ulcers on the glans penis. His right knee is warm and tender, and there is a significant amount of palpable synovial fluid. The remainder of the examination findings are unremarkable.

1. What other forms of rheumatic disease need to be considered when Reiter's syndrome is suspected, and what diagnostic tests or procedures should be performed to rule them out?
2. What are some of the clinical or laboratory characteristics of Reiter's syndrome that help to differentiate it from rheumatoid arthritis?
3. What are the four types of skin lesions seen in patients with Reiter's syndrome?
4. The back disease in patients with Reiter's syndrome is characterized by what radiographic findings?
5. What is the therapy for Reiter's syndrome?

Case Discussion

1. *What other forms of rheumatic disease need to be considered when Reiter's syndrome is suspected, and what diagnostic tests or procedures should be performed to rule them out?*

In a patient suspected of having Reiter's syndrome, septic arthritis also needs to be considered. The findings yielded by joint aspiration, which includes examination of the fluid for cell count with differential, together with Gram's staining and culture, can clinch the diagnosis of a nongonococcal bacterial septic joint. Gonococcal arthritis is another possible diagnosis. Beside examination of synovial fluid, the evaluation should include urethral or cervical, blood, pharyngeal, and perirectal cultures. Crystal-induced arthritis is diagnosed by the finding of crystals in the synovial fluid. Both SLE and rheumatoid arthritis also need to be considered. Serologic testing for ANA and rheumatoid factor is performed to assess for these disorders. A routine complete blood count and a full chemistry profile, including liver function tests, should also be performed to search for a systemic disease that may present with joint findings similar to those seen in the setting of Reiter's syndrome. Reiter's syndrome can be associated with HIV infection.

2. *What are some of the clinical or laboratory characteristics of Reiter's syndrome that help to differentiate it from rheumatoid arthritis?*

An asymmetric arthritis that predominates in the lower extremity is a characteristic of Reiter's syndrome. In addition, sacroiliitis afflicts 20% to 30% of patients, the syndrome is associated with HLAB27 (80% of patients), and patients frequently have an enthesopathy along with Achilles tendinitis or sausage digits (dactylitis).

3. *What are the four types of skin lesions seen in patients with Reiter's syndrome?*

The skin lesions of Reiter's syndrome include keratoderma blennorrhagicum (psoriasiform lesions on the plantar surface of the heel and metatarsal heads), painless mouth ulcers, hyperkeratotic nodules on the soles and palms, and circinate balanitis (serpiginous ulceration of the glans penis).

4. *The back disease in patient's with Reiter's syndrome is characterized by what radiographic findings?*

The back radiographic study of a patient with Reiter's syndrome may show asymmetric and bulky syndesmophytes. This is in contrast with ankylosing spondylitis, in which the syndesmophytes are usually symmetric and flowing. In Reiter's syndrome, sacroiliitis, if present, is often unilateral and asymmetric.

5. *What is the therapy for Reiter's syndrome?*

Patients with Reiter's syndrome are first treated with NSAIDs (typically indomethacin), together with appropriate antibiotics during the acute phase if urethritis or cervicitis occurs. If the disease progresses despite NSAID treatment, sulfasalazine or methotrexate may be of value for managing the inflammatory arthritis. Intraarticular corticosteroids may be helpful, but systemic corticosteroids are usually ineffective. Physical therapy consisting of heat, ultrasound, and range-of-motion exercises may be important in all patients with Reiter's syndrome.

Suggested Readings

Arnett FC. Seronegative spondyloarthropathies: reactive arthritis (Reiter's syndrome) and enteropathic arthritis. In: Klippel JH, ed. *Primer on the rheumatic diseases*, 11th ed. Atlanta: Arthritis Foundation, 1997, p. 184.

Fan PT, Tak Yan Yu D. Reiter's syndrome. In: Kelley WN, Harris ED Jr, Ruddy S, Sledge CB, eds. *Textbook of rheumatology*, 5th ed. Philadelphia: WB Saunders, 1997, p. 983.

Rheumatoid Arthritis

1. What four characteristics of rheumatoid arthritis help to distinguish it from osteoarthritis?

2. What constitutional symptoms may be seen in rheumatoid arthritis?

3. What are three characteristic physical findings in rheumatoid arthritis?

4. What five diseases may mimic rheumatoid arthritis?

5. Which serologic tests may be useful in the diagnosis of rheumatoid arthritis?

Discussion

1. *What four characteristics of rheumatoid arthritis help to distinguish it from osteoarthritis?*

   Unlike osteoarthritis (noninflammatory), patients with rheumatoid arthritis (inflammatory) experience morning stiffness lasting more than 30 minutes, plus gel phenomenon (worse stiffness after rest), symmetric joint disease, characteristic involvement of the hands and feet, and an intermittent or waxing and waning course.

2. *What constitutional symptoms may be seen in rheumatoid arthritis?*

   Most patients experience generalized malaise or fatigue. Occasionally weight loss, low-grade fever, or mild lymphadenopathy may be present.

3. *What are three characteristic physical findings in rheumatoid arthritis?*

   Physical findings encountered in the setting of rheumatoid arthritis may include swelling and warmth of one or more joints, typically in a symmetric distribution, tenderness on palpation of the swollen joints, and the presence of nontender subcutaneous nodules (rheumatoid nodules) over the extensor surface of the forearm, Achilles tendon, and digits of the hands.

4. *What five diseases may mimic rheumatoid arthritis?*

   Rheumatoid arthritis may be mimicked by SLE and other connective tissue diseases such as mixed connective tissue disease, scleroderma, and polymyalgia rheumatica, polyarticular gout or pseudogout, the arthritis of subacute bacterial endocarditis, the arthritis secondary to malignancy, and the seronegative spondyloarthropathies. Diagnosis is based on the history, physical examination, or laboratory findings.

5. *Which serologic tests may be useful in the diagnosis of rheumatoid arthritis?*

   A complete blood count may be useful in the diagnosis of rheumatoid arthritis if it shows an anemia of inflammatory disease or a low white blood cell count (neutropenia). An elevated ESR may suggest the presence of an acute inflammatory disease. ANAs are found in 25% of patients with rheumatoid arthritis, usually in a low titer and with a negative ANA profile. Rheumatoid factor is detected in 85% of patients with rheumatoid arthritis.

Case   A 38-year-old woman is seen because of pain and swelling in the joints of her hands, as well as in her wrists, elbows, and knees. Her symptoms have been intermittent over the past 3 years, but recently have worsened and become more prolonged. The pain and swelling have been accompanied by hand stiffness in the morning, frequently lasting for 2 hours or more, and she has noted return of the stiffness later in the day after periods of inactivity. She also complains of progressively worsening fatigue and lack of energy. She denies experiencing, recently or in the past, rash, photosensitivity, alopecia, oral ulcers, or symptoms of Raynaud's phenomenon. She experiences left wrist pain that radiates to her elbow and into her fingers that is worse in the morning and occasionally wakes her at night.

On physical examination, swelling, warmth, and tenderness are noted in several MCP and PIP joints bilaterally. Her wrists are slightly swollen and tender to palpation, especially in the region of the ulnar styloid processes. Her elbows exhibit slight tenderness to palpation and mild flexion contractures bilaterally. Small effusions are present in both knees. Tenderness is elicited over several MTP joints in both feet. Tinel's sign is elicited over the left wrist and Phalen's test reproduces the patient's left wrist and forearm pain. Decreased sensation to light touch is noted over the left first to third fingers. Examination of the skin reveals the presence of several subcutaneous nodules over the proximal extensor aspects of both forearms.

1. What is the primary pathophysiologic process in rheumatoid arthritis?
2. What are four characteristic radiographic findings in rheumatoid arthritis, and what are the mechanisms responsible for their development?
3. What are the four most common extraarticular manifestations of rheumatoid arthritis?
4. The natural history of the joint disease in patients with rheumatoid arthritis assumes what three patterns?
5. What is the treatment for rheumatoid arthritis?

Case Discussion

1. *What is the primary pathophysiologic process in rheumatoid arthritis?*

    The joint disease in rheumatoid arthritis begins as an inflammation in the synovium and involves the infiltration of macrophages and lymphocytes. Fibroblasts then proliferate and grow over the cartilage; this inflammatory proliferative synovitis is known as *pannus*. The subsequent joint destruction that may take place is secondary to this proliferative synovitis, which is capable of destroying cartilage and bone.

2. *What are four characteristic radiographic findings in rheumatoid arthritis, and what are the mechanisms responsible for their development?*

    The soft tissue swelling seen on radiographic studies in patients with rheumatoid arthritis is due to edema in the soft tissues surrounding an inflamed joint. Joint space narrowing results from the loss of articular cartilage, which, in turn, results from destruction by enzymes produced by the proliferative synovitis. Juxtaarticular osteopenia is due to the loss of calcium in bones surrounding the inflammatory arthritis and results from the effects of prostaglandins and interleukin-1, which are released by the inflamed synovium. Marginal erosions are produced by the proliferative synovitis as it extends into the subchondral bone at the joint margins.

3. *What are the four most common extraarticular manifestations of rheumatoid arthritis?*

The four most common extraarticular manifestations of rheumatoid arthritis comprise subcutaneous nodules (rheumatoid nodules), carpal tunnel syndrome, interstitial lung disease, and Felty's syndrome (splenomegaly and neutropenia in the setting of rheumatoid arthritis).

4. *The natural history of the joint disease in patients with rheumatoid arthritis assumes what three patterns?*

The natural history of rheumatoid arthritis may consist of a single episode, although in retrospect some of these cases may have been a viral-induced, self-limited polyarthritis; repeated episodes of active disease interspersed with periods of inactivity; or a waxing and waning progressive course with no disease-free intervals.

5. *What is the treatment for rheumatoid arthritis?*

The initial treatment for rheumatoid arthritis consists of medications, heat, specific exercises, and physical therapy. These initial medications include ASA or other NSAIDs. Many patients also respond well to low doses of oral corticosteroids. Early in the disease in most patients, treatment with disease-modifying medications is initiated, and these agents include gold (administered either orally or by injection), hydroxychloroquine, sulfasalazine, and methotrexate. Therapies directed against the actions of tumor necrosis factor, interleukin-1, and lymphocyte function are being developed. When joints become severely damaged due to chronic rheumatoid arthritis, reconstructive orthopedic surgical procedures may be performed to help restore function.

Suggested Readings

Anderson RJ. Rheumatoid arthritis: clinical and laboratory features. In: Klippel JH, ed. *Primer on the rheumatic diseases*, 11th ed. Atlanta: Arthritis Foundation, 1997, p. 161.

Harris ED Jr. Clinical features of rheumatoid arthritis. In: Kelley WN, Harris ED Jr, Ruddy S, Sledge CB, eds. *Textbook of rheumatology*, 5th ed. Philadelphia: WB Saunders, 1997, p. 898.

Harris ED Jr. Treatment of rheumatoid arthritis. In: Kelley WN, Harris ED Jr, Ruddy S, Sledge CB, eds. *Textbook of rheumatology*, 5th ed. Philadelphia: WB Saunders, 1997, p. 933.

Paget SA. Rheumatoid arthritis: treatment. In: Klippel JH, ed. *Primer on the rheumatic diseases*, 11th ed. Atlanta: Arthritis Foundation, 1997, p. 168.

Scleroderma

1. What three different rheumatic diseases are suggested by a predominance of skin findings?
2. Raynaud's phenomenon may occur in association with what four rheumatic diseases?
3. Dysphagia or heartburn may predominate in what two rheumatic diseases?
4. What features characterize the CREST syndrome?

5. What is the difference between limited and diffuse scleroderma or systemic sclerosis?

Discussion

1. *What three different rheumatic diseases are suggested by a predominance of skin findings?*

   A predominance of skin findings in a patient with a suspected rheumatic disease suggests a diagnosis of SLE, dermatomyositis, or scleroderma. The skin findings in each of these diseases, however, are distinct, which allows their differentiation.

2. *Raynaud's phenomenon may occur in association with what three rheumatic diseases?*

   Raynaud's phenomenon (a cold-induced blanching or cyanosis of the fingers or toes) may be seen in the settings of SLE (20%), scleroderma (90%), mixed connective tissue disease (70%), or polymyositis/dermatomyositis (20%). When the phenomenon occurs alone, without an associated connective tissue disease, it is called *Raynaud's disease*.

3. *Dysphagia or heartburn may predominate in what two rheumatic diseases?*

   Dysphagia (discomfort when swallowing food) and heartburn are esophageal abnormalities that may occur in the setting of either scleroderma or dermatomyositis and polymyositis. In scleroderma, the lower portion of the esophagus is involved; in dermatomyositis or polymyositis, the muscles in the pharynx and upper third of the esophagus may be involved.

4. *What features characterize the CREST syndrome?*

   The CREST syndrome is a clinical variant of scleroderma that is characterized by *c*alcinosis, *R*aynaud's phenomenon, *e*sophageal dysmotility, *s*clerodactyly, and *t*elangiectases. Patients with the syndrome may experience a more benign course than those with more widespread scleroderma that involves other internal organs.

5. *What is the difference between limited and diffuse scleroderma or systemic sclerosis?*

   In limited systemic sclerosis (CREST), fibrotic skin disease is limited to the hands and forearms, feet, neck, and face. Pulmonary hypertension can occur. In diffuse systemic sclerosis, fibrotic skin involves the fingers, hands, arms, legs, and typically the trunk and face. Pulmonary (interstitial lung disease), renal, gastrointestinal, and cardiac involvement can occur.

Case   A 65-year-old white woman seeks medical attention because of progressive symmetric skin tightening that has involved the digits, hands, and forearms during the past 3 months. These skin changes are painless and associated with mild pruritus. During the past 6 months, she has also noted the onset of cold sensitivity, especially when handling objects in the refrigerator, with multiple fingers becoming cold, pale, and numb. She also reports generalized fatigue, dyspnea on exertion, and a decrease in exercise tolerance without claudication. She denies chest pain, palpitation, or paroxysmal nocturnal dyspnea, but has noticed symmetric swelling in both lower extremities. She has noted a 10-pound (4.5-kg) weight loss in the past 6 months, which she has attributed to decreased food intake because of the heartburn and dysphagia provoked by eating.

Physical examination reveals a blood pressure of 170/100 mm Hg, pulse of 110 beats per minute, temperature of 37°C, and respiratory rate of 18 breaths per minute. The woman appears younger than her stated age; she lacks the normal forehead wrinkling and she has a "pursed-lips" appearance. A few scattered facial telangiectases are noted. Her skin is very tight and cannot be easily lifted from over the dorsum of the hands, fingers, and lower forearms. There are very small punctate healed ulcerations on several fingertips. Nail findings are unremarkable. Her muscle strength is normal and there is no evidence of synovitis. Chest examination reveals symmetric dry rales that are limited to the lower third of the posterior lung bases. On cardiac examination, no gallops, murmurs, or rubs are heard, but the pulmonic second sound (P_2) is loud and fixed splitting is noted. Her jugular venous pressure is slightly elevated, and there is 1+ pitting edema over both lower extremities.

1. What are three ANA-related characteristics commonly seen in patients with scleroderma?
2. What four radiographic findings may be seen in patients with scleroderma?
3. What are some of the complications stemming from the esophageal or small intestinal involvement in scleroderma?
4. What cardiac and renal problems may arise in patients with scleroderma?
5. What is the therapy for patients with scleroderma?

Case Discussion

1. *What are three ANA-related characteristics commonly seen in patients with scleroderma?*

   More than 95% of patients with scleroderma show positivity for ANAs. Anti-centromere antibodies may be found in patients with the CREST syndrome (50% to 95%), whereas anti-topoisomerase I (Scl-70) antibodies may be identified in patients with diffuse scleroderma (20% to 40%).

2. *What four radiographic findings may be seen in patients with scleroderma?*

   Radiographic abnormalities that may be found in patients with scleroderma include wide-mouth diverticula of the colon on barium enema, pulmonary interstitial fibrosis, loss of distal digital tufts, and subcutaneous calcifications, particularly in the hands.

3. *What are some of the complications stemming from the esophageal or small intestinal involvement in scleroderma?*

   The lower esophageal involvement that can occur in patients with scleroderma may lead to heartburn caused by acid reflux, and ultimately esophageal strictures may develop. Involvement of the small intestine may lead to loss of motility with malabsorption, secondary to bacterial overgrowth.

4. *What cardiac and renal problems may arise in patients with scleroderma?*

The hearts of patients with scleroderma may be affected by patchy fibrosis, which is manifested by conduction disturbances and arrhythmias on electrocardiograms. In the event of renal involvement, patients may have hypertension with mild proteinuria that sometimes leads to a renal crisis (rapid loss of kidney function progressing to renal failure).

5. *What is the therapy for patients with scleroderma?*

There are no known medications that can alter the natural course of scleroderma, although penicillamine is being evaluated in this regard. Aggressive skin care is helpful in preventing breakdown and local infection. Gastroesophageal reflux typically requires therapy with a gastric acid (proton) pump inhibitor. Broad-spectrum antibiotics may be used if diarrhea arises as a result of small intestinal involvement. An angiotensin-converting enzyme inhibitor should be used in hypertensive patients with scleroderma in an effort to prevent further renal damage and possible renal crisis by reversing underlying hyperreninemia.

Suggested Readings

Seibold JR. Scleroderma. In: Kelley WN, Harris ED Jr, Ruddy S, Sledge CB, eds. *Textbook of rheumatology*, 5th ed. Philadelphia: WB Saunders, 1997, p. 1133.

Steen VD. Systemic sclerosis and related syndromes: treatment. In: Klippel JH, ed. *Primer on the rheumatic diseases*, 11th ed. Atlanta: Arthritis Foundation, 1997, 273.

Wigley FM. Systemic sclerosis and related syndromes: clinical features. In: Klippel JH, ed. *Primer on the rheumatic diseases*, 11th ed. Atlanta: Arthritis Foundation, 1997, p. 267.

Synovial Fluid Analysis and Septic Arthritis

1. What are the characteristics of a noninflammatory synovial effusion?

2. What are the characteristics of an inflammatory synovial effusion?

3. What are some of the characteristics of a septic (or infected) synovial fluid?

4. What are some clinical situations that would suggest or support the diagnosis of septic arthritis?

5. What are the clinical characteristics of the joint disease that affects patients with gonococcal arthritis?

Discussion

1. *What are the characteristics of a noninflammatory synovial effusion?*

Noninflammatory synovial fluid is highly viscous, straw colored to yellow, and transparent with a white blood cell count of 200 to 2000 cells/μL, with less than 25% polymorphonuclear leukocytes. Synovial fluid culture is negative.

2. *What are the characteristics of an inflammatory synovial effusion?*

Inflammatory synovial fluid is of low viscosity, yellow and translucent to turbid, with a white blood cell count of 2,000 to 75,000 cells/μL, with greater than 50% polymorphonuclear leukocytes, although cell counts in excess of 75,000 can occur. Synovial fluid culture is negative.

3. *What are some of the characteristics of a septic (or infected) synovial fluid?*

Septic synovial fluid is of variable viscosity and turbid, with a white blood cell count often exceeding 100,000 cells/μL with more than 90% polymorphonuclear leukocytes. Synovial fluid culture is often positive. Any synovial fluid white blood cell count of over 50,000 cells/μL should raise the suspicion of infection.

4. *What are some clinical situations that would suggest or support the diagnosis of septic arthritis?*

Septic arthritis may be suggested when a disproportionately warm and swollen joint develops acutely in a patient who has chronic rheumatoid arthritis or an underlying abnormal joint, or has recently undergone intraarticular aspiration and injection or an orthopedic procedure. In addition, septic arthritis should be considered in a patient with diabetes, renal or hepatic failure, or malignancy who presents with a swollen joint, as well as in an intravenous drug abuser. In the latter instance, infection of the sternoclavicular, acromioclavicular, sacroiliac joints, or intervertebral discs can also occur.

5. *What are the clinical characteristics of the joint disease that affects patients with gonococcal arthritis?*

The joint disease in disseminated gonococcal infection often starts as a migratory polyarthralgia and then becomes a monoarthritis. It is associated with a tenosynovitis of the hands, wrists, ankles, or knees. A dermatitis (maculopapular or vesicular) is often present on the lower extremities or trunk.

Case

A 52-year-old woman is seen in the emergency room because of an acutely painful and swollen right knee. The patient has a 10-year history of rheumatoid arthritis that has not responded well to multiple medications. For the past 6 months, she has been taking ibuprofen, azathioprine (100 mg daily), prednisone (10 mg daily), and hydrochlorothiazide. Despite this regimen, she continues to experience 2 hours of morning stiffness with swelling, erythema, and pain in multiple small joints of her hands, wrists, knees, and ankles. She is now unable to bear weight on the right leg. A low-grade fever also developed.

On physical examination, the patient's temperature is found to be 39°C and her blood pressure is 150/100 mm Hg. She appears both acutely and chronically ill, with mild swelling of multiple MCP and PIP joints, as well as both wrists and ankles. Her right knee is held in 10 degrees of flexion and it cannot be moved because of severe pain. The knee exhibits a large effusion and is diffusely tender, and there is erythema around the entire joint. Joint aspiration is performed and 20 mL of opaque, yellow fluid is removed that shows low viscosity. The white blood cell count in the synovial fluid aspirate is 75,000/μL with 80% polymorphonuclear leukocytes. There are questionable gram-positive cocci on Gram's stain of the synovial fluid. The fluid is cultured for organisms.

1. What are three synovial fluid findings typically encountered in rheumatoid arthritis?
2. What are the possible causes of a bloody synovial fluid?
3. What are the characteristics of monosodium urate or calcium pyrophosphate crystals when visualized by polarized microscopy?
4. What diseases predispose to the development of gram-negative joint infections?
5. What diagnostic tests should be performed on all synovial fluid aspirates, regardless of the suspected diagnosis?

Case Discussion

1. *What are three synovial fluid findings typically encountered in rheumatoid arthritis?*

   Synovial fluid findings commonly seen in patients with rheumatoid arthritis may consist of a loss of viscosity, a low glucose concentration, and a white blood cell count of 2,000 to 75,000 cells/μL. Again, any synovial fluid white blood cell count greater than 50,000 cells/μL should raise the suspicion of infection.

2. *What are the possible causes of a bloody synovial fluid?*

   Some causes of a hemarthrosis include trauma, iatrogenic (postprocedure) causes, bleeding diatheses, over-anticoagulation, tumors, pigmented nodular synovitis, Charcot's joint, scurvy, hemangiomas, and intense inflammatory disease.

3. *What are the characteristics of monosodium urate or calcium pyrophosphate crystals when visualized by polarized microscopy?*

   Monosodium urate crystals are needle-like and negatively birefringent (yellow when parallel to the long axis of the red compensator). In contrast, calcium pyrophosphate crystals are rhomboid and positively birefringent (light blue when parallel to the long axis of the red compensator). Both forms of crystals may be found in phagocytic cells from synovial fluid.

4. *What diseases predispose to the development of gram-negative joint infections?*

   Gram-negative joint infections are more common in patients with predisposing chronic diseases such as diabetes, chronic renal failure, chronic liver disease, or malignancy. Gram-negative septic arthritis also can occur in intravenous drug abusers.

5. *What diagnostic tests should be performed on all synovial fluid aspirates, regardless of the suspected diagnosis?*

   A total white blood cell count with differential, Gram's staining and culture, and a crystal examination should be performed on all synovial fluid aspirates.

Suggested Readings

Goldenberg DL. Bacterial arthritis. In: Kelley WN, Harris ED Jr, Ruddy S, Sledge CB, eds. *Textbook of rheumatology*, 5th ed. Philadelphia: WB Saunders, 1997, p. 1435.

Hasselbacher P. Arthrocentesis, synovial fluid analysis, and synovial biopsy. In: Klippel JH, ed. *Primer on the rheumatic diseases*, 11th ed. Atlanta: Arthritis Foundation, 1997, p. 98.
Mahowald ML. Infectious disorders: septic arthritis. In: Klippel JH, ed. *Primer on the rheumatic diseases*, 11th ed. Atlanta: Arthritis Foundation, 1997, p. 196.

Systemic Lupus Erythematosus

1. Which rheumatic diseases may manifest polyarticular arthritis?
2. What clinical features suggest a diagnosis of SLE?
3. What are three clinical characteristics of SLE that help to differentiate it from rheumatoid arthritis?
4. What abnormal laboratory results suggest a diagnosis of SLE?
5. Besides SLE, ANAs are commonly found in what other diseases?

Discussion

1. *Which rheumatic diseases may manifest polyarticular arthritis?*

In general, chronic polyarticular arthritis (five or more joints involved) can occur in rheumatoid arthritis, SLE, diffuse systemic sclerosis, seronegative spondyloarthropathies, polyarticular gout, calcium pyrophosphate deposition disease, sarcoid, vasculitis, polymyalgia rheumatica, osteoarthritis, and occasionally in inflammatory myopathies.

2. *What clinical features suggest a diagnosis of SLE?*

For the purposes of clinical studies, any person having 4 or more of the following 11 criteria is considered to have SLE: malar rash, discoid rash, photosensitivity, oral ulcers, arthritis, serositis, renal disorder, neurologic disorder, hematologic disorder, immunologic disorder (anti-DNA, anti-Smith, false-positive test for syphilis), and ANA.

3. *What are three clinical characteristics of SLE that help to differentiate it from rheumatoid arthritis?*

Systemic lupus erythematosus differs from rheumatoid arthritis in that the joint disease is milder and nonerosive, and renal and skin disease are more common.

4. *What abnormal laboratory results suggest a diagnosis of SLE?*

Almost all patients with SLE demonstrate elevated serum levels of ANA. However, this test is not specific for SLE. Other laboratory abnormalities in SLE can include anti–double-stranded DNA antibodies, anti-Smith nuclear antibodies, false-positive test for syphilis, low serum complement levels, prolonged partial thromboplastin time, anti-phospholipid antibodies, cytopenias, and active urine sediments.

5. *Besides SLE, ANAs are commonly found in what other diseases?*

Antinuclear antibodies can be found in rheumatoid arthritis (25%), Sjögren's syndrome (96%), scleroderma (95%), mixed connective tissue disease (93%), polymyositis/dermatomyositis (50%), and drug-induced lupus (100%). More patients on procainamide (90%) or hydralazine (30% to 50%) demonstrate an asymptomatic positive ANA than acquire drug-induced lupus (10% to 30%).

Case   A 28-year-old white woman is seen because of a 2-month history of painful joints and fatigue. She states that the joint pain affects her hands, wrists, feet, ankles, and knees and is associated with some joint swelling and 2 to 3 hours of morning stiffness. Over the past 3 to 4 months, the patient has noted gradually increasing fatigue and has had three or four episodes of rash over her face and neck. During the past summer, she states that she had a similar rash, which was precipitated by exposure to the sun. She has also noted that prolonged sun exposure results in increasing fatigue and a flu-like syndrome. Two weeks ago, she noted her ankles tend to swell at the end of the day. Past medical history reveals that 8 months ago she had an episode of pleuritic chest pain that lasted 8 to 10 days and was treated by her family doctor with indomethacin, followed by gradual resolution.

Physical examination reveals a tired-looking woman who is in no acute distress. Her temperature is 38.2°C, her blood pressure is 140/100 mm Hg, and her pulse is 96 beats per minute and regular. On examination of the skin, an erythematous rash is noted over her cheeks that extends into the "V" region of the neck. Several shallow ulcers are found in her mouth. Joint examination reveals minimal swelling of the wrists and MCP joints. Pulmonary and cardiac findings are normal, except for 1+ to 2+ pitting edema in the pretibial area bilaterally.

1. What are the two most common mechanisms of tissue damage in patients with SLE?
2. Besides the joints and skin, what other organs are commonly affected in patients with SLE?
3. What serologic tests and diagnostic procedures may be helpful in the management of lupus nephritis?
4. What are three possible causes of peripheral edema in patients with SLE?
5. What is the therapy for SLE?

Case Discussion

1. *What are the two most common mechanisms of tissue damage in patients with SLE?*

Tissue damage in patients with SLE may be caused by antibodies to cell surface components or by the presence of soluble immune complexes in the circulation. Antibodies to platelets, white blood cells, or red blood cells may induce thrombocytopenia, leukopenia, or anemia, respectively. Anti-phospholipid antibodies may induce venous or arterial thromboses, recurrent fetal loss, or thrombocytopenia. Soluble immune complexes in the circulation may deposit in blood vessels or along basement membranes in the skin or kidneys, resulting in vasculitis, dermatitis, or glomerulonephritis.

2. *Besides the joints and skin, what other organs are commonly affected in patients with SLE?*

Other organs that may be affected in the setting of SLE include the central and peripheral nervous systems, lungs, heart, kidneys, and gastrointestinal system, as well as the formed elements of the blood and serous membranes.

3. *What serologic tests and diagnostic procedures may be helpful in the management of lupus nephritis?*

Low serum complement levels or high titers of antibodies to double-stranded DNA may precede flares of renal disease. A kidney biopsy may aid in the management of patients with lupus nephritis, particularly when the severity of the disease appears to be changing, the disease is refractory to high-dose prednisone therapy, and cytotoxic therapy with intravenous bolus cyclophosphamide therapy is being considered.

4. *What are three possible causes of peripheral edema in patients with SLE?*

Peripheral edema in a patient with SLE may be due to renal disease with nephrotic syndrome, congestive heart failure secondary to cardiac involvement, or peripheral venous thrombosis stemming from the formation of anticardiolipin antibodies.

5. *What is the therapy for SLE?*

Patients with SLE are managed according to the extent and severity of their organ involvement. Patients with mild disease consisting of arthritis, skin, and non-life-threatening blood or other organ involvement may be treated with NSAIDs, antimalarials such as hydroxychloroquine, and low-dose corticosteroids if necessary. Patients with more severe organ involvement, particularly of the central nervous system and kidneys, may be treated with high doses of corticosteroids and oral azathioprine or intravenous cyclophosphamide. Other therapies may be used for the amelioration of specific organ involvement.

Suggested Readings

Gladman DD, Urowitz MB. Systemic lupus erythematosus: clinical and laboratory features. In: Klippel JH, ed. *Primer on the rheumatic diseases*, 11th ed. Atlanta: Arthritis Foundation, 1997, p. 251.

Lahita RG. Clinical presentation of systemic lupus erythematosus. In: Kelley WN, Harris ED Jr, Ruddy S, Sledge CB, eds. *Textbook of rheumatology*, 5th ed. Philadelphia: WB Saunders, 1997, p. 1028.

Vasculitis

1. Vasculitis should be suspected in patients presenting with any combination of what five clinical manifestations?

2. What four characteristics may be used to identify specific types of vasculitis?

3. What serologic tests or diagnostic procedures should be performed in patients with suspected vasculitis?

4. What more extensive procedures may be of value in helping to establish the diagnosis of a specific form of vasculitis?

Discussion

1. *Vasculitis should be suspected in patients presenting with any combination of what five clinical manifestations?*

    Vasculitis comprises a heterogeneous group of diseases characterized by inflammatory changes in the blood vessels. Vasculitis should be suspected in patients presenting with a skin rash, arthralgias or arthritis, peripheral neuropathy, hematuria, or anemia. In addition, patients commonly have fever, anorexia, weight loss, weakness, or fatigue.

2. *What four characteristics may be used to identify specific types of vasculitis?*

    Forms of vasculitis differ in terms of the type and size of the blood vessels involved as well as in the histologic appearance of a biopsy specimen of a blood vessel. Forms of vasculitis can also be differentiated on the basis of the nature and extent of organ involvement, and on the presence or absence of hematuria or proteinuria. The vasculitides can be classified as follows:

    Vasculitides affecting large, medium-sized, and small vessels:

    Takayasu's arteritis: aortic arch and its branches, can involve any part of the aorta; more claudication of upper than lower extremities, central nervous system events; granulomatous panarteritis.

    Giant cell arteritis: temporal arteries, vessels originating from the aortic arch, other arteries less common; temporal headache, jaw claudication, scalp tenderness, visual loss; giant cell arteritis with disruption of the internal elastic lamina.

    Vasculitides affecting predominantly medium-sized and small vessels:

    Polyarteritis nodosa: small and medium-sized arteries; may affect any organ, but skin, joints, peripheral nerves, gut, and kidney are most commonly involved; focal but panmural necrotizing arteritis with a predilection for involvement at the vessel bifurcation.

    Wegener's granulomatosis: small and medium-sized arteries; upper respiratory tract (sinuses), lungs, and kidneys, may affect other organs; pauci-immune, necrotizing, granulomatous arteritis usually associated with serum cytoplasmic–antineutrophil cytoplasmic antibodies (c-ANCA).

    Churg-Strauss syndrome: small arteries and venules; asthma, eosinophilia, multiorgan involvement—lungs, skin, peripheral nerves, gut, heart, renal (rare); necrotizing extravascular granulomas and vasculitis of small arteries and venules, eosinophils present in early stage.

    Vasculitides affecting predominantly small vessels:

    Henoch-Schönlein purpura: arterioles and venules; palpable purpuric skin lesions lower extremities, arthritis, abdominal pain, hematuria; leukocytoclastic (neutrophilic perivascular/transmural infiltrate) or necrotizing vasculitis often with IgA deposition.

    Hypersensitivity angiitis: arterioles and venules; palpable purpuric skin lesions, arthralgias, systemic symptoms may be present, usually secondary to an immune response [drugs, bugs (infections), connective tissue disease, malignancy]; leukocytoclastic vasculitis.

Microscopic polyangiitis: arterioles, capillaries, and venules; pulmonary hemorrhage, glomerulonephritis, palpable purpura, peripheral neuropathy, joint and abdominal pain; pauci-immune, necrotizing vasculitis, serum perinuclear-ANCA (p-ANCA) common.

3. *What serologic tests or diagnostic procedures should be performed in patients with suspected vasculitis?*

The diagnostic evaluation of a patient with suspected vasculitis should include a chest radiographic study, a complete blood count with differential, liver function tests, creatinine and urinalysis, tests for the presence of ANAs, ANCAs and rheumatoid factor, cryoglobulins, and biopsy of a skin lesion or an involved organ. In some types of vasculitis, complement levels may be low secondary to consumption.

4. *What more extensive procedures may be of value in helping to establish the diagnosis of a specific form of vasculitis?*

More extensive diagnostic procedures for establishing the diagnosis of a specific form of vasculitis include arteriography of the mesenteric vessels if a tissue biopsy is inaccessible, and an electromyogram with evaluation of nerve conduction velocities to evaluate a peripheral neuropathy or a mononeuritis multiplex.

Case   A 45-year-old white man seeks medical care because of hemoptysis of 1 week's duration. He has not felt well for approximately 4 months and has lost 10 pounds (4.5 kg) over this time. He has been receiving various antibiotics for the treatment of chest radiographic abnormalities thought to represent pneumonia. Although these changes have varied in presentation, they have not disappeared. A few weeks earlier, he noted some bloody nasal discharge. He started coughing up blood 1 week ago but attributed it to his bloody nose. The patient also complains that his left knee has been hurting and that red spots have appeared on his arms and legs. He denies fever, purulent sputum, allergies or asthma, known tuberculosis, or chest pain.

On physical examination, erythema is noted on the medial portion of the patient's right eye. There is a curious depression in his upper nose (saddle-nose deformity), bloody discharge in his nasal cavity, a painless ulcer on his soft palate, and a slightly warm and swollen left knee. Chest findings are normal. There are many small, red, raised lesions on the skin of his extremities that are painless.

1. What are three possible diagnoses in this patient?

2. What five diagnostic studies or procedures might be of value in this patient?

An open lung biopsy is performed and the specimen shows the histologic features of Wegener's granulomatosis.

3. What constitutes appropriate therapy for this patient with Wegener's granulomatosis?

4. What three specific findings yielded by physical examination or diagnostic testing strongly suggest a diagnosis of periarteritis nodosa?

5. What are some of the clinical characteristics of temporal arteritis that help to distinguish it from other forms of vasculitis?

Case Discussion

1. *What are three possible diagnoses in this patient?*

   Three possible diagnoses in this patient are Churg-Strauss syndrome (allergic granulomatosis), Wegener's granulomatosis, or a lung tumor.

2. *What five diagnostic studies or procedures might be of value in this patient?*

   A slit-lamp examination of the eyes, computed tomography scan of the sinuses and chest, nasopharyngeal examination with biopsy, skin biopsy, bronchoscopy with biopsy, or open lung biopsy would all be helpful in the evaluation of this patient's disorder. An ANCA should be ordered because most patients with systemic Wegener's granulomatosis are c-ANCA positive.

3. *What constitutes appropriate therapy for this patient with Wegener's granulomatosis?*

   Appropriate therapy for Wegener's granulomatosis includes both high doses of corticosteroids and oral cyclophosphamide.

4. *What three specific findings yielded by physical examination or diagnostic testing strongly suggest a diagnosis of periarteritis nodosa?*

   Periarteritis nodosa is supported by the finding of painful subcutaneous nodules, a mesenteric angiogram showing vasculitic changes particularly at vessel bifurcations, and a positive hepatitis B surface antigen (15% of patients) or hepatitis C antibody. Again, a biopsy of an affected organ showing a focal but panmural necrotizing arteritis is most helpful.

5. *What are some of the clinical characteristics of temporal arteritis that help to distinguish it from other forms of vasculitis?*

   Temporal arteritis (giant cell arteritis) is characterized by temporal headaches, visual blurring or loss, fatigue, jaw claudication, scalp tenderness, and enlarged, tortuous, and tender temporal arteries, as well as by the possible coexistence of polymyalgia rheumatica.

Suggested Readings

Hunder GC. Vasculitis: clinical and laboratory features. In: Klippel JH, ed. *Primer on the rheumatic diseases*, 11th ed. Atlanta: Arthritis Foundation, 1997, p. 294.

Valente RM, Hall S, O'Duffy JD, Conn DL. Vasculitis and related disorders. In: Kelley WN, Harris ED Jr, Ruddy S, Sledge CB, eds. *Textbook of rheumatology*, 5th ed. Philadelphia: WB Saunders, 1997, p. 1079.

Subject Index

Note: Page numbers followed by *t* indicate tabular material.